ESSENTIALS OF
NURSING ADULTS

Sara Miller McCune founded SAGE Publishing in 1965 to support the dissemination of usable knowledge and educate a global community. SAGE publishes more than 1000 journals and over 800 new books each year, spanning a wide range of subject areas. Our growing selection of library products includes archives, data, case studies and video. SAGE remains majority owned by our founder and after her lifetime will become owned by a charitable trust that secures the company's continued independence.

Los Angeles | London | New Delhi | Singapore | Washington DC | Melbourne

ESSENTIALS OF
NURSING ADULTS

EDITED BY

KAREN ELCOCK, WENDY WRIGHT, PAUL NEWCOMBE AND FIONA EVERETT

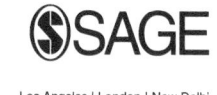

Los Angeles | London | New Delhi
Singapore | Washington DC | Melbourne

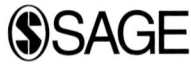

Los Angeles | London | New Delhi
Singapore | Washington DC | Melbourne

SAGE Publications Ltd
1 Oliver's Yard
55 City Road
London EC1Y 1SP

SAGE Publications Inc.
2455 Teller Road
Thousand Oaks, California 91320

SAGE Publications India Pvt Ltd
B 1/I 1 Mohan Cooperative Industrial Area
Mathura Road
New Delhi 110 044

SAGE Publications Asia-Pacific Pte Ltd
3 Church Street
#10-04 Samsung Hub
Singapore 049483

Editor: Alex Clabburn
Development editor: Nina Smith
Editorial assistant: Jade Grogan
Assistant editor, digital: Chloe Statham
Production editor: Martin Fox
Copyeditor: Clare Weaver
Proofreader: Philippa May
Indexer: Gary Kirby
Marketing manager: Tamara Navaratnam
Cover design: Wendy Scott
Typeset by: C&M Digitals (P) Ltd, Chennai, India
Printed in the UK

Editorial arrangement © Karen Elcock, Wendy Wright, Paul Newcombe and Fiona Everett 2019

Foreword © Jane Salvage 2019

Chapter 1 © Karen Elcock and Paul Newcombe 2019
Chapter 2 © Andrew Lloyd and Simon Chippendale 2019
Chapter 3 © Karen Elcock and Omar Mansaray 2019
Chapter 4 © Robert Jenkins and Ruth Northway 2019
Chapter 5 © Julie Gambin and Ronnie Meechan-Rogers 2019
Chapter 6 © Sally Dowling and Jo Williams 2019
Chapter 7 © Winifred Mcgarry 2019
Chapter 8 © Wendy Wright and Fiona Everett 2019
Chapter 9 © Jacqueline Chang and Laura Belton 2019
Chapter 10 © Lucie Llewellyn and Lee Peng Lui 2019
Chapter 11 © Ann Kettyle 2019
Chapter 12 © Steven Beach 2019
Chapter 13 © Ronnie Meechan-Rogers and Kris Paget 2019
Chapter 14 © Claire Chalmers and Heather Gourlay 2019
Chapter 15 © Lindsay Gillman 2019
Chapter 16 © Caroline Adam 2019
Chapter 17 © Margaret Brown and Trudi Marshall 2019
Chapter 18 © Janette Barrie, Sheila Steel and Diane Loughlin 2019
Chapter 19 © Angela Quigley 2019
Chapter 20 © Margaret Brown and Helen Fox 2019

Chapter 21 © Robert Stanley 2019
Chapter 22 © Maura Dowling and Elizabeth Meade 2019
Chapter 23 © Anthony Duffy 2019
Chapter 24 © Rachel Bowater and Sarah Leyland 2019
Chapter 25 © Meghan Bateson, Fiona Everett and Wendy Wright 2019
Chapter 26 © Chris Jones and Emma Bond 2019
Chapter 27 © Sue Szczepanska 2019
Chapter 28 © Cathy Poole and Sue Woodcock 2019
Chapter 29 © Mark Molesworth and Moira Lewitt 2019
Chapter 30 © Emily Carne and Nicky Owen 2019
Chapter 31 © Julie Santy-Tomlinson and Kathryn Lewis 2019
Chapter 32 © Maura Dowling, Mary B Kelly and Teresa Meenaghan 2019
Chapter 33 © Andrew Evered and Lyn Bazley 2019
Chapter 34 © Debbie Rainey and Deirdre McGrath 2019
Chapter 35 © Debbie Rowberry 2019
Chapter 36 © Ruth Taylor and Nancy Fontaine 2019
Chapter 37 © Karen Elcock 2019
Chapter 38 © Marie Cerinus and Claire McGuire 2019
Chapter 39 © Helen Walker 2019

First published 2019

Library of Congress Control Number: 2018938121

British Library Cataloguing in Publication data

A catalogue record for this book is available from the British Library

ISBN 978-1-4739-7419-7
ISBN 978-1-4739-7420-3 (pbk)
ISBN 978-1-5264-5017-3 (pbk and ieb)

At SAGE we take sustainability seriously. Most of our products are printed in the UK using responsibly sourced papers and boards. When we print overseas we ensure sustainable papers are used as measured by the PREPS grading system. We undertake an annual audit to monitor our sustainability.

CONTENTS

FOREWORD

JANE SALVAGE

A lot has changed since I began my nursing training in 1976 – much of it for the better. I already had a degree, in English literature, and setting foot in my school of nursing in London was like stepping back in time. It was a stand-alone institution on a big hospital campus, most of the students were young, white British school leavers, very few of our teachers were graduates, and the teaching methods were traditional. Many of our textbooks were dry tomes of anatomy and physiology that we had to mug up and regurgitate in essays and exams.

The intervening decades have seen huge progress in nursing education, as demonstrated by this state-of-the art textbook. Nothing illustrates that more clearly than Part 5, 'Being a Professional Adult Nurse'. Of course nurses still need to master that medical knowledge, but this alone is not sufficient. Today's nurses also need to become competent in nursing practice, leadership, management and decision-making, their entire careers underpinned with lifelong learning and continuing professional development.

I couldn't escape from my school of nursing fast enough, though with the wisdom of hindsight I can see that it was not all bad. My experiences in the school and our local hospitals and community had set me alight – I wanted the world of nursing and healthcare to change, and to change fast. I became a nursing activist and wrote a book called *The Politics of Nursing* that advocated sweeping reforms (Salvage, 1985). It made me famous – or perhaps infamous – and I never looked back.

My subsequent career in nursing took me to completely unexpected places, literally – from mental health nursing workshops in Mongolia to editing *Nursing Times*, teaching nursing students at Kingston University and training global nursing leaders. More by accident than design, I became the head nurse at the European regional office of the World Health Organization. Working in countries where nursing had even lower status and poorer quality education than the United Kingdom, I began to see how much progress British nursing had made, and how much more there was still to do.

Above all, perhaps, I learned how well educated, empowered nurses are needed more than ever to solve global health problems. These are challenging times, for the planet, for our societies and for the health of nations, with major implications for nurses – a global profession of some 23 million women and men. From caring for older people to halting infectious disease epidemics, reducing mother and child deaths and tackling and mitigating the health effects of climate change, the issues we confront are remarkably similar worldwide.

The value of nursing to health and society has barely been explored or quantified outside its own professional circles, but that is beginning to change. For example, I recently contributed to an influential report by British parliamentarians that highlights the 'triple impact' of nursing worldwide: better health, greater gender equality, and stronger economies (APPG, 2016). It shows that investing in nursing brings rich returns and rewards.

Now is the moment, but wide social forces still present many obstacles. Our archetypal female profession is still widely perceived as doing women's work, with many men (and some women) taking the view that it requires little in the way of particular skills or training, at home or at work. Worldwide, most senior medics, managers and policy-makers are still men and their behaviours are often rooted in sexist assumptions and attitudes. Yet the evidence shows that front-line staff can lead and own the changes needed to ensure high quality care, and there is an ever-growing body of research to prove it.

Nurses in many countries, including the UK, are better educated, more competent and more confident than ever before.

Global awareness is growing of nurses' massive actual and potential contribution to improving health, creating gender equality and strengthening economies. This is the moment to shift the paradigm, to be taken seriously, when the old certainties and ways are being shaken to the core by economic crisis, climate change, insecurity, a deep desire for stronger social solidarity, and the rising clamour of women's voices. Armed with the high quality professional knowledge, skills and attitudes exemplified by this textbook, nurses can, do and will change the world.

REFERENCES

All Party-Parliamentary Group on Global Health (APPG) (2016) *Triple Impact: How developing nursing will improve health, promote gender equality and support economic growth.* Available at: www.appg-globalhealth.org.uk

Salvage, Jane (1985) *The Politics of Nursing.* London: Heinemann Nursing.

Jane Salvage is Writer-in-Residence at Kingston University and St George's, University of London, UK, and an independent nursing consultant.

GUIDE TO YOUR BOOK

We are the student panel for this book.
We've road tested the features for this book and the additional online resources available in the interactive eBook to make sure that they work for you. We hope you enjoy this book and the online resources, and that it helps you to succeed in your degree and future career.

NADINE, EMILY AND EMMA – THE SAGE STUDENT PANEL

 '**VOICES** from people working or studying in this field really helped me to understand how the healthcare system is evolving, showing how diverse nursing is and how peers manage different situations. They add a practical real-life context to your own learning and practice.'

 'I found the **ONLINE VIDEO LINKS** really good for visualising what was being discussed to give yourself a better insight and understanding. They are well worth watching!'

 '**KNOWLEDGE LINKS** encouraged me to reflect on the knowledge I was acquiring and the information I need to revise. I found it helped plan for revision and writing assignments, pointing to important further information or materials that come up time and time again throughout the course.'

'CASE STUDIES help broaden and deepen your knowledge and visualise how changes are being put into practice. I found them invaluable in supporting research, assignments and revision. They encourage critical analysis of complex situations.'

'The ACTIVITIES AND ONLINE ANSWERS will help you to consolidate knowledge and understanding of what you have read. I found that active participation deepened my understanding and supported my revision.'

'THE ONLINE EXAMPLES OF DIFFERENT BOOKS, JOURNALS AND WEBSITES further expanded my knowledge about specific programmes and helped me to find data relevant to my local practice.'

'The ONLINE SELF-ASSESSMENT QUESTIONS allow you to check your knowledge to see if there is anything missing. It will provoke you to engage more with topics that you might not have fully understood and it will help knowledge to "stick".'

'CRITICAL THINKING STOP POINTS help you to question your own ethics and beliefs, and put them into context within a constantly evolving field. They encouraged me to stop reading and self-reflect on my learning, and my strengths and weaknesses, as well as highlighting key information.'

'WHAT'S THE EVIDENCE? These are great for referencing and provoke ideas for further research, as evidence-based practice is so important when working as registered nurses.'

'CHAPTER SUMMARY I found these short synopses of the chapters supported me in synthesizing complex information and concepts, providing useful soundbites to cement my learning.'

Not a fan of eBooks?
The interactive eBook provides the most seamless way to move between your textbook and the digital resources, but your can also access the resources at:

https://study.sagepub.com/essentialadultnursing

NOTES ON THE EDITORS AND CONTRIBUTORS

EDITORS

Karen Elcock is Head of Programmes for Pre-registration Nursing and Deputy Head of School at Kingston University and St George's, University of London. By background an adult critical care nurse, she has worked in nurse education for over 30 years. Her publications in journals and books cover a wide range of nursing topics with a particular focus on practice education and she is a seasoned speaker at national conferences. She is on the international editorial panel for Nurse Education in Practice and a reviewer for the Journal of Advanced Nursing. Karen is also a role model for women in higher education as part of the Aurora Leadership Foundation for Higher Education and a mentor on the university Equality Mentoring Scheme for female staff.

Fiona Everett is currently a Nurse Lecturer within pre-registration and master's level nursing programmes with teaching, co-ordination and research supervision responsibilities. Fiona has a wide range of clinical experience including adult nursing, midwifery, district nursing and research project management within primary care.

She has particular interests in clinical skills, dementia care and developing contemporary support mechanisms in nurse education. She has published in these areas in nursing journals and has disseminated her work at national and international conferences.

She is also an editor and author for SAGE publications in relation to the Essentials of Nursing Practice and Essential Clinical Skills for Nurses: Step by Step.

Fiona is the co-creator of 'Class in a Bag', which is a portable educational resource that enables the delivery of health promotion in a diverse range of environments to suit individual needs. (Winner of Scotland's Dementia Awards, 2016, Best Educational Initiative)

Paul Newcombe is Associate Professor in Adult Acute Care and BSc Nursing Course Leader at Kingston University and St George's, University of London. Paul's clinical background is in Emergency Nursing, Acute Medicine and Trauma, having worked in Oxford, London and Australia. Paul teaches across pre- and post-registration nursing courses and at both undergraduate and postgraduate level. He has a particular interest in developing high-fidelity simulation to help student nurses learn how to manage deteriorating patients. Paul has also staged an annual series of extra-curricular and cultural events with students, staff and local artists in celebration of International Nurses' Day. He is the co-editor of Emergency Nursing at a Glance.

Wendy Wright is an Adult Nursing Lecturer in the pre-registration and the master's level nursing programmes and is currently the BSc Adult Nursing Programme Lead. Wendy has a wide range of acute clinical experience including infectious diseases, stroke and elderly assessment and rehabilitation. Wendy's interests include clinical skills education for student nurses, dementia, the frail older Adult and the student experience, with a particular interest in the development of Class in A Bag (CIAB) which has developed from the initial research of Dementia through the eyes of a child. She has published in these areas in nursing journals and has presented at national and international conferences.

She is also an editor and author for SAGE publications in relation to *Essentials of Nursing Practice* and *Essential Clinical Skills for Nurses*.

CONTRIBUTORS

Caroline Adam, Lecturer in Adult Health at the University of the West of Scotland. Particular interests: clinical skills and simulation, dementia awareness and practice learning.

Janette Barrie, Nurse Consultant for Long Term Conditions and National Clinical Lead for Anticipatory Care Planning with Living Well in Communities, Healthcare Improvement Scotland, Edinburgh.

Meghan Bateson, Nurse Lecturer, University of the West of Scotland.

Mr Lyn Bazley, RN (Adult). Former Dermatology Unit Manager and Senior Photo Therapist for Abertawe Bro Morgannwg University Health Board.

Steve Beach MSc, BSc (Hons), RN, FHEA. Head of Nursing – Corporate. East Sussex Healthcare NHS Trust.

Laura Belton, Advanced Nurse Practitioner managing patients with long-term conditions in her local community of Kingston.

Emma Bond, Specialist Vascular Nurse at Glan Clwyd Hospital in Wales, and past president of the Society of Vascular Nurses.

Rachel Bowater, Senior Lecturer in Intensive Care (Nursing), at Kingston and St George's Joint Faculty of Health, Social Care and Education

Dr Margaret Brown, Senior Lecturer and Deputy Director, Alzheimer Centre for Policy and Practice, University of the West of Scotland.

Emily Carne, Advanced Nurse Practitioner and Lead Clinical Nurse Specialist in Immunology and Allergy, Immunodeficiency Service and Specialist Allergy Service for Wales.

Dr Marie Cerinus, former Director of NMAHP Practice Development, NHS Lanarkshire.

Claire Chalmers, RGN and qualified district nursing sister, currently Senior Lecturer at the University of the West of Scotland.

Jacqueline Chang, Senior Lecturer in Adult Nursing, Kingston University and St George's, University of London. Specialising in palliative care, Jacqueline has 20 years nursing experience.

Simon Chippendale, Staff Nurse, Silver Ward, Oncology; Worcestershire Royal Hospital, Worcester

Dr Maura Dowling, Senior Lecturer in Nursing, Programme Director for the Masters/Postgraduate Diploma in Oncology and Haematology Nursing at the National University of Ireland, Galway, Ireland.

Dr Sally Dowling, Senior Lecturer in the Department of Nursing and Midwifery at the University of the West of England, Bristol.

Anthony Duffy, MSc, BSc (Hons), RN, RNT, ITEC, MBPsS, FHEA. Senior Lecturer, Department of Nursing, College of Human and Health Sciences, Swansea University.

Andrew Evered, MSc Social Research, Dip Nursing, PGCE, RNT, RN, SFHEA. Senior Lecturer and Senior Academic Mentor, College of Human and Health Sciences, Swansea University.

Nancy Fontaine, Chief Nurse at Norfolk and Norwich Hospitals University Foundation Trust and Visiting Professor of Nursing, Anglia Ruskin University, University of Essex.

Helen Fox, Nurse Consultant for Old Age Psychiatry/Alzheimer's Scotland. NHS Lanarkshire.

Julie Gambin, a Registered Nurse for 24 years, currently working for an NHS Trust as Patient Safety Coordinator investigating serious patient safety incidents and complaints.

Lindsay Gillman, Associate Professor of Midwifery, Faculty of Health, Social Care and Education, Kingston University and St George's, University of London.

Heather Gourlay, RGN, holds a Specialist Practitioner Qualification in Infection Control. She is Head of Infection Prevention and Control at Golden Jubilee Foundation in Glasgow.

Dr Robert Jenkins, Registered Learning Disability Nurse, independent trainer, examiner and consultant. He is currently developing a number of distance learning courses.

Chris Jones was, until his retirement, a Senior Lecturer at Edge Hill University, where he taught cardiovascular subjects including an online course in vascular disease.

Mary B Kelly, Advanced Nurse Practitioner in Haematology, Dublin Mid Leinster Region, Ireland for 12 years. Also runs haematology telephone clinics and myeloma support group.

Ann Kettyle, Associate Professor, School of Nursing, Faculty of Health, Social Care and Education, Kingston University & St Georges, University of London.

Kathryn Lewis, Trauma Research Nurse, Kadoorie Centre, Oxford University Hospitals NHS Foundation Trust, Oxford.

Moira Lewitt, MBChB, MMedEd, PhD, FLF, FRACP, FRCP, PFHEA. Professor, Interprofessional Learning and Practice at the University of the West of Scotland.

Sarah Leyland, Practice Educator in General ICU at St George's University Hospitals NHS Foundation Trust.

Lucie Llewellyn, MSc, BSc (Hons), RN (Adult), FHEA, Senior Lecturer, Course Director FdSc Healthcare Practice (Nursing Associate), Kingston University and St George's, University of London.

Andy Lloyd, Lecturer in Nursing, Health and Social Care Department, University of Gloucestershire.

Diane Loughlin, retired from UWS on Hogmanay 2016. Since then she has been involved in some NHS projects and currently considering consultancy work.

Lee Peng Lui, Senior Lecturer at Kingston University and St Georges, University of London. Module leader on perioperative courses and also practising clinically. Main area of clinical work is in anaesthetics.

Omar Mansaray, Senior Lecturer in Mental Health Nursing, Kingston University, London. Special interest in child and adolescent mental health.

Trudi Marshall, Associate Director of Nursing, NHS Lanarkshire.

Winifred McGarry, Lecturer in Adult Nursing at the University of the West of Scotland. Particular interests: simulation, clinical skills, colorectal cancer, health promotion and dementia.

Deirdre McGrath, currently a Lecturer in Education – Nursing at Queen's University Belfast. Her key teaching areas are in relation to pathophysiology and nursing care.

Clare McGuire, Lecturer in Specialist Community Public Health Nursing (Health Visiting), University of the West of Scotland.

Elizabeth Meade, Registered Advanced Nurse Practitioner in Oncology, Midland Regional Hospital Tullamore, HSE Dublin Mid Leinster, Ireland.

Ronnie Meechan-Rogers, Adult and Mental Health nurse. Head of Education for the Institute of Clinical Sciences at the University of Birmingham.

Teresa Meenaghan, Registered Advanced Nurse Practitioner in Haematology, Galway University Hospital, managing patients for review with myeloma, idiopathic thrombocytopenia purpura, bloods and review post chemotherapy.

Mark Molesworth, Senior Lecturer in Adult Nursing at the University of the West of Scotland.

Mandy Nichols-Davies, Registered Nurse, and Head of Nursing at Hywel Dda University Health Board.

Ruth Northway, Professor of Learning Disability Nursing, School of Care Sciences, University of South Wales.

Nicky Owen, Nurse Lecturer in the School of Healthcare Sciences, Cardiff University, with an involvement in pre-registration and Masters level programmes. She is also a mentor for the Postgraduate Education for Health Professionals programme.

Kris Paget, Senior Lecturer in Adult Nursing, Faculty of Health, Social Care and Education; Kingston University and St George's, University of London.

Cathy Poole, MSc, PG Dip, NMC Lecturer / Practice Educator Registered Adult and Child Nurse, currently works as the Training and Education Manager for Fresenius Medical Care, largest dialysis company in the world.

Angela Quigley, Lecturer in Mental Health Nursing, School of Health, Nursing and Midwifery, University of the West of Scotland, Hamilton Campus.

Debbie Rainey, MA ed BA (Hons) Healthcare Management, RGN. Nurse Lecturer and Academic Lead for Clinical Practice at Queens University Belfast.

Debbie Rowberry, Lecturer in Adult Nursing at Swansea University. Debbie also has 23 years of clinical experience in a variety of medical areas.

Julie Santy-Tomlinson, Senior Lecturer in Nursing at the School of Health Sciences, Faculty of Biology, Medicine and Health, The University of Manchester.

Robert Stanley, Senior Lecturer in Learning Disability Nursing at Kingston University and St George's, University of London Joint Faculty.

Sheila Steel BA, RGN. Associate Improvement Advisor for Anticipatory Care Planning (ACP), Living Well in Communities (LWiC) and Healthcare Improvement Scotland, Edinburgh

Dr Sue Szczepanska, Lead Lecturer Practitioner in Acute Care at Epsom & St Helier NHS Trust, supporting qualified and student nurses in education within these areas.

Ruth Taylor, Senior Pro Vice Chancellor and Dean of the Faculty of Health, Education, Medicine, and Social Care at Anglia Ruskin University.

Dr Helen Walker, Senior Lecturer in Mental Health at the University of the West of Scotland and Consultant Nurse for the Forensic Network.

Dr Jo Williams, Senior Lecturer (Mental Health) in the Department of Nursing and Midwifery at the University of the West of England, Bristol.

Sue Woodcock, Head of Nursing, Renal Services (UK) Ltd. RGN, BSc, MA, NMC Teacher Stage 4, Fellow HEA.

ACKNOWLEDGEMENTS

The editors and SAGE would like to thank all the students, patients/service users and nurses who contributed their stories to the book and online resources. The book is much richer for your contribution.

We would also like to thank all the lecturers and students who helped to review this book's content, design and online resources to ensure it is as useful as possible.

LECTURERS

Helen Ashwood, Staffordshire University

Simone Bedford, University of Sunderland

Kim Bezzant, University of Southampton

Darren Brand, University of Brighton

Dianne Burns, University of Manchester

Alison Cork, University of Greenwich

John Costello, University of Manchester

Mary Crawford, King's College London

Kevin Crimmon, Birmingham City University

Jane Dundas, Kingston University

Laura Green, University of Bradford

Pamela Holland, Sheffield Hallam University

Regina Holley, University of West London

Fiona-Jean Howson, Edinburgh Napier University

Angela Hudson, UWE Bristol

Sharon Jones, University of Plymouth

Mhairi Kidd, The University of the west of Scotland

Niall McLaughlin, Canterbury Christ Church University

Teresa McMahon, University of Greenwich

Nicola Morrell-Scott, Liverpool John Moores University

Jane Nicol, University of Worcester

David Reid, University of Sheffield

Catherine Savin, University of Salford

Steven J Walden, University of South Wales

Nikki Welyczko, De Montfort University

THE STUDENT PANEL

Emily Davis

Emma Lyndon

Nadine Wylie

PUBLISHER'S ACKNOWLEDGEMENTS

The authors and publisher are grateful to all third parties for permission to reproduce the following material:

Figure 2.1 The Person-centred nursing framework, McCormack, B. and McCance, T. (2010). *Person-Centred Nursing; Theory and practice*. Chichester: Wiley-Blackwell.

Figure 2.2 The House of care, Collins A. (2014). *Measuring What Really Matters: Towards a coherent measurement system to support person-centred care*. London: The Health Foundation. Reproduced with permission of the Coalition for Collaborative Care.

Figure 3.1 The 6Cs, Department of Health and NHS Commissioning Board (2012) *Compassion in Practice: Nursing, Midwifery and Care Staff – Our Vision and Strategy*. Available at: http://www.eng land.nhs.uk/wp-content/uploads/2012/12/compassion-in-practice.pdf.

Table 3.1 Key skills for values-based practice, Woodbridge K, Fulford, K.W. (2004). *Whose Values? A Workbook for Values-based Practice in Mental Health Care*. London: The Centre for Mental Health, formerly the Sainsbury Centre for Mental Health.

Table 3.2 Alignment of the revalidation model with the four themes of the Code, Royal College of Nursing (2017). *Revalidation Requirements: Reflection and reflective discussion*. Available at: https://www.rcn.org.uk/professional-development/revalidation/reflection-and-reflective-discussion.

Figure 4.1 Safeguarding principles, Department of Health (DH) (2011). *Safeguarding Adults: The role of health service practitioners*. London: Department of Health.

Figure 4.3 Nursing and Midwifery Council (NMC) (2017). *Raising and Escalating Concerns: Guidance for nurses and midwives*. London: NMC. Available at: https://www.nmc.org.uk/standards/guidance/raising-concerns-guidance-for-nurses-and-midwives/.

Figure 6.1 Hierarchy of evidence, Ellis, P. (2013). *Evidence-based Practice in Nursing* (2nd ed.). Exeter: Learning Matters.

Figure 7.2 Prochaska and DiClemente's Transtheoretical Stages of Change Model (1982). Reproduced with permission of the American Psychological Association.

Table 8.2 NMC Standards of Proficiency, Nursing and Midwifery Council (2018a) Standards of Proficency for Registered Nurses. London: NMC.

Table 9.2 National Early Warning Score (NEWS) 2: Standardising the assessment of acute-illness severity in the NHS. Updated report of a working party. London: RCP, 2017. Reproduced with permission of the Royal College of Physicians.

Figure 11.12 Three-Step Ladder, World Health Organization (1986) *WHO's Pain Relief Ladder.* Available at: http://www.who.int/cancer/palliative/painladder/en/.

Figure 19.2 Two-continuum model of mental health, Scottish Government (2007) *Towards a mentally flourishing Scotland.* Available at: http://www.gov.scot/Resource/Doc/201215/0053753.pdf.

NICE comprehensive assessment, National Institute for Care Excellence (NICE) (2006) Dementia: supporting people with dementia and their carers in health and social care. [Online] Available: http://www.nice.org.uk/guidance/cg42.

Table 20.2 Dementia, Delirium and Depression: A quick guide, *Acute Care Dementia* (Learning Resource) (2011). Edinburgh: NHS Scotland. Available at: http://www.nes.scot.nhs.uk/media/350872/acute_dementia_interactive_2011.pdf.

Figure 23.5 Trajectories to death in residential care homes during the last month of life, Barclay, S., Froggatt, K., Crang, C., Mathie, E., Handley, M., Iliffe, S., Manthorpe, J., Gage, H. and Goodman, C. (2014). Living in uncertain times: Trajectories to death in residential care homes. *British Journal of General Practice*, 64 (626): e576–e583. Reproduced with permission under the terms of the Attribution 3.0 Unported (CC BY 3.0) license.

Table 24.1 Clinical features of asthma and COPD (NICE 2010) NICE (2010) National Institute for Health and Care Excellence. Chronic obstructive pulmonary disease in over 16s: diagnosis and management.

Table 24.2: NICE (2017) Asthma: diagnosis, monitoring and chronic asthma aims to improve patient diagnosis and control of symptoms. National Institute for Health and Care Excellence. Asthma: diagnosis, monitoring and chronic asthma management.

Figure 24.7 Asthma management (BTS and Sign 2016). Reproduced from BTS/SIGN British Guideline on the management of asthma, with kind permission of the British Thoracic Society.

Figure 24.8 Asthma management for adults (BTS and Sign 2016). Reproduced from BTS/SIGN British Guideline on the management of asthma, with kind permission of the British Thoracic Society.

Table 28.1 Renal imaging, Schmitz, P.G. and Maddukuri, G. (2015). Kidneys, Ureters, and Bladder Imaging. Medscape. Available at: http://emedicine.medscape.com/article/2165400-overview.

Table 29.1 The 3Ps and the 4Ts, Diabetes UK (2017) *'Do you know the 4 Ts of Type 1 diabetes'.* London: Diabetes UK. Available at: https://www.diabetes.org.uk/get_involved/campaigning/4-ts-campaign.

Table 30.2 Al-Herz W, Bousfiha, A. et al. (2014). Immunodeficiency Diseases: An Update on the Classification from the International Union of Immunological Societies Expert Committee for Primary Immunodeficiency. *Frontiers in Immunology*; 5:162. Adapted from the original and reproduced with permission under the Creative Commons Attribution License (CC BY).

Figure 30.4 Jolles, S. et al. (2015). Current treatment options with immunoglobulin G for the individualization of care in patients with primary immunodeficiency disease. *Clinical Experimental Immunology*. Feb; 179(2): 146–160. John Wiley & Sons.

Figure 32.1 Blood Composition, Thibodeau, A., Patton, K. (2004) *Anatomy and Physiology.* (6th ed.). New York: Elsevier.

Figure 35.1 Macro-nutrients and Micro-nutrients, Kozier, B., Erb, G., Berman, A., Snyder, A., Harvey, S., Morgan Samuel, H. (2012). *Fundamentals of Nursing: Concepts, Process and Practice* (2nd ed.). Pearson Education Limited, England.

Figure 36.1 Most common sources of workplace conflict, Chartered Institute of Personnel and Development (2008). *Leadership and the Management of Conflict at Work*, page 2. London: Chartered Institute of Personal Development.

Fig. 37.1 A cognitive continuum of five modes of clinical judgement and ten perceptions of decision-making in nursing, Standing, M. (2017). *Clinical Judgement and Decision Making in Nursing* (3rd ed.) Exeter: Learning Matters. Reproduced with kind permission of Mooi Standing.

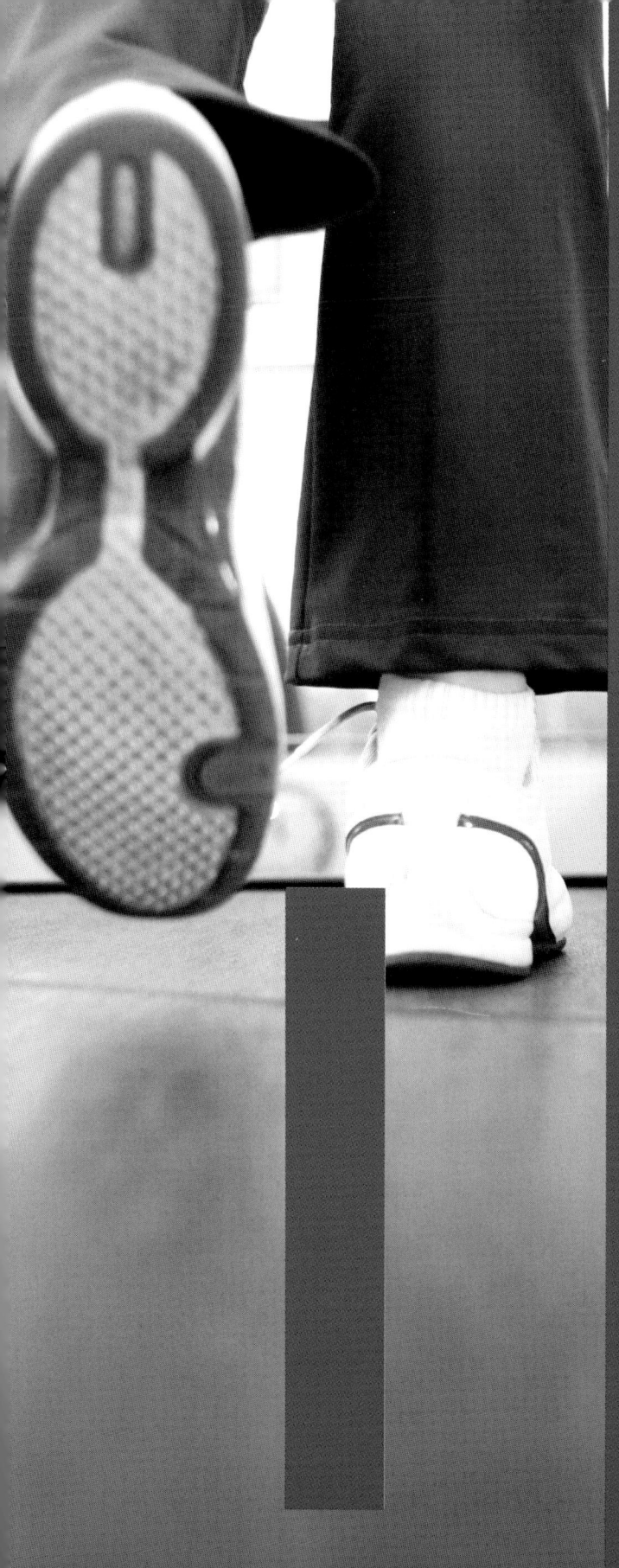

PRINCIPLES OF NURSING ADULTS

THE CHANGING WORLD OF HEALTHCARE

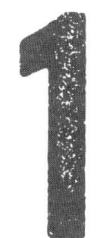

PAUL NEWCOMBE AND KAREN ELCOCK

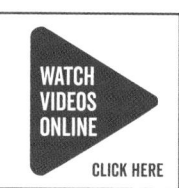

--- **THIS CHAPTER COVERS** ---

- The impact of a growing and ageing population and the increase in long-term conditions
- The impact of lifestyle choices and a shifting focus to prevention
- Changing expectations of healthcare

- New care models, increasing use of technology and changes in professional roles
- Nursing in a global context.

> Nursing has changed significantly since I qualified in the 1980s, back then nurses did not even give IV drugs, now I work in a GP surgery running my own clinics and am a nurse prescriber.
>
> **Ali, GP practice nurse**

INTRODUCTION

As Ali points out above, working in healthcare means that you are going to be exposed to constant change. Each UK government makes changes to the structure of our healthcare systems and processes in an attempt to continue to deliver a first-class service within financial constraints. Nurses are at the front line of care delivery and so inevitably feel the impact of these changes. The role of the nurse has changed significantly over the last 30 years and nurses now perform a wide range of skills that were once only undertaken by doctors. This blurring of boundaries is also occurring within nursing with an expectation that nurses both understand the needs of clients in all fields of practice and are able to respond to these needs. This makes sense as you will meet adults with both physical and mental health problems, and children and people with learning disabilities in both community and hospital settings, and you will need to recognise and provide care for all their needs. Being an adult nurse is exciting as it offers such a diverse range of job opportunities in hospitals, the community, the independent and voluntary sectors across the UK and in other countries. This chapter will look at some of the key policies that have influenced how care is structured and delivered and the drivers behind them. It will explore the changes in professional roles and the increased use of Information Technology and how both are transforming how and where care is delivered. Examples of care models being used across the UK will be given and we will finish with a discussion of the global context of care, recognising that some of you may decide to work abroad in the future.

THE IMPACT OF A GROWING AND AGEING POPULATION

The first, most important and constant change in healthcare is the rapidly growing population. The current world population is over 7.5 billion and it is growing at about 1% per year (83 million people). UK population growth is a little slower at 0.6%, but at 64.6 million people, the current UK population is 15% bigger than in 1975, with half of this growth occurring since 2005. This UK growth is due to increased immigration, an increased birth rate and increased life expectancy. The direct impact on nursing is a greater demand for healthcare services, which arguably haven't fully kept pace. Nurses must also address the needs of an increasingly diverse population and, particularly for adult nurses, the needs of an ageing population.

By 2031, minority ethnic groups will make up 15% of some parts of the UK and 37% of the population in London. Increased diversity offers enormous enrichment to the UK; however, it also presents huge challenges. A changing population brings changing healthcare needs. For example, some ethnic groups have much higher rates of conditions such as diabetes and communicable diseases like HIV, whereas others have lower rates of cancer. More than 100 languages are spoken in many parts of the UK (250 or more in London), with 2% of the population unable to speak English well or at all. As an adult nurse, you will need to address this communication barrier in order to provide culturally competent care (Douglas et al., 2014).

The UK's ageing population, while partly due to a surge in birth rate after the Second World War – so-called Baby Boomers – is also attributable to improved health outcomes. People are not only living longer, but they also have an increased 'healthy life expectancy' (the number of years without illness/disability). However, the number of older adults (>65 years) is expected to account for almost 25% of the UK population by 2046 (Table 1.1). This means that there will be gradually less adults of working age to support those reaching state pension age. This has obvious financial implications but will also impact on the supply and demand of the nursing workforce.

While many older adults are leading healthy lives, most will increasingly seek the services of healthcare providers as they grow older. More than 40% of people admitted to acute hospitals are over 65 years old and length of stay increases with age.

Table 1.1 Age distribution of the UK population, 1976 to 2046 (projected)

	0 to 15 years (%)	16 to 64 years (%)	Aged 65 and over (%)	UK population
1976	24.5	61.2	14.2	56,216,121
1986	20.5	64.1	15.4	56,683,835
1996	20.7	63.5	15.9	58,164,374
2006	19.2	64.9	15.9	60,827,067
2016	18.9	63.1	18.0	65,648,054
2026	18.8	60.7	20.5	69,843,515
2036	18.0	58.2	23.9	73,360,907
2046	17.7	57.7	24.7	76,342,235

Source: Office for National Statistics (2017)

1. Population estimates data are used for 1996 to 2016, while 2014-based population projections are used for 2026 and 2036.

Additionally, a number of other factors arise:

- Increased frailty, incidence of falls and subsequent neck of femur fractures
- Increased disability, including sight and hearing loss, resulting in reduced ability to carry out activities of daily living (ADL) independently
- Increased malnutrition
- Increased incontinence
- Increased incidence of mental health problems, such as depression and dementia
- Increased loneliness and social isolation
- Increased burden on unpaid family carers, many of whom are older adults themselves.

Age UK (2018)

SEE ALSO
CHAPTER 31

SEE ALSO
CHAPTER 19

SEE ALSO
CHAPTER 20

THE IMPACT OF LONG-TERM CONDITIONS

Another factor that increases with age is the incidence of long-term conditions (LTC). More than 40% of over 65s and more than half of over 75s have a LTC compared with a third of the general UK population. These are diseases for which there is no cure, but which require ongoing treatment in order to manage the impact on the individual. This is a huge economic burden on the NHS and will also make up a large part of your work as an adult nurse. Examples of LTCs include: diabetes; respiratory disease, such as chronic obstructive pulmonary disease (COPD); cardiovascular disease, such as hypertension, stroke, coronary heart disease and heart failure; neurological disease, such as Parkinson's; musculoskeletal disease, such as arthritis; and cancer. There is also a huge overlap between LTC and mental health (MH) problems: a third of people with a LTC also have MH problems, predominantly depression and anxiety. Similarly, while a fifth of the UK population have a MH problem, nearly a half of these also have a LTC (The Kings Fund, 2013). As a result, the physical and psychological care of people encountered by adult nurses must always be inextricably linked.

SEE ALSO
CHAPTER 18

SEE ALSO
CHAPTER 19

PREPARATION FOR PRACTICE PLACEMENTS 1.1

When you prepare for a new placement, you should always research the population you will be caring for. You can access the healthcare organisations' websites, but also those of the local council, for example.

What are the demographics (age, ethnicities, socioeconomic profile, incidence of long-term conditions, etc.)? Is this similar to what you have experienced before? Do you need to do any further reading around particular groups you may encounter? Will there be any communication or cultural issues you can prepare for?

THE IMPACT OF LIFESTYLE CHOICES

Although awareness about healthy lifestyles is much greater in the UK today, there is still a general increase of avoidable risk factors as a result of individual health behaviours. Furthermore, there is an increase in health inequalities: while the most advantaged groups are getting healthier, the most disadvantaged Britons are becoming more unhealthy. There is a seven-year difference in life expectancy between the lowest and the highest socioeconomic groups. The North–South divide also still persists. The most significant risk factor is obesity – caused by inactivity and poor diet. Two-thirds of people do not take enough exercise or eat the recommended amount of fruit and vegetables. Intake of refined sugar and 'fast food' is also far too high. More than a quarter of the UK is classed as obese, and a half to two-thirds is considered overweight, with numbers continuing to rise. Obesity increases the risk of having at least one LTC, particularly cardiovascular disease, type II diabetes, arthritis and cancer. It also reduces life expectancy by about 10 years.

Smoking is another health behaviour with significant risks to health. It causes cancer, heart and respiratory disease and is the greatest preventable cause of death, reducing life expectancy by about 10 years. Although smoking rates have almost halved in the last 40 years, still around a fifth of the population are regular smokers. Finally, excessive alcohol intake is the other key risk factor for poor physical and mental health, with a fifth to a quarter of people drinking more than the recommended safe limits. There has been a dramatic increase in admission to hospital due to alcohol-related illness in recent years. Other lifestyle choices impacting on the health of the UK population are illicit drug use, which increases the incidence of mental health problems; and unsafe sexual behaviour, which increases the risk of unwanted pregnancies and transmissible infections (HIV/STIs). Having multiple unhealthy behaviours further increases the risk of poor health and mortality. Encouragingly, young people are showing reduced rates of smoking, drinking and illicit drug use, although 80% are still considered to have a poor diet (The Kings Fund, 2013).

SHIFTING THE FOCUS TO PREVENTION

As a result of these patterns there is huge shift towards focusing on public health and preventative healthcare. The UK's public health departments (in England, Wales, Scotland and Northern Ireland) each set priorities for promoting healthier lifestyles, preventing ill health and reducing health inequalities. These are addressed through working with local and national government, the NHS and the voluntary sector. Legislation, health education, screening and preventative services are examples of relevant activities. Promoting health is a core proficiency for all registered nurses and you will need to be able to support individuals to make informed choices and prevent ill health (NMC, 2018).

SEE ALSO
CHAPTER 7

ACTIVITY 1.1: CRITICAL THINKING

Visit the website for your country's public health department and access its strategic plan (see Reports under Go Further at the end of the chapter).

- What are the priorities for promoting health?
- How will this impact on your role as an adult nurse?
- How do these relate to your own health?

CHANGING EXPECTATIONS OF HEALTHCARE

Another key influence on the changing healthcare landscape is the greater expectations held by the people who use the services, including around dignity, respect and satisfaction. The public are also much better informed about health issues now due to the availability of information online. As a result, patients demand greater engagement and involvement in decision-making about their own care (The King's Fund, 2013). Fortunately, this complements the aims of the NHS, which requires patients to take more responsibility for their own health. Nurses, even more than before, need to work in partnership with their patients. Healthcare is also becoming more personalised as we move away from a standardised approach. Diagnostics are becoming much more specific and are facilitating targeted treatments. Patients are considered to be the greatest untapped resource in the NHS. New ways of working, alongside new technologies, are being employed to empower patients and promote independence; expert patients are at the centre of some care models, being supported to self-manage their own care. Peer-to-peer support is also increasingly important for information exchange and promotion of wellbeing.

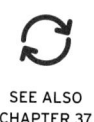

SEE ALSO
CHAPTER 37

NEW CARE MODELS

The NHS is now 70 years old and still cherished in the UK for the principles upon which it was founded – universal healthcare for all, free at the point of delivery. However, it has changed very little since it was first set up and now needs to adapt to a rapidly changing world. NHS England's *Five Year Forward View* (NHS England et al., 2014) set out plans for the structural changes and service redesign required to address the priorities now and for future generations. It identifies a 'triple challenge' – better health, transformed quality of care delivery and sustainable finances. The most significant element of this strategy represents a seed change in the approach to UK health policy. *Five Year Forward View* firmly rejects the concept that 'one size fits all'. For the first time, services are being actively encouraged to grow organically in response to local need. In order to achieve this, organisations must first remove existing barriers between themselves, including:

- Providers vs commissioners
- Primary/community vs acute care

- Health vs social care
- Physical vs mental health.

The New Care Models programme (NHS, 2016) is focused on supporting the improvement and integration of services that are aimed at addressing the health and care needs of a local population. It is supported by a partnership of the NHS, Care Quality Commission (CQC), Health Education England (HEE), NHS Improvement, Public Health England and the National Institute of Health and Care Excellence (NICE). In 2015, organisations and partnerships were invited to apply to become a 'Vanguard' – a group of people leading the way in new developments and ideas. The job of the Vanguards is to develop a blueprint for the future of NHS and social care services, and to inspire the rest of the health and care system. Their innovative approaches must produce changes which are both effective and which develop at pace. So far, 50 Vanguards have been selected to redesign whole health and care systems in five different areas, but all with a focus of shifting care from acute to primary/ community care:

- Integrated primary and acute care systems (PACS) – joining up GP, community, hospital and mental health services
- Multispecialty community providers (MCP) – moving specialist care out of hospitals into the community; bringing care closer to home and reducing travel for patients
- Enhanced health in care homes (EHCH) – offering older people living in care homes better, joined-up health, care and rehabilitation services
- Urgent and emergency care (UEC) – new approaches to improve the coordination of services and reduce pressure on A&E departments; reducing confusion for the public
- Acute care collaborations (ACC) – linking local hospitals together to improve their clinical and financial viability, reducing variation in care and efficiency.

Services covered by Vanguards have already demonstrated successes, such as slower growth in emergency admissions and reduced length of hospital stays. This is particularly significant in the over 75s who are more likely to experience a cycle of emergency admissions, delayed discharges and unplanned readmission (NHS England, 2017). Vanguards are sharing their learning and spreading good practice by developing frameworks which set out the key ingredients and steps required to set up the model elsewhere. Case Study 1.1 describes a new care model set up in Scotland.

——— GO FURTHER ———

WEBLINK: KINGS FUND PAPER

Read more about how integrated care is being delivered across Scotland, Wales and Northern Ireland. Read the Kings Fund paper *Integrated care in Northern Ireland, Scotland and Wales: Lessons for England.* Available at: www.kingsfund.org.uk/sites/default/files/field/field_publication_file/integrated-care-in-northern-ireland-scotland-and-wales-kingsfund-jul13.pdf

Another key strategy for health service reform alongside Vanguards is the development of 44 Sustainability and Transformation Partnerships (STP). These are partnerships between the NHS and local authorities, providers and commissioners, patients and the public, with responsibility for improving health, wellbeing and care for a local population. Evolved versions of STPs are called Accountable Care Systems (ACS), which are fully integrated models of services and funding. An ACS is awarded the power and freedom to plan care provision for the area it covers. These can evolve further still into an Accountable Care Organisation (ACO). An ACO is more complex and time consuming to create but offers simplified governance and decision-making and maximises efficiencies from available funding. These new collaborative business models allow informal partnerships to become formalised, but present new challenges as financial, contractual and managerial relationships are renegotiated (Collins, 2016). However, the Five Year Forward View set out a commitment to support local diverse solutions rather than central reorganisation. It is clear that there is no turning back on this journey towards high-quality, fully integrated and efficient care.

CASE STUDY 1.1

Tayside has combined its older people locality model that aligns consultant geriatricians in the acute sector to GP practices, with an enhanced community support service.

The Tayside model aims to:

- Prevent older people at risk of an unplanned hospital admission being admitted by identifying them and giving them an enhanced level of support at home before they reach crisis point
- Facilitate patients' discharge from acute hospital to home or to a more homely setting, such as a community hospital.

The enhanced community support service is delivered by a multidisciplinary team (MDT) at GP practice level. The patient's assessment is led by the GP while the enhanced care package tends to be coordinated by either an advanced nurse practitioner specialising in medicine for the elderly or a senior district nurse with time protected for the assessment of frail people and care coordination. The MDT, which also involves nurses, community pharmacists, allied health professionals, community mental health staff and social workers, meet weekly to discuss patients currently receiving the enhanced service and to identify others who could benefit from the service. The teams also have links with the voluntary sector.

From Audit Scotland (2016: 9)

- What is the above a perfect example of?

CASE STUDY 1.1
ANSWER

INCREASING USE OF TECHNOLOGY

> In my three years of training I have seen medication rounds change from paper format drug charts to using the EPMA (Electronic, Prescribing & Medicines Administration) system. At times I felt like this was a step backwards as doctors, pharmacists and nurses got used to a new way of working and a new system, but it definitely seems to have its benefits; it is a lot quicker for obtaining the right medication for the patient in an accurate, rapid and precise manner.
>
> **Louise, 3rd year adult student nurse**

Since the beginning of the twenty-first century we have entered the digital age. Technology is now as pervasive in healthcare as it is in the rest of our lives, however, the effective use of technology in healthcare is considered to be 10 years behind other sectors. Nevertheless, there is huge potential to transform the quality and efficiency of patient care as some of the current challenges are addressed. It is anticipated that we will then enter a new era of healthcare, where the use of technology will result in 30% of current processes being done differently.

Imison et al. (2016a) propose seven areas of opportunity for digital healthcare:

1. More systematic, high-quality care
    In order to reduce the variability of care between clinicians, technology can be used to develop protocols with embedded decision-support, which supplements, rather than replaces clinical judgement. Nurses can use this to work more autonomously in isolated settings. Safer drugs administration can also be achieved through e-prescribing and automated dispensing.
2. More proactive and targeted care
    A good example of this is the use of vital signs monitoring and predictive analysis to generate real time early warning scores to pre-empt risk of patient deterioration. These systems are commonly used in acute hospital settings but are increasingly recognised as important in the community.
3. Better-coordinated care
    Fully integrated, accessible electronic health records allow different professionals to communicate with each other more effectively. Mobile access to data in real time is of particular benefit to those working in the community.
4. Improved access to specialist expertise
    Telehealth and electronic communication can remove geographical barriers between patients and healthcare professionals. This can reduce A&E attendances, face-to-face consultations and improve referrals. Specialist support can also be provided to remote locations.
5. Greater patient engagement
    Through the use of shared electronic health records (as above), patients have increased opportunities for self-managed care. The Internet of Things (IoT) – connected devices such as wearable technology, apps, telehealth and online communities can all be employed to empower patients and put them at the centre of their care.
6. Improved resource management
    Healthcare can borrow tools from other sectors to improve productivity and efficiency through enhanced resource management. Capacity can be better matched to demand through tools such as e-rostering and patient flow management.
7. System improvement and learning
    The development of new technology systems needs to be iterative. Large amounts of data are generated ('big data'), which can be processed with tools such as predictive analysis to create and refine algorithms. Continuous improvement can then take place.

To keep pace with this technological revolution, nurses must develop and maintain their digital literacy. This is defined by Health Education England (HEE) (2017) as the capabilities that prepare someone for working, living, learning, participating and thriving in a digital society.

HEE identify six domains that define the skills, attitudes, values and behaviours you will need to achieve digital literacy (see Figure 1.1).

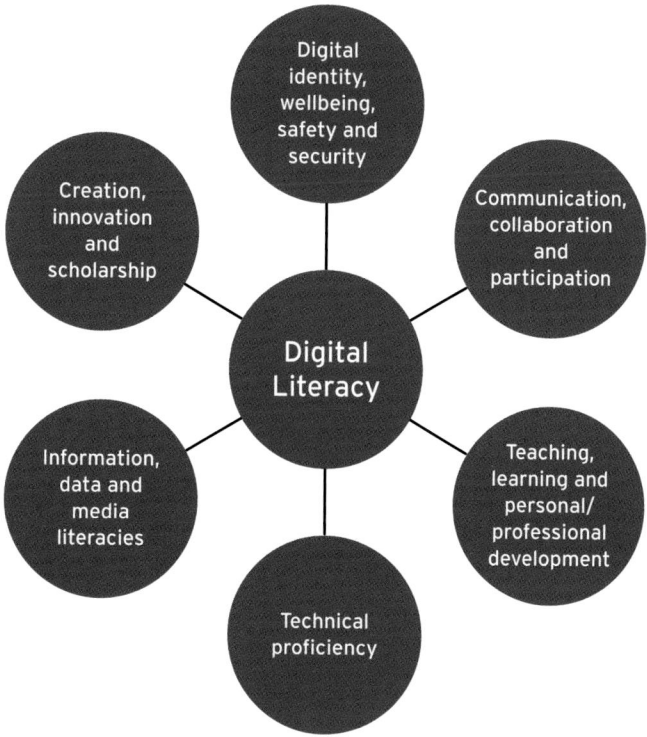

Figure 1.1   The 6 domains for digital literacy

CRITICAL THINKING STOP POINT 1.1

Are you comfortable with new technology? Are there any areas you need to improve on? If so, what can you do to achieve this?

CHANGES IN PROFESSIONAL ROLES

In order to deliver these new services, professional roles are also evolving to keep pace with the changing needs of the population. So, what does this mean for you as an adult nurse? It is clear so far that nurses will need to be increasingly flexible and responsive. Constant adaptation to the changing landscape is now a given. There will be more roles, which require nurses to work in, or close to, people's homes, and outside of hospital settings. That said, the need for hospitals will never completely disappear – people will always need surgery, specialist treatment and critical care, for example, which can only be delivered safely and effectively in a hospital environment. However, working across these traditional boundaries will become more commonplace. All nurses will need an increased primary care focus as patients are supported to stay at home for longer and live more independently. Nurses will also need to take a greater role in preventative healthcare, educating the public to take greater responsibility for their health. This will involve working in partnership with patients, making best use of emerging technology and implementing new care models. Within this, nurse-led services will become increasingly common and will offer nurses greater responsibility for managing both care and services. The UK is looking to other health systems around the world to examine the impact of new nursing roles (Case Study 1.2).

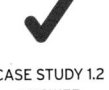

CASE STUDY 1.2
ANSWER

CASE STUDY 1.2: THE BUURTZORG APPROACH

Founded in the Netherlands in 2006/07, Buurtzorg is a unique district nursing system which is internationally renowned for being entirely nurse-led and cost effective. Before Buurtzorg, home care services in the Netherlands were fragmented with patients being cared for by multiple practitioners and providers. Ongoing financial pressures within the health sector led to home care providers cutting costs by employing a low-paid and poorly skilled workforce. They were unable to properly care for patients with complex needs and this led to a decline in patient health and satisfaction. Buurtzorg's answer to this problem was to give its district nurses far greater control over patient care. Nurses lead the assessment, planning and coordination of patient care. The model consists of small self-managing teams with a maximum of 12 professionals including nurses and allied health professionals such as occupational therapists. These teams coordinate care for a specific catchment area.

The Buurtzorg service:

- provides a holistic assessment of an individual's needs, including their medical, personal and social care needs, that feeds into a care plan
- identifies networks of informal care and assesses ways to involve these carers in the individual's treatment plan
- identifies any other formal carers and helps to coordinate care between providers
- delivers a range of care from basic nursing to palliative care
- supports clients in their home
- promotes self-care and independence.

A range of health providers are successfully implementing the Buurtzorg approach in the UK.

(RCN, 2016)

Google Buurtzorg UK and find out where this model is being implemented in the UK.

Extending the skills of nurses and developing more advanced roles is also inevitable, although this has always been a controversial subject. Nursing worries about its loss of identity and core role in the provision of care, whereas colleagues, such as doctors, worry about the erosion of their territory. However, bearing in mind there was a time when nurses weren't allowed to take a blood pressure, evolution of the profession has come a long way. Furthermore, this reshaping and development of the existing workforce is considered central to the success of service improvement (Imison et al., 2016 b). Nurses are expected to take on more advanced skills, such as history-taking, physical assessment, diagnosis, clinical decision-making, requesting investigations, prescribing, referral and case management (HEE, 2016). They will need to undertake further education, which takes time and resources. There are also likely to be fewer doctors and more support staff, meaning nurses will have an even greater leadership and coordination role.

Advanced Clinical Practitioner (ACP) or Advanced Nurse Practitioner (ANP) roles have grown organically within the health service, both for nurses and allied health professionals (AHPs – e.g. physiotherapists, pharmacists and paramedics). The roles are difficult to define, mean different things in different settings and currently have no formal regulatory framework. However, ACP/ANPs have been successfully deployed across both primary and secondary care areas, including general practice, minor injury and illness, urgent and emergency care, long-term conditions, mental health, paediatrics and general surgery. ACP/ANPs are experienced and highly educated registered nurses who manage the complete clinical care of their patients, not focusing on any sole condition. In Scotland, ANPs have advanced-level capability across four pillars of practice (Scottish Government, 2017):

- Clinical practice
- Facilitation of learning
- Leadership
- Evidence, research and development.

These roles offer benefits for both patients and nurses (Table 1.2).

Table 1.2 Benefits of ACP roles

Benefits of ACP for patients	Benefits of ACP roles for nurses
Improved access to services	New career opportunities
More frequent follow-up care	Improved staff satisfaction
Reduced hospital admissions	Improved learning and development for other staff
Increased patient satisfaction	
More timely care	
Lower length of stay	
Better continuity of care	

Source: Imison et al., 2016b

WHAT'S THE EVIDENCE? 1.1

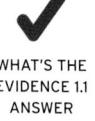

WHAT'S THE EVIDENCE 1.1 ANSWER

Read the following article, which explores the consultation preferences for seeing or speaking to a GP or a nurse.

Paddison, C.A.M., Abel, G.A., Burt, J., Campbell, J.L., Elliott, M.N., Lattimer, V. and Roland, M. (2017) What happens to patient experience when you want to see a doctor and you get to speak to a nurse? Observational study using data from the English General Practice Patient Survey. *BMJ Open*, 2018;8:e018690. doi: 10.1136/bmjopen-2017-018690 Available at: http://bmjopen.bmj.com/content/8/2/e018690

(Continued)

(Continued)

- Why do you think patients may prefer to see a GP rather than a nurse?
- What are the benefits of seeing a nurse rather than a GP?
- How can we ensure that patients have confidence and trust in the nurse when they are given an appointment with a nurse rather than the GP?

NURSING IN A GLOBAL CONTEXT

Across Europe and the rest of the world, nursing is identified as playing a key role in tackling public health challenges and in delivering safe, high-quality, effective and efficient services. Health 2020, the European policy framework, cites the importance of nursing in improving health and wellbeing, reducing inequalities and ensuring sustainable people-centred systems (WHO, 2015). Comparing the UK to the rest of the world, and Europe in particular, allows policy makers to assess the quality of healthcare provided nationally. Across 27 internationally available and validated indicators, the UK's healthcare system is found to be better than average in some areas, but requires significant improvement in others, such as cardiovascular disease and cancer. While there is progress being made in the majority of these areas it is worrying that the UK performs worse than most countries in more than half of the indicators (Kossarova et al., 2015).

Increased globalisation over the last half century has changed the world in which we live beyond all recognition. Improvements in transport, communication, free trade and cheap labour have resulted in greater interconnectedness, immigration and cultural exchange. We must now think about population health from a global perspective. The top priority for the World Health Organization (WHO, 2018) is 'health for all' – ensuring universal health coverage which is equitable and affordable. However, there is a long way to go: one in 17 of the world's population still lack access to essential health services. Statistics such as these draw many nurses towards working in international development. Humanitarian or aid work can be hugely rewarding, but also very demanding. Experience and maturity are important, so taking knowledge and learning gained in the UK is essential. Undertaking an international elective placement during your nurse training is a great way to get started.

CONCLUSION

This chapter has considered some of the key areas that illustrate the changing world of healthcare. From changing demographics to disease patterns, health services must evolve at scale and pace to keep up with the population they serve. Ham and Brown (2015) emphasise that this results in a complex, uncharted and messy healthcare environment. However, in order to succeed, nurses must embrace the unpredictability and uncertainty. Nurses need to be flexible, adaptable, agile, responsive, risk-takers, open to experimentation and, above all, willing to try and fail.

CHAPTER SUMMARY

- The healthcare landscape is constantly changing.
- The population is growing, getting older and requires care for long-term conditions.
- Prevention of ill health is becoming increasingly important.

- Service redesign offers creative and more efficient solutions to address growing demand.
- The role of the nurse is evolving to adopt new leadership and coordination responsibilities, more advanced skills, new technologies and a global perspective.

GO FURTHER

Go to https://study.sagepub.com/essentialadultnursing for a further case study related to this chapter. If you are using the interactive ebook, simply click on the book icon in the margin to go straight to the resource.

CASE STUDY: DIGITAL MONITORING

Journal Articles

Go to https://study.sagepub.com/essentialadultnursing for further free online journal articles related to this chapter. If you are using the interactive ebook, simply click on the book icon in the margin to go straight to the resource.

FURTHER READING: JOURNAL ARTICLES

- Pearce, L. (2018) Digital literacy part 1: You can be an e-nurse. *Nursing Standard*. Available at: https://rcni.com/nursing-standard/features/digital-literacy-part-1-you-can-be-e-nurse-126751 (accessed 15/02/18)

Reports

- Government Office for Science (2016) *Future of an Ageing Population*. Available at: www.gov.uk/government/uploads/system/uploads/attachment_data/file/535187/gs-16-10-future-of-an-ageing-population.pdf (accessed 15/02/18)
- NHS England (2016) *Leading Change, Adding Value: A framework for nursing, midwifery and care staff*. Available at: www.england.nhs.uk/wp-content/uploads/2016/05/nursing-framework.pdf
- NHS Health Scotland (2012) *A Fairer Healthier Scotland. A strategic framework for action 2017–2022*. Available at: www.healthscotland.scot/publications/a-fairer-healthier-scotland-a-strategic-framework-for-action-2017-2022
- Public Health Agency (Northern Ireland) (2014) *Making Life Better: A Whole System Strategic Framework for Public Health 2013–2023*. Available at: www.health-ni.gov.uk/sites/default/files/publications/dhssps/making-life-better-strategic-framework-2013-2023_0.pdf
- Public Health England (2016) *Strategic Plan for the Next Four Years: Better outcomes by 2020*. Available at: www.gov.uk/government/uploads/system/uploads/attachment_data/file/516985/PHE_Strategic_plan_2016.pdf
- Public Health Wales (2017) *Our Strategic Plan 2017–2020*. Available at: www.wales.nhs.uk/sitesplus/documents/888/Integrated%20Medium%20Term%20Plan%202017-2020%20v1.pdf

Weblinks

Go to https://study.sagepub.com/essentialadultnursing for further weblinks related to this chapter. If you are using the interactive ebook, simply click on the book icon in the margin to go straight to the resource.

FURTHER READING: WEBLINKS

For the latest information on what is happening in each of the four countries of the UK see:

- **England** www.england.nhs.uk
- **Northern Ireland** www.health-ni.gov.uk
- **Scotland** www.scot.nhs.uk
- **Wales** www.wales.nhs.uk

ACE YOUR ASSESSMENT

Revise what you have learned by visiting https://study.sagepub.com/essentialadultnursing

- Test yourself with multiple-choice and short-answer questions
- Do the chapter activities in the book and check your answers online

REFERENCES

Age UK (2018) *Later Life in the United Kingdom*. Available at: www.ageuk.org.uk/globalassets/age-uk/ documents/reports-and-publications/later_life_uk_factsheet.pdf?dtrk=true (last accessed 15 February 2018).

Audit Scotland (2016) *Changing Models of Health and Social Care: Case studies and supplementary materials*. Available at: www.audit-scotland.gov.uk/uploads/docs/report/2016/nr_160310_ changing_models_care_supp1.pdf (last accessed 15 February 2018).

Collins, B. (2016) *New Care Models: Emerging innovations in governance and organisational form. The King's Fund*. Available at: www.kingsfund.org.uk/sites/files/kf/field/field_publication_file/New_ care_models_Kings_Fund_Oct_2016.pdf (last accessed 15 February 2018).

Douglas Rosenkoetter, M., Pacquiao, D.F., Callister, L.C., Hattar-Pollara, M., Lauderdale, J., Milstead, J., Nardi, D. and Purnell, L. (2014) Guidelines for implementing culturally competent nursing care. *Journal of Transcultural Nursing*, 25(2): 109–21.

Ham, C. and Brown, A. (2015) *The Future is Now. The King's Fund*. Available at: www.kingsfund.org. uk/reports/thefutureisnow/ (last accessed 15 February 2018).

Health Education England (2017) *Improving Digital Literacy*. Available at: https://www.hee.nhs. uk/sites/default/files/documents/Improving%20Digital%20Literacy%20-%20HEE%20and%20 RCN%20report.pdf (last accessed 15 February 2018).

Imison, C., Castle-Clarke, S., Watson, R. and Edwards, N. (2016a) *Delivering the benefits of digital health care. Nuffield Trust*. Available at: www.nuffieldtrust.org.uk/files/2017-01/delivering-the-benefits-of-digital-technology-web-final.pdf (last accessed 15 February 2018).

Imison, C., Castle-Clarke, S. and Watson, R. (2016b) *Reshaping the workforce to deliver the care patients need*. Available at: www.nuffieldtrust.org.uk/files/2017-01/reshaping-the-workforce-web-final.pdf (last accessed 15 February 2018).

Kossarova, L., Blunt, I. and Bardsley, M. (2015) *QualityWatch. Focus on: International comparisons of healthcare quality*. The Health Foundation and the Nuffield Trust. Available at: www.qualitywatch. org.uk/sites/files/qualitywatch/field/field_document/QW%20International%20comparisons%20 %28final%29_disclaimer_update.pdf (last accessed 15 February 2018).

NHS England, Public Health England, Health Education England, Monitor, Care Quality Commission, NHS Trust Development Authority (2014) *Five Year Forward View*. Available at: www. england.nhs.uk/wp-content/uploads/2014/10/5yfv-web.pdf (last accessed 15 February 2018).

NHS England (2016) *New Care Models: Vanguards – developing a blueprint for the future of NHS and care services*. Available at: www.england.nhs.uk/wp-content/uploads/2015/11/new_care_models.pdf (last accessed 15 February 2018).

NHS England (2017) *Next Steps on The NHS Five Year Forward View*. Available at: www.england.nhs.uk/ wp-content/uploads/2017/03/NEXT-STEPS-ON-THE-NHS-FIVE-YEAR-FORWARD-VIEW.pdf (last accessed 15 February 2018).

Nursing and Midwifery Council (2018) *Standards of Proficiency for Registered Nurses* Available at: www. nmc.org.uk/ (last accessed 15 February 2018).

Office for National Statistics (2017) *Overview of the UK Population July 2017*. Available at: www.ons. gov.uk/peoplepopulationandcommunity/populationandmigration/populationestimates/articles/ overviewoftheukpopulation/july2017 (last accessed 15 February 2018).

RCN (2016) *The Buurtzorg Nederland (home care provider) model: Observations for the United Kingdom (UK)*. Available at: www.rcn.org.uk/about-us/policy-briefings/br-0215 (last accessed 15 February 2018).

Scottish Government (2017) *Transforming Nursing, Midwifery and Health Professions' (NMaHP) Roles: Pushing the boundaries to meet health and social care needs in Scotland*. Available at: www.nes.scot. nhs.uk/media/4031450/cno_paper_2_transforming_nmahp_roles.pdf (last accessed 15 February 2018).

The King's Fund (2013) *Time to Think Differently*. Available at: www.kingsfund.org.uk/projects/time-think-differently (last accessed 15 February 2018).

World Health Organization (WHO) (2015) *European Strategic Directions for Strengthening Nursing and Midwifery Towards Health 2020 goals*. Available at: www.euro.who.int/__data/assets/ pdf_file/0004/274306/European-strategic-directions-strengthening-nursing-midwifery-Health2020_en-REV1.pdf?ua=1 (last accessed 15 February 2018).

World Health Organization (WHO) (2018) *WHO Priorities*. Available at: www.who.int/dg/priorities/ en/ (last accessed 15 February 2018).

PERSON-CENTRED CARE

ANDY LLOYD AND SIMON CHIPPENDALE

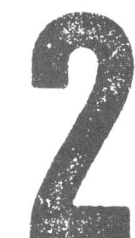

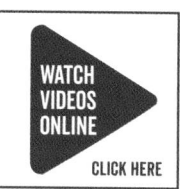

WATCH VIDEOS ONLINE
CLICK HERE

--- **THIS CHAPTER COVERS** ---

- The history of person-centred care (PCC)
- Holistic PCC models
- Shared decision making

- The importance of dignity
- The House of Care.

> " She always seems to know what mood I'm in.
>
> **Arthur, patient** "

> " When you attend the clinic for the first time it is like being cast up on a foreign shore – everything is strange and they speak a foreign tongue (medical terms). Being put at ease is a great help. Empathy is everything – you can become friends with your nursing staff, then having the 'craic' plus the relief from pain makes your trips to clinic something to look forward to and not a thing to dread! A bond forms between you and your nurse which is worth as much if not more than your treatment, because you know they will be there when needed. It also stops you from straying off the wagon because you don't want to let them down after all the effort they have made on your behalf.
>
> **Ken, liver transplant recipient** "

> " While on placement in my second year of my nursing degree, I experienced some good communication to meet patient needs, working alongside my mentor. The patient that we were caring for had learning disabilities and their communication verbally was limited. This led to the patient not being able to verbalise their needs. The patient had carers with them and they were happy to communicate for the patient. But my mentor made a simple communication board to aid communication from the patient directly. This ensured that the patient was involved fully in the care that we were providing for them.
>
> **Molly, student nurse** "

INTRODUCTION

Person-centred care is not so much a specific and prescriptive model that organises care for an individual person, as an *approach* to nursing care. There is potential for person-centredness in almost every interaction between you and your patients. As a philosophy of care, it promotes respect, shared decision making, empowerment and enablement, and respect for autonomy.

You may already feel that providing person-centred care is your natural inclination. You may be one of many who are drawn to nursing as a career because you want to improve other people's lives (Rhodes et al., 2011). This altruistic outlook is often aligned with the principles of person-centred care. As nurses, we put our patients' interests at the heart of everything we do. As such, it is important for you to seek out, listen to, and act in accordance with their wishes, when it is appropriate and practicable to do so. Once you have established the patient's needs in this way, you are in a better position to offer individualised, compassionate care.

Person-centred care (PCC) is not just a personal philosophy for practitioners, but is also increasingly a methodology underpinning many strands of health and social care.

The late Tom Kitwood defined person-centredness, as applied in dementia care, in this way:

> … a standing or status that is bestowed upon one human being by others, in the context of relationship and social being. It implies recognition, respect and trust. (Kitwood, 1997: 8)

SEE ALSO
CHAPTER 37

The importance and value of PCC is that it ensures people are central partners in decisions about their health and care. This approach can improve quality of care, and help make funding go further. It can be successful only through the adoption, integration and engagement of its core principles by all professionals and managers across the various care services that an individual might access.

ACTIVITY 2.1
ANSWER

ACTIVITY 2.1: REFLECTIVE PRACTICE

Think of occasions when you have assessed a person's needs and planned their care. Reflect on examples where:

- Your assessment went well.
- Your assessment did not go so well.

What factors seemed to make the difference to these encounters?

THE HISTORY OF PERSON-CENTRED CARE

The concept of *person-centred care* (PCC) is not new. The first person-centred care approach derived from the holistic work of Swiss physician Paul Tournier, published in 1940. His writing focused upon supporting an individual person through integrative therapeutic approaches within medicine, psychology and pastoral care, and a combined response to meeting individual needs (Cox et al., 2007).

This egalitarian approach to care was not widely in use in the post-war years, when healthcare systems, particularly in Europe, adopted a socialised, one-size-fits-all model. Bucking this trend, Virginia Henderson advocated approaches to nursing care, which were patient-centred, with assessment involving negotiation and empathic understanding of the patient's needs, and interventions aimed at restoring independence as quickly as possible (Henderson, 1955). This approach reflected the concept of individualised care.

By the 1990s, some local authorities in the UK began to personalise the commissioning of community care services. At this time, a number of equivalent terms were used interchangeably (individualised, holistic, patient-centred and person-centred care). There was an evolution in terminology, the use of which, to some extent, was dependent upon context. The change from patient-centred to person-centred reflects a recognition of a person's intrinsic worth as a human being, above and beyond their status as a patient in need of care.

The importance of a person-centred approach to care developed further in the early twenty-first century, as modernisation of health and social care shifted focus more generally towards the individual. This was partly in response to a wide consultation exercise, following publication of a Government white paper entitled *Our Health, Our Care, Our Say* (Department of Health, 2006). The paper called for reforms which would better meet individual needs, and put people in control of their own care provision.

In response to the neglectful culture which had been in evidence at the Mid Staffordshire NHS Foundation Trust between January 2005 and March 2009, the final report of the subsequent public inquiry (Francis, 2013) focused national attention on putting patients at the centre of decision making, improving quality of care and enhancing the patient experience within the NHS. The realisation that there was a lack of patient-centredness within the NHS acted as a catalyst for wide-ranging change, towards the development of a 'policy of personalisation' (Manthorpe and Samsi, 2016). This is in keeping with a general trend towards PCC approaches across the Western world, with hopes of achieving **population health management** and reduced capital expense in healthcare (Capko, 2014).

ACTIVITY 2.2: CRITICAL THINKING

ACTIVITY 2.2
ANSWER

Consider how these changing approaches to care across the Western world might impact upon service provision in your local area.

- Do you think care might be delivered differently in the future?
- How might you prepare for these changes?

HOLISTIC PCC MODELS

A focus on holistic care is arguably a factor distinguishing nursing models from the standard medical model, with an emphasis on patient experience rather than upon the disease process in one body system (Aggleton and Chalmers, 2000: 28–9). That's not to say that doctors are immune from person-centred practices, but it may be fair to say that the traditional medical approach has not always embraced holistic principles. Efforts are underway to remedy this through a greater emphasis on teaching communication skills and a person-centred approach in medical schools (English, 2016).

There have been many approaches used to implement PCC in practice, all of which have been constructed upon three main pillars: communication, partnership and health promotion (Constand et al., 2014). A widely used PCC model of nursing is the Person-Centred Nursing Framework (by McCormack and McCance, 2010). It was derived from a combination of conceptual frameworks, developed in collaboration with healthcare practitioners and then tested within an acute hospital setting (McCormack and McCance, 2006). The model combines an holistic assessment of the care needs of an individual person, with subsequent enablement, support and provision provided within the boundaries of existing services. The conceptual framework is represented in Figure 2.1.

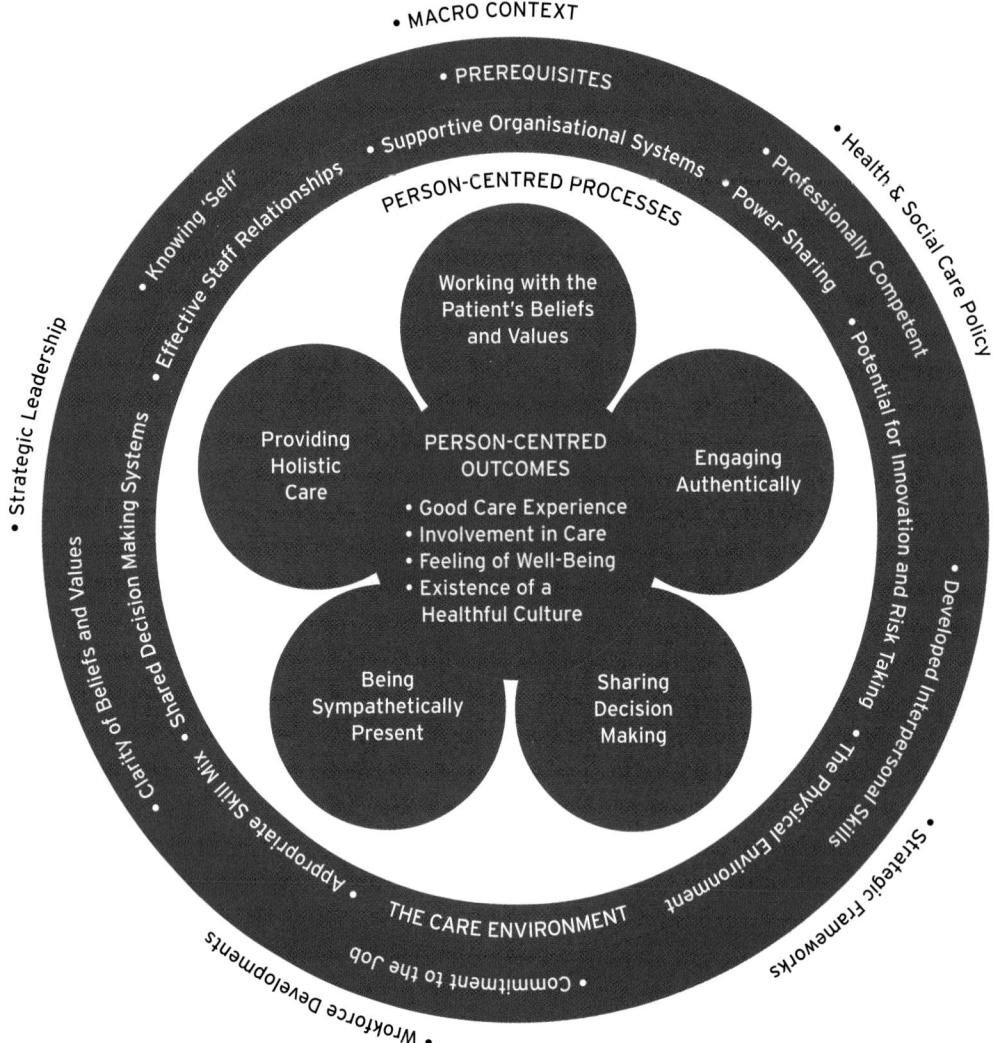

Figure 2.1 The Person-Centred Nursing Framework

McCormack and McCance (2016) *Person-centred Practice in Nursing and Health Care: Theory and Practice.* Wiley Blackwell. © John Wiley & Sons 2016.

The hoped-for person-centred outcomes are in the centre. To achieve them, you must first move through the surrounding circles. These are the fundamental *pre-requisites* enabling PCC.

The outermost concentric circle represents your personal attributes as a nurse: your interpersonal skills, professional competency, commitment to your work and self-awareness of your own values and beliefs. Your ability to provide good person-centred care hinges upon you developing a high degree of **emotional intelligence**.

The inner concentric circle represents the care environment, in both a physical and cultural sense. The recognition and promotion of PCC should be embedded within your workplace culture. There must be robust processes enabling shared decision making, enhancing and supporting your patient's ability to actively involve themselves in decisions about their own care. The focus should be shifted away from mere task-oriented care delivery. (Task-orientation can become the reality within many care environments, even while they claim to uphold person-centred values.)

ACTIVITY 2.3: REFLECTIVE PRACTICE

Examine Figure 2.1 depicting a person-centred approach to care.

* Consider how the model might apply to a care environment you have recently worked in.
* What qualities that facilitate PCC have you noticed in the staff ?
* Does the care environment have a Philosophy of Care standard promoting PCC?
* What barriers do you think exist within the care environment impeding PCC from taking place?

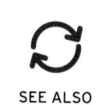

ACTIVITY 2.3
ANSWER

Other important factors include the multidisciplinary team's skill mix, the quality of the relationships within it, as well as the flexibility to innovate and take risks. If, during your practice, you realise that there is a need to innovate, or problem-solve in a creative way, then you need to be able to exercise a degree of autonomy. However, often the scope for this can be quite limited. Creative innovation may prove inconsistent with the safety culture that has resulted from the Mid Staffordshire scandal. Strategic approaches to nursing, arising from NHS England's *Five Year Forward View* (2014), place a high value on person-centred innovation, while simultaneously calling for the uniform adoption of best practice nationally (NHS England, 2016). This may create an uncomfortable dichotomy for healthcare staff.

SEE ALSO
CHAPTER 5

The centre of Figure 2.1 contains the care processes delivering the desired person-centred outcomes. This is where you can be most effective in providing PCC, by being respectful, and making best use of your communication and empathy skills. The authors describe the importance of a nurse having a 'sympathetic presence', engaging with patients meaningfully to provide holistic care (McCormack and McCance 2010). A mutual understanding of values and beliefs between you and your patient is enhanced through dialogue relevant to care, including, where appropriate, personally held matters such as spirituality, religious values and sexuality. This helps to engender a foundation of trust between you, supporting the vital process of shared decision making.

SEE ALSO
CHAPTER 3

ACTIVITY 2.4: LEADERSHIP AND TEAM-WORKING

Read Molly's story from the beginning of the chapter. What does this tell us about the role of communication in providing person-centred care? Additionally, what do we learn about the nurse's role within the broader care team?

ACTIVITY 2.4
ANSWER

SHARED DECISION MAKING

Person-centred care promotes the inclusion of patients in decisions about their own care. By promoting the principles of person-centred care, and raising awareness about choice, you can enhance the capacity for 'shared decision making'. Achieving success rests upon a mutual sharing of values, beliefs and perspectives between you and your patient.

SEE ALSO
CHAPTER 37

Enabling people to take part in decision making about their care is a crucial aspect of PCC. Traditionally, a person presenting with an illness adopts a patient role, essentially handing over decision-making responsibility to the doctors and nurses charged with their care. The adoption of this role can range from profoundly important, life-changing decisions (e.g. whether to operate), to whether it's alright to leave the ward for ten minutes to buy a newspaper.

This conditioning puts the patient into a passive role where they may significantly amend their behaviour and decision-making capabilities in order to satisfy the perceived expectations of healthcare professionals. Loss of personal power within a situation can degrade a person's dignity. It is vital for you to be aware of this and consciously promote the dignity of those you care for. To achieve this, you should show people respect, and take their values into account when providing care. PCC aims to re-empower individuals who come into contact with the healthcare system, so that they can become a central decision maker in their own care.

ACTIVITY 2.5
ANSWER

ACTIVITY 2.5: REFLECTIVE PRACTICE

Consider a recent situation where someone in your care was faced with an important decision.

- Do you think they were well supported in coming to their decision?
- What efforts were made to provide information and to gain insight into that person's opinions?
- Did the decision properly reflect the person's values and beliefs?

A word of caution: be aware that there can be considerable risks to such an approach, however benevolent and appealing it may seem. Medical practice is a complicated world full of jargon. Decisions often hinge upon a nuanced approach to complex evidence-based frameworks, built upon years of professional expertise and experience. As a result, it is sometimes unreasonable in healthcare to expect a lay person to get up to speed with everything they need to know to make a wise choice. To facilitate good decisions, you need to provide succinct, targeted information to enable your patient to make informed decisions about their care. You must be able to back up any advice with reliable evidence.

Patients have a tendency to overestimate the benefits of medical tests, treatments and screening. At the same time, they underestimate the potential harm that such interventions can cause. As a result, if you discuss tests and treatments with a patient, as part of shared decision making, you need to cover the benefits and harms of a particular intervention (preferably based upon quantifiable evidence), as well as correct any misconceptions.

Arguments have been presented questioning whether patient choice can truly be implemented within the NHS, given the social model which lies at the heart of its traditional values (Fotaki, 2014). Despite the institutional difficulties which the NHS faces in bringing PCC into its everyday processes, you can make a difference through supporting your patients to make informed choices.

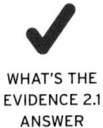

WHAT'S THE
EVIDENCE 2.1
ANSWER

WHAT'S THE EVIDENCE? 2.1

Healthcare professionals and patients tend to agree that being treated with dignity and respect is a fundamental attribute of good care. However, measuring outcomes in PCC can prove challenging for researchers. Many of the standard methods of measuring the effectiveness of the work of nurses don't really reflect the complexity of what's going on in practice. This is especially the case when attempting to evaluate person-centred nursing.

Search the nursing literature for research providing evidence for the effectiveness, or otherwise, of PCC. Do you think what you have found provides a sufficiently strong evidence base for PCC?

It is part of your role to communicate relevant and up-to date knowledge, within the bounds of your accumulated knowledge and experience. Sometimes, when confronted with new information about disease, diagnostic tests or intended treatments, patients will feign understanding, while remaining confused and unsettled. If you recognise that this might be taking place, you can remedy the situation through your use of good communication skills, thereby enhancing mutual understanding and supporting emotions.

It is important that you are prepared to take the time to listen and learn, with an approach that is friendly, inquisitive and empathetic (Hashim, 2017). If you can, try to pick up what is *not* being said. A climate of honesty, openness and respect will always nurture good care. It will help you to be supportive of patients as they grapple with new information, and make informed decisions.

By offering choice, you need to recognise the risk of the 'wrong' decision being arrived at. You should be prepared to act as a 'moral agent', advocating on behalf of your patient and their family, even if you may not personally agree with the choices they make. This requires from you a well-developed sense of self-belief and inner confidence.

A key factor in PCC is for you to know how to maximise an individual's autonomy and enable choice based upon current reliable evidence (McCormack and McCance, 2010). But PCC also acknowledges times when your patient might prefer simply to let you act on their behalf, becoming passive in decisions about their own care. You should also be prepared to respect this wish, even if you're in the midst of providing appropriate information, options and time.

CASE STUDY 2.1: KEN

Re-read Ken's story provided at the beginning of this chapter. Consider the importance of empathy, dignity and respect in Ken's battle with liver cirrhosis. What part did honesty play in his recovery?

CASE STUDY 2.1
ANSWER

THE IMPORTANCE OF DIGNITY

Definitions of dignity vary, but essentially it is the quality of being worthy of respect. This may include self-respect, but most importantly it is the value of being respected by others. Within a healthcare environment, where illness and loss of basic mental or physical function may jeopardise that respect, it is vitally important for the individual affected to feel that they are valued and important (Matiti and Baillie, 2011: 13).

SEE ALSO
CHAPTER 3

The value that is placed upon dignity by both care givers and service users is reflected in UK legislation relating to healthcare. Dignity and respect feature strongly within the NMC's *Code* (2015), which aims to embody the principles of PCC. The *Code* provides guidance on what to do if you think that the care within a setting is not person-centred or values-based. Your local care providers will also have policies in place to enable their staff, and students placed in their settings, to raise concerns. It is incumbent upon you to uphold the values discussed in this chapter, and always treat the patients in your care with dignity, respect and compassion.

ACTIVITY 2.6: CRITICAL THINKING

Can you think of which national and international laws pertain to human dignity? Then look up the professional code of conduct relevant to your practice.

ACTIVITY 2.6
ANSWER

- Read the section pertaining to dignity and respect.
- Critically consider how these passages relate to your personal approach to care.

Person-centred care is particularly vital when working with people whose identity, or 'personhood', is in danger of becoming lost. Examples may be people living with dementia, or having learning disabilities (Thompson et al., 2008). Other examples may include people suffering from the long-term consequences of a major stroke, loss of consciousness, brain damage, or other neurological disorders where cognitive capacity, or a sense of personal identity, has been lost.

SEE ALSO
CHAPTER 4

The Mental Capacity Act (Great Britain, 2005) sets out the legal framework for how decisions are to be made in the interests of people who lack the capacity to make those decisions for themselves. This includes decision making about how to protect themselves from abuse. Those to whom the legislation might apply could include people suffering with dementia, learning disabilities and some mental health problems. Everyone working with and/or caring for an adult who may lack capacity to make decisions must comply with this Act and its Codes of Practice, which include the Deprivation of Liberty Safeguards (DoLS).

Loss of social functioning can exacerbate a sense of disengagement, isolation and loneliness, particularly when someone is being cared for outside of their normal, familiar environment. The same difficulties may also occur when vulnerable people are placed within an unfamiliar context (e.g. a hospital ward) where expectations are placed upon them to behave in a certain way, but their cognitive function is not sufficient to meet that expectation. This often leads to fear, confusion, a loss of dignity, and capacity to function independently.

As providers of care, it is important for you to relate to the person in front of you, and not the *patient role* they might feel obliged to play. By doing so, you're providing *person*-centred care, rather than merely *patient*-centred care. Simply put, you need to get to know the people in your care, and leave any temptation to judge them at the door.

This is facilitated by highly developed inter personal skills, particularly communication, awareness and powers of observation (Hinchliff and Rogers, 2008). Nonetheless, this can often prove challenging, especially in cases where personhood is undermined by disease, disability or environment. Assumptions can be made about what is in the best interests of that person. Choice can be denied because it is either too difficult to achieve, or too time-consuming a process to undertake.

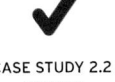

CASE STUDY 2.2
ANSWER

CASE STUDY 2.2: JOHN

You receive a phone call at work from the sister of one of your patients, John. He has been left with long-term cognitive impairment following a stroke, which has recently extended. His sister, Elizabeth, speaks with an air of authority. She informs you that she is a journalist for a national newspaper. Elizabeth works long hours some distance away and explains that she is unable to visit in person. She says communication with hospital staff has often been a problem because of this. As John's next of kin, Elizabeth wants to be involved in decision making about his care. She explains that she has provided support and guidance to John in the past, and that he always accepts her advice. However, John is not currently in the position to give his consent to this.

- Which local policies might you need to take into account when discussing matters over the phone?
- How might you go about safely involving Elizabeth in decisions about John's care?
- Can you imagine a scenario where this situation might need to be escalated, and to whom?

The person-centred approach builds partnerships. It helps to empower patients and the involvement of their families, even when the decisions they arrive at might not fit with received opinion. PCC values the uniqueness of the individual, and finds worth in each person, irrespective of whether the affliction they suffer with may potentially deny them their 'personhood'.

THE HOUSE OF CARE

PCC places emphasis on the relationship of care around four key principles:

1. Dignity, respect and compassion
2. Coordination of care
3. Personalised care and interventions
4. Enabling care.

This requires not just a change in approach by the individual practitioner, but also the active support of the healthcare system (Collins, 2014). The 'House of Care' (Figure 2.2) amply illustrates the PCC approach to care, whereby engagement and communication is fostered between service providers and the person receiving care.

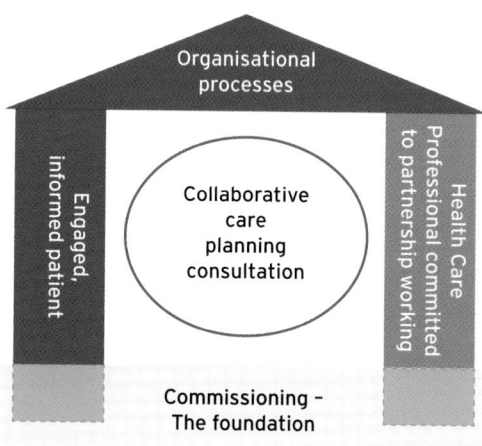

Figure 2.2   The House of Care

Reproduced with permission of the Coalition for Collaborative Care.

SEE ALSO
CHAPTER 18

The House of Care is a coordinated person-centred delivery system for people suffering with long-term conditions (Coulter et al., 2013).

It provides a framework helping you to mould your practice to benefit the health and wellbeing of a variety of patients in different settings (Taylor, 2015).

The House's diagrammatic components are composed of the following:

- The roof represents the organisational and administrative processes.
- The left-hand wall represents an informed and involved patient.
- The right-hand wall represents an enabling workforce, committed to working in partnership with one another.
- The foundation represents the commissioning processes and services.
- At the centre of the House of Care is a truly collaborative care-planning consultation.

Multidisciplinary and multi-agency approaches are essential for this to work in practice, creating strong and viable partnerships.

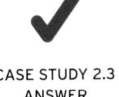

CASE STUDY 2.3
ANSWER

CASE STUDY 2.3: JOHN

People suffering with long-term conditions sometimes require complex packages of care to maintain their quality of life. Consider John's situation. He has received long-term care twice a day to maintain his independence at home following his stroke. His sister, who lives some distance away, has provided additional support over the phone, and through occasional visits. Unfortunately, John's stroke has been extended, threatening his independence, and curtailing his capacity to make decisions. Using a person-centred approach, consider what the next steps might be in his care, and who might get involved in the decision-making process.

Person-centred approaches to care also recognise the importance of 'peer support'. This innovation has the potential to improve healthcare experiences and outcomes among people with long-term physical and mental health conditions, promoting self-management within a supportive community, as well as providing much needed emotional and social support (National Voices, 2015). The use of social media shows great promise, helping to bring people suffering with similar long-term conditions together in mutually supportive networks. The establishment of these virtual patient communities can empower people, build autonomy and facilitate health promotion, all of which are underlying principles of PCC (Amann et al., 2016).

Proposals for the provision of a more person-centred healthcare system have been put forward by The Health Foundation (Collins, 2014). It argues for a service that supports and empowers people to make their own informed decisions about healthcare, and to successfully manage their own health and social care – or to reject the care provided. As a result of new legislation (Great Britain, 2014), personal budgets became mandatory for all eligible users from April 2015. This new system of working put many adults coping with long-term social care needs in charge of their own care budgets, facilitating person-centred choice.

Shortly afterwards, the National Audit Office published a review of personalised commissioning in adult social care in England (National Audit Office, 2016). Despite acknowledging a paucity of official data suggesting improved outcomes, it found widespread support for the concept of personalised commissioning, with most service users reporting that they had benefited from the change.

CHAPTER SUMMARY

- Person-Centred Care is a vitally important approach to nursing care. As well as defining and describing PCC, we explored one model of person-centred nursing in detail.
- PCC emerged from a cultural shift towards individualisation, an increasing emphasis on holistic care, as well as healthcare scandals where patients were badly let down by the providers of their care.
- The values of dignity and respect are bound up in the person-centred approach to care.
- PCC ensures people are central partners in decisions about their own health, and their care.
- Providing choice, through shared decision making, allows innovation in nursing, but also recognises that patients may make choices that you don't always agree with.
- The healthcare system must actively support the principles of PCC to enable nurses to practise it effectively.

GO FURTHER

Books

- Binnie, A. and Titchen, A. (1999). *Freedom to Practise: The development of patient-centred nursing.* Oxford: Elsevier.
  This book provides practical guidance for implementing PCC into your practice.
- Brooker, D. (2007). *Person-centred Dementia Care: Making services better.* London: Jessica Kingsley Publishers Ltd.
  An alternative framework for PCC.
- McCormack, B. and McCance, T. (2010). *Person-Centred Nursing; Theory & Practice.* Chichester: Wiley-Blackwell.
  A comprehensive framework for the use of PCC in nursing.

Journal Articles

FURTHER READING: JOURNAL ARTICLES

Go to https://study.sagepub.com/essentialadultnursing for further free online journal articles related to this chapter. If you are using the interactive ebook, simply click on the book icon in the margin to go straight to the resource.

- Baillie, L. (2007) The impact of staff behaviour on patient dignity in acute hospitals. *Nursing Times*, 103 (34): 30-1.
  There are many practical lessons to be learned from previous mistakes. Awareness of these can promote PCC.
- Chenoweth, L. , Stein-Parbury, J., Lapkin, S. and Wang, Y. (2015) Organisational interventions for promoting person-centred care for people with dementia. *Cochrane Database of Systematic Reviews*, Issue 11. Art. No.: CD011963.
  Although this article simply provides a protocol for reviewing organisational interventions in dementia care, it contains a useful précis of PCC.
- Constand, M., MacDermid, J.C., Dal Bello-Haas, V. and Law, M. (2014) Scoping review of patient-centred care approaches in healthcare. *BMC Health Services Research*, 14: 27.
  Much of the evidence supporting PCC in the literature focuses upon communication.

Weblinks

FURTHER READING: WEBLINKS

Go to https://study.sagepub.com/essentialadultnursing for further weblinks related to this chapter. If you are using the interactive ebook, simply click on the book icon in the margin to go straight to the resource.

- The Health Foundation (2017) *Person-centred Care Resource Centre.* London: The Health Foundation. Available at: http://personcentredcare.health.org.uk/
  The Health Foundation has produced a significant online resource centre about PCC.
- Sieff, Adrian (2013) *A Portal for Resources and Learning on Person-centred Care.* London: The Health Foundation. Available at: www.health.org.uk/newsletter/portal-resources-and-learning-person-centred-care
  This article, about the various PCC resources available online, is aimed at care providers and clinicians.
- Skills for Health (2017) *Person-Centred Approaches: Empowering people in their lives and communities to enable an upgrade in prevention, wellbeing, health, care and support.* Bristol: Skills for Health. Available at: www.skillsforhealth.org.uk/images/pdf/Person-Centred-Approaches-Framework.pdf
  This framework helps develop the skills, knowledge and attitudes of the health and social care workforce to put PCC into practice.

ACE YOUR ASSESSMENT

Revise what you have learned by visiting https://study.sagepub.com/essentialadultnursing

- Test yourself with multiple-choice and short-answer questions
- Do the chapter activities in the book and check your answers online

REFERENCES

Aggleton, P. and Chalmers, H. (2000) *Nursing Models and Nursing Practice* (2nd ed.). Basingstoke: Palgrave.

Amann, J., Zanini, C. and Rubinelli, S. (2016) What online user innovation communities can teach us about capturing the experiences of patients living with chronic health conditions. A scoping review. *PloS One*, 11 (6): pe0156175.

Capko, J. (2014) The patient-centred movement. *The Journal of Medical Practice Management*, 29 (4): 238–42.

Collins A. (2014) *Measuring What Really Matters; Towards a coherent measurement system to support person-centred care*. London: The Health Foundation.

Constand, M., MacDermid, J.C., Dal Bello-Haas, V. and Law, M. (2014) Scoping review of patient-centred care approaches in healthcare. *BMC Health Services Research*, 14: 27.

Coulter, A., Roberts, S. and Dixon, D. (2013) *Delivering Better Services for People with Long-term Conditions: Building the house of care*. London: King's Fund.

Cox, J., Campbell, A. and Fulford, B. (2007). *Medicine of the Person; Faith, science and values in health care provision*. London: Jessica Kingsley Publishers.

Department of Health (2006) *Our Health, Our Care, Our Say: A new direction for community services*. London: Department of Health.

English, J. (2016) Training doctors for person-centred care. *Journal of the Association of American Medical Colleges*, 91 (3): 294–6.

Fotaki, M. (2014) *Choice and the NHS: What market-based patient choice can't do for the NHS: The theory and evidence of how choice works in health care*. London: Centre for Health and the Public Interest. Available at: https://chpi.org.uk/wp-content/uploads/2014/03/What-market-based-patient-choice-cant-do-for-the-NHS-CHPI.pdf (last accessed 6 June 2018).

Francis, R. (2013) *Report of the Mid Staffordshire NHS Foundation Trust Public Inquiry*. London: The Stationery Office.

Great Britain (2005) *Mental Capacity Act*. London: HMSO.

Great Britain (2014) *Care Act*. London: HMSO.

Hashim, M.K. (2017) Patient-centred communication: Basic skills. *American Family Physician*, 95 (1): 29–34.

Henderson, V. (1955) *Principles and Practice of Nursing*. New York: Macmillan.

Hinchliff, S. and Rogers, R. (2008) *Competencies for Advanced Nursing Practice*. London: Hodder Arnold.

Kitwood, T. (1997) *Dementia Reconsidered: The person comes first*. Milton Keynes: Open University Press.

Manthorpe, J. and Samsi, K. (2016) Person-centred dementia care: Current perspectives. *Clinical Interventions in Aging*, 11: 1733–40.

Matiti, M.R. and Baillie L. (2011) *Dignity in Healthcare*. London: Radcliffe Publishing.

McCormack, B. and McCance, T. (2006) Development of a framework for person-centred nursing. *Journal of Advanced Nursing*, 56 (5): 472–9.

McCormack, B. and McCance, T. (2010) *Person-Centred Nursing; Theory & Practice*. Chichester: Wiley-Blackwell.

National Audit Office (2016) *Personalised Commissioning in Adult Social Care*. London: National Audit Office, Department of Health and local authorities, pp 4–12. Available at: www.nao.org.uk/wp-content/uploads/2016/03/Personalised-commissioning-in-adult-social-care-update.pdf (last accessed 6 June 2018).

National Voices (2015) *Peer Support: What is it and does it work?* London: National Voices & Nesta.

NHS England (2014) *Five Year Forward View*. London: NHS England. Available at: www.england.nhs.uk/ourwork/futurenhs/ (last accessed 6 June 2018).

NHS England (2016) *Leading Change, Adding Value: A framework for nursing, midwifery and care staff*. London: NHS England. Available at: www.england.nhs.uk/wp-content/uploads/2016/05/nursing-framework.pdf (last accessed 6 June 2018).

Nursing and Midwifery Council (NMC) (2015) *The Code for Nurses and Midwives*. London: NMC.

Rhodes, M., Morris, A. and Lazenby, R. (2011) Nursing at its best: Competent and caring. *Online Journal of Issues in Nursing*, May 2011, 16 (2).

Taylor, A. (2015) *Building the House of Care: How health economies in Leeds and Somerset are implementing a coordinated approach for people with long-term conditions*. London: The Health Foundation. Available at: http://personcentredcare.health.org.uk/sites/default/files/resources/buildingthehouseofcare_0.pdf (last accessed 6 June 2018).

Thompson, J., Kilbane, J. and Sanderson, H. (2008) *Person Centred Practice for Professionals*. Maidenhead: McGraw-Hill.

PROFESSIONAL VALUES

KAREN ELCOCK AND OMAR MANSARAY

3

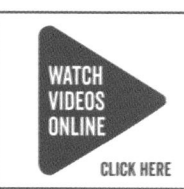

WATCH VIDEOS ONLINE

CLICK HERE

THIS CHAPTER COVERS

- The meaning of professional values in the context of adult nursing care
- Why professional values have become an important focus in nursing
- The development of professional values in adult nursing
- Values-based practice
- How professional values are demonstrated through the nurse revalidation process.

> "
> My professional values have developed through placements, my communication, both verbal and non-verbal. I have also learnt the difference between hearing and listening to the patient. I have learnt about empathy and how to be patient.
>
> **Jodine Weekes, 1st-year adult student nurse**
> "

> "
> The 6Cs have been a major part of my nursing journey with each one being equally important. The more time you spend with your patients, their carers and relatives, the more you realise that the 6Cs can be initiated throughout all your nursing interactions.
>
> **Louise, 3rd-year adult student nurse**
> "

INTRODUCTION

Professional values are the cornerstone of our professional practice. For students, there will always be a strong focus on the need to develop the knowledge and practical skills to deliver safe and effective care. However, the importance of those softer skills that demonstrate caring and compassion cannot be underestimated, nor how our personal and professional values influence their development. Jodine above encapsulates the importance of these softer skills beautifully in her reflection on her learning so far in her first year. Healthcare scandals in recent years have led the NMC, GMC, universities and healthcare and social care employers to emphasise the importance of an individual's professional values. While patients value technical competence and knowledgeable nurses, they prioritise the importance of them having the appropriate professional values (Griffiths et al., 2012). This chapter, therefore, will explore what we mean by professional values and how they may influence your approaches to care. We will look at how healthcare scandals have led to a series of changes in nursing including, recruitment; the development of the NMC's *The Code* (NMC, 2015); influenced your curriculum; changed approaches to clinical practice; the introduction of revalidation and significant changes in how concerns are raised in practice. You will have looked at the *Code* and the 6Cs (Department of Health and NHS Commissioning Board, 2012) in year one so it is worth revisiting these again as they underpin much of this chapter.

THE MEANING OF PROFESSIONAL VALUES IN THE CONTEXT OF ADULT NURSING CARE

The nursing profession carries with it great privilege and responsibility. Nursing provides an incredibly meaningful and fulfilling role in supporting people in difficult and vulnerable periods in their lives. Being a member of the nursing profession proclaims something about who we are as individuals and people tend to make assumptions and have high expectations about our character, believing nurses to have a caring, compassionate, hardworking and trustworthy disposition. These characteristics are woven into our identity as people.

Values are central to our practice and we need a thorough awareness and understanding of how they influence our practice and their impact on the care that we provide to patients. Baillie and Black (2014: p.2) suggest that values are generally defined as 'beliefs or principles that influence behaviour' and go on to describe how our work is governed at its core by standards, beliefs and principles which underpin our attitudes and so guide and influence our professional behaviour. As professionals, we need to understand patients' needs, empathise and display humanity, maintain dignity, and demonstrate compassion and kindness. We are also expected to demonstrate leadership, evidence-based knowledge and skills, and raise concerns as soon as we believe patients are at risk (NMC, 2015).

HOW ARE PROFESSIONAL VALUES RELATED TO PERSONAL VALUES?

As we have already discussed, professional values are necessary to reinforce our professional identity and performance. Our practice as nurses must exemplify the integration of both the core standards of professional nursing and our inherent personal values in our clinical practice. As nurses, we are expected to be aware of our professional values and apply them to our decision making and clinical practice. As we adopt the professional values of the organisations we work for, we should also be aware of our own values, beliefs and attitudes as they may vary from the NHS and organisational standards we must follow in our professional practice. This can cause dissonance for us if the two are in conflict when caring for patients: examples are provided in the Go Further box.

GO FURTHER

The NMC identifies two areas where nurses and midwives can lawfully have conscientious objection (termination of pregnancy and technological procedures to achieve conception and pregnancy). Outline the actions you must take if this applies to you. See the NMC website for more information. www.nmc.org.uk/standards/code/conscientious-objection-by-nurses-and-midwives/

WEBLINK: NMC STANDARDS

Personal values are described by Carvalho et al. (2011) as the starting point for morality and ethics. They explain that these three concepts of values, morals and ethics can be seen to interact with and relate to each other. These values are rooted in the environments and the families that we were raised in and, for some, their spiritual or religious point of view. These influences determine our attitudes towards certain issues and the sort of person we are, and why we respond to people and events in our life as we do. As we grow, these values will develop and continue to evolve all through our lives. It is not surprising, therefore, that Shahriari et al. (2013) in reviewing the literature to identify the ethical values for nurses found that, while there were values common globally, there were also differences in the definition of some values. These were ones that had been influenced by economic status and social, cultural and religious beliefs.

Caring for patients presenting with a variety of physical and psychological health and complex social care needs, coupled with the many financial and structural challenges in the NHS and the growing demand for healthcare means, that providing high-quality nursing care can be complicated, resulting in ethical dilemmas in caring for patients. Alongside this we live in increasingly culturally diverse communities and our practices may be challenged by patients who have lifestyles or health beliefs that we may disagree with (Leininger and McFarland, 2002). In addition, we may have difficulties with some treatment strategies that challenge our personal and professional values. The guiding principles we can apply in these circumstances are to maintain a broad, objective and open attitude about each patient and avoid seeing all patients alike. By following these principles, we can open ourselves to learning about the way others view health and illness and enable relationships that are therapeutic (Leininger and McFarland, 2002).

GO FURTHER

Madeleine Leininger developed the theory of transcultural nursing which focuses on the importance of understanding that different cultures have different values, beliefs and practices and how nurses can identify and address these differences in order to deliver culturally competent care. A good introduction to her work can be found here: https://nurseslabs.com/madeleine-leininger-transcultural-nursing-theory/

WEBLINK: MADELEINE LEININGER

Our professional values must be used as our reference point when confronted with ethical concerns. Where we find our personal and professional values are in conflict we must use resources such as clinical reflection, mentor support and clinical supervision to find solutions to alleviate the stress this may cause and the impact it may have on the care that we provide.

As you start your journey into nursing, getting acquainted with the NMC's *The Code,* the *Standards of Proficiency* (NMC, 2018), the 6Cs and the *NHS Constitution* (DH, 2015) will increase your knowledge about expectations regarding your professional practice and will guide your understanding of the professional nurse's responsibilities to patients and the organisations they work for. This will enable us to take pride in our profession and work hard to safeguard its reputation, employing good clinical skills in practice and demonstrating exemplary behaviour.

CRITICAL THINKING STOP POINT 3.1

Write down any personal values or beliefs that may come into conflict with the professional values expected of you.

VALUES FRAMEWORKS IN NURSING

The NMC's *The Code* (NMC, 2015) describes principles that patients and their carers should expect from the care we provide and standards that nurses should follow in their professional practice. The *Code* sets out values and principles within four themes: prioritise people; practise effectively; preserve safety; and promote professionalism and trust. As nurses, we are expected to follow these standards in relation to our personal and professional behaviour and performance, which are important in making sure we safeguard the health and wellbeing of the public.

Nursing values are also described in the 6Cs for nursing, midwifery and care staff (Figure 3.1). The 6Cs – care, compassion, courage, communication, commitment and competence – are a set of core values drawn up by the Chief Nursing Officer for England, Jane Cummings, and the Department of Health's Chief Nursing Adviser, Viv Bennett, in 2012 (Department of Health and NHS Commissioning Board, 2012). They apply to both clinical and non-clinical staff who work in the NHS. The 6Cs reinforce the core values and beliefs that underpin nursing practice and emphasise placing patients at the centre of the care we provide.

The 6Cs and the NMC's *Code* underpin the NMC *Standards of Proficiency for Registered Nurses* (NMC, 2018) which acknowledge the public's expectation *that registered nurses possess the values and personal attributes of being caring, empathetic and compassionate* and makes clear the need for nurses to recognise the diversity of the people they will care for and so take into account the differing beliefs and values they hold.

In addition, the NHS in all four countries of the UK has each declared its own common values in line with the recommendations by Francis (2013). You may be familiar with them as they have been used to underpin recruitment processes to nursing programmes and to posts in the NHS, but it is worth taking time to review them again by undertaking Activity 3.1.

ACTIVITY 3.1
ANSWER

ACTIVITY 3.1: REFLECTIVE PRACTICE – COMMON VALUES

You will find the values for healthcare in each country available on the Internet. Look up the relevant document below for your country:

NHS England The NHS Constitution for England (2015)
Northern Ireland Quality 2020 (2011)
NHS Scotland 2020 Workforce Vision, Everyone Matters (2013)
NHS Wales Values and Standards of Behaviour Framework (2016)

1. What do these values mean to you?
2. Are there are any values you feel are missing and if so why?

A summary of the NHS values can be found at https://study.sagepub.com/essentialadultnursing

Care	• Care is our core business and that of our organisations, and the care we deliver helps the individual person and improves the health of the whole community. Caring defines us and our work. People receiving care expect it to be right for them, consistently, throughout every stage of their life.
Compassion	• Compassion is how care is given through relationships based on empathy, respect and dignity – it can also be described as intelligent kindness, and is central to how people perceive their care.
Communication	• Communication is central to successful caring relationships and to effective team working. Listening is as important as what we say and do and essential for 'no decision about me without me'. Communication is the key to a good workplace with benefits for those in our care and staff alike.
Commitment	• A commitment to our patients and populations is a cornerstone of what we do. We need to build on our commitment to improve the care and experience of our patients, to take action to make this vision and strategy a reality for all and meet the health, care and support challenges ahead.
Courage	• Courage enables us to do the right thing for the people we care for, to speak up when we have concerns and to have the personal strength and vision to innovate and to embrace new ways of working.
Competence	• Competence means all those in caring roles must have the ability to understand an individual's health and social needs and the expertise, clinical and technical knowledge to deliver effective care and treatments based on research and evidence.

Figure 3.1   The 6Cs (DH & NHS Commissioning Board, 2012)

Reproduced with permission under the Open Government Licence.

PREPARATION FOR PRACTICE PLACEMENTS

In addition to the core NHS values for each country you will find that each healthcare organisation will have published their own values, which are linked to the common NHS values, on their website. It is a good idea prior to each placement to find out what these values are for your placement provider and they are also useful as you prepare your application for your first post.

CRITICAL THINKING STOP POINT 3.2

Keep a reflective diary that links your learning in practice to key professional values. This evidence can be used for your assessment in practice, course assignments and for future job applications/ interviews.

WHY PROFESSIONAL VALUES HAVE BECOME AN IMPORTANT FOCUS IN NURSING

The increased focus on professional values in nursing in recent years arose following a series of healthcare scandals which revealed poor standards of care across a range of healthcare settings (Keogh, 2013), with the failings at Mid Staffordshire NHS Foundation Trust (Francis, 2010, 2013) having the most significant repercussions. The first Francis Inquiry (2010) found that patients were deprived of many of the fundamental elements of care (food, drink, hygiene, toileting, privacy in care, death with dignity) and raised concerns regarding what was viewed as a decline in compassionate care by nurses as well as other healthcare workers. The two Francis reports along with the report on Winterbourne View (DH, 2012) identified a lack of the core values, skills and behaviours required by nurses and healthcare staff to deliver compassionate care, and a work culture where poor care was neither challenged nor concerns raised (Sykes and Durham, 2014).

The second Francis Report (2013) made several recommendations with a specific focus on values: the need for common values, the need to recruit both students and staff with the right values and training standards that ensured nurses were prepared to deliver compassionate care (see Figure 3.2).

You may feel at this stage that you are drowning in different views on values, so for a very different perspective on values in healthcare see the What's the Evidence? box.

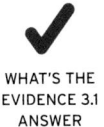

WHAT'S THE
EVIDENCE 3.1
ANSWER

WHAT'S THE EVIDENCE? 3.1

Read Chapter 1, The Values Delusion in Seedhouse, D. (2017) *Thoughtful Health Care. Ethical Awareness & Reflective Practice*. London: Sage.

- David provides a very provocative view on the over emphasis on values and how useful (or not) they are to us in healthcare.
- What are your views?

Regardless of whether you agree with David or not, values are endemic in healthcare and now heavily influence how both students and qualified nurses are recruited using values-based recruitment, the content of your course, your assessment in practice and the NMC requirement for you to revalidate with them every three years to maintain your registration with them.

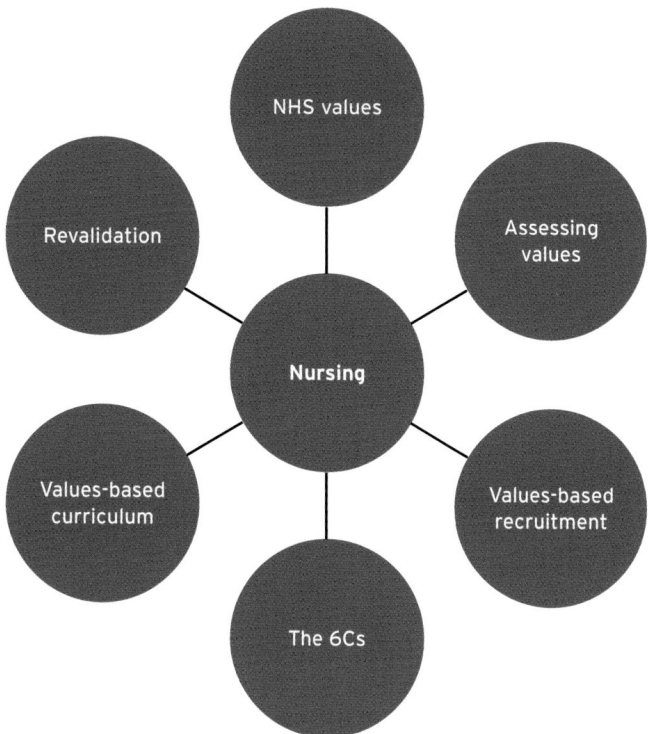

Figure 3.2 The increasing emphasis on values in nursing

THE DEVELOPMENT OF PROFESSIONAL VALUES IN ADULT NURSING

The NMC expect all students to meet the professional values and behaviours that are set out in the *Code* (NMC, 2015) and that these will be developed through learning in both university and placement settings. You will already have a set of values developed by your culture, society, religion/spiritual beliefs, ethnicity and family and many of these may align closely with nursing's professional values, while others may be modified by your experiences on the course and out in practice. The development of your professional values will be influenced in a number of ways.

Professional socialisation and the learning of values

While recruitment of students using values-based recruitment methods may select those who exhibit the right values, maintenance and development of those values through their programme and once qualified is essential. Students learn about professional values in university but it is the practice environment that has the greatest impact on the professional socialisation of students (Rejon and Watts, 2014; Hall, 2013). It is there that students learn how to apply the values they have learnt about in university to the real world of practice. Professional socialisation is a process whereby individuals learn about and adopt the skills, behaviours, roles, attitudes and values of the profession they are joining (Dinmohammadi et al., 2013). Professional socialisation can be both positive and negative with Mackintosh (2006) finding that the negative consequences can result in a loss 'of humanistic concern' (p. 953), that is, the ability to care about the individual. There are a number of consequences of negative professional socialisation on students, with Mackintosh (2006) and Thomas et al. (2012) identifying the loss of, or reduction in, the caring ability of the nurse and the continuation of poor or ritualised practice. These areas were also found in the inquiries led by Francis (2010, 2013). Curtis et al. (2012) describe the dissonance that students experience as they try to balance the wish to deliver compassionate care against the need to fit in by not challenging the status quo. The nurses that students work with are, therefore, highly influential in the socialisation process. While some students will have the courage to challenge poor care and the resilience to maintain and further develop the required values and behaviours, others may adopt the prevailing culture and model the poor practices they see (Hall, 2013) and in turn influence future nursing students that they come in contact with.

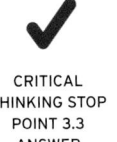

CRITICAL
THINKING STOP
POINT 3.3
ANSWER

CRITICAL THINKING STOP POINT 3.3

- How often have you seen poor care and said nothing?
- Why have you not raised concerns?

The reasons for staff not raising concerns are many and it is likely that, as a student, you have been concerned about the impact on your placement and your practice assessment or becoming known as a 'trouble-maker' in the organisation you are placed in. These were all issues identified by Francis in his report *Freedom to Speak Up* (2015), which has led to improvements in support to both students and staff in practice settings through the development of new roles such as Whistleblowing champions or Freedom to Speak Up Guardians.

GO FURTHER

WEBLINK:
NMC RAISING
CONCERNS

Look at the NMC Raising Concerns webpage, which provides guidance on raising concerns and useful case studies and videos. www.nmc.org.uk/standards/guidance/raising-concerns-guidance-for-nurses-and-midwives/

VALUES-BASED PRACTICE

To be effective in our practice as nurses it is necessary to understand the importance of the role of values and appreciate that we hold both common and different values as individuals to other people. The values of patients and other people we work with will vary widely, and we may find that the values that some individuals view as important may be different to ours.

As society continues to change rapidly and the people we care for come from a range of diverse backgrounds with diverse values, we will increasingly find patients with different values from us. We will also find that patients are more knowledgeable and clear about the care they expect from services. We cannot take for granted that we share the same values in all respects when we make decisions about patient care, where complex and conflicting values may sometimes be in play.

Nursing practice in its core is founded on the principles of a sound evidence base to support effective decision making. Increasingly, the role of values, as well as evidence, is used to support all clinical decision making. The centrality of values in healthcare makes the role of value-based practice not only relevant but also inseparable from clinical decision making (Petrova et al., 2006).

Values-based practice is the theory and skills base for effective healthcare decision making where different and sometimes potentially conflicting values are in play (Fulford, 2008). What this really means is that healthcare staff aim to work in a positive and constructive way with a diversity of values, putting the values and views of patients and carers at the centre of everything we do, and understanding and using our own values and beliefs in a positive way to effectively support decisions we make in the care that we provide (Woodbridge and Fulford, 2004). It is only when these three elements are integrated (evidence-based practice, person-centred care and values-based practice) that clinicians and patients form a therapeutic relationship and, in turn, produce good care outcomes (Sackett et al., 2000).

SEE ALSO
CHAPTER 37

There are many complex and conflicting values which impact on decisions about care that we provide. Complex issues, such as balancing the cost-effectiveness of treatment, quality-of-life issues, and views on the sanctity and prolongation of life, to give a few examples, all impact on treatment decisions in healthcare. One recent example is that of baby Charlie Gard (see Case Study 3.1).

SEE ALSO
CHAPTER 2

SEE ALSO
CHAPTER 6

CASE STUDY 3.1: BABY CHARLIE GARD

CASE STUDY 3.1
ANSWER

Baby Charlie Gard was one month old when he was taken ill and diagnosed with an exceptionally rare genetic condition which causes progressive muscle weakness and brain damage. Great Ormond Street Hospital where he was being cared for went to court and asked the Judge to rule that life support treatment should stop because Charlie could only breathe through a ventilator and was fed through a tube rendering the view that his quality of life was poor and that he should be allowed to die with dignity. The Judge concluded that life-support treatment should end and said a move to a palliative care regime would be in Charlie's best interests. Charlie's parents took their case through the Court of Appeal, the UK Supreme Court and the European Court of Human Rights with no success. The parents returned to the High Court to present fresh evidence about a new, untested experimental treatment for a similar condition in America that they believed could prolong the then 11-month-old Charlie's life. The parents had raised £1.3million to pay for the treatment. By the time a decision was made that this treatment should be considered Charlie's condition had deteriorated significantly and he had suffered irreversible brain damage such that Charlie's parents ended their legal fight over treatment for their terminally-ill son as it had been too late to treat Charlie due to the length of the legal battle with the hospital. Charlie Gard died soon after he was moved to the hospice after his life-support was withdrawn. (Mendick, 2017)

- If you had to make the decision, what personal values would influence your decision about Charlie?
- How do these conflict with professional values around best interests for Charlie?

This is just one example of complex decision making in healthcare. The clinical team and the parents, in deciding what to do regarding treatment, appeared to share the values of respect and best interests but the meaning was understood very differently from the clinicians'/parents' perspectives. What then ensued was the apparent conflict in values between Charlie's parents who wanted to prolong Charlie's life and the hospital's decision, which was based on research evidence and Charlie's best interest – which focussed on the complex question of Charlie's quality of life if his life was prolonged.

Values-based practice utilises a framework for practice, which includes four key clinical skills: awareness, reasoning, knowledge and communication skills. These are summarised in Table 3.1.

Table 3.1 Key skills for values-based practice

- **Awareness of values** includes awareness of the **diversity of values,** awareness of one's **own values** as well as the values of others, and awareness of **positive values** (StAR values, i.e. strengths, aspirations and resources) as well as negative values (such as needs and difficulties).
- **Reasoning about values** includes any of the established methods of ethical reasoning (such as principles reasoning, case-based reasoning (casuistry), or **utilitarianism**) when used to improve understanding of the values, bearing on a given situation (to **'widen our values horizons'**) rather than (directly) to decide what is right.
- **Knowledge of values** covers tacit (or craft) knowledge as well as knowledge derived from research; and it includes the skills for **knowledge retrieval** from electronic databases.
- **Communication skills** include skills for **eliciting values** (including **strengths,** as in ICE-StAR) and skills of conflict resolution.

(Woodbridge and Fulford, 2004)

Values-based practice offers a fresh skills-based approach to working with complex and conflicting values in nursing and it fully complements and supports evidence-based approaches and person-centred care. Nurses should be aware of values and their role in influencing the experience of nursing practice, and undertake training in this approach already used in mental healthcare to enhance their practice. The use of reflection on difficult situations you have encountered in practice is a valuable tool to help you explore your own values and how they may be in conflict with others. Reflection is also an important skill that you will need to use once qualified in order to revalidate with the NMC every three years.

HOW PROFESSIONAL VALUES ARE DEMONSTRATED THROUGH THE NURSE REVALIDATION PROCESS

As discussed earlier, the NMC *Code* (2015) is a set of standards designed to guide our practice as nurses and support our professional development in ensuring our practice is safe and effective; that we put the interests of patients and service users first; and promote trust in the public throughout our practice. The NMC introduced a new framework called revalidation, to enable nurses to demonstrate that they practise safely and effectively and are meeting the standards set out in the *Code* and can therefore maintain their registration with the NMC.

The process of revalidation gives assurance for our continuing fitness to practise beyond the point of initial registration. Nurses must complete and submit reflections on feedback from our colleagues and patients once every three years to demonstrate that we are engaging in continuing professional training and development and are continuing to meet the requirements of our registration as nurses.

Nurse revalidation was introduced by the NMC following recommendations from the Francis reports in 2010 and 2013. Revalidation's true value lies in the opportunity it offers for reflection and reviewing how we apply our practice against the requirements of the *Code*. It is important to note that many fitness to practise cases are concerned with a broad range of poor professional conduct linked to practice, so it is crucial that we understand the role of revalidation in our continuing fitness to practise. Analysis of fitness to practise data indicate that professional conduct is much more frequently a concern than competence (NMC, 2017) and therefore there is a need to raise awareness of professional values as an important aspect in our practice as nurses.

The structure of the revalidation process is directly aligned to the values and behaviours set out in the four main domains of the NMC *Code* – to prioritise people, practise effectively, preserve safety and promote professionalism and trust. These values provide signposting and act as reference points for our professional behaviour. As nurses, we will need to be very familiar with the *Code* and understand how it can be used to support our practice and promote trust in the public.

The requirements for completing the revalidation process include: providing evidence of 450 practice hours; 35 hours of CPD including 20 hours of participatory learning; five pieces of practice-related feedback; five written reflective accounts on practice; reflective discussion about your practice; a health and character declaration; proof of professional indemnity arrangement and a confirmation from an experienced colleague or manager that you have met the revalidation requirements.

The four main values in the *Code* and how to address them in the revalidation process are described in Table 3.2 below.

Table 3.2 Alignment of the revalidation model with the four themes of the *Code*

- **Prioritise people** by actively seeking and reflecting on any direct feedback received from patients, service users and others to ensure that we can fulfil their needs.
- **Practise effectively** by reflecting on our professional development with our colleagues, identifying areas for improvement in our practice and undertaking professional development activities.
- **Preserve safety** by practising within our competency for the minimum number of practice hours, reflecting on feedback, and addressing any gaps in our practice through CPD.
- **Promote professionalism and trust** by providing feedback and helping other NMC colleagues reflect on their professional development, and being accountable to others for our professional development and revalidation.

As you progress in your nursing career it is important to familiarise yourself with the *Code* and be reminded of the principles that constitute safe and effective nursing care, involving the aspects of values, behaviour, attitude and approach that underpin good care. There are significant benefits for revalidation for nurses, patients and their families as it will support and complement the requirements of reflection in helping to improve our practice, satisfy the continuing fitness to practise requirements and generate professionalism in our practice and trust in those that we care for.

GO FURTHER

WEBLINK: NMC REVALIDATION PROCESS

Look at the NMC revalidation website for more information on the revalidation process. http://revalidation.nmc.or.g.uk/

CHAPTER SUMMARY

- Concerns around the professional values held by nurses have become a major focus for the NMC, educators and employers following healthcare scandals in the UK.
- Values are developed over time and influenced by economic status and social, cultural and religious beliefs.
- Professional values may differ from personal values and are developed through socialisation into nursing and healthcare practices.
- There is a range of professional frameworks to guide us including the NMC Code.
- Values-based practice offers an approach that encourages everyone involved in patient care decisions to put the patient's own values at the centre of decision making.
- The revalidation process ensures that we continue to reflect on our values and how we enact them in everyday practice.

GO FURTHER

CASE STUDY:
CONFLICT

Go to https://study.sagepub.com/essentialadultnursing for a further case study related to this chapter. If you are using the interactive ebook, simply click on the book icon in the margin to go straight to the resource.

Books

- Baillie, L. and Black, S. (2014) *Professional Values in Nursing.* London: Taylor and Francis Group.
  A practical easy-to-read book that covers a range of areas which will ensure you embed professional values in your practice.
- Fulford, K., Peile, E. and Carroll, H. (2012) *Essential Values-Based Practice: Clinical Stories Linking Science with People.* Cambridge: Cambridge University Press.
  Offers concrete examples of how values-based practice can be enacted based on real-life stories.
- Gault, I., Shapcott, J., Luthi, A. and Reid, G. (2017) *Communication in Nursing and Healthcare: A guide for compassionate practice.* London: Sage.
  This book will help you develop the communication skills needed to demonstrate compassionate care in a wide range of healthcare settings and applied to a range of client groups.
- Seedhouse, D. (2017) *Thoughtful Health Care. Ethical Awareness & Reflective Practice.* London: Sage.
  A thought-provoking book which offers a critical view on our fixation on values.

Journal Articles

FURTHER
READING:
JOURNAL
ARTICLES

Go to https://study.sagepub.com/essentialadultnursing for further free online journal articles related to this chapter. If you are using the interactive ebook, simply click on the book icon in the margin to go straight to the resource.

- Jimenez-Lopez, F., Roales-Nieto, J., Seco, G.V. and Peeciado, J. (2016) Values in nursing students and professionals: An exploratory comparative study. *Nursing Ethics,* 23(1): 79–91.
  An interesting article that shows how values are changing in nursing with different generations.
- Smith, P. (2014) 'The State we're in': nursing in the 21st Century – a view from Scotland. *Journal of Research in Nursing,* 19(7-8): 606-18.
  A fascinating article which explores many issues for nursing in Scotland.

Weblinks

FURTHER
READING:
WEBLINKS

Go to https://study.sagepub.com/essentialadultnursing for further weblinks related to this chapter. If you are using the interactive ebook, simply click on the book icon in the margin to go straight to the resource.

- NMC Raising concerns
  www.nmc.org.uk/standards/guidance/raising-concerns-guidance-for-nurses-and-midwives/
  An excellent website for students providing guidance, resources for workshops and case studies.
- The Collaborating Centre for Values-based Practice
  https://valuesbasedpractice.org/
  An excellent website with lots of information and resources to help you understand VBP.
- The Arts in Nursing
  The Art of Caring www.artofcaring.org.uk/
  Caring Words www.caringwords.mmu.ac.uk/
  Both these websites offer different ways of using the arts in nursing and so offer an alternative way to think about what nursing is and the values you hold.

ACE YOUR ASSESSMENT

✔

Revise what you have learned by visiting https://study.sagepub.com/essentialadultnursing

- Test yourself with multiple-choice and short-answer questions
- Do the chapter activities in the book and check your answers online

REFERENCES

Baillie, L. and Black, S. (2014) *Professional Values in Nursing*. London: Taylor and Francis.

Carvalho, S., Reeves, M. and Orford, J. (2011) *Fundamental Aspects of Legal, Ethical and Professional Issues in Nursing* (2nd ed.) London: Quay Books.

Curtis, K., Horton, K. and Smith, P. (2012) Student nurse socialisation in compassionate practice: A Grounded Theory study. *Nurse Education in Practice*, 32: 790–5.

Department of Health (2012) *Transforming Care: A national response to Winterbourne View Hospital. Department of Health Review: Final Report.* Available at: www.gov.uk/government/publications/winterbourne-view-hospital-department-of-health-review-and-response (last accessed 6 June 2018).

Department of Health and NHS Commissioning Board (2012) *Compassion in Practice: Nursing, Midwifery and Care Staff – Our Vision and Strategy.* Available at: www.england.nhs.uk/wp-content/uploads/2012/12/compassion-in-practice.pdf (last accessed 6 June 2018).

Department of Health (2015) *The NHS Constitution for England.* Available at: www.gov.uk/government/publications/the-nhs-constitution-for-england (last accessed 6 June 2018).

Department of Health, Social Services and Public Safety (2011) *Quality 2020. A 10-Year Strategy to Protect and Improve Quality in Health and Social Care in Northern Ireland.* Available at: www.health-ni.gov.uk/sites/default/files/publications/dhssps/q2020-strategy.pdf (last accessed 6 June 2018).

Dinmohammadi, M., Peyrovi, H. and Mehrdad, N. (2013) Concept analysis of professional socialization in nursing. *Nursing Forum*, 48(1): 26–34.

Francis, R. (2010) *Independent Inquiry into Care Provided by Mid Staffordshire NHS Foundation Trust January 2005 – March 2009.* Available at: www.midstaffspublicinquiry.com/previous-independent-inquiry (last accessed 6 June 2018).

Francis, R. (2013) *The Mid Staffordshire NHS Foundation Trust Public Inquiry.* Available at: www.midstaffspublicinquiry.com/report (last accessed 6 June 2018).

Francis, R. (2015) *Freedom to Speak Up: An independent review into creating an open and honest reporting culture in the NHS.* Available at: www.gov.uk/government/groups/whistleblowing-in-the-nhs-independent-review (last accessed 6 June 2018).

Fulford, K.W.M. (2008) Values based practice: A new partner to evidence based practice and a first for psychiatry? *Mens Sana Monographs*, 6: 10–21.

Griffiths, J., Speed S., Horne, M. and Keeley, P. (2012) 'A caring professional attitude': What service users and carers seek in graduate nurses and the challenge for educators. *Nurse Education Today*, 32 (2): 121–7.

Hall, J. (2013) Developing a culture of compassionate care—The midwife's voice? *Midwifery* 29, 269–71.

Keogh, B. (2013) *Review into the Quality of Care and Treatment Provided by 14 Hospital Trusts in England: overview report.* London: NHS England.

Leininger, M. and McFarland, M. (2002) *Transcultural Nursing: Concepts, theories, research, and practice* (3rd ed.). New York: McGraw-Hill.

Mackintosh, C. (2006) Caring: The socialisation of pre-registration student nurses: A longitudinal qualitative descriptive study. *International Journal of Nursing Studies, 43:* 953–62.

Mendick, R (2017) Charlie Gard: The tragic case of a too short life. *The Telegraph.* Available at: www.telegraph.co.uk/news/2017/07/28/charlie-gard-tragic-case-short-life/ (last accessed 6 June 2018).

NHS Scotland (2013) *Everyone Matters: The 2020 Workforce Vision.* Available at: www.gov.scot/Topics/Health/NHS-Workforce/Policy/2020-Vision (last accessed 6 June 2018).

NHS Wales (2016) *Values and Standards of Behaviour Framework.* Available at: www.wales.nhs.uk/governance-emanual/values-and-standards-of-behaviour-framew (last accessed 6 June 2018).

Nursing and Midwifery Council (2015) *The Code. Professional standards of practice and behaviour for nurses and midwives.* Available at: www.nmc.org.uk/standards/code/ (last accessed 6 June 2018).

Nursing and Midwifery Council (2017) *Annual Fitness to Practise Report 2016–2017.* Available at www.nmc-uk.org (last accessed 6 June 2018).

Nursing and Midwifery Council (2018) *Standards of Proficiency for Registered Nurses.* Available at www.nmc-uk.org (last accessed 6 June 2018).

Petrova, M., Dale, J. and Fulford, K.W. (2006) Values-based practice in primary care: Easing the tensions between individual values, ethical principles and best evidence. *British Journal of General Practice,* 56(530): 703–9.

Rejon, C.J. and Watts, C. (2014) *Supporting Professional Nurse Socialisation: Findings from evidence reviews.* Royal College of Nursing: London. Available at: https://my.rcn.org.uk/__data/assets/pdf_file/0007/553165/professional-attitudes-behaviours-socialisation-review.pdf (accessed 19 September 2017).

Royal College of Nursing (2017) *Revalidation Requirements: Reflection and reflective discussion.* Available at: www.rcn.org.uk/professional-development/revalidation/reflection-and-reflective-discussion (last accessed 6 June 2018).

Sackett, D.L., Straus, S.E., Scott Richardson, W., Rosenberg, W. and Haynes R.B. (2000) *Evidence-Based Medicine: How to Practice and Teach EBM* (2nd Ed.). Edinburgh: Churchill Livingstone.

Shahriari, M., Mohammadi, E., Abbaszadeh, A. and Bahrami, M. (2013) Nursing ethical values and definitions: A literature review. *Iranian Journal of Nursing and Midwifery Research*, 18(1): 1–8.

Sykes, C. and Durham, W. (2014) Embedding NHS values: a framework and learning tool to support practice. *Nursing Management,* 20(9): 31–7.

Thomas, J., Jack, B.A. and Jinks, A.B. (2012) Resilience to care: A systematic review and meta-synthesis of the qualitative literature concerning the experiences of student nurses in adult hospital settings in the UK. *Nurse Education Today, 32:* 657–64.

Woodbridge, K., and Fulford, K.W. (2004) *Whose Values? A Workbook for Values-based Practice in Mental Health Care.* London: The Sainsbury Centre for Mental Health.

SAFEGUARDING ADULTS AT RISK OF HARM

4

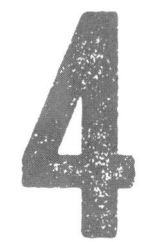

ROBERT JENKINS, RUTH NORTHWAY AND MANDY NICHOLS-DAVIES

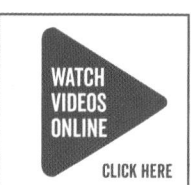

WATCH VIDEOS ONLINE
CLICK HERE

THIS CHAPTER COVERS

- Definitions of safeguarding and abuse
- The principles that underpin safeguarding
- The legal context of safeguarding
- The ethical context of safeguarding

- The professional implications of safeguarding
- Preparing for clinical placements.

> "
> I just feel it shouldn't happen, but it does ... it's actually abusing your human rights basically, and we all have human rights.
>
> Sean, participant in Northway et al. (2013)
> "

INTRODUCTION

As the quote from Sean (a young man with learning disabilities) at the beginning of this chapter indicates, abuse occurs and this is contrary to our human rights. As nurses it is essential that we are aware of how people can be safeguarded from abuse and (where abuse does occur) that we are able to respond in a timely and appropriate manner. Indeed, our professional Code requires that we take all reasonable steps to safeguard people who are vulnerable or at risk of harm (Nursing and Midwifery Council [NMC], 2015): safeguarding is, therefore, a central role of nurses. This chapter will build on the knowledge gained in the first year of your course to increase your awareness of safeguarding and the principles that underpin it, explore the legal, ethical and professional issues associated with safeguarding in nursing practice, and encourage you to consider how this knowledge and understanding can assist you when working within clinical settings. Given the importance of safeguarding you will also find that it is a theme running through other chapters in this book.

CRITICAL THINKING STOP POINT 4.1

Before reading further take a few minutes to think about what you currently understand by the term 'safeguarding' in relation to working with adults.

DEFINITIONS OF SAFEGUARDING AND ABUSE

The Care Act (2014) defines safeguarding as upholding an adult's right to live in safety, free from abuse and neglect. Historically, UK policy focused on the 'protection' of vulnerable adults but the change to 'safeguarding' has placed greater emphasis on prevention of abuse and neglect. There has been a move away from being 'reactive' once abuse has taken place towards a proactive, preventative model that recognises that citizens who are at risk of abuse or neglect must have their rights, wishes and feelings respected (Social Services and Well-being (Wales) Act, 2014).

Safeguarding is often referred to as an 'umbrella' term to include concepts of promoting wellbeing, welfare and protection from harm. It includes a continuum of support encompassing the prevention of abuse and neglect through to responding when abuse or neglect is suspected. The NHS and other care providers must, therefore, have safeguards in place (for example, leadership, policies, procedures and a competent workforce through staff training and supervision) to both prevent and respond to abuse and neglect. The DH (2011) emphasises that the NHS and individual practitioners have a key role in safeguarding which includes working with patients and/or their carers to reduce and manage risks and to ensure effective and person-centred care. This requires inter-professional and inter-agency working.

Adult safeguarding policy and legislation has also moved away from referring to people as 'vulnerable adults'. This is in recognition that people should not be labelled as 'vulnerable' since such terminology implies weakness and places the 'cause' of the abuse with them (Spencer-Lane, 2010). Current thinking recognises that it is the situation or context they are in, and the action or inaction by another person/people, which places them at risk of abuse or neglect. Therefore, safeguarding policy and legislation now refer to adults at risk of harm.

Vulnerability, however, remains an important concept that we need to understand and the DH (2011) proposes that it is affected by the following factors:

- Personal circumstances (including but not limited to disability or ill health)
- Risks from the environment (including levels of social contact, a lack of adaptations to meet individual needs and the quality of care)

- Resilience factors (including access to support networks, personal strengths and coping mechanisms).

People in need of safeguarding may live in their own home or in a residential or nursing home and include those in private hospitals and those in receipt of care in the NHS. It is, therefore, important that professionals are able to identify people who may be at risk of or suffering abuse or neglect and the signs of abuse or neglect.

Abuse and neglect can take many forms and most national policies and legislation will refer to the well-established categories of abuse – namely physical, sexual, emotional/psychological, financial and neglect. Some countries within the UK include other types of abuse such as institutional and discriminatory abuse. Further information regarding indicators of the different types of abuse are provided online.

Other forms of abuse include domestic violence, female genital mutilation, hate crime, forced marriage, human trafficking and slavery. Local safeguarding policies and procedures will provide more detail on the types of abuse and these should be accessible through your NHS Trust/Health Board intranet and the relevant Local Authority Internet pages.

THE PRINCIPLES THAT UNDERPIN SAFEGUARDING

Earlier it was highlighted that safeguarding was concerned with promoting the right to live in safety and free from abuse and neglect: to achieve this aim we need guidance or a set of principles to inform practice such as those identified by DH (2011) in Figure 4.1 below.

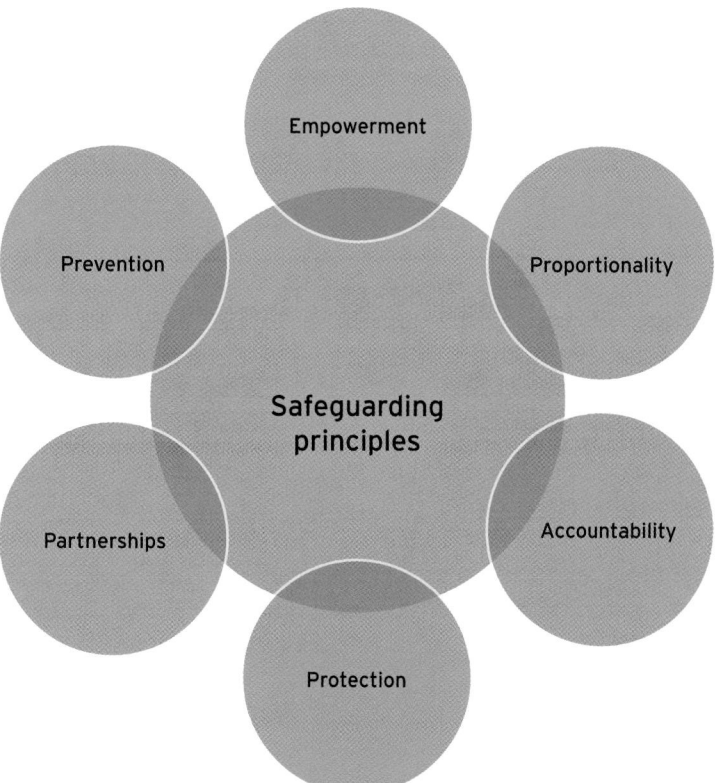

Figure 4.1 Safeguarding principles (DH, 2011)

Reproduced with permission under the terms of the Open Government Licence.

A brief explanation of each of the six principles is provided below:

Empowerment – Supporting and encouraging individuals to make their own decisions as well as safeguarding themselves from harm. Issues relating to capacity and consent need to be considered.

Prevention – It is better to take action or adopt approaches that reduce the likelihood of harm occurring rather than waiting for abuse to occur before responding.

Proportionality – Positive risk taking should be a measured approach in relation to a proposed action or activity. A comprehensive risk assessment is a crucial component of this principle.

Protection – Those adults deemed to be most at risk of harm are supported and protected.

Partnership – Working together including the individual at risk, professionals, carers, families, communities, services and agencies.

Accountability – Professionals, agencies and services should be transparent in their actions and held to account for their actions or omissions.

ACTIVITY 4.1: LEADERSHIP AND MANAGEMENT

Imagine that you are managing a clinical area (this could be a hospital ward, a community nursing team or a nursing home). How would you seek to ensure that the principles of safeguarding discussed above are upheld by your team? Why is team working important in relation to safeguarding?

SEE ALSO CHAPTER 3

As well as the above principles there are four levels of safeguarding which can be applied to practice (Northway and Jenkins, 2017) (See Figure 4.2). At an *individual* level, you have personal responsibility to safeguard people you support. As a student or registered nurse you must adhere to the professional *Code* (NMC, 2015) in which there are a number of themes that refer both implicitly and explicitly to the nurse's safeguarding role (for example, practising safely). You can also see the six safeguarding principles threaded throughout the *Code* and you may wish to reflect on this. These responsibilities also apply to the *Professional* level. The NMC regulates the nursing profession to ensure that registered nurses have the necessary skills, competence and knowledge in order to safeguard individuals in their care. They achieve this through setting standards for the training and education of nurses while they study at university. All registered nurses now have to demonstrate how they have kept themselves updated and reflected on their practice through the process of revalidation (NMC, 2018).

GO FURTHER

WEBLINK: REVALIDATION – WHAT TO DO

For more information on revalidation see http://revalidation.nmc.org.uk/what-you-need-to-do .

At an *organisational* level, the NHS, for example, has a responsibility to safeguard all who use the many services it provides. This has not always been a high priority for the NHS but recent reports regarding poor care and abuse (for example, Francis, 2013; Andrews and Butler, 2014) have changed this.

Policies, procedures and training in regards to safeguarding have been implemented in an attempt to prevent such abuses recurring. However, history suggests that abuse scandals tend to be repeated in spite of the numerous inquiries and serious case reviews (Northway and Jenkins, 2017).

The final level is *societal*. The wider public and communities have an important role in safeguarding adults at risk of harm in society. Public services, housing, transport and public health initiatives all play a part in supporting individuals and communities. Positive media campaigns can also help to shape public perceptions and reduce negative attitudes towards groups of people who may be at risk of abuse and neglect.

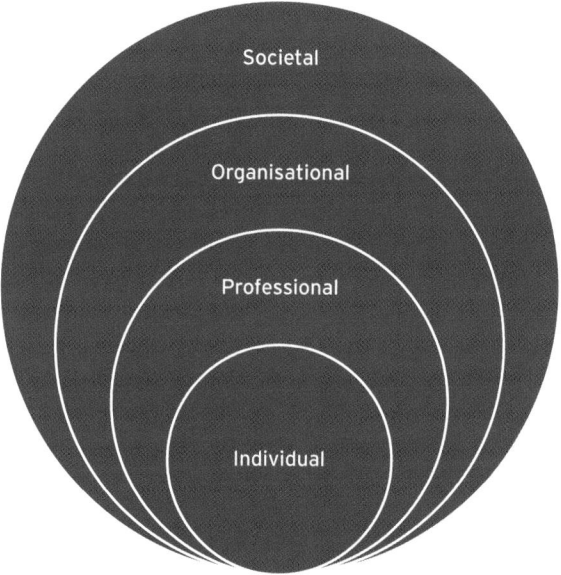

Figure 4.2   Levels of safeguarding (Northway and Jenkins, 2017)

CASE STUDY 4.1: JAMAL

Jamal is a 26-year-old man who loves to listen to music, interact with other people and to have a lot of activities. He has profound and multiple learning disabilities and while he has only limited verbal communication skills, he can make his needs known quite well through gestures or through changes in his behaviour. For example, if he does not like something (like orange juice or other people touching his head) he will scream, start to get agitated, and sometimes injures himself. He requires assistance with all aspects of daily living and so lives in a house with two other young men who have similar needs. They are supported 24 hours a day by a team of social care staff. Jamal's parents have regular contact with him.

Jamal is soon to be admitted to your ward for surgery. It is likely that he is going to have to be in hospital for 2-3 days.

Imagine that you are working on the ward that Jamal is going to be admitted to.

1. How can you work with other people before, during and after his admission to ensure that he is safeguarded?
2. Who will you need to work with?

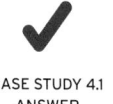

CASE STUDY 4.1
ANSWER

THE LEGAL CONTEXT OF SAFEGUARDING

Law sets out rules that are legally binding on a community such as citizens of a country. These rules may be 'positive' (they set out legal obligations to do or not do something with sanctions being applied if they are not obeyed) or 'normative' (where they state what a person should or should not do but sanctions are not applied for non-compliance) (Griffith and Tengnah, 2014). Increasing devolution of responsibility for law making to the four countries within the UK means that differences in legislation between the nations are increasing. For this reason the NMC (2015) reminds us of the importance of working within the laws of the country in which we are practising. In addition, our legal system operates on the basis of case law whereby a judgement in one case becomes the basis for future judgements: this means that the exact interpretation of the law changes over time and it is important that we keep ourselves up to date with relevant legal developments. This chapter can only provide you with an introduction to some safeguarding legislation and you are advised to make use of the resources at the end of the chapter and online to increase your knowledge further.

While safeguarding children has operated within a legal framework for a number of years, safeguarding adults has only more recently been addressed via legislation. Initially, growing awareness of the need to protect adults who may be vulnerable to abuse and neglect was addressed via policy guidance within England (DH, 2000) and Wales (Wales Social Service Inspectorate, 2000). Such guidance, however, does not have the same force as legislation and sanctions are not readily available when it is not followed. Scotland was the first of the UK countries to develop specific legislation concerned with safeguarding adults: the Adult Support and Protection (Scotland) Act 2007. England (via the Care Act 2014) and Wales (via the Social Services and Well-being (Wales) Act 2014) have more recently developed their own adult safeguarding legislation. At the time of writing, Northern Ireland was still in the process of finalising legislation but updated policy guidance had been published (DHSSPS and Department of Justice, 2015).

There are similarities between these different laws but also differences in terms of the powers available within individual countries. Each country has taken the approach that those who are covered by the provisions of the legislation are those adults who meet the stated definitions of being an adult at risk of harm due to a range of circumstances and who are unable to safeguard themselves from such harm. Each places a responsibility on local authorities to make enquiries where there is cause to suspect that an individual is at risk of harm and to work in partnership with other agencies (including health services). In Scotland the legislation allows (if certain conditions are met and procedures followed) for local authorities to enter premises if they believe an adult is at risk, to interview them in private, to examine their records, to request a medical examination, to remove the individual for the purpose of assessment and to apply for orders that ban alleged perpetrators from contact with the individual at risk. The powers in England and Wales are more limited – for example, in Wales local authorities can apply for an order allowing entry to premises to access an individual at risk of harm for the purpose of assessment but there are no powers to remove that individual.

Other legislation relevant to safeguarding adults includes the Mental Capacity Act (MCA) (2005) in England and Wales, which addresses issues related to the assessment of capacity and consent. To safeguard the right of individuals to make their own decisions concerning their lives, this legislation starts from the assumption that people have such capacity. However, where someone has a mental impairment and may not be able to make an informed decision concerning an aspect of their care or treatment, then their capacity to make that specific decision should be assessed. If they are found to have capacity then their decision must be respected, even if others consider it unwise. For example, someone with a known history of mental health problems may withhold consent for a blood transfusion that medical staff feel is needed to treat their health condition. If they are assessed as having capacity to make that decision at that point in time then this has to be respected even if the doctor feels that decision is unwise. However, if at the time they are asked to make that decision they lack capacity due to the presence of a psychosis that leads them to believe that the doctors are seeking to poison them, then best interests procedures must be followed to ensure that decisions are made in the best interests of the individual concerned.

The Mental Capacity Act (MCA) 2005 also contains provision for people to be prosecuted if they ill-treat or wilfully neglect an individual who lacks capacity. This provides a mechanism by which legal sanctions can be applied to people who are found to have abused or neglected adults who lack mental capacity.

A further provision within the MCA that is relevant to safeguarding is the Deprivation of Liberty Safeguards (also referred to as DoLS). Some people who lack capacity to consent to care and treatment may place themselves at harm if they refuse such support. Think back, for example, to the case of Jamal discussed earlier in this chapter – if he becomes agitated during his admission and seeks to leave the ward what can be done to safeguard him from harm? In such a scenario it may be necessary to prevent him from leaving but it is contrary to Article 5 of the European Convention on Human Rights to deprive anyone of their liberty. Where an individual lacks capacity the MCA, therefore, allows professionals to deprive someone of their liberty where it is deemed to be in their best interests but it also specifies the procedures that need to be followed and the safeguards that must be in place.

GO FURTHER

The Mental Capacity Act

For further information regarding the MCA please follow the links below:

The Mental Capacity Act Code of Practice: www.gov.uk/government/publications/mental-capacity-act-code-of-practice

WEBLINKS

Revised guidance concerning the Deprivation of Liberty Safeguards following the Cheshire West decision - this document explores the implications in different clinical settings:

www.gov.uk/government/uploads/system/uploads/attachment_data/file/485122/DH_Consolidated_Guidance.pdf

---

THE ETHICAL CONTEXT OF SAFEGUARDING

Barker (2011) suggests that ethics involves both a set of principles and a system of moral values: it is concerned with what we feel are the right actions to take in situations and why we believe that these actions are right. A 'principles' approach to ethics is often used in nursing and the framework commonly cited is that offered by Beauchamp and Childress (2013) who identify four key ethical principles:

Autonomy – respecting people's capacity to make their own decisions and to control their own lives

Non–maleficence – avoiding doing harm

Beneficence – seeking to do good

Justice – being concerned with issues of fairness and equality.

Earlier in this chapter we introduced you to the principles that underpin safeguarding (DH, 2011) and you will have noticed some similarities between those and the ethical principles identified by Beauchamp and Childress (2013): autonomy is linked with empowerment, non-maleficence with protection, and justice with accountability. Indeed, safeguarding in general may be seen as being concerned with beneficence. However, you may also have noticed that there can be times when, in the context of safeguarding, there can be tension between one principle and another. Think, for example, of an older patient who is admitted to your ward following a fall but who also has numerous older bruises that are not consistent with falls. When you ask them about these older bruises they say that one of the carers who visits them at home often treats them very roughly and sometimes slaps them. However, they say that they don't want you to say anything to anyone else as they know that the carer is having a hard time financially and they really need their job. Your patient has full mental capacity, you want to respect their autonomy and maintain confidentiality, but at the same time you know that your patient is being harmed and that other people supported by the same carer may also be at risk (the principle non-maleficence is not being upheld).

In such circumstances you may feel that you are faced with an ethical dilemma, which Ellis (2015) describes as feeling that there are two (or more) equally correct ways of acting. However, in the situation described it is clearly not possible to both respect your patient's autonomy and protect them (and possibly other people) from harm. We need, therefore, to be very clear about our decision making and be able to provide a clear rationale for our actions (what Barker [2011] would view as being able to say why we feel certain actions are right).

Many frameworks have been proposed to help us resolve ethical dilemmas and promote clearer decision making. One developed specifically to assist nurses in relation to safeguarding issues is the GUARD framework offered by Northway and Jenkins (2017). This has five elements to guide you through the process of ethical decision making and you may wish to use it to consider the case scenario of Louise below:

- **G**athering information concerning the situation
- **U**nderstanding this information
- **A**ssessing alternative courses of action and identifying a response
- **R**esponding using an appropriate strategy
- **D**etermining the effectiveness.

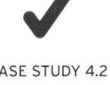

CASE STUDY 4.2
ANSWER

CASE STUDY 4.2: LOUISE

You are visiting Mrs Lucas, an older woman with dementia who lives with her daughter Louise and Louise's young family. Louise is the sole carer for her mother who has early onset dementia and whose behaviour can be difficult to manage at times as she needs constant supervision to ensure that she does not put herself into situations of risk. Mrs Lucas can get very agitated and, at times, can be both verbally and physically aggressive towards Louise who she sees as stopping her from doing things.

The reason for your visit was to dress a wound on Mrs Lucas' leg but while there you become concerned about the welfare of Simon, the youngest child in the family. Simon is 8 years of age and is usually at school when you visit. However, today he is home and has some noticeable bruising to his arms. Louise breaks down and says that she hit him the previous day as she had 'lost it' when he asked for something at a time when she was trying to prevent her mother from leaving the house. She asks you not to report her to anyone as she is worried that Simon might be taken away from her but felt that she needed to tell someone. Although you can sympathise with Louise you say that you will need to discuss the situation with your manager.

1. What are your legal responsibilities within this scenario?
2. What are your ethical responsibilities within this scenario?
3. Are there any tensions between these two areas?

THE PROFESSIONAL IMPLICATIONS OF SAFEGUARDING

Frontline health professionals have an important role in safeguarding. For example, they may witness incidents of harm and they may receive disclosures of abuse or neglect from patients. Failing to provide safe and effective care or not responding to safeguarding concerns can also have professional implications. Professional responsibility and accountability are fundamental to safeguarding (McGarry et al., 2015) and it is integral that nurses and other healthcare professionals know how to identify actual/potential abuse and neglect and how to respond to it. The NMC *Code* (2015) sets out clearly its expectations of registered nurses both in terms of their own competence and conduct and their responsibility to respond to safeguarding concerns. The NMC has evidence of nurses who put patients and/or the public at risk through their personal conduct or professional conduct and incompetence (see Go further below).

GO FURTHER

WEBLINK: FITNESS FOR PRACTICE CASES

You can view Fitness for Practice cases on the NMC website via the following link: www.nmc.org.uk/concerns-nurses-midwives/hearings-and-outcomes/

It is essential that nurses and other health professionals raise concerns at the time of an incident or disclosure so that it may be responded to in the most appropriate way to both safeguard the individual and others who may also be at risk of abuse or neglect. Think, for example, of the case study of Louise discussed earlier in this chapter. The *Code* (NMC, 2015) is explicit about a nurse's accountability in ensuring patients and the public are protected by working within the limits of the competence and exercising the professional 'duty of candour', and includes raising concerns immediately if a person is 'vulnerable' or at risk and needs extra support and protection. The NMC (2017) has further guidance for nurses and midwives in raising concerns that sets out broad principles to aid decision making in the public interest (see Figure 4.3).

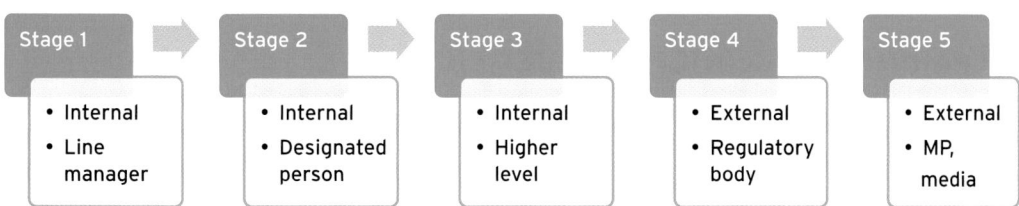

Figure 4.3 Raising and escalating concerns process (NMC, 2017)

Reproduced with permission of the Nursing and Midwifery Council. Available at: www.nmc.org.uk/standards/guidance/raising-concerns-guidance-for-nurses-and-midwives/

The above process requires the nurse to raise their concerns with their line manager in the first instance. If this is not possible because the line manager is unavailable or they fail to address it adequately, then it is taken to the next level. If you feel your concern has still not been dealt with properly then it should be taken to the highest level internally within the organisation (stages 1–3). You should always take further advice before raising the concern externally (stage 4) and whistleblowing to the media in the final stage (5) should only ever be considered after all the other avenues and stages have been exhausted. Ash (2016) highlights that whistleblowing is not without risks and can leave the whistle-blower feeling very isolated, anxious, angry and with other negative feelings. However, it can also make you and the patient feel empowered as their concerns and yours are being addressed and potential harm minimised or eliminated.

WHAT'S THE EVIDENCE? 4.1

Clarke (2015) undertook two focus groups with first year student nurses (13 students in total) who had undertaken placements in nursing homes in order to explore their experiences of such placements. Some examples of poor practice and inadequate leadership emerged along with the complex nature of raising concerns about observed poor practice. Clarke concludes that the study findings revealed both challenges and opportunities for students and educational institutions and that educational providers need to equip students with the necessary knowledge and skills to raise concerns not only as students but as future qualified nurses. How prepared do you feel to raise concerns if you observe what you feel is poor care or abuse while on placement?

'Safeguarding can be at times a difficult issue when you are a student nurse, nevertheless it is important. Raising concerns in a potentially new environment amongst a group of potential strangers is indeed daunting, as you will be trying your best to fit in. However, safeguarding is a shared responsibility amongst healthcare professionals at all stages in their career, including the student nurse. As soon as you take on the role of a student nurse you must understand it is your duty to ensure the safety of patients, and as a student it should be made clear who you can turn to in order to discuss any possible issues in practice.'

Rhianydd, 3rd-year student nurse

PREPARING FOR CLINICAL PLACEMENTS

Starting a new placement can be a daunting and emotional experience for any student nurse. One way to overcome the possible stresses is to prepare well, especially in regards to safeguarding. There are a number of steps that will help you achieve this. First, you need to be sure that you are fit and healthy to be in the practice learning environment. A student who is unwell and/or feels disempowered is not in the best position to support, empower and safeguard others. Second is to have background knowledge of safeguarding issues, policies and procedures. This chapter provides some direction but additional reading will be required to give you a greater understanding of the topic area. Third is to have a discussion with your mentor on the safeguarding-related competencies that you may be able to achieve while on the clinical placement.

A key requirement of any nurse is the ability to speak out when you have a concern or report abusive practice. The last section highlighted the process for doing so but this can be very difficult. Raising a concern is never easy but now nurses have no option but to do so; a confident, empowered and knowledgeable student working in an environment that encourages openness to question practice should be more likely to raise a concern (Northway and Jenkins, 2017; Ash, 2016).

CHAPTER SUMMARY

- Safeguarding is concerned with ensuring that people's human rights are upheld and that they are not abused or neglected. It is everyone's responsibility.
- It has both proactive (preventative) and reactive (responding to abuse) elements.
- There are many different types of abuse and neglect.
- Safeguarding requires that we have a good understanding of both the relevant legal and ethical issues.
- We have a professional responsibility to safeguard people and to raise concerns in a timely and appropriate manner where people are at risk of harm.

GO FURTHER

CASE STUDY: PROFESSIONAL VALUES

Go to https://study.sagepub.com/essentialadultnursing for a further case study related to this chapter. If you are using the interactive ebook, simply click on the book icon in the margin to go straight to the resource.

Books

- Brammer, A. (2014) *Safeguarding Adults*. Basingstoke: Palgrave Macmillan.
  Although aimed primarily at social workers it provides further information concerning legislation relevant to safeguarding adults.
- Northway, R. and Jenkins, R. (2017) *Safeguarding Adults in Nursing Practice* (2nd ed.). London: Learning Matters/Sage.
  This provides you with a more in depth exploration of safeguarding adults and the associated legal, ethical, professional and research issues.
- Wate, R. and Boulton, N. (2015) *Multiagency Safeguarding in a Public Protection World: A handbook for protecting children and vulnerable adults*. Hove: Pavilion.
  This provides an introduction to safeguarding both children and adults with a particular focus on inter-agency working.

Journal articles

FURTHER READING: JOURNAL ARTICLES

Go to https://study.sagepub.com/essentialadultnursing for further free online journal articles related to this chapter. If you are using the interactive ebook, simply click on the book icon in the margin to go straight to the resource.

- Ion, R., Smith, K., Moir, J. and Nimmon, S. (2016) Accounting for actions and omissions: A discourse analysis of student nurse accounts of responding to instances of poor care. *Journal of Advanced Nursing*, 72 (5): 1054-64.
  This paper explores how student nurses talk about raising (or not raising) concerns about poor care and the factors that influence their decision making.
- Lauder, W. and Roxburgh, M. (2012) Self-neglect consultation rates and comorbidities in primary care. *International Journal of Nursing Practice*, 18: 454-61.
  This paper explores the issue of self-neglect in primary care settings. They conclude that nurses need to be aware of the different ways it can present and to develop self-management interventions.
- Rees, C.E., Monrouxe, L.V. and McDonald, L.A. (2014) 'My mentor kicked a dying woman's bed ...' Analysing UK nursing students' 'most memorable' professionalism dilemmas. *Journal of Advanced Nursing*, 71 (1): 169-80.
  This article explores dilemmas (including some safeguarding issues) experienced by nursing students within clinical settings.

Weblinks

Go to https://study.sagepub.com/essentialadultnursing for further weblinks related to this chapter. If you are using the interactive ebook, simply click on the book icon in the margin to go straight to the resource.

- www.nspcc.org.uk/
  While adult nurses are primarily concerned with safeguarding adults a good knowledge of safeguarding children is also required. This link takes you to the NSPCC website and a range of resources including information regarding the legal position in different parts of the UK.
- www.scie.org.uk/adults/safeguarding/
  This link takes you to the safeguarding section of the Social Care Institute of Excellence website.
- https://www.rcn.org.uk/library/subject-guides/safeguarding
  This link takes you to the safeguarding section of the RCN website.

ONLINE
QUIZZES

ACE YOUR ASSESSMENT

Revise what you have learned by visiting https://study.sagepub.com/essentialadultnursing

- Test yourself with multiple-choice and short-answer questions
- Do the chapter activities in the book and check your answers online

REFERENCES

Andrews, J. and Butler, M. (2014) *Trusted to Care. An Independent Review of the Princess of Wales Hospital and Neath Port Talbot Hospital at Abertawe Bro Morgannwg University Health Board.* Stirling: Dementia Services Development Hospital.

Ash, A. (2016) *Whistle Blowing and Ethics in Health and Social Care.* London: Jessica Kingsley Publishing.

Barker, P. (2011) Ethics. In Search of the good life. In Barker, P. (ed) *Mental Health Ethics. The Human Context.* London: Routledge, pp. 5–30.

Beauchamp, T.L. and Childress, J.F. (2013) *Principles of Biomedical Ethics* (7th ed.). Oxford: Oxford University Press.

Clarke, P. (2015) Student nurses on placement – collaborators or challengers? *Journal of Adult Protection*, 17 (5): 287–95.

Department of Health (DH) (2000) *No Secrets: Guidance on developing and implementing multi-agency policies and procedures to protect vulnerable adults from abuse.* London: The Stationery Office.

Department of Health (DH) (2011) *Safeguarding Adults: The role of health service practitioners.* London: Department of Health.

Department of Health, Social Services and Public Safety and the Department of Justice (2015) *Adult Safeguarding: Prevention and Protection in Partnership.* Belfast: Northern Ireland Office.

Ellis, P. (2015) *Understanding Ethics for Nursing Students.* London: Learning Matters/Sage.

Francis, R. (2013) *The Mid Staffordshire NHS Foundation Trust Public Inquiry.* Available at: www.midstaffspublicinquiry.com/report (last accessed 6 June 2018).

Griffith, R. and Tengnah, C. (2014) *Law and Professional Issues in Nursing* (3rd ed.). London: Learning Matters/Sage.

McGarry, J., Baker, C., Wilson, C., Felton, A. and Banerjee, A. (2015) Preparation for safeguarding in UK pre-registration graduate nurse education. *The Journal of Adult Protection,* 17 (6): 371–9.

Northway, R. and Jenkins, R. (2017) *Safeguarding Adults in Nursing Practice* (2nd ed.). London: Learning Matters/Sage.

Northway, R., Melsome, M., Flood, S., Bennett, D., Howarth, J. and Thomas, B. (2013) How do people with intellectual disabilities view abuse and abusers? *Journal of Intellectual Disabilities,* 17 (4): 361–75.

Nursing and Midwifery Council (NMC) (2015) *The Code. Professional Standards of Practice and Behaviour for Nurses and Midwives.* London: NMC.

Nursing and Midwifery Council (NMC) (2017) *Raising and Escalating Concerns: Guidance for nurses and midwives.* London: NMC.

Nursing and Midwifery Council (2018) *Revalidation.* Available at: http://revalidation.nmc.org.uk/ (last accessed 18 May 2018).

Spencer-Lane, T. (2010) A statutory framework for safeguarding adults? The Law Commission's consultation paper on adult social care. *The Journal of Adult Protection,* 12 (1): 43–9.

Wales Social Services Inspectorate (2000) *In Safe Hands: Protection of Vulnerable Adults in Wales.* Wales: The National Assembly for Wales.

STATUTES

Adult Support and Protection (Scotland) Act 2007
Care Act 2014
Mental Capacity Act 2005
Social Services and Well-being (Wales) Act 2014

PATIENT SAFETY

JULIE GAMBIN AND RONNIE MEECHAN-ROGERS

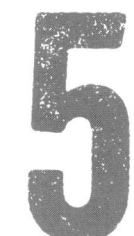

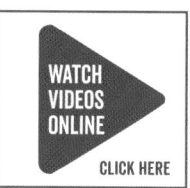

WATCH VIDEOS ONLINE
CLICK HERE

THIS CHAPTER COVERS

- A brief history of patient safety
- The Current National Quality Agenda
- The legal implications of incidents
- Recognising and reporting adverse events/ incidents

- Investigating and reporting serious incidents and Never Events.

> This is a story of appalling and unnecessary suffering of hundreds of people. They were failed by a system which ignored the warning signs and put corporate self interest and cost control ahead of patients and their safety ... At every level there was a failure to communicate known concerns adequately to others, and to take sufficient action to protect patients' safety and wellbeing from the risks arising from those concerns.
>
> Sir Robert Francis QC (2013)

INTRODUCTION

The quote by Sir Robert Francis QC at the start of this chapter refers to the appalling events that took place at Mid Staffordshire Hospitals NHS Foundation Trust. This chapter aims to outline what roles and responsibilities you, your colleagues and employers have in maintaining a patient's safety and assessing risk to ensure another scandal like Mid Staffs never takes place again. We will also discuss how healthcare organisations can improve the quality of care provided and what happens when things go wrong.

What is good quality care? The answer will vary on who you ask – be it the patient, their family, the commissioner, the manager, the healthcare professional or the media. The World Health Organization (WHO) says it encompasses:

Safe. Delivering health care which minimises risks and harm to service users, including avoiding preventable injuries and reducing medical errors

Effective. Providing services based on scientific knowledge and evidence-based guidelines.

Timely. Reducing delays in providing and receiving health care.

Efficient. Delivering health care in a manner that maximizes resource use and avoids waste.

Equitable. Delivering health care that does not differ in quality according to personal characteristics such as gender, race, ethnicity, geographical location or socioeconomic status.

People-centred. Providing care that takes into account the preferences and aspirations of individual service users and the culture of their community.

(WHO, 2006: 9)

A BRIEF HISTORY OF PATIENT SAFETY IN THE UNITED KINGDOM

Adapted from a presentation by the Health Foundation (2013).

1855 Florence Nightingale published a study of mortality of soldiers in military hospitals (Nightingale, 1858).

1948 NHS came in to being providing care to all.

1960 to 1980 Several public inquiries into failures which led to patients' deaths.

1995 NHS litigation authority (NHSLA) was established to manage claims against the NHS.

2000 Sir Liam Donaldson, Chief Medical Officer publishes a DH report *An organisation with a memory*. This outlines that there is a lot of really good care provided; however, there are some serious failures and many of these failures happen over and over again and sound familiar. These could be avoided if lessons could be learned.

2008 WHO safe surgery checklist introduced which identifies set tasks to minimise avoidable harm.

2013 There is a national inquiry into Mid Staffordshire NHS Foundation Trust. The investigation was triggered by families and media concerns about poor care and increasing mortality rates in emergency patients. The Francis Inquiry uncovered appalling conditions, inadequate care, suffering and excess deaths. It identified failures in care, in regulation and in openness. The inquiry made 290 recommendations (Francis, 2013). Following this Professor Don Berwick said, 'The NHS should continually and forever reduce patient harm by embracing wholeheartedly an ethic of learning' and called for a need to embed the voice of the patient (The National Advisory Group on the Safety of Patients in England, 2013).

As you can see, patient safety has been increasingly recognised as the cornerstone of high-quality healthcare and the pace of change has been rapid over the last 60 years.

Key Reports that influenced the current NHS Quality Agenda 2014 to present

In 2014 NHS England published its *Five Year Forward View*, which is underpinned by the three basic pillars of quality: safety, effectiveness and the patient experience of care.

The NHS Constitution: The NHS belongs to us all (DH, 2015) sets out the principles and values of the NHS and what it pledges to achieve. It also details the rights of patients and staff and also their responsibilities.

THE CURRENT NATIONAL QUALITY AGENDA

Following publication of the *Five Year Forward View* (NHS England, 2014), many Trusts have made a quality commitment, which should aim to reduce harm, improve patient experience and improve clinical effectiveness mirroring the national agenda. There is now a greater focus on safety themes rather than individual incidents.

Collaborative working and learning with other organisations is being encouraged with new government bodies such as NHS Improvement (formerly NPSA) sharing learning from incidents. The Healthcare Safety Investigation Branch (HSIB) was established in 2017 as an independent organisation which will investigate up to 30 safety incidents each year and share what is learnt across the whole healthcare system.

Trust boards (post-Francis) need to be aware of what's going on, with accountability from floor to the board. In practice, this means Trusts may have various director level committees set up to scrutinise internal investigations, with increased visible presence, i.e. walkabouts to meet staff and patients, and regular 'Meet the boss' events and briefings and so on.

There is now increased recognition of the 'second victim' in incidents/accidents, these second victims are the staff involved. Support from peers and managers is vital when an error has occurred to restore confidence and promote learning.

A revised *Never Event Framework* was published in January 2018 (NHS Improvement, 2018) and the Duty of Candour is now enshrined in law which means NHS organisations are mandated to be open and honest to patients when things go wrong. There are heavy financial penalties if they fail to inform patients or if they fail to do so in a timely way. Staff are also being encouraged to speak up about concerns and every NHS Trust should now have a Freedom to Speak Up Guardian (NHS Improvement, 2016).

Alongside the changes above, there is now a move towards more reliance on electronic systems for recording observations, prescribing and dispensing medications, ordering tests and investigations and recording findings. The systems include alerting key staff of abnormal results.

THE LEGAL IMPLICATIONS OF INCIDENTS

First, don't be afraid to speak up/report an adverse event, an unsafe act or unsafe practices or environments. It is your legal and professional duty to do so. The Health and Social Care Act 2012, Health and Social Care (Safety and Quality) Act 2015 and the Nursing and Midwifery Council's professional *Code* (NMC, 2015) mandate that that you must speak up and report adverse events. You are the patient's advocate; therefore, it's your duty to protect those in your care and to promote their wellbeing. Additionally, in common law you have a duty to protect yourself and your colleagues and any other persons within your working environment.

TOP TIPS FOR ENSURING YOU STAY WITHIN THE LAW

- Accurate contemporaneous documentation: document clearly what happened, what you did, what you observed, remedial steps you took, who you informed.
- Keep your written record factual, do NOT include your opinion.
- Everything to be legibly written, signed and dated.
- NEVER share passwords or log-on details or smart cards or devices assigned to you.
- If involved in an incident write your own reflective notes as soon as possible.
- Remember, there are valuable lessons from near misses.
- If unsure whether you can/cannot disclose information always seek advice from the on-call manager or patient safety team.
- Don't be afraid to say sorry. This shows compassion and acknowledges a person's distress.

The law and being open and honest with our patients/service users

In everyday life when something goes wrong, when we are injured or are disadvantaged by a mistake, the principal thing that the people affected want is an open and honest explanation, an apology and things to be put right, and to be reassured that steps will be taken to prevent a reoccurrence – this holds true within the healthcare setting as well. A thorough open investigation can provide this reassurance and may restore an individual's or the organisation's reputation. Our professional duty is outlined in *The Professional Duty of Candour* (NMC and GMC, 2015). This means we have a legal obligation to inform relatives/patients when an organisation is investigating a patient's care when things have gone wrong. This is the responsibility of a patient's Consultant or Ward Sister or Matron (each Trust may have their own local policy for this).

RECOGNISING AND REPORTING ADVERSE INCIDENTS

There are a number of different incident reporting systems in the UK. A number of these are moving towards being a cloud-based service (staff will have an app on their phone to make it easier to report) and this service can link with other hospital systems, which essentially means it can pull lots of different data about the one patient from many different systems in the hospital. So, an investigator will see the demographics of blood results, radiology reports, outputs from morbidity and mortality reviews, complaints, claims and thematic data.

Matrons look at ward metrics and audits via **safety thermometers** and incident reporting systems. Advanced reporting systems can be configured to display the number of incidents and types of incidents at ward and departmental level. This helps managers identify hot spots and so direct resources and plan care appropriately. The range of data available is vast; Table 5.1 lists some of these.

Dealing with error

Errors are where an intended or untended action leads to an unexpected event. This can be positive or negative. In his excellent book *The Human Contribution: Unsafe acts, accidents and heroic recoveries* (2008)

Table 5.1 Examples of quality and safety data

- Patient experience data, e.g. message to Matron
- Patient satisfaction survey and staff surveys including Friends and Family Test
- Complaints and compliments
- Mortality data, readmission figures and length of stay data
- Quarterly and yearly reports including number of Serious Untoward Incidents and costs of claims
- Care Quality Commission (CQC) Reports

James Reason describes many different types of error and different ways of classifying error. These range from absent minded 'slips' such as putting the coffee jar in the fridge instead of the milk to intentional rule violations such as deliberately taking a shortcut by missing a step in the process to get the task finished more quickly.

CRITICAL THINKING STOP POINT 5.1

How often have you taken a short cut such as not washing your hands as per policy?

Reason (2000) also explains what causes people to make errors and describes various error prevention models, such as the person model, the legal model and the sequential accident model which uses the domino effect to describe where one accident leads to another. James Reason developed the *Swiss Cheese Model* of error causation. The model has been updated since its introduction and been challenged and adapted to suit a variety of industries.

In brief, this model likens the defensive barriers such as physical safeguards and administrative controls that stand between a potential hazard and an actual error happening to a pile of slices of Swiss cheese. Akin to Swiss cheese slices these barriers have holes in; his error theory states that holes in the cheese represent latent (hidden) failures and other holes represent active failures (Figure 5.1). These holes, unlike in cheese, are in motion, constantly changing, opening and closing. If a failure occurs,

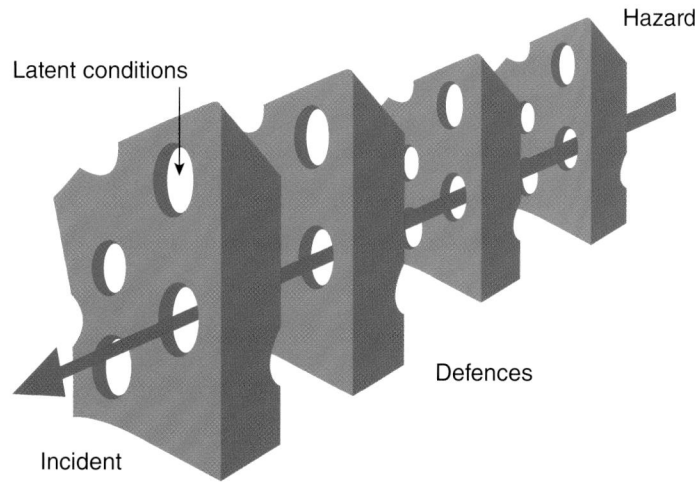

Figure 5.1 The 'Swiss cheese' model of error causation

the next barrier (or slice) blocks the hazard passing through the hole from reaching patients, but when by chance all the holes line up the hazard cannot be prevented from progressing and an adverse event then happening to the patient (Reason, 2000).

The following scenario looks at what happens when Joe comes into hospital and the series of events that take place due to a series of errors.

CASE STUDY 5.1: PATIENT SCENARIO

Joe is a patient who is unknown to the hospital and arrives without his family. He is hard of hearing and doesn't hear the nurse ask if he has any allergies. Joe is muttering to himself while the nurse is admitting him. The nurse misinterprets this as a verbal response and as confirmation that he has no allergies. Information about Joe's allergy is not recorded in his notes. The doctor looks at Joe's chart and forgets to ask or check this with Joe. The doctor prescribes a medication, which Joe is allergic to. Medication reconciliation is normally carried out by the pharmacist each day, unfortunately they were absent and Joe's medication and allergy status wasn't checked by pharmacy team. The same nurse checks the medication and patient's identity and administers the medication and then goes to lunch as planned. The patient goes into a cardiac arrest and dies.

Can you identify some of the safeguards that should have been in place to prevent this error?

Modern healthcare organisations are using a blend of system perspective models of error and human factors science to identify overt and hidden deviations in the system and the contributory factors at an individual team and organisational level. The focus now is to strive to find system and process errors rather than appoint individual blame, as this is where the big wins can be found. This approach will potentially save many lives in comparison to blaming one individual. Blaming the individual does not fix the problem long term and discourages open and honest reporting. Individuals will eventually move on and if the system is not fixed the error could happen again when somebody new is in post.

HUMAN FACTORS SCIENCE

This is the study of the interrelationship between humans, the tools and equipment they use in the workplace, and the environment in which they work (Kohn et al., 1999). All humans make errors in the normal course of their daily lives. Human factors science examines how we can make it easier for staff to avoid making errors. It recognises that humans are fallible, and errors increase when staff are hungry, tired and stressed.

WHAT ARE COMMON CONTRIBUTORY FACTORS TO ERRORS IN HEALTH CARE?

The NPSA published a framework of contributory factors in 2010. This list of common causes of errors is segmented into nine themes as shown in Figure 5.2.

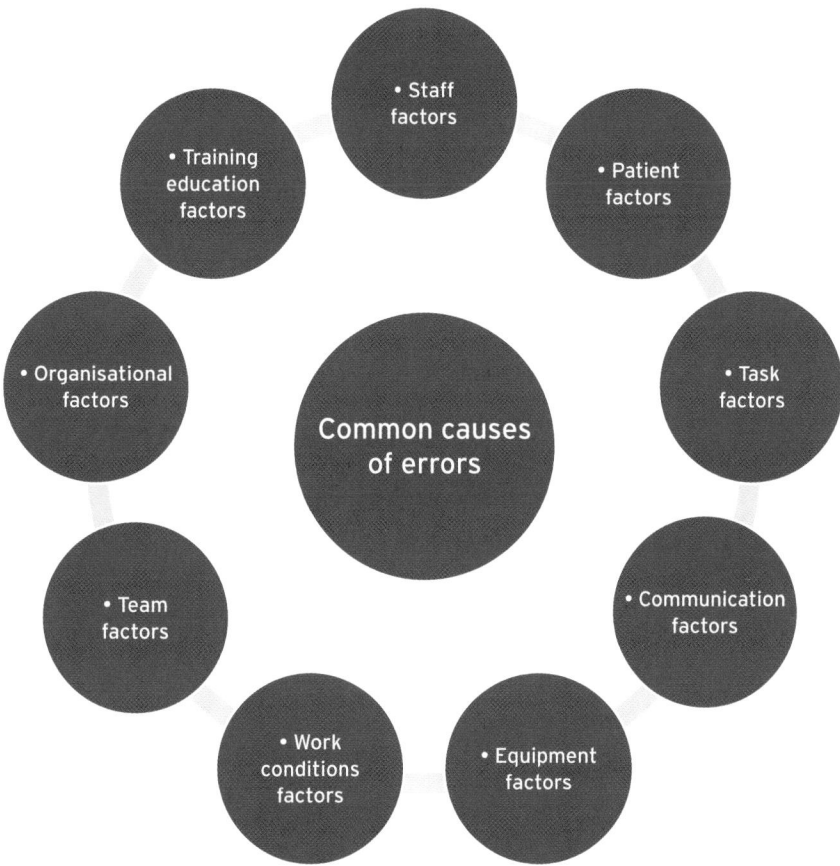

Figure 5.2 Common causes of errors

Each of these are then segmented into different components: for an example, see Table 5.2, which provides a summary from the NPSA Framework (NPSA, 2010) and shows the possible components which may contribute to an error arising from a piece of equipment.

Table 5.2 Contributory Factors Classification Framework – Equipment

Equipment	Components
Displays	• Incorrect information/feedback available • Inconsistent or unclear information • Illegible information • Interference/unclear equipment display
Integrity	• Poor working order • Inappropriate size • Unreliable • Ineffective safety features/not designed to fail safe • Poor maintenance programme • Failure of general services (power supply, water, piped gases, etc.)

(Continued)

Table 5.2 (Continued)

Equipment	Components
Positioning	• Correct equipment not available • Insufficient equipment/emergency backup equipment • Incorrectly placed for use • Incorrectly stored
Usability	• Unclear controls • Not intuitive in design • Confusing use of colour or symbols • Lack of or poor-quality user manual • Not designed to make detection of problems obvious • Use of items which have similar names or packaging • Problems of compatibility

Reproduced with permission under the terms of the Open Government Licence.

WHAT TYPE OF HARMS COMMONLY OCCUR IN THE CLINICAL SETTING?

Types of harms that commonly occur in an acute hospital:

- Hospital acquired pressure ulcers
- Venous thromboembolism
- Hospital acquired infections
- Falls
- Overdose of high-risk medications – heparin/potassium/insulin
- Patient deterioration due to:

    o   failure to act on results (often due to poor reporting/communication processes)
    o   failure to spot deteriorating patient (often due to poor compliance with observations)
    o   failure to spot Red Flag Sepsis (often due to attributing symptoms to another cause)

- Staff accidents – sharps injuries, verbal abuse.

In addition, electronic systems are being increasingly used for recording observations, requesting tests, making referrals and prescribing drugs. These systems have their own risks such as:

- mis-selection when using drop-down boxes
- people sharing sign-in passwords
- things getting missed due to staff having to navigate multiple screens or systems rather than a paper chart
- equipment failure or lack of equipment (not enough computers)
- systems being vulnerable to power outages and malicious IT attacks
- personal data being possibly vulnerable due to hacking or theft of hardware.

So how do you prevent accidents from happening and what can we do to put things right when something goes wrong for those in our care?

RESPONDING TO ADVERSE EVENTS

On witnessing or becoming aware of an actual or potential adverse event you have a duty as a nurse to act to minimise actual harm. This may include summoning emergency help, moving staff or patients out of danger or providing first aid emergency treatment. Once the immediate danger or threat has passed, all evidence of the adverse event should be recorded and secured. If patients or their representatives require explanation, an apology or reassurance you should facilitate this to happen.

In the case of serious incidents, records should be secured, if equipment is involved it should be taken out of service and secured, and names of visitors or contractors should be recorded. In the case where a crime is suspected the police should be called and the scene should be preserved.

Finally, you must report the event.

> To err is human, to cover up is unforgivable, and to fail to learn is inexcusable. (Sir Liam Donaldson Speaking at the launch of the World Alliance for Patient Safety in Washington DC on 27 October 2004)

HOW ARE ADVERSE EVENTS REPORTED?

Most NHS Trusts now have electronic reporting systems, which will be monitored by the patient safety team (PST). The common systems in use are Datix and Ulysses reporting systems, and these also feed into the national reporting and learning system (NRLS) which, as stated earlier, use the information to inform national strategy and disseminate alerts to all healthcare providers nationally on newly emerging dangers or threats.

The incident reporting forms have a series of drop-down boxes to gather basic details and free text sections to describe the event. It is important that your report is purely factual and does not contain hearsay or opinion. As well as providing the very basic details, the reporter will be asked the type of incident and the severity as they see it at the time of reporting. This is how you ensure that you and your colleagues learn from this. It is a legal, professional and moral duty to report all incidents.

TYPES OF INCIDENTS (AS CLASSIFIED USING A STANDARD REPORTING SYSTEM)

PSI (Patient safety incident) This is any adverse event that has directly affected a patient.

PPSI (Prevented patient safety incident) This is where staff have intervened to prevent an incident. These incidents are very important to report. They are free lessons and, if shared, potentially prevent numerous adverse events.

Accident This category is applied to anybody else other than the patient, e.g. staff and visitors, contractors and delivery personnel. This category should also be used to report staff abuse, both verbal or physical.

Prevented accident/near miss As above, except that this is where a non-patient adverse event was prevented.

Equipment property incident This includes damage, theft, loss of your workplace equipment and theft of personal property that you have brought into the workplace.

Following investigation, the level of harm originally reported may be changed in light of further information. For example, a nurse may report a patient who has fallen over as having suffered no harm if when examined initially there was no apparent injury; however, the patient may develop a subdural bleed or sustained fracture that only becomes obvious some hours later.

Levels of harm can be described as:

None Incident occurred but no harm sustained.

Minor harm is described as harm only requiring very basic treatment, such as small scratches/cuts/minor bruises.

Moderate harm is that which results in requiring further care or treatment or prolongs a patient's stay in hospital for over 8 days. Moderate harm is non-permanent. Such harm will require a formal investigation.

Major harm is harm that is permanent in nature and will require a comprehensive formal investigation.

Death This category is chosen when an adverse incident directly causes the death of one or more patients.

Some harm that happens to our patients is unavoidable; for example, recognised complications in surgery, a simple fall where all risks have been assessed and appropriate measures to prevent fall are in place. However, it is not the responsibility of staff reporting an incident to determine this. If you believe harm has occurred or there is a strong possibility it could have occurred, you must report it.

**ACTIVITY 5.1
ANSWER**

ACTIVITY 5.1: CRITICAL THINKING

Read the scenarios below and categorise what sort of incident has occurred and grade the incident in terms of harm.

1. A Staff Nurse arrives on shift. The ward should have three Staff Nurses on duty and four Healthcare Assistants. The Deputy Sister has rung in to say her car has broken down and two of the Healthcare Assistants have rung in sick. The Staff Nurse has taken charge of the ward a couple of times before, but she is concerned so she rings her Matron who informs her that unfortunately there is no one else available to cover or lend support. The Staff Nurse makes a plan and ensures all the patients have basic assistance and are comfortable, she prioritises which vital observations and treatments need performing and persuades the housekeeper to stay behind and help. The Deputy Sister arrives three hours later. The Staff Nurse at the end of her shift completes an incident form about the unsafe staffing level.
2. A Staff Nurse was assisting an elderly rather tall patient to walk to the toilet. He had been assessed as requiring the assistance of one, he was making good recovery post hip replacement and was looking forward to being discharged home in the next few days. As they were walking along he collapsed on top of the nurse and she felt a sudden pain in her back. She quickly recognised, however, that the patient was in cardiac arrest and called for help and resuscitation was commenced. The resuscitation was continued for 20 minutes but was sadly futile. The nurse took the following 10 days off work to recover from her back injury.
3. An elderly man of frail appearance was admitted to a busy assessment ward in the early hours of the morning. The nurses noted he was of frail appearance, independently mobile and not confused in anyway, his vital observations were recorded, and he had a NEWS score of zero. The plan was for him to have a chest x-ray and to be assessed by the

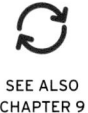

SEE ALSO
CHAPTER 9

medical team. After a very brief assessment by the medical staff and a short discussion with nursing staff the doctors ordered the x-ray. The request indicated he was a chair transfer and no escort was deemed necessary. While awaiting the x-ray the gentleman grew weary and got into bed. A porter arrived and taking pity on the gentleman decided to take him to x-ray on his bed with the help of another porter who happened to be leaving the ward. They raised the bedrails, which was standard procedure in hospital when transporting patients. Once in the x-ray department the procedure was delayed as a number of emergencies took precedence. The patient was in a bed in a small corridor and by this time the patient wanted to go to the toilet. He asked several staff to lower the bedrails, but they declined to do as they later reported they did not feel it was safe to do so. In desperation the patient climbed over the cot sides and fell landing on his hip and sustaining a fracture to his right neck of femur.

What are the lessons to be learnt?

As we have said, it is a nurse's legal, professional and moral duty to speak up and report any incident or situation that could cause, or has caused, harm. As nurses we are obliged to cooperate and assist with any complaint or incident investigation. Finally, you need to know that your opinion is equally valid. As a new starter you are a fresh pair of eyes and may be able to identify actions or behaviours that are unsafe, which staff familiar with the environment may not notice. Staff familiar with routine tasks who then take shortcuts may not recognise the potential danger that a student or newly qualified nurse is more likely spot. In addition to reporting electronically, nursing staff should also inform their Ward manager/Matron/clinical supervisor, or they can also call the corporate patient safety team, union or education lead.

What happens next after an incident is reported?

A common misconception from frontline staff is that they report an incident and nothing changes. In fact, all the data that is reported helps build a picture that the organisation and NHS, nationally, can use to make really effective changes and improvements. The value of feeding back to the reporter is becoming more recognised and is a very valuable means of strengthening an organisation's safety culture.

The electronic reporting system will flag the incident to various senior members of staff who will be responsible for investigating the incident and acting to prevent a reoccurrence. The unit manager and Heads of service will be notified of and review all incidents and will investigate and check the grading and the level of actual harm caused. They will then be able to determine the risk of it reoccurring and this will determine the seriousness of the incident and what level of response is required. They will identify any necessary actions and feedback to staff and close the incident once the investigation is completed for minor and no harm incidents.

If the incident is graded moderate/major/death, an alert is also automatically sent through to the patient safety team to verify grading and consider a corporate level investigation. Depending on the type of incident the police or coroner may be contacted. If a police investigation is required, this takes precedence over any internal inquiry. If a corporate investigation is agreed upon then these proceed using a **Root Cause Analysis (RCA)** process.

WHAT IS A SERIOUS INCIDENT?

A serious incident is an incident that has the potential to cause or actually causes significant or permanent harm or impacts on the ability of the organisation to provide its normal level of service. Examples of these are:

- a fire on the ward
- death of patient due to an avoidable fall
- permanent harm or death from a delayed diagnosis or poor delivery of care.

WHAT IS A NEVER EVENT?

A 'Never Event', as the name suggests, is an adverse event that should never occur if the correct barriers/safeguards are in place. All Never Events are externally reportable, even if they result in no actual harm. If a Never Event occurs there are financial penalties for the organisation/Trust concerned and it can cause a loss of organisational reputation and often attracts negative media attention. The *Never Events Framework* is republished yearly and lists all the different types of event that should never occur.

———————————— GO FURTHER ————————————

WEBLINKS

The NHS Improvements website https://improvement.nhs.uk/resources/never-events-policy-and-framework/ provides information on both the *Never Events Framework* and the latest list of Never Events.

Similar information can also be found on the Healthcare Improvements Scotland website: www.healthcareimprovementscotland.org/our_work/governance_and_assurance/learning_from_adverse_events.aspx, The Patient Safety Wales website: www.patientsafety.wales.nhs.uk/patient-safety-reports and the Department of Health in Northern Ireland web page on Safety and quality standards circulars: www.health-ni.gov.uk/topics/safety-and-quality-standards/safety-and-quality-standards-circulars

Examples of Never Events are:

- fall from an unrestricted window
- scalding of a patient
- misplacement of feeding tube
- wrong site surgery, e.g. wrong knee, wrong eye, wrong patient
- the unintended retention of a foreign object post-surgery, e.g. surgical swabs, temporary packing (that should be removed) and guidewires in central lines, wrong strength ocular lens or mismatched prosthesis
- administration of medical air to a patient you are intending to administer oxygen to.

To prevent these events organisations should have restrictions in place to prevent windows opening wide enough for patients to fall through, water temperature in sinks, baths and showers should be restricted so it is not hot enough to scald and is externally controlled. Kitchens and kettles are out of bounds to patients. There should be a process in place and training for staff, so they can verify that a nasogastric tube is in the patient's stomach before the feed commences. Even if mistakes turn out to be beneficial to the patient they are still Never Events because adequate barriers should have been in place to ensure that they never occurred.

INVESTIGATING AND REPORTING SERIOUS INCIDENTS AND NEVER EVENTS

The Serious Incident Framework sets out the standards and timeframes for these investigations. The incidents are reported onto a secure national database, which is monitored by regional commissioners. The Serious Incident Framework is due to be republished in late 2018 following consultation on redesigning the reports and improving investigations.

Once reported, the lead investigator and investigation chair form an investigation team. The team consists of senior staff who have not been directly involved in the incident – this ensures objectivity. The team participants vary depending upon the type of incident that has occurred. Teams typically include matrons, consultants, managers, pharmacists, therapists and facilities managers. IT analysts are used to support the investigation and the team should also include a patient representative.

The investigation starts by agreeing the terms of reference (scope of investigation); this should be discussed and agreed with the patient or their representatives. Following this, statements from interviews are gathered, medical/nursing notes are scrutinised as well as other patient data such as blood tests, x-rays, recent audits and metrics. Equipment is inspected, and the site visited if relevant. CCTV footage and phone call recordings may be examined. There is also a retrospective look at similar incidents that may have occurred.

A Root Cause Analysis meeting is then held, and after the purpose and scope of the investigation is agreed, the team discuss the evidence in front of them including what happened, and what contributed to the incident. The members of the team then agree a set of actions to prevent a reoccurrence and disseminate learning. The team use tools to critically analyse what happened, and what the root cause or causes were. They also look at what contributed to the event and determine what barriers can be put in place to prevent a future reoccurrence.

The overwhelming majority of healthcare staff come to work to do a good job and promote the health of the patients in their care. However, investigation leads and teams are mindful that there may be staff acting maliciously and there are decision tools to help investigators objectively determine what further appropriate action should be if they do determine an individual is at fault. This may include referral to occupational health, human resources, external professional statutory bodies or the police.

How to prevent future reoccurrence

Following the investigation, a report and action plan is then written. Action plans need to be SMART. This acronym has several slightly different variations, which can be used to determine S – specific, M – measurable, A – attainable, R – relevant and T – time bound actions. These actions should be developed and owned by the clinical team. All actions from serious incidents and Never Events should be monitored to completion by the patient safety team and reviewed by the Trust board.

Selecting effective actions/strong barriers

The effectiveness of the actions can be graded using a hierarchy of interventional effectiveness (Figure 5.3).

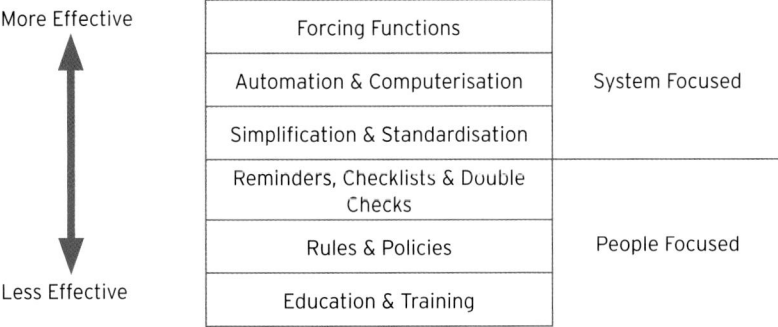

Figure 5.3   **A hierarchy of interventional effectiveness**
Adapted from McDaniel (2012)

This diagram demonstrates clearly that actions such as training and writing rules are less effective in preventing staff from making an error than physical barriers. An example is that of oral syringes which are purposely designed so they cannot fit into an intravenous cannula port. Investigation teams are being encouraged to number actions in line with this hierarchy to encourage critical thinking of the effectiveness of their action plan.

Sharing the learning

The investigation report and recommendations and lessons learnt from these investigations are shared with the patient and/or their representatives, with the staff involved and across the organisation at divisional and corporate level boards and committees. Additionally, the report is shared with relevant external bodies and it is uploaded to NHS commissioners who will usually provide comment and feedback and ensure the incident is shared nationally.

Within the organisation lessons need to be shared in an engaging way; for example, face-to-face events, internet-linked mini video teaching sessions. There is also a web-based staff safety portal which provides staff with a range of interactive resources and newsletters. Information about serious incidents and Never Events should be routinely built into corporate teaching sessions, e.g. staff briefings by the Chief Executive Officer (CEO).

The patient and/or family should be supported throughout the investigatory process signposted to professional support or advocacy as necessary. They will usually meet with the organisation at the end of the investigation to discuss the report, after which they may decide to seek compensation or take legal action.

Investigations (complaints or incidents) should not seek to attribute blame on individuals. It's all about learning as an organisation, finding the system and process errors that allowed the adverse incident to happen. Serious Investigations should include patients' views and participation; some Trusts are now using patient partners to provide an alternative viewpoint.

ACTIVITY 5.2: REFLECTIVE LEARNING

Do you know where to find out information about the incidents that have occurred on your ward/ unit/clinical management groups or directorate?

Are these incidents discussed at team meetings? Should they be?

If you witnessed unsafe practices what would you do? Who would you seek support from?

CHAPTER SUMMARY

- The importance of ensuring patient safety has a long history but received national attention following the scandals at Mid Staffordshire NHS Foundation Trust.
- In response to the Francis Report the government has published a number of new policies and established new bodies to guide and support healthcare organisations to improve quality and reduce risk.
- A Duty of Candour requires healthcare organisations and staff to be open and honest to patients and families when things go wrong.
- A range of mechanisms now exists to identify and report risks that allow an organisation to direct resources appropriately. Reporting also allows a national picture to be developed which informs national strategy and enables alerts to be disseminated nationally where required.
- The Serious Incident Framework provides guidance on the process and procedures to identify serious incidents and ensure that they are investigated thoroughly. A key outcome is the learning that takes place to prevent similar incidents occurring again.

GO FURTHER

Go to https://study.sagepub.com/essentialadultnursing for a further case study related to this chapter. If you are using the interactive ebook, simply click on the book icon in the margin to go straight to the resource.

CASE STUDY: PATIENT SAFETY

Books

Fisher, M. and Scott, M. (2013) *Patient Safety and Managing Risk in Nursing*. London: Sage/Learning Matters.

Journal Articles

Go to https://study.sagepub.com/essentialadultnursing for further free online journal articles related to this chapter. If you are using the interactive ebook, simply click on the book icon in the margin to go straight to the resource.

FURTHER READING: JOURNAL ARTICLES

- Samra, R., Car, J., Majeed, A., Vincent, C. and Aylin, P. (2016) How to monitor patient safety in primary care? Healthcare professionals' views. *Journal of the Royal Society of Medicine Open*, 7(8): 1-8. http://journals.sagepub.com/doi/pdf/10.1177/2054270416648045 A study which identifies safety monitoring strategies in primary care in north west London.
- Woodward S. (2015) Implementing change: Lessons from the patient safety movement. *Journal of Infection Prevention*, 17(2): 79-82. http://journals.sagepub.com/doi/10.1177/1757177415600243 A useful overview of patient safety.

Weblinks

Go to https://study.sagepub.com/essentialadultnursing for further weblinks related to this chapter. If you are using the interactive ebook, simply click on the book icon in the margin to go straight to the resource.

FURTHER READING: WEBLINKS

- NHS Improvement https://improvement.nhs.uk/ A website with useful resources to improve the quality of care in Trusts.
- Ihub supporting health and social care http://ihub.scot/

This is Healthcare Improvement Scotland's Improvement Hub, supporting health and social care organisations to redesign and continuously improve services – with lots of resources.

- Healthcare Safety Investigation Branch
  www.hsib.org.uk/
  A new website which provides information on investigations into incidents in healthcare.

ONLINE
QUIZZES

———————————— ACE YOUR ASSESSMENT ————————————

Revise what you have learned by visiting https://study.sagepub.com/essentialadultnursing

- Test yourself with multiple-choice and short-answer questions
- Do the chapter activities in the book and check your answers online

REFERENCES

Department of Health (2015) *The NHS Constitution: The NHS belongs to us all.* Available at: www.gov.uk/government/uploads/system/uploads/attachment_data/file/480482/NHS_Constitution_WEB.pdf (last accessed 10 February 2018).

Francis, R (2013) Press Statement on the publication of the Mid Staffordshire NHS Foundation Inquiry. Available at: http://webarchive.nationalarchives.gov.uk/20150407084231/www.midstaffspublicinquiry.com/report (last accessed 8 March 2018).

Health and Social Care Act 2012. Available at: www.legislation.gov.uk/ukpga/2012/7/contents/enacted (last accessed 8 March 2018).

Health and Social Care (Safety and Quality) Act 2015. Available at: www.legislation.gov.uk/ukpga/2015/28/pdfs/ukpga_20150028_en.pdf (last accessed 8 March 2018).

Kohn L.T., Corrigan J.M. and Donaldson M.S. (eds) (1999) *To Err is Human - building a safer health system.* Washington, DC: Committee on Quality of Health Care in America, Institute of Medicine, National Academy Press.

McDaniel, C. (2012) *Hierarchy of Effectiveness.* Available at: www.cassiemcdaniel.com/blog/hierarchy-of-effectiveness-process/ (last accessed 12 February 2018).

National Patient Safety Agency (2010) *Root Cause Analysis Investigation tools. Contributory Factors Classification Framework.* Available at: https://www.npeu.ox.ac.uk/downloads/files/pmrt/3_Contributory%20Factors%20Classification%20Framework.pdf (last accessed 5 February 2018).

NHS England (2014) *Five Year Forward View.* Available at: www.england.nhs.uk/five-year-forward-view/ (last accessed 10 February 2018).

NHS Improvement (2016) *Freedom to Speak Up: Raising concerns policy for the NHS.* Available at: https://improvement.nhs.uk/resources/freedom-to-speak-up-whistleblowing-policy-for-the-nhs/ (last accessed 8 March 2018).

NHS Improvement (2018) *Never Events Policy and Framework* (revised January 2018). Available at: https://improvement.nhs.uk/documents/2265/Revised_Never_Events_policy_and_framework_FINAL.pdf (last accessed 18 May 2018).

Nightingale F. (1858) *Notes on matters affecting the health, efficiency, and hospital administration of the British Army [electronic resource]: founded chiefly on the experience of the late war.* Available at: https://archive.org/details/b20387118 (last accessed 5 February 2018).

Nursing and Midwifery Council (2015) *The Code. Professional standards of practice and behaviour for nurses and midwives.* Available at: www.nmc-uk.org (last accessed 6 June 2018).

Nursing and Midwifery Council & General Medical Council (2015) *Openness and Honesty When Things go Wrong: The professional duty of candour.* Available at: www.nmc.org.uk/standards/guidance/the-professional-duty-of-candour/ (last accessed 8 March 2018).

Reason J. (2000) Human error: models and management. *British Medical Journal,* 320(7237): 768–70.

The Health Foundation (2013) *Patient Safety Timeline.* Available at: www.health.org.uk/patient-safety-timeline (last accessed 5 February 2018).

The National Advisory Group on the Safety of Patients in England (2013) *A Promise to Learn – a commitment to act: improving the safety of patients in England.* Available at: www.gov.uk/government/publications/berwick-review-into-patient-safety (last accessed 5 February 2018).

World Health Organization (2006) *Quality of Care: A Process for Making Strategic Choices in Health Systems.* Geneva: WHO.

RESEARCH AND EVIDENCE-BASED PRACTICE IN NURSING

6

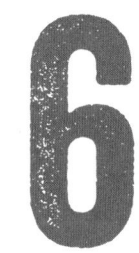

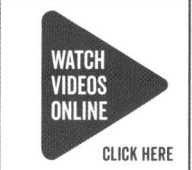
WATCH VIDEOS ONLINE — CLICK HERE

SALLY DOWLING AND JO WILLIAMS

--- **THIS CHAPTER COVERS** ---

- What is Evidence-Based Practice (EBP)?
- Why is EBP important to nursing adults?
- What are the different types of research evidence and how might they be used in practice?

- What are the key skills needed for EBP in adult nursing?

> "
> Registered nurses take the lead in providing evidence based, compassionate and safe nursing interventions; care and support to people of all ages in a range of care settings. They ensure that any nursing care they delegate is of a consistently high standard. They work in partnership with people, families and carers to evaluate whether the goals of care have been met in line with their wishes, preferences and desired outcomes.
>
> **NMC, 2018**
> "

INTRODUCTION

Evidence-Based Practice (EBP) is an important and relevant topic for all nurses, whether in training, newly qualified or experienced. The quote above highlights the expectations of the NMC in relation to EBP; we will also discuss other drivers. There are many books covering these issues in more detail but in this chapter we aim to specifically discuss EBP in relation to nursing adults and to remind you of some of the key skills needed. We will outline the different sorts of evidence available and discuss the 'hierarchy of evidence' and how this is used. We will show you how to develop a clinical question and search for the right evidence, and introduce you to the steps involved in appraising evidence, giving you links to other resources to help you develop these skills. Throughout the chapter we will give you examples, showing you how to use and apply evidence in practice. This chapter is not about how to *do* research but, rather, about how to *use* research in your practice.

WHAT IS EVIDENCE-BASED PRACTICE?

EBP is how we ensure our patients are given the best care possible. It is how we justify and explain what we do, to ourselves, our colleagues and our patients; how we work with those we care for to plan and deliver effective care that has a clear rationale and which makes the best use of the resources we have.

The EBP movement has its origins in Evidence-Based Medicine (EBM) and the work of David Sackett and colleagues; their definition was originally framed in relation to medicine but now recognises the broader nature of EBP:

> [Evidence-based practice is] the conscientious and judicious use of current best evidence in conjunction with clinical expertise and patient values to guide health care decisions. (Sackett, 2000: 71)

Since the early days of EBM in the 1990s, using evidence to inform decisions has become good practice in many areas of health and social care, as well as in policy making. We all use evidence in our daily lives, using information from different sources to aid decision making. Nurses work to make their practice evidence-based because they want to do the best for their patients and know that what they are doing is supported by good evidence.

Later in this chapter we talk about the different types of research evidence nurses draw on in planning the best care for their patients, but it's important to remember that 'evidence' doesn't just mean reports from research studies, published in peer-review journals. Nurses draw on many different types of evidence in their clinical decision making and most definitions of EBP acknowledge this:

> EBP is a problem-solving approach to the delivery of health care that integrates the best evidence from well-designed studies and patient care data, and combines it with patient preferences and values and nurse expertise. (Melnyk et al., 2009: 51)

We have given you two examples here but there are a number of different definitions of EBP; they all draw on the same main elements – the use of up-to-date evidence to inform decisions, as well as how those *giving* care, work together with those *receiving* care, to make decisions. The *experience* of the healthcare professional (as shown in their professional judgement and decision making) as well as the *preferences* of the patient are, therefore, also taken into account. This is important because EBP has moved us away from *'doing it like this because we've always done it like this'*; health professionals are able to draw on a wealth of experience of what works for their patients and why – both individually and as members of teams. To do this, nurses use a range of skills including listening, assessment, planning and teamwork, discussed in other chapters in this book

The three components of EBP: using research (and other) evidence; professional experience and judgement, and the patients' preferences are all equally important but we are focusing here on the skills needed to find and assess research evidence. Later definitions of EBP (Dawes et al., 2005) also recognise that this takes place within limited resources and that this might influence decisions made.

SEE ALSO
CHAPTER 9

SEE ALSO
CHAPTER 37

SEE ALSO
CHAPTER 38

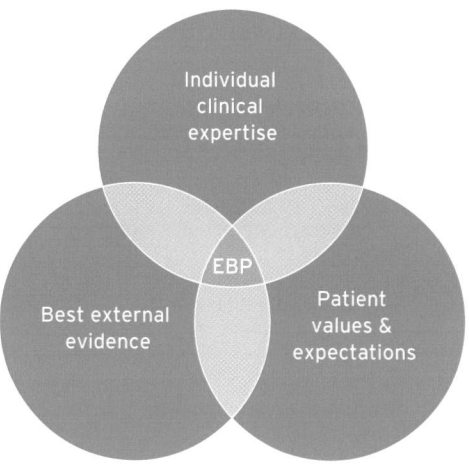

Figure 6.1   An evidence-based (EBP) triad

Adapted from Florida State University (2013)

The NMC *Code* states nurses must '*Always practice in line with the best available evidence*' (NMC, 2015) and be accountable for what they do; this is very important but is not the only driver for EBP. Nurses are accountable for what they do in law and so they must be able to explain and justify decisions they have made about their practice. Nurses are also responsible to the organisations they work for (via local clinical governance mechanisms) but also through national monitoring bodies such as the Care Quality Commission (CQC) and standards such as Essence of Care (DH, 2010). Practising in an evidence-based culture helps to minimise poor care and reduces the chance of failings in care such as those documented in the Francis Report (2013).

SEE ALSO
CHAPTER 37

Finding evidence to support clinical decision making is based around the idea of a 'hierarchy of evidence' – acknowledging that some study designs produce stronger evidence than others (see Table 6.1). This can be useful when thinking about issues where the strength of the evidence is very important (in pharmaceutical treatment decisions, for example).

The idea of a hierarchy minimises the value of some forms of knowledge, which might also be very important in certain types of patient care or in complex situations. Aveyard and Sharp (2017) argue we should structure a hierarchy of evidence in relation to the clinical/research question being asked; if the question is about *experiences* or *feelings* then **qualitative research** would be near the top of the hierarchy as these studies would provide the best evidence. If the question is about which is the best *treatment* for a condition, then **randomised controlled trials** (RCTs) or systematic reviews of RCTs would be near the top as they would provide the best (strongest) evidence.

The move towards EBP has influenced both medical and nursing training and practice but it has been criticised (Greenhalgh et al., 2014; Rizzo Parse, 2014). One criticism is the focus on finding the *best* evidence when sometimes there simply isn't enough evidence from high-quality studies to use. Another

Table 6.1   Hierarchy of evidence (adapted from Ellis, 2013)

Strongest	Type of evidence	
	Description	Formally called
	The combined results of a number of studies which use a very strict experimental design where there is random allocation of individuals to the treatment they will receive.	Systematic review of randomised controlled trials (RCT).
	The combined results of a number of studies which use a very strict experimental design but individuals are not allocated to treatment by random methods.	Systematic review of non-randomised trials.
	The results of one study which uses a very strict experimental design where there is random allocation of individuals to the treatment they will receive.	A randomised controlled trial (RCT).
	The results of one study which uses a very strict experimental design, but individuals are not allocated to treatment by random methods.	A non-randomised trial.
	The combined results of a number of studies which examine the links between causes and effects.	Systematic reviews of correlational or observational studies.
	The results of one study which examines the links between causes and effects.	A correlational or observational study.
	The combined results of a number of studies that describe an event or experience.	Systematic reviews of descriptive or qualitative studies.
	The results of one study that describes an event or experience.	A descriptive or qualitative study.
Weakest	The understanding and interpretations of a group of people who are experienced in a specific area.	Opinions of authorities or expert committees.

is that it is not always possible – or sensible – to use the results from research studies based on groups of people (such as RCTs) to determine the care of an individual. Finally, it is argued that practitioners do not have the training, time and resources to be good at EBP. These issues are still being debated but the inclusion of EBP modules in undergraduate nurse training is one way of addressing the last point.

GO FURTHER

See Mullen and Streiner (2004) for a more detailed discussion.

HOW DO WE KNOW THAT EBP WORKS?

A good example in nursing of how EBP has made a difference is infection control; how effective handwashing can reduce and prevent the spread of infection. The National Institute for Health and Care Excellence (NICE) highlighted how basic hygiene protocols (handwashing/hand decontamination) may be overlooked by *some* health professionals, which threatens patient safety. NICE (2012) reported that 1 in 16 people being treated by the NHS contracted a hospital acquired infection, such as **meticillin-resistant Staphylococcus aureus** (MRSA). By utilising a range of methods and tools to gather evidence, including research and audit, the outcomes to reduce infection were implemented through education (staff, patients, carers and visitors) and policies and procedures, ensuring a more up-to-date approach to handwashing and decontamination.

SEE ALSO
CHAPTER 14

ACTIVITY 6.1 CRITICAL THINKING

- What are the areas of evidence that make up the 'EBP triad'? Thinking about your experience in practice, identify examples where we have research evidence that a treatment option works but where patients would prefer nurses to use alternative treatments.
- Can you think of some barriers to implementing EBP in clinical practice? What might make it difficult for you and your colleagues to find and use the best current evidence in your care?

ACTIVITY 6.1
ANSWER

WHY IS EBP IMPORTANT TO NURSING ADULTS?

There are a number of ways in which *all* nurses are required to use evidence in their practice. However, there may be some nurses who also hold a dual role as a 'practitioner-researcher' and for these people, research may be a much more overt part of their work. Others may carry out reviews or other pieces of research, gather data or generate evidence as part of their work in clinical practice. Examples might include looking at the length of admission for patients who have suffered a stroke, or ways in which service provision can be improved, such as waiting times for treatment, or how service user and carer involvement can enhance service provision. Nurses may gather evidence for audits (for example, handwashing practices; this is common and you may have experience of this) or evaluations of care or aspects of care. Nurses who undertake research are most likely to study topics relevant to the profes-sional (in this case, clinical) setting; determined and influenced by the nursing/clinical agenda and the concerns of the setting.

Even if you are not involved in research in any organised or formal way, the requirement on you to make decisions about care *'on the basis of the best evidence available'* and to *'make sure that any infor-mation or advice given is evidence-based'* (NMC, 2015) means that you need to think about how you use evidence, including research evidence, in your practice. This includes how you seek out, find and assess evidence, and we discuss this later. The Case Study below gives an example of one way in which EBP is important to nursing adults. EBP relates to every aspect of nursing adults in hospital and com-munity settings – whether it is decisions about treatment plans, pressure ulcer prevention or end of life care; you need to think about how you *know* that what you are doing is providing the best and most effective care for your patients.

CASE STUDY 6.1: MARY

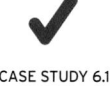

CASE STUDY 6.1
ANSWER

Mary is 84 years old. She has a diagnosis of type 2 diabetes, which is diet managed. Her husband Peter died three years ago following a stroke. Mary lives alone in a bungalow in a rural community, where she and Peter moved to following their retirement 25 years ago. Before retiring, Mary worked

(Continued)

SEE ALSO
CHAPTER 20

SEE ALSO
CHAPTER 29

(Continued)

as a nurse, then a midwife, in a busy city. During her midwifery career she delivered many babies and enjoyed overseeing the development of a midwifery-led birthing unit in the community where she worked. Mary has three adult children: Jane (56), Robert (53) and Sarah (50). All her children are married with children of their own; Mary is the proud grandmother to seven grandchildren. Mary's children live some distance away; Sarah lives 20 miles away travelling by car once a week to visit her mum. Jane and Robert visit once a month. Mary has been an active member of her community including helping set up and run the village playgroup and volunteering at the local school to support children learning to read. Family and friends regularly visit Mary to check she is okay but they are becoming increasingly concerned her memory is worsening and she is not managing her diabetes and diet well, as she forgets if she has eaten and what she ate. The nurses caring for Mary need to consider what evidence would be useful to help care for Mary and manage the risks associated with type 2 diabetes and the potential onset of dementia.

Question – what evidence is available to help you understand the link between type 2 diabetes and the onset of vascular dementia, and what can nurses do to support and treat patients with these diagnoses?

CRITICAL THINKING STOP POINT 6.1

Reflection:

- Reflect on an aspect of care that you have provided for a patient recently; it can be something that seems quite routine. Think about how you knew what to do. How did you know what you were doing was in the best interest for your patient? What evidence did you use to do this? Think widely.
- Can you think of a time when you have participated in or have observed research being undertaken in practice? (This may involve audits or service evaluation.)
- What happened? Did practice change as a consequence of this work?

WHAT ARE THE DIFFERENT TYPES OF RESEARCH EVIDENCE AND HOW MIGHT THEY BE USED IN PRACTICE?

What is evidence and how do nurses recognise what evidence 'looks like'? What kind of evidence is available to nurses? Nurses are involved in a range of decision-making processes drawing on a diverse selection of evidence to assist with these, and with subsequent nursing interventions. We noted earlier on in this chapter that evidence doesn't just mean 'research studies'; evidence that comes from the health professional's experience and taking into account patient preferences is also very important. You may have heard the term *anecdotal evidence*; this is often based on what people tell each other, rather than facts, although it may still include, for example, elements of good practice. Basing practice on anecdotal evidence is risky as it may be unreliable or even untrue. However, where there is absence of substantial evidence to support a particular approach to treatment or a specific intervention, nurses may draw on anecdotal evidence as well as on their clinical experience. In the absence of scientific evidence, anecdotes or personal testimonies should not be relied upon on their own and you should always try and find other sources of evidence to support your decision making.

Although we recognise the value of professional experience and other points of view, here we are going to focus on evidence that comes from *research studies* and outline some of the forms that this might take. Different types of research evidence can be used to support different sorts of decisions; we talked about this earlier in the chapter in relation to the hierarchy of evidence. One important distinction to make when you start to look at research evidence is between **primary** and **secondary** research. Primary research presents the results from studies where the data has been collected for the purposes of that research project; secondary data uses data that was originally collected for another purpose and it is collated, reviewed or re-analysed.

An example of primary research would be a study comparing the use of two different types of pressure ulcer assessment tools, where the data reported on has been collected and analysed by the researchers who designed the study. A systematic review of studies looking at pressure ulcer assessment tools would be an example of secondary research. The researchers would find primary studies undertaken by other people and analyse the results of the studies all together (sometimes using a statistical technique called **meta-analysis**).

Primary studies are very important as they may report on new knowledge or explanations, but secondary research is also very important as the analysis of many studies can provide much more robust evidence. They can be very useful for busy professionals in practice as they gather together recent evidence and review it; this saves time as well as helping those who might not be confident or have the skills to do this themselves. **Systematic reviews** use a specific methodology – there are also other, weaker, forms of secondary evidence such as literature reviews (of articles in peer-reviewed journals), clinical guidelines and protocols (Aveyard and Sharp, 2017; Moule et al., 2017).

WHAT ARE THE MAIN TYPES OF PRIMARY EVIDENCE YOU MIGHT FIND TO USE IN YOUR PRACTICE?

Answers to research questions are usually generated in either numbers (quantitative) or words (qualitative), or a combination of both (**mixed methods research**). The methods used to answer research questions will be clearly related to the type of question being asked. Quantitative research seeks to answer questions such as 'How many patients are affected by this?', 'Is this treatment better than that treatment?' and 'How many people with this condition go on to develop this complication?' In other words, quantitative research is about things that can be *counted* or measured and the results can be expressed in numbers or analysed statistically. Quantitative studies are usually either **observational** (cohort or case-control studies) or **experimental** (RCTs). Quantitative research often uses methods that produce results that can be generalised to similar populations.

Qualitative research seeks to answer questions like 'What is it like to care for a partner who has had a stroke?' or, 'What is the experience of young men living with a stoma?' Qualitative research finds out about feelings and experiences (through observation, interviews or focus groups) and the results (often called 'findings') are expressed in words. The analysis of these looks at themes, patterns and commonalities. Qualitative research often uses small groups of participants and the results are not generalisable, although the findings can be transferable (helping us to understand the experience of similar groups of people). There are a number of different qualitative approaches you may come across. The most common, **phenomenology, ethnography and grounded theory**, are derived from **anthropology, sociology and psychology**; all aim to understand more about experiences within social and healthcare settings (Polit and Beck, 2014). Ultimately, EBP aims to ensure care is patient focused and clinically and cost effective (DH, 2014).

Mixed methods research is increasingly used by nursing researchers, particularly those undertaking evaluations of services or practice, or wanting to explore different aspects of an issue (Moule et al., 2017). A combination of qualitative and quantitative research methods uses different sources of data to answer questions, for example, to evaluate a new service providing support for people with dementia and their carers/families. A combination of in-depth interviews with service users, carers and practitioners, alongside some measurable outcomes (such as attendance numbers, presenting problems, take-up of different professional services offered), might be used to provide a picture of the service and inform future developments.

HOW WILL I KNOW WHAT SORT OF EVIDENCE I NEED TO LOOK FOR?

This very much depends on what you are trying to achieve in practice. For example, you may be employed as a practice nurse and trying to understand how many people adhere to their medication treatment regime, enabling the effective management of raised blood pressure and cholesterol levels (for instance, the use of statins), or perhaps you are working in an inpatient older adult care setting, trying to gauge the experience and impact of being a carer for a relative with a diagnosis of dementia. Each of these examples requires different sources and types of evidence in order to understand the issue in question.

The first example requires you to understand the effectiveness of a treatment approach; the best way to establish this is to locate a study (or series of studies) where different treatment options have been directly compared to one another, ideally an RCT or a systematic review of RCTs. Experimental comparison studies where participants are allocated to treatment, intervention or control, or placebo groups, using a randomised sampling mechanism, are recognised as the gold standard of research, creating an unbiased distribution of confounders and enabling statistical analysis. However, you might also want to look at qualitative studies, to understand more about the experience of being on these treatments and why people do or do not adhere to them (for example, because of resistance to accepting treatment or side effects of the medication).

The second example regarding individuals' personal experiences of being a carer is unlikely to be answered by looking for RCTs, but is more likely to be answered by asking people about their feelings and experiences; you would need to search for qualitative studies that had used in-depth interviews or focus groups to gain rich and insightful data (Moule et al., 2017).

ACTIVITY 6.2
ANSWER

ACTIVITY 6.2: CRITICAL THINKING

- Think about the example regarding individuals' personal experiences of being a carer. How might you go about finding out what this experience is like? What sort of questions would you ask? Once you have thought about what questions to ask, think about how you might approach gathering the information (the method) and why you would use this particular method.
- Think about an area in practice that involves supporting patients and carers (for example, dementia care). Find three recent research articles (ideally less than 5 years old) which relate to your chosen area of practice and the experience of carers. These can be quantitative, qualitative or mixed methods. Read each article and make some notes. Why did you choose these articles? What was the method used in each? What were the results/outcomes? Could I use the evidence generated from these articles in practice and if so how?

WHAT ARE THE KEY SKILLS NEEDED FOR EBP IN ADULT NURSING?

How do you go about using EBP in your adult nursing practice, either as a student or as a qualified practitioner? What skills do you need to search for and find the evidence to help you in caring for your patients? There are a number of commonly accepted steps in doing this. We can only describe these briefly here but we have given you some references to sources where you can find fuller descriptions, as well as other ideas about how you can get help and support. First, you need to know what it is you are seeking evidence about (what is your clinical question?) and then you need the skills to search for the best evidence to help you answer that question. You need to know how to choose among the evidence you find and how to assess (appraise) it to see how useful it will be to you, in your clinical setting. Finally, you need to be able to apply the evidence in your practice – to use it to provide your patient/client with the best possible care.

Developing your question is a very important step; if you are not clear exactly what it is you need to know it is hard to search for the evidence. Some questions derive from immediate patient care situations – *'What is the best dressing to use on this type of wound?'* or *'What is the most effective tool to assess my patient's risk of pressure sores?'* Others may be more related to specific aspects of your patients' journey or experience, for example, in relation to discharge planning. Whatever your question, it is important to use it as the first step in finding 'current' and 'best evidence' as stated in the definitions quoted above. A well-formulated question will make the task of searching for and finding evidence much more straightforward (see Table 6.2 below).

CRITICAL THINKING STOP POINT 6.2

A good question needs to be focused and clear.

There are a number of tools that can help you with this – one of the most well known is the acronym PICOT. Using this can make sure that your question (and therefore your subsequent search) addresses all the important elements. Exactly how you use PICOT will depend on whether the issue you are interested in is likely to be addressed by quantitative or qualitative research.

Table 6.2 Developing a good question using PICOT

Population	Who is it you are interested in? All patients? Patients with a particular health problem, experience or illness?
Intervention/**I**ssue	What are you interested in doing/finding out about? This could be a treatment or other type of intervention, or it could relate to experiences or perceptions.
Comparison/ **C**ontext	Comparison will only apply in studies with a control or comparison group – but you need to know if you are interested in this sort of quantitative study. For qualitative studies you might be interested in the context in which the research took place or which might impact on experiences.
Outcome	What is measured in relation to what happened to the people in the studies?
Time	Is there a time element? Before and after treatment? During the stay in hospital? There might not be a time element in the studies you are interested in.

When you have refined the question you can begin to search for the evidence. This does not just mean searching for papers published in peer-review journals but this is always a good place to start; remember that we are looking for the *best* and *most current* evidence. If you have a well-constructed question this should form the basis for your search but before you can start you need to decide *where* you are searching. Sometimes, a search using an Internet search engine like Google might help you to get some ideas about how other people are talking/writing about your issue, but in order to do a systematic literature search and if you are looking for published, peer-reviewed journal articles, then this means searching within databases. Databases are large collections of published material, organised in a way that makes it possible to search within them using a range of criteria.

There are many good databases used by nurses to find evidence to support their practice (see Table 6.3), including the British Nursing Index (BNI), Cumulative Index to Nursing and Allied Health (CINAHL) and MEDLINE. If you are unfamiliar with database searching it is always a good idea to speak to a librarian in your university or hospital library – ask them to show you how to find the different databases (and how to choose between them), as well as how to get started on a search if you are still unsure.

Table 6.3 Databases of health-related literature

British Nursing Index (BNI): A UK nursing and midwifery database, including articles from medical, allied health and management titles. For core UK nursing and midwifery, it is the most up-to-date resource available.

CINAHL (Cumulative Index to Nursing and Allied Health): The most commonly used database in nursing, providing access to a wide range of general nursing and allied health literature and indexing almost all English-language publications in these fields.

MEDLINE: A database created by the National Library of Medicine providing medical information on medicine, nursing, the healthcare system and other fields from more than 4,800 journals. A good source of information relating to treatment evaluation and explanation.

Embase: A biomedical and pharmaceutical database indexing over 3,500 international journals with selective coverage for nursing. A further good source of information relating to treatment evaluation and explanation.

AMED (Allied and Complementary Medicine Database): A database created by the Health Care Information Service of the British Library covering journals in complementary medicine, palliative care and the allied health professions. Citations can help to inform work relating to rehabilitation and inter-professional working.

ASSIA (Applied Social Sciences Index and Abstracts): An indexing and abstracting tool covering health, social services, psychology, sociology and providing an inclusive source of social science and health information from more than 500 journals. Good for finding literature related to social issues, sociology and social care.

PsycINFO: A database of literature predominantly in psychology but also in the related disciplines of medicine, nursing, psychiatry, sociology, pharmacology and physiology. An excellent source of citations relating to psychological adaptation, mental health issues and communication.

The Cochrane Library: An electronic publication providing high quality evidence to inform care from all perspectives and at all levels. Papers bring together research findings from different research studies with similar research aims to explore the strength of evidence for specific interventions.

Once you have conducted your search (and perhaps repeated it in a range of databases, remembering to keep records of what you find and how you found it), you will need to decide whether the evidence you have found is going to be useful to you in your practice. You may not have found many papers, or you may have found a lot – but reading the abstracts will help you to find the most relevant ones. You can then access the full text of the papers (via the journal website or your institution's library pages) so that you can read them in full, and appraise them.

Appraisal of research (sometimes called *critical appraisal*) is the process of assessing the strengths and weaknesses of the evidence you have found, helping you decide how relevant and useful it is to your clinical situation. Appraisal is not just about *reading* the research but about *evaluating* it too, interpreting it and applying it to your context. It's about considering how the research was undertaken (were the methods appropriate to answer the question? were they rigorous? reproducible?), how the findings are explained and interpreted (the strength of the evidence, the reliability) and how they are reported (trustworthiness and validity) as well as about how issues such as ethics, strengths and limitations are discussed. You will also want to think about how generalisable (quantitative studies) or transferable (qualitative studies) the results and findings are. A part of this is thinking about how useful the results will be for you, in your setting and with your patient group.

There are a number of critical appraisal tools that can help with the process, by giving a structure to focus the appraisal, often in the form of a series of questions that you can ask of your evidence. Becoming familiar with one or more of these, and using them to help you think about the research papers you are finding, can help you to become more critical and to think in more depth about what you are reading.

GO FURTHER

WEBLINK: CRITICAL APPRAISAL TOOLS

Examples of critical appraisal tools can be found at: www.casp-uk.net/appraising-the-evidence

---

Before you are able to appraise the literature it's important that you are confident about the *type* of research you are looking at: if you are not sure, re-read the previous section to clarify your understanding. Getting the results of your work into practice and using what you have found to improve care is not always straightforward. Time (to search for and appraise evidence, and then to implement any changes identified) is not always available, colleagues may not be convinced of the need for change and other issues may take priority. Sometimes, presenting the need for change to a team can require assertiveness and persistence. A range of skills identified in other chapters in this book will help with this; in addition, you will increasingly work alongside other nurses who, like you, have been trained to think and work in this way.

SEE ALSO CHAPTER 37

SEE ALSO CHAPTER 38

ACTIVITY 6.3

ACTIVITY 6.3 ANSWER

- Thinking about the different skills needed to implement EBP, can you identify the ones that you feel confident about, and those which will need more practice? Write yourself a brief plan to improve your skills. How can you get help? Who from? When will you be able to do this?
- Find three different critical appraisal tools. Find one research paper in an area you are interested in. Is it quantitative, qualitative or mixed method research? Use the appraisal tools to assess the paper. Which one did you find easiest to use, and why?

CHAPTER SUMMARY

- There are different definitions of EBP available but most include using up-to-date evidence combined with patient preferences and practitioner experiences to provide the best possible care.
- There are a number of drivers for EBP, including the NMC Code and ideas of quality, safety and value for money.
- EBP is important to all adult nurses, not just those who carry out research themselves. Using evidence to inform practice is important in all settings in which registered nurses work.
- Different types of research are used to answer questions about practice and service delivery. This may be primary or secondary research. Primary research methods include quantitative, qualitative and mixed methods studies. Being able to identify different research methods is an important skill in EBP.
- The key EBP skills needed in adult nursing include being able to search for and appraise the most relevant evidence, being able to identify a clear question and to structure a search of relevant databases. A number of tools are available to help appraise the quality and usefulness of any evidence found.
- Using evidence in practice involves asking questions and searching for potential answers, in addition to how the evidence can be used, with patients and other health professionals, in improving care in both hospital and out of hospital settings.

GO FURTHER

CASE STUDY: EVIDENCE-BASED TRIAL

Go to https://study.sagepub.com/essentialadultnursing for a further case study related to this chapter. If you are using the interactive ebook, simply click on the book icon in the margin to go straight to the resource.

Books

- Aveyard, H. and Sharp, P. (2017) *A Beginner's Guide to Evidence-Based Practice in Health and Social Care* (3rd ed.). Maidenhead: Open University Press.
  This is a straightforward guide to EBP, which draws on a range of examples from health and social care to illustrate the issues.
- Moule, P., Aveyard, H. and Goodman, M. (2017) *Nursing Research: An introduction* (3rd ed.). London: Sage.
  A comprehensive introduction to research for nurses. This is very useful to provide an understanding of common research methods, when and how they are used. An excellent glossary of terms will help novice appraisers of research studies.
- Greenhalgh, T. (2017) *How to Implement Evidence Based Healthcare*. Oxford: Wiley Blackwell.
  Informative text for students, clinicians and researchers focused on evidence-based medicine and healthcare, implementation science, applied healthcare research, and those working in public health, public policy and management.

Journal Articles

FURTHER READING: JOURNAL ARTICLES

Go to https://study.sagepub.com/essentialadultnursing for further free online journal articles related to this chapter. If you are using the interactive ebook, simply click on the book icon in the margin to go straight to the resource.

- Emanuel, V., Day, K., Diegnan, L. and Pryce-Miller, M. (2011) Developing evidence-based practice among students. *Nursing Times,* 107 (49/50): 21–3.
- Greenhalgh, T., Snow, R., Ryan, S., Rees, S. and Salisbury, H. (2015) Six 'biases' against patients and carers in evidence-based medicine. *BMC Medicine*, 13 (1): 200. (Published online 2015 Sep 1, doi: 10.1186/s12916-015-0437-x)

- Hewitt-Taylor, J., Heaslip, V. and Rowe, N.E. (2013) Applying research to practice: exploring the barriers. *British Journal of Nursing*, 21(6): 356–9. (Published online 2013 August 16, doi: http://dx.doi.org/10.12968/bjon.2012.21.6.356)
- Mullen, E.J. and Streiner, D.L. (2004) The evidence for and against evidence-based practice. *Brief Treatment and Crisis Intervention*, 4: 111–21.

Weblinks

FURTHER READING: WEBLINKS

Go to https://study.sagepub.com/essentialadultnursing for further weblinks related to this chapter. If you are using the interactive ebook, simply click on the book icon in the margin to go straight to the resource.

- www.nmc.org.uk/standards/code/
  This takes you to the NMC page where you can read the *Code* in full, including the section which relates specifically to EBP, as well as access a range of other resources.
- www.cochrane.org
  Information about the work of the Cochrane Collaboration, which provides high-quality resources for those working in healthcare; includes access to the Cochrane Library (database of systematic reviews).
- www.evidence.nhs.uk
  This provides access to NICE guidance and standards as well as a range of other high-quality evidence in health, social care and public health.

ACE YOUR ASSESSMENT

ONLINE QUIZZES

Revise what you have learned by visiting https://study.sagepub.com/essentialadultnursing

- Test yourself with multiple-choice and short-answer questions
- Do the chapter activities in the book and check your answers online

REFERENCES

Aveyard, H. and Sharp, P. (2017) *A Beginner's Guide to Evidence-Based Practice in Health and Social Care* (3rd ed.). Maidenhead: Open University Press.

Dawes, M., Davies, P., Gray, A., Mant, J., Seers, K. and Snowball, R. (2005) *Evidence-Based Practice: A primer for health care professionals* (2nd ed.). Edinburgh: Elsevier Churchill Livingstone.

Department of Health (2010) *Essence of Care, 2010: Benchmarks for the Fundamental Aspects of Care*. Available at: www.gov.uk/government/uploads/system/uploads/attachment_data/file/216691/dh_119978.pdf (last accessed 7 February 2017).

Department of Health (2014) *Five Year Forward View*. Available at: https://www.england.nhs.uk/wp-content/uploads/2014/10/5yfv-web.pdf.

Ellis, P. (2013) *Evidence-Based Practice in Nursing* (2nd ed.). Exeter: SAGE/ Learning Matters.

Florida State University (2013) *Definition of Evidence-Based Medicine*. Available online: http://med.fsu.edu/indexcfm?page=medicalinformatics.ebmTutorial (last accessed 13 February 2017).

Francis, R. (2013) *Report of the Mid Staffordshire NHS Foundation Trust Public Inquiry*. Available at: http://webarchive.nationalarchives.gov.uk/20150407084003/www.midstaffspublicinquiry.com/report (last accessed 8 February 2017)

Greenhalgh, T., Howick, J. and Maskrey, N. (2014) Evidence based medicine: A movement in crisis? *British Medical Journal*, 348 doi: 10.1136/bmj.g3725.

Melnyk B.M., Fineout-Overholt, E., Stillwell, S. and Williamson, K.M. (2009) Igniting a spirit of inquiry: An essential foundation for Evidence Based Practice. *American Journal of Nursing*, 109(11): 49–52.

Moule, P., Aveyard, H. and Goodman, M. (2017) *Nursing Research: An introduction* (3rd ed.). London: Sage.

Mullen, J. and Streiner, E. (2004) The evidence for and against Evidence-Based Practice. *Brief Treatment and Crisis Intervention*, 4(2): 111–21.

National Institute for Health and Care Excellence (2012) *Healthcare-associated infections: prevention and control in primary and community care.* Available at: www.nice.org.uk/guidance/cg139/chapter/1-guidance (last accessed 1 March 2017).

NMC (2015) *The Code: Professional standards of practice and behaviour for nurses and midwives.* Available at: www.nmc.org.uk/globalassets/sitedocuments/nmc-publications/nmc-code.pdf (last accessed 10 February 2017).

NMC (2017) *Standards of Proficiency for Registered Nurses.* NMC (2018) Standards of Proficiency for Registered Nurses. Available at: https://www.nmc.org.uk/standards/standards-for-nurses (last accessed 3 October 2017).

Polit, D. and Beck, C. (2014) *Essentials of Nursing Research: Appraising evidence for nursing practice* (8th ed.). Philadelphia, PA: Lippincott Williams and Wilkins.

Rizzo Parse, R. (2014) Evidence-based practice in nursing: Here or gone with the wind of disenchantment? (editorial). *Nursing Science Quarterly*, 27(3): 189.

Sackett, D.L. (2000) *Evidence-Based Medicine: How to practice and teach EBM.* Edinburgh: Churchill Livingstone.

HEALTH PROMOTION

7

WINIFRED MCGARRY

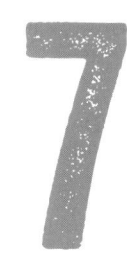

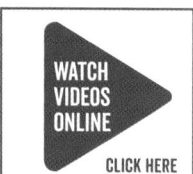
WATCH VIDEOS ONLINE — CLICK HERE

THIS CHAPTER COVERS

- The concept of health promotion
- Health inequalities
- Models and approaches to health behaviour change

- Health behaviour change: motivation, action, prompts and cues
- Steps to initiate a behaviour change discussion.

> I am conscious that for some weeks now, my bowel habit has changed. Sometimes I'm constipated and sometimes I have diarrhoea with a little blood ... It's a bit embarrassing and I am reluctant to visit my GP. I am a 45-year-old lorry driver, married with 5-year-old twin boys. I live in a 'run down' area and try to do my best for the boys so I work long hours. Usually when I get home I just want to relax, have a beer and watch TV. At the weekends, I like to take the boys to watch the football and pick up a burger as a treat on the way home. I have seen the adverts on TV about bowel cancer ... I know people who have died of this. I am really worried about how my wife will cope with the twins if something happens to me.
>
> **Bill, patient**

> Now that I am in my final year of my nursing programme, I am only just beginning to understand the difficulties some people have, deciding to make changes to their lifestyle. I can see the benefit of health promotion and realise now that unless someone wants to change their health behaviours, they won't. I know that change is difficult and understand that my role is to encourage them to take small steps towards healthier life choices.
>
> **Amaka, student nurse**

This chapter will explore the concept of health promotion and discuss techniques that will help you engage with people, individually and within communities, who want to make changes in their own health behaviours and perhaps those around them. This chapter will introduce steps that will enable you to initiate an effective behaviour change discussion. It would be beneficial for you to revisit your coursework relating to health promotion models before reading this chapter.

INTRODUCTION

The Nursing and Midwifery Council's professional *Code* highlights the importance of 'promoting well-being, preventing ill health and meeting the challenging health and care needs of people during all life stages' (NMC, 2015, Clause 3.1).

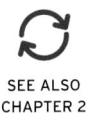

SEE ALSO
CHAPTER 2

The above clause emphasises that health promotion and the prevention of ill health is an important role of the nurse, professionally and ethically. The challenge, however, is not just in the delivery of health promotion advice, but more on *how you* as a nurse *involve* the individual to explore their own lifestyle choices and, through a **person-centred approach** to health promotion, support individuals to make changes in their own health behaviours to improve health and wellbeing. Nurses, like you, are becoming more involved in partnership working, reaching out to a range of community groups to promote health messages within their own local environments. This includes youth work, local councils, schools and involvement with community initiatives. At the heart of all this activity is shared health promotion theory and principles and there is an emerging focus on using health behaviour change methods to help people change and improve their own health.

Bill, in the patient's voice at the beginning of this chapter, is clearly anxious about his symptoms, which resonate closely with the Department of Health, Be Clear on Cancer mass media campaign (DH, 2012) and the Scottish Government Bowel Cancer Screening campaign (The Scottish Government, 2013) to support earlier diagnosis and treatment of bowel cancer. Such campaigns help raise awareness of the symptoms of bowel cancer and encourage the public to participate in the bowel cancer screening process. The symptoms of bowel cancer, however, are vague and can mimic many other bowel complaints; therefore, it is important that the general health promotion advice given to Bill is appropriate and well informed. To do this, you must have an understanding of the progression of colorectal disease to ensure that Bill is advised appropriately.

THE CONCEPT OF HEALTH PROMOTION

The concept of health promotion is not new to the nursing profession. As nurses, we consider the idea of health promotion central to the prevention of ill health, the maintenance of health and the recognition of optimum health and wellbeing. In real terms, however, we need to think more about *how* we talk and engage with individuals and *how* we work with them to help them make decisions about lifestyle choices that can improve their health and wellbeing. This can often prove to be a challenge when we consider, in real terms, the relatively small contact time we have with our patients to achieve this. Therefore, it is important that nurses develop partnerships and work together with external agencies who will have a longer-term relationship with individuals who want to continue the process of change to a healthier lifestyle.

What is health?

The word '*health*' is complex and means different things to different people. It originates from the Old English word '*hael*', which means '*wholeness*' or '*being whole*'. This early definition suggests that health is concerned with the *whole* person and is reflected in the World Health Organization definition as 'a state of complete physical, mental and social wellbeing, not merely the absence of disease or infirmity' (WHO, 1946). This original definition, however, has been criticised as being idealistic and limited, as it is unrealistic for any one individual to assume total fulfilment. Subsequently, the WHO updated its definition in 1986, stating that health 'is a resource for everyday life, not the objective of living, making it a positive concept, emphasising social and personal resources, as well as physical capabilities' (WHO, 1986: 1). This updated definition of health places emphasis on the social and personal resources that can enable the attainment of health rather than focusing on the enablement of complete health and absence of disease. This definition, therefore, is deemed more practical and achievable in terms of delivering holistic person-centred care.

What is health promotion?

The World Health Organization defines health promotion as 'the process of enabling people to increase control over and to improve their health' (WHO, 1986: 1). This definition was modified slightly in WHO's Bangkok Charter for Health Promotion in a Globalised World to 'the process of enabling people to increase control over their health and its determinants and thereby improve their health' (WHO, 2005: 1). Health promotion, therefore, moves beyond a focus on individual behaviour towards changing the wider social and environmental conditions and systems that affect health (NICE, 2007). As such, person-centred health promotion needs to consider individual circumstances and the factors that determine their health.

What is health education?

Health education is any combination of learning experiences designed to help individuals and communities improve their health, by increasing their knowledge or influencing their attitudes (WHO, 2016). Health education is one strategy of health promotion and is focused on helping people learn and use health-enhancing skills. This may be accomplished through face-to-face contact with individuals or groups within a community or it may be by implementing government initiatives relating to public health.

HEALTH INEQUALITIES

It is well published that almost half of the burden of illness in developed countries is associated with poor diet, low levels of physical activity, smoking and cardiovascular disease (Buck and Frosini, 2012). This tells us that the behaviours we have towards our health and the poor lifestyle choices we make are leading to the development of disease. Furthermore, existing conditions may be exacerbated by the health behaviours we adopt. The Dahlgren-Whitehead rainbow model of health (1992) illustrates that many health issues can be determined by social factors. It explains that economic, environmental and social inequalities can determine an individual's risk of becoming ill, their ability to prevent illness and their access to health treatments. The social and economic factors that we are surrounded by can influence the lifestyle choices we make. Figure 7.1 below shows that individuals are placed at the centre and surrounding them are the various layers of influences on health, such as individual lifestyle factors, community influences, living and working conditions and more general social conditions.

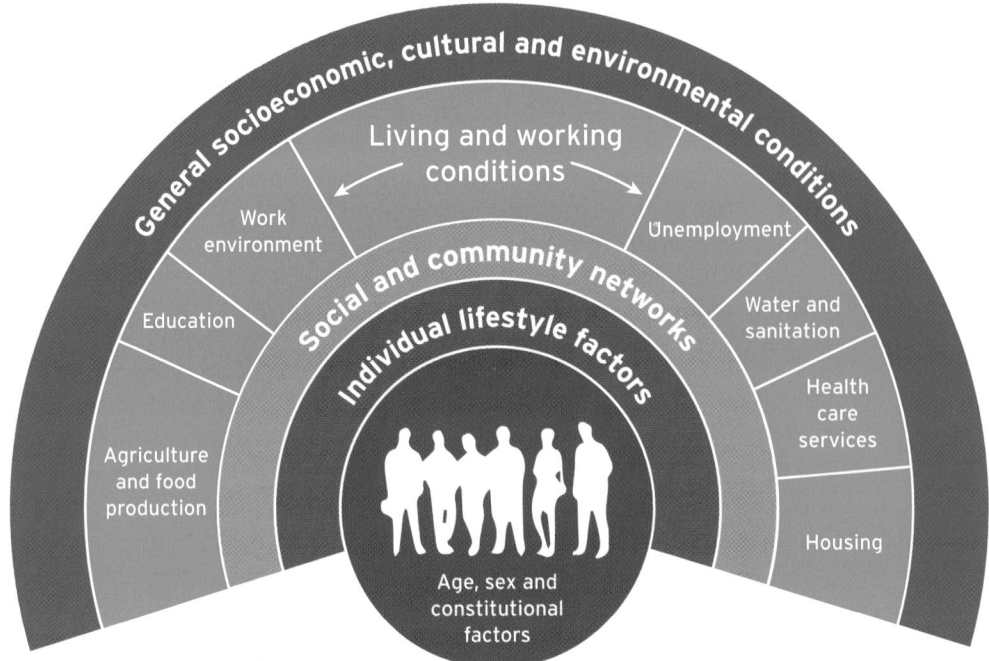

Figure 7.1   The determinants of health (Dahlgren and Whitehead, 1992)

GO FURTHER

WEBLINK:
DAHLGREN-
WHITEHEAD
RAINBOW
MODEL

A more detailed explanation of the **Dahlgren-Whitehead rainbow model of health** can be found at: www.open.edu/openlearn/health-sports-psychology/health/factors-influence-health-introduction/content-section-1

CRITICAL
THINKING
STOP POINT 7.1
ANSWER

CRITICAL THINKING STOP POINT 7.1

Consider Bill's scenario. Evaluate the social and environmental conditions that impact positively or negatively on his health behaviour.

What factors of the Dahlgren-Whitehead model of health do you think he may be able to modify? Can you relate this to yourself?

NHS Health Scotland (2015) defines health inequalities as unfair and avoidable differences in people's health across social groups and between different population groups. Inequalities in health arise because of inequalities in society, that is, the conditions in which people are born, grow, live, work and age. Reducing health inequalities is about fairness and social justice and to address this does not require a separate health agenda but action across the whole of society. The Commission on Social Determinants of Health (2008) examined health inequalities from a global perspective and concluded that 'social injustice is killing on a grand scale'. In response to this, the *Fair Society, Healthy Lives,*

(The Marmot Review) set out key areas that needed to be improved to make a significant impact in reducing health inequalities in England (Marmot, 2010). Recently updated, The Marmot Indicators 2015 are a new set of indicators of the social determinants of health, health outcomes and social inequality that broadly correspond to the six policy recommendations proposed in *Fair Society, Healthy Lives*:

- Give every child the best start in life
- Enable all children, young people and adults to maximise their capabilities and have control over their lives
- Create fair employment and good work for all
- Ensure healthy standard of living for all
- Create and develop healthy and sustainable places and communities
- Strengthen the role and impact of ill health prevention.

If we try to apply the principles of the Marmot review to Bill's situation, it is important that we, as nurses, consider creative ways to engage Bill to make better lifestyle choices to improve his own health and help influence the lifestyle choices of those around him. If someone has grown up in a particular environment and adopted similar lifestyle habits as the people they are surrounded by, then changing a particular health behaviour can be challenging.

CASE STUDY 7.1: ENGAGING OTHERS IN HEALTH PROMOTION

To help address the recommendations above, the University of the West of Scotland has formed partnerships with local council education departments. Students provide a range of age-specific healthy lifestyle information to school children ranging from 4 to 17 years. This activity addresses the outcomes of the Scottish Government's Curriculum for Excellence (2010) while responding to the needs of the undergraduate pre-registration nursing programmes, developing graduate skills such as team working, decision making and communication. Evidence supports that changing children's attitudes of health, through involvement and active engagement within an educational setting, is highly effective in influencing mental and social wellbeing (Paton et al., 2000). An example of this is when children are taught about the long-term benefits of physical activity, responding to the Department of Health's Start Active, Stay Active report (2011), which presents guidelines on the volume, duration, frequency and type of physical activity required across the life course to achieve general health benefits (DH, 2011). Students also promote the benefits of physical activity with a variety of community groups, engaging people from all ages across the lifespan.

Furthermore, students teach children aged 9 years and upwards about the sensitive topic of dementia. Here, children learn through interactive workshops about the brain, reminiscence and assistive technologies. This awareness encourages children to consider ways that they can help support someone living with the condition. Joshua, the child voice in Case Study 7.2, feels confident to make suggestions that may make a difference to his gran's friend, such as reminiscence therapy, using photographs to evoke fond memories from the past. This type of intervention with children not only helps prepare them for citizenship, but helps foster caring and compassionate attitudes for the vulnerable person.

CASE STUDY 7.2: JOSHUA

'Today in school, I learned that some people develop a condition called dementia. I am sad that there is no cure for dementia but I learned about ways that I can help someone living with the condition. My gran's friend has dementia and I have told her about 'reminiscence'. This helps the person with dementia remember about things that have happened in their lives, from when they were young and can make them feel happy.'

Think about your own programme of study.

- Do you think there is scope for you to engage in health promotion activities with school children or community groups?
- What would you promote and who would this benefit?

ACTIVITY 7.1
ANSWER

ACTIVITY 7.1: CRITICAL THINKING

Follow the link below to help answer the following questions:

www.gov.uk/government/uploads/system/uploads/attachment_data/file/216370/dh_128210.pdf

- What is physical activity?
- What do the guidelines say about the type and amount of physical activity people should take to benefit their health and prevent disease?
- What does the report say about the relationship between physical activity and mental health?
- What groups within our society are less likely to engage in physical activity? How might you encourage these groups to participate?

ACTIVITY 7.2
ANSWER

ACTIVITY 7.2: REFLECTIVE PRACTICE

Imagine if Bill's children were involved in a health promotion activity at school and were made aware of the impact of inactivity and health – how do you think they might feel?

Having reflected on Bill's scenario, can you think of ways that might encourage him to participate more in physical activity?

GO FURTHER

The following links will help you put what you have learned into context:

WEBLINKS

The Right to Health: Tackling inequalities. NHS Health Scotland (2015): www.healthscotland.com/uploads/documents/24729-Concertina%20Leaflet%20Spreads.pdf

Health Inequalities and Population Health (2012): www.nice.org.uk/advice/lgb4/chapter/support-for-planning-review-and-scrutiny

Inequalities in Life Expectancy: Changes over time and implications for policy (2015): www.kingsfund.org.uk/sites/files/kf/field/field_publication_file/inequalities-in-life-expectancy-kings-fund-aug15.pdf

MODELS AND APPROACHES TO HEALTH BEHAVIOUR CHANGE

There are many models and theories of health promotion that have relevance to health behaviour change (for further details, please see Nutbeam et al., 2010; Di Clemente et al., 2009; and Connor and Norman, 2005). You may have been introduced to some of these earlier in your programme of study, but it may be helpful for you to revisit. For the purpose of this chapter, however, we will consider the following health promotion models with a focus on health behaviour change:

- The Social Cognitive Theory
- The Health Belief Model
- The Transtheoretical Model of Change

The social cognitive theory

Bandura (1995) posits that people learn from one another, via observation, imitation, and modelling. Bandura (1977) believes in the correlation between behaviour and consequence and that observational learning could not occur unless cognitive processes were active. These mental factors intervene with the learning process to determine whether a new response is acquired. This suggests that individuals do not just replicate behaviour without some degree of consideration. Bandura proposed four mediational processes for this theory:

1. Attention (the extent to which we are exposed/ notice the behaviour)
2. Retention (how well the behaviour is remembered)
3. Reproduction (the ability to reproduce the behaviour)
4. Motivation (the will to perform the behaviour).

This approach acknowledges the role that thought processes play in deciding if a behaviour should be imitated or not.

The health belief model

This model can be used to explain health-related decision making. Based on pioneering work by Lewin (1951) this model was originated by Hochbaum (1958) and developed by Rosenstock (1966, 1974) to

Table 7.1 Application of the health belief model

Belief	Action	
In personal susceptibility to a negative event (condition or problem)	If the person thinks they are likely to suffer from a particular condition/problem, they will make attempts to change their health behaviour	
That the event is serious (consequences significant enough to try to avoid)	If the person thinks the consequences of having a condition/problem is serious, they will make attempts to change their health behaviour	Motivation to change health behaviour is key
That the recommended preventative measure will be effective in reducing the negative event	If the person thinks their actions will reduce their risk of suffering from a condition/problem, they will make attempts to change their health behaviour	
That the recommended measure will not entail too heavy a cost	If the person thinks the benefits outweigh the cost, they will make attempts to change their health behaviour	

(Adapted from Becker, 1975 cited in Nutbeam and Harris, 2004)

explain variations in the utilisation of preventative medical services. The model proposes that decision making depends on the individual believing that a particular course of action will result in the likelihood of a valued outcome being achieved. Table 7.1 illustrates how the model can be applied:

These beliefs suggest that, in general, people will not follow advice if they do not believe it will work for them. In addition, acting on what they believe will depend on how motivated they are to change their health behaviours.

Prochaska and DiClemente's transtheoretical model of change

This model makes the assumption that individuals move through a series of stages, but may relapse at any time (see Figure 7.2). This model is also known as the **Cycle of Change:**

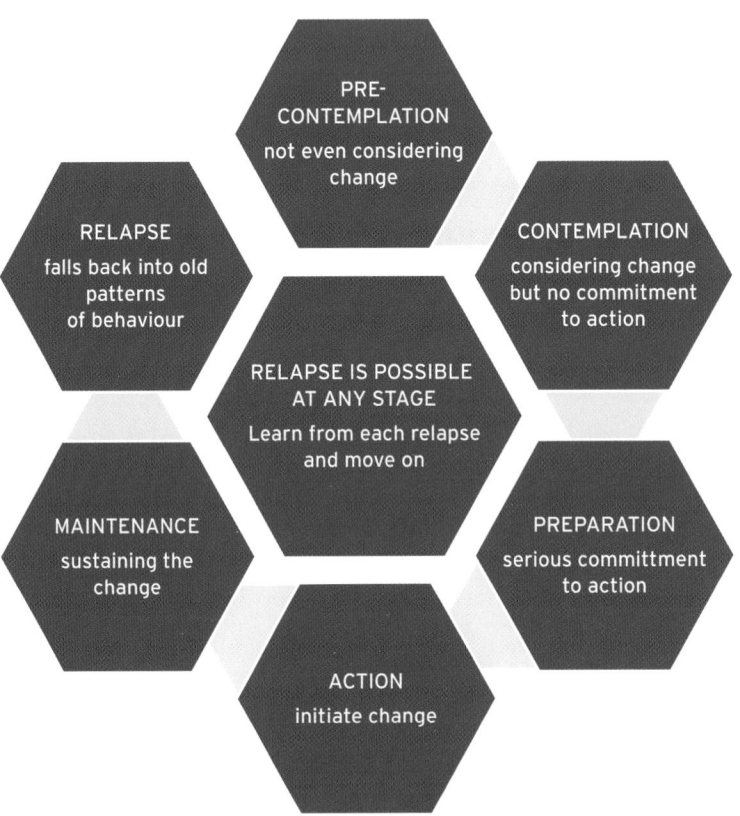

Figure 7.2 Prochaska and DiClemente's Transtheoretical Stages of Change Model (1982)

Reproduced with permission of the American Psychological Association.

This model allows you to judge the stage that a person has reached and develop an intervention, which will enable them either to move on to the next stage of the cycle or return from relapse. It can be effective on a *one- to-one* or *group* situation and is particularly effective in smoking cessation or weight loss programmes.

HEALTH BEHAVIOUR CHANGE: MOTIVATION, ACTION, PROMPTS AND CUES

The UK government has made a public commitment to improve the health and wellbeing of the population and reduce health inequalities. Furthermore, it acknowledges that changing the behaviours of a population will require interventions delivered at individual, household, community and population levels (NICE, 2007; Marmot, 2010).

The theories previously discussed suggest that individuals need to be ready and they need to be motivated to want to make changes in their current health behaviour. The motivation to change has to be maintained by the individual throughout the change process and external motivational support helps the individual to sustain them. Furthermore, the evidence suggests that if someone is not ready to initiate health behavioural changes, it may be detrimental to the person to continue the health-promoting conversation until they are ready.

> There is nothing more frightening than having a pain in your chest that won't go away. I tried to stop smoking a few years back, but to be honest, I thought it would never happen to me. I thought I had indigestion and didn't want to bother anyone … The doctors said that I was lucky! None of us are invincible and if I'd known I would be lying here in a hospital bed aged 48, I would have quit the cigarettes long ago.
>
> **Joe, patient**

CRITICAL THINKING STOP POINT 7.2

Consider Joe in the patient's voice above.

- What health promotion advice would you offer him now?
- How do you know that he is ready to make changes in his current health behaviour?
- Can you suggest why he may have been unsuccessful in his attempts to stop smoking before now?

Since there are several models of human behaviour available, and little evidence to recommend any particular one, a review carried out by NICE, Behavioural Change at Population, Community and Individual Levels (NICE, 2007) concluded that training programmes or interventions should be based on **competencies and skills** rather than any particular model. This emphasises that when you are working with someone to help them make better lifestyle choices you will use different behaviour change techniques, depending on what suits the individual at that time. The Health Behavioural Competency Framework (2010) describes the **route MAP** to behaviour change, which can be used to structure and inform person-centred health behavioural interventions. This tool incorporates the principles of behaviour change models and describes three routes to behaviour:

1. **M**OTIVATION (develop motivation)
2. **A**CTION (support actions)
3. **P**ROMPT (prompt behaviours)

MOTIVATION

Motivation comes from the person's decision and readiness to make a change in their current health behaviour. If you acknowledge and explore the advantages and disadvantages of change (or no change) with the person, it will help you assess if they are ready and committed to start the change process. Acceptance that a change is necessary is key and if the person is not fully committed to start the change process, then it may be helpful to revisit this stage before moving on.

Motivational interviewing

This is a counselling approach that can be used to explore a person's motivation to change. It allows you to explore with the individual any potential ambivalence and barriers to behaviour change. The use of open-ended questions allows the individual to freely express how they feel about change and your ability to listen to the person is key (Powell and Thurston, 2008).

The underpinning principles of motivational interviewing are the ability to:

- express empathy through reflective listening
- acknowledge and explore the person's resistance to change, rather than opposing it
- discuss the person's goals in relation to their current behaviour
- avoid conflict
- refer to other agencies for specialist advice and support.

Sometimes, a brief, person-centred conversation, carried out in a supportive way, can encourage self-belief that health behaviour change is possible.

CRITICAL THINKING STOP POINT 7.3

Reflection

Think back to a time where you were in clinical practice.

- Can you think of an example where motivational interviewing with a patient or family member would have been helpful?
- Do you see the opportunity for this approach to behaviour change in future practice?

ACTION

It is sometimes difficult to make intentions turn into actions. However, when a person is ready to make a change in their health behaviour, it is important that you work together to discuss what they are aiming to change, why they want to make the change and plan SMART goals and objectives to help achieve the desired behaviour. If the goals you set are unrealistic, the person will fall at the first hurdle. If you think about Bill's lack of physical exercise – do you think it would be achievable for him to visit a gym three nights per week to help him become healthier? Sometimes, taking small steps to making change is more manageable and in the long term more likely to be sustained over a longer period. Remember the cycle of change and that the person may relapse at any point during the process. With this in mind, it is important to anticipate potential barriers and agree ways to overcome or avoid them. It is also helpful to encourage self-monitoring behaviour – this allows the person to take ownership of the change process and provides them with further motivation to believe they can succeed.

PROMPTS AND CUES

As previously mentioned, the UK government is committed to improve the health and wellbeing of the population (NICE, 2007) and that for health behaviour change to be effective, it should be targeted at population, community and individual levels. This is effected by the use of prompts and cues. For example, since October 2015, it has been illegal to smoke in a car carrying anyone under the age of 18 in England and Wales (The Smoke-free (Private Vehicles) Regulations, 2015). This law was made to protect children from the unavoidable dangers that tobacco smoke presents to their health and wellbeing. At a national level, people are reminded through public health awareness campaigns that second-hand smoke is dangerous, particularly for children in a confined space, such as a car. TV adverts are targeted at communities during peak family viewing times to remind people of the potential harm they could be exposing their own children to through smoking. This exposure leads children to ask questions and sometimes can prompt people to consider their own health behaviours and begin to contemplate change.

CRITICAL THINKING STOP POINT 7.4

- Are you aware of any other national or local health promotion campaigns?
- Consider how this campaign has impacted on you as an individual or others you know.
- In what way do you think this campaign was successful?

STEPS TO INITIATE A BEHAVIOUR CHANGE DISCUSSION

The NHS Health Scotland (2016) Discussion Flowchart describes the process of a health behaviour intervention. Figure 7.3 suggests five steps of a planned intervention and provides an explanation of how this may be applied in practice. The use of Open questions, Affirmations, Reflections and Summaries (OARS) (Miller and Rollnick, 2013) is useful to develop rapport with your patient and helps you to build a therapeutic relationship. At any point during the discussion, it may be appropriate to stop the conversation. The person may feel that the change discussion is moving too fast and feel pressured into making a change when they are not ready. If this happens, it is important to exit the discussion but signpost the person or refer them for further help and support when they are ready to move on with the change conversation.

The student voice, Amaka, introduced at the beginning of this chapter, is confident to apply the techniques highlighted to help people take the necessary small steps to make changes in their own health behaviours. Through effective discussion we can establish if the person (or group) is ready to make change and if so we too can begin to apply this learning to develop and sustain healthier lifestyle choices.

ACTIVITY 7.3

Can you apply the flowchart to Bill or Joe's scenario? Answers will be available on the companion website.

ACTIVITY 7.3
ANSWER

Process of discussion	Application to practice
Raise the issue	Ensure that the person is comfortable to talk to you about their health behaviour
	Ensure that the environment is conducive to start the conversation
Explore current awareness	Ask the person what they know about the impact of their current behaviour
	Gauge their understanding and correct any inaccuracies in the information they have
	Give them the facts and ask how they feel about the information you have given
	Screening tools may be a useful resource
Summarise information	Recap on the information that the person has told you to make sure you understand exactly what they have said
	Is your interpretation of what they have told you correct?
Listen for signs of readiness to change	Listen for verbal cues that the person is ready to change... Examples of readiness may include:
	I want ... I can ... I need ... I will ...
Choose a suitable approach	Depending on the person's readiness to change, use the route MAP to support them

RAPPORT AND EMPATHY (OARS)

EXIT STRATEGY/ SIGNPOST/ REFER

Figure 7.3 Discussion Flowchart

Source: adapted from NHS Scotland's Discussion Flow Chart (2016)

CHAPTER SUMMARY

- There are many models and theories of health promotion that have relevance to health behavioural change.
- The provision of information and advice alone is not enough.
- It is important that we develop different behaviour change techniques, tailored to meet the needs of the person who wants to make a change in their health behaviour.
- There are external factors that can influence the choices we make.
- Small steps to change behaviour can make a difference and we need to be realistic in what we are aiming to achieve.
- If the person is not ready to make changes in their current health behaviour, they won't, and motivation to change is key.
- It is important to develop our communication skills to help motivate someone to make a change in health behaviour through motivational interviewing.

GO FURTHER

Books

- Green, J., Tones, K., Cross, R. and Woodall, J. (2015) *Health Promotion: Planning and Strategies* (3rd ed.). London: Sage.
  A definitive text on health promotion covering both the knowledge-base and the process of planning, implementing and evaluating successful health promotion programmes.

- Naidoo, J. and Wills, J. (2016) *Foundations for Health Promotion* (4th ed.). London: Elsevier.
  This is a comprehensive, user-friendly book, discussing the foundations of health promotion practice using relevant examples, activities and discussion points.
- Rollnick, S., Mason, P. and Butler, C. (2010) *Health Behavior Change* (2nd ed.). London: Elsevier.
  This book presents an interesting method which can be used to help patients change their behaviour in both hospital and community settings.

Journal Articles

FURTHER READING: JOURNAL ARTICLES

Go to https://study.sagepub.com/essentialadultnursing for further free online journal articles related to this chapter. If you are using the interactive ebook, simply click on the book icon in the margin to go straight to the resource.

- Benyon, K. (2014) Health literacy. *InnovAiT: Education and inspiration for general practice*, 7(7): 437–40.
  https://doi.org/10.1177/1755738014532627
  This article aims to improve knowledge, awareness and understanding of health literacy and suggests ideas for everyday practice.
- Linke, S.E., Robinson, C.J. and Pekmezi, D. (2013) Applying psychological theories to promote healthy lifestyles. *American Journal of Lifestyle Medicine*, 8(1): 4–14.
  https://doi.org/10.1177/1559827613487496
  Explores psychological theories and models and describes their application to various public health issues and behaviours.

Weblinks

FURTHER READING: WEBLINKS

Go to https://study.sagepub.com/essentialadultnursing for further weblinks related to this chapter. If you are using the interactive ebook, simply click on the book icon in the margin to go straight to the resource.

- Health Behaviour Change: Competency Framework: Competencies to deliver interventions to change lifestyle behaviours that affect health (2010):
  www.healthscotland.com/documents/4877.aspx
- Visit NICE pathway–Behaviour change Public health guidance (PH6) (2007):
  www.nice.org.uk/guidance/ph6
- Visit NICE pathway - Behaviour change: Individual approaches Public health guideline (PH49) (2014):
  www.nice.org.uk/guidance/ph49
- Visit Approaches to health behaviour change:
  https://elearning.healthscotland.com/pluginfile.php/41000/mod_resource/content/17/course/course83616.html
- Visit Motivating behaviour change:
  https://www.eufic.org/en/healthy-living/article/motivating-behaviour-change

ACE YOUR ASSESSMENT

ONLINE QUIZZES

Revise what you have learned by visiting https://study.sagepub.com/essentialadultnursing

- Test yourself with multiple-choice and short-answer questions
- Do the chapter activities in the book and check your answers online

REFERENCES

Bandura, A. (1977) *Social Learning Theory*. Englewood Cliffs, NJ: Prentice Hall.

Bandura, A. (1995) cited in Davies, M. and MacDowall, W. (2006) (eds) *Health Promotion Theory*. Berkshire: Open University Press.

Becker (1975) cited in Nutbeam, D. and Harris, E. (2004) *Theory in a Nutshell*. Sydney: McGraw Hill.

Buck, D. and Frosini, F. (2012) *Clustering of Unhealthy Behaviours Over Time: Implications for policy and practice*. London: Kings Fund.

Commission on Social Determinants of Health (2008) *CSDH Final Report: Closing the gap in a generation: Health equity through action on the social determinants of health*. Geneva: World Health Organization.

Connor, M. and Norman, P. (eds) (2005) *Predicting Health Behaviour: Research and practice with social cognition models* (2nd ed.). Maidenhead: Open University Press.

DiClemente, R.J., Crosby, R.A. and Kegler, M.C. (eds) (2009) *Emerging Theories in Health Promotion Practice and Research*. San Francisco, CA: John Wiley and Sons.

Department of Health (DH) (2012) *Be clear on cancer campaigns 2012/13 - Supporting earlier diagnosis of cancer*. Available at: http://connect.qualityincare.org/oncology/awareness_and_early_diagnosis/case_studies/be_clear_on_cancer_campaigns_201213_supporting_earlier_diagnosis_of_cancer#contacts

Hochbaum, G.M. (1958) *Public Participation in Medical Screening Programs: A socio-psychological study*. Washington, DC: Public health service publication No. 572, US Government Printing Office.

Lewin, R.W. (1951) *Field Theory in Social Science*. New York: Harper.

Marmot, M. (2010) *Fair Society, Healthy Lives (The Marmot Review)*. London: The Marmot Review. Available at: www.instituteofhealthequity.org/resources-reports/fair-society-healthy-lives-the-marmot-review (last accessed 6 June 2018).

Miller, W.R. and Rollnick, S. (2013) *Motivational Interviewing: Helping People Change* (3rd ed.). New York: Guilford Press.

National Institute for Health and Clinical Excellence (2007) *Public Health Guidance 6. Behaviour Change: General Approaches*. Available at: www.nice.org.uk/PH6 (last accessed 6 June 2018).

NHS Health Scotland (2015) *Health inequalities*. Available at: http://www.healthscotland.scot/health-inequalities

NHS Health Scotland (2016) Introduction of the Scottish Government Healthier Scotland, Health Behaviour Change Level 2. Available at: https://elearning.healthscotland.com/enrol/index.php?id=411

Nursing and Midwifery Council (NMC) (2015) *The Code. Professional standards of practice and behaviour for nurses and midwives*. NMC: London.

Nutbeam, D., Harris, E. and Wise, M. (2010) *Theory in a nutshell: A practical guide to health promotion theories* (3rd ed). London: McGraw-Hill

Powell, K. and Thurston, M. (2008) *Commissioning training for behaviour change interventions: evidence and best practice in delivery*. Chester: Centre for Public Health Research, University of Chester.

Rosenstock, I.M. (1966) Why people use health services. *Millbank Memorial Fund Quarterly*, 44:94–124.

Rosenstock, I.M. (1974) Historical origins of the health belief model. *Health Education Monographs*, 2: 1–8.

The Smoke-free (Private Vehicles) Regulations 2015. Available at: https://www.legislation.gov.uk/uksi/2015/286/contents/made (last accessed 6 June 2018)

World Health Organization (WHO) (1946) *Constitution*. Geneva: WHO.

World Health Organization (WHO) (1986) *Ottowa Charter for Health Promotion. First international conference on health promotion, 17–21 November, Ottowa*. Copenhagen: WHO Regional Office for Europe.

World Health Organization (WHO) (2005) *The Bangkok Charter for Health Promotion in a Globalization World*. Geneva: WHO. Available at: www.who.int/healthpromotion/conferences/6gchp/bangkok_charter/en/ (last accessed 6 June 2018).

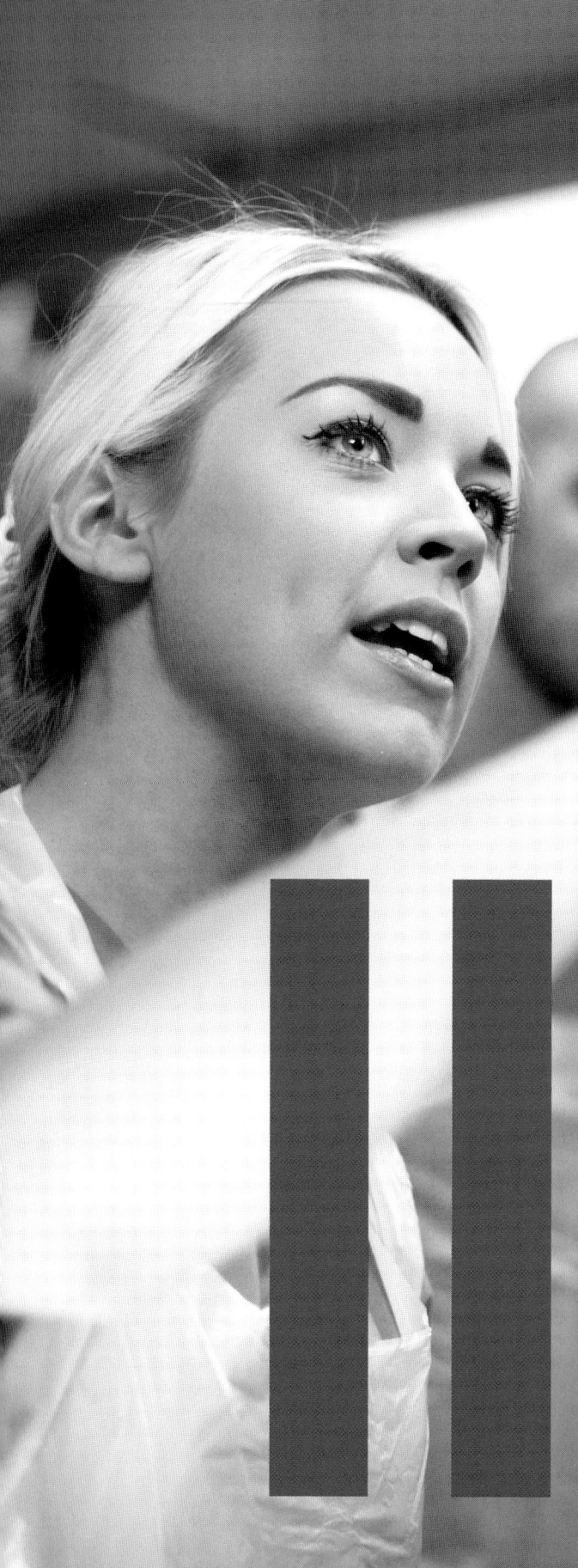

ASPECTS OF NURSING ADULTS

THE FUNDAMENTALS OF CARE IN NURSING ADULTS

8

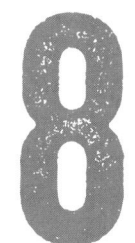

WENDY WRIGHT AND FIONA EVERETT

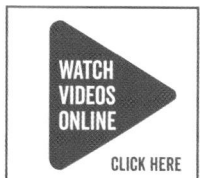

WATCH VIDEOS ONLINE — CLICK HERE

THIS CHAPTER COVERS

- A definition of what constitutes high-quality care
- A summary of fundamental standards and how they contribute to care delivery
- The significance of the NMC standards of proficiency in relation to your preparation for registration
- The importance of the NMC Code in relation to your practice.

> My name is Gordon, I am 25 years old and I am a professional rugby player. Unfortunately, I sustained a shoulder injury while tackling one of my opponents, which meant that I had to undertake a period of initial immobilisation of my shoulder joint, followed by physiotherapy to stabilise and strengthen the joint and surrounding muscles.
>
> This experience made me realise how important it was for me to receive accurate assessment and monitoring of my injury, tailored symptom control, health promotion and management. An individualised care plan was put in place for me, which enabled me to focus on my recovery and a phased return to professional rugby. Thanks to this care and attention, by skilled professionals, I am able to continue playing the sport that I love.
>
> **Gordon, patient**

> As part of my nursing programme, I undertook a module in my first year entitled 'Fundamental Skills', which introduced me to nursing skills. However, I soon began to realise that in order to deliver care, that was safe and effective, I required to develop a comprehensive knowledge and understanding of all of the facets involved in the delivery of contemporary care: what patient-centred care means, the importance of professional values, safeguarding, patient safety, research and evidence-based practice in nursing and professional, legal and ethical principles and policy.
>
> **Kirsty, Adult Nursing Student**

INTRODUCTION

In order to become a safe and effective practitioner who is fit for practice and purpose at the point of registration, your practice should be underpinned by fundamental nursing, professional, legal and ethical standards. You must also develop knowledge and understanding of the common and complex health conditions that can affect adults.

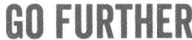

GO FURTHER

WEBLINK:
CQC
FUNDAMENTAL
STANDARDS

To ensure that you have a clear definition of what fundamental standards of care are please refer to the Care Quality Commission, *The Fundamental Standards* (CQC, 2015) on its website: https:// www.cqc.org/ what-we-do/how-we-do-our-job/fundamental-standards

You will already have engaged in a variety of learning activities as part of your nursing programme, including exploring professional, legal and ethical aspects of care delivery and the pathophysiology of some of the conditions that can affect adults, and the needs and potential challenges that may arise when living with these conditions. You will also have experience in the delivery of relevant care through simulation and/or direct patient care, which should enable you to link theory to practice.

Also key to the provision of safe and effective care is the ability to assess, plan, implement and evaluate care delivery and to manage the challenges that face patients. Ensuring that your interventions are evidence based contributes to the quality of care delivered. It is, therefore, more than likely that you will be continually developing your literature searching and critiquing skills in order to define, refine and source robust, contemporary evidence which underpins nursing interventions and management of care.

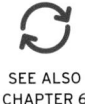

SEE ALSO
CHAPTER 5

You will also be engaged in developing your knowledge and understanding in relation to person-centred care and discharge, which entails placing the patient at the centre of the care being delivered. Developing your knowledge of health promotion is another important aspect of your learning, which has the potential to enable patients to increase control over and to improve their health.

SEE ALSO
CHAPTER 6

Competent assessment, supported by critical thinking and problem-solving skills in collaboration with the patient and your mentor and/or other team members will also contribute to the delivery of safe and effective care. This should ensure that patients are treated with dignity and respect, consent to and receive safe care or treatment that he/she needs by appropriately trained professionals, as these are all integral aspects of safeguarding.

SEE ALSO
CHAPTER 4

The essential skills and knowledge required to nurse adults is complex, but through your active participation and application in both theory and practice and through robust support mechanisms, your university and practice learning environments should prepare you appropriately for registration.

This chapter will start with a definition of what constitutes high-quality care and provide a summary of fundamental standards and how they contribute to care delivery. Specific focus will be placed on the NMC and the significance of its standards of proficiency in relation to your preparation for practice and the NMC Code (NMC, 2015) in relation to how it must underpin your practice.

WHAT CONSTITUTES HIGH-QUALITY CARE?

If you were asked to define what constitutes high-quality care, what factors would you take into consideration? NHS England (2014), for example, proposes high-quality care for all, now and for future generations. Their intention is, therefore, to provide support, which is compassionate, inclusive and responds to suggestions for improvement. Ultimately, the goals of contemporary health policy across the UK are very similar as their intention is to enable all citizens to have greater control of their individual circumstances and ultimately promote health and wellbeing across the lifespan. As a student nurse, you are part of a team of professionals who will make a contribution to achieving this goal.

Quality in healthcare provision is made up of many constituent parts, where each part is considered as vitally important. Care should be clinically effective, which means that the right person does the right thing in the right way at the right time in the right place with the right result. The care delivered should also, therefore, be evidence based, safe and person-centred, which should result in a positive experience for the patient, their family and carers.

In order to provide high-quality care as part of your programme of study you will be encouraged to develop your critical thinking skills. If you think critically and reflect about what you do, this will enable you to identify what works well and what doesn't and then take the necessary steps to contribute to developing the former and reforming the latter. This could involve, for example, a discussion with your mentor or senior nurse, which would enable you to demonstrate application of your critical thinking skills and make a contribution to the delivery of high-quality care.

The provision of high-quality care is, therefore, the goal of all healthcare professionals, which is also underpinned by reducing inequalities in access to health services and the outcomes of care. In striving for high-quality healthcare provision all patients, irrespective of individual circumstances, for example, isolation, poverty or vulnerability, should be treated as equals with dignity and respect.

ACTIVITY 8.1: CRITICAL THINKING

The following are some examples of the policies that have been published in regard to the delivery of high-quality care within the UK. Access and read through the policies, which are most relevant to your geographical area of practice.

Scotland

Scottish Government (2010) *The Healthcare Quality Strategy for NHS Scotland*
Healthcare Improvement Scotland (2011) *Healthcare Quality Standard: Assuring person centered, safe and effective care: clinical governance and risk management*
Scottish Government (2016) *National Clinical Strategy for Scotland*

England

National Institute for Health and Care Excellence (2018) *Quality Standards*
Department of Health (2012) *NHS Constitution for England*
Care Quality Commission (2013) *Raising Standards, Putting People First*
NHS England (2014) *Five Year Forward View*

Northern Ireland

Department of Health, Social Services and Public Safety (DHSSPS) (2006) *The Quality Standards for Health and Social Care*
DHSSPS (2011) *Quality 2020: A 10-year strategy to protect and improve quality in health and social care in Northern Ireland*
DHSSPS (2011) *Transforming Your Care*

Wales

Welsh Government (2010) *Doing Well, Doing Better. Standards for health services in Wales*
Welsh Government (2011) *Together for Health*

(Continued)

> (Continued)
>
> Welsh Government (2012) *Achieving Excellence. The quality delivery plan for the NHS in Wales*
> Welsh Government (2012) *Working Differently – Working Together*
>
> - Write down the key points you have learned from reading your chosen policy.
> - Have you seen this policy being implemented in practice?
> - If not, how might you respond to an instance where you believe that high-quality care has not been delivered?

Equally important to the delivery of care is the measurement of care. If care is not measured it is unlikely that achievement of goals and ultimately quality can be evaluated. Across the UK, a variety of frameworks are utilised. These frameworks are designed to measure:

- prevention of premature death
- successful early diagnosis and management of health issues
- enhancing quality of life for people living with long-term conditions, preventing complications and the need for hospital admission
- effective management of ill health or injury, which promotes recovery and maximum independence
- positive experience of care, which is underpinned by dignity and respect
- patient safety and protection from avoidable harm.

There are also designated organisations that regulate and inspect the delivery of care across the UK:

Scotland: The Care Inspectorate (SCSWIS)

England: The Care Quality Commission (CQC)

Northern Ireland: The Regulation and Quality Improvement Authority (RQIA)

Wales: The Care and Social Services Inspectorate Wales (CSSIW)

Regulation and inspection of the quality of care by an independent body are important in ensuring that patients receive high-quality care. Inspection reports can be accessed for each of the organisations responsible for each of the geographical regions of the UK. Their websites provide valuable information for both members of the public and professionals and are designed to promote change and innovation and support improvement and signposting of good practice. Awareness and utilisation of these resources can support you to enhance your knowledge and understanding of high-quality care and in supporting the delivery of such care.

Table 8.1 provides a summary of fundamental standards, which inform and define the expectations of the delivery of quality care from the following bodies:

- the Care Quality Commission (2015)
- the fundamentals of care cited by the NMC (2015) Code
- the Healthcare Quality Strategy for NHS Scotland (2010) based on the Institute of Medicine's (2001) six dimensions of quality care.
- the 6 Cs from the Compassion in Practice, Nursing, Midwifery and Care Staff, Our Vision and Strategy (DH and NHS Commissioning Board, 2012)
- the ten commitments from Leading Change, Adding Value (DH and NHS Commissioning Board 2016)
- the Royal College of Nursing's Principles of nursing practice (2018).

All of these documents demonstrate a similar focus and similar integral elements, which are considered necessary in the delivery of high-quality care.

Table 8.1 Summary of Fundamental Standards

NMC The Code (2015) Professional Standards of practice and behaviour for nurses and midwives	Care Quality Commission (2015)	Healthcare Quality Strategy NHS Scotland (2010) (based on the six dimensions of healthcare quality, Institute of Medicine)	6 Cs from the Compassion in Practice, Nursing, Midwifery and Care Staff, Our Vision and Strategy (2012)	RCN's principles of Nursing Practice (2018)	Leading Change, Adding Value (2016) 10 commitments to support action of nursing midwifery and care staff
Prioritise people	~ Care and treatment must be appropriate and reflect service users' needs and preferences	Person-centred: providing care that is responsive to individual personal preferences.	**Care** Caring defines us and our work	Principle A Dignity, equality, diversity and humanity	We will
~ Treat as individuals and uphold dignity	~ Service users must be treated with dignity and respect	Equitable: providing care that does not vary in quality	**Compassion** Care based on empathy, respect and dignity	Principle D Advocacy, empowerment and patient centred care	promote a culture where improving the population's health is a core component of the practice of all nursing, midwifery and care staff
~ Listen to people and respond to preferences and concerns	~ Consent				work with individuals, families and communities to equip them to make informed choices and manage their own health
~ Act in the best interests of people at all times	~ Nutrition and hydration needs must be met				be centred on individuals experiencing high value care
~ Respect right to privacy and confidentiality	Compliance with the fundamental standards				work in partnership with individuals, their families, carers and others important to them
					lead and drive research to evidence the impact of what we do

(Continued)

Table 8.1 (Continued)

NMC The Code (2015) Professional Standards of practice and behaviour for nurses and midwives	Care Quality Commission (2015)	Healthcare Quality Strategy NHS Scotland (2010) (based on the six dimensions of healthcare quality, Institute of Medicine)	6 Cs from the Compassion in Practice, Nursing, Midwifery and Care Staff, Our Vision and Strategy (2012)	RCN's principles of Nursing Practice (2018)	Leading Change, Adding Value (2016) 10 commitments to support action of nursing midwifery and care staff
Practice effectively ~ Always practice in line with the best available evidence ~ Communicate clearly ~ Work cooperatively	~ Sufficient numbers of suitably qualified, competent, skilled and experienced staff ~ Fit and proper persons required ~ Safe care and treatment ~ Protected from abuse and improper treatment	Effective: providing services based on scientific knowledge. Efficient: avoiding waste, including waste of equipment, supplies, ideas and energy Timely: reducing waits and delays	**Competence** Expertise, clinical and technical knowledge to deliver effective care and treatments based on research evidence **Communication** Central to successful caring relationships and to effective team working	Principle E Communication Principle F Evidence-based practice, education, technical skills, clinical reasoning Principle G Interdisciplinary and multi-agency working; team working, continuity of care	have the right education, training and development to enhance our skills, knowledge and understanding have the right staff in the right places and at the right time champion the use of technology and informatics to improve practice, address unwarranted variations and enhance outcomes
Preserve safety ~ Recognise and work within the limits of your competence ~ Be open and candid ~ Raise concerns immediately	~ Premises and equipment must be clean, secure, suitable and used properly ~ Complaints appropriately investigated and action taken	Safe: avoiding injuries to patients from healthcare that is intended to help them	**Courage** Enables us to do the right thing for the people we care for, speak up if we have concerns	Principle B Ethical and legal integrity, accountability, responsibility Principle C Safety of patients, visitors and staff	increase the visibility of nursing and midwifery leadership and input in prevention actively respond to what matters most to our staff and colleagues
Promote professionalism and trust ~ Uphold the reputation of your profession at all times ~ Provide leadership			**Commitment** to build on and improve care and patient experiences.	Principle H Leadership which contributes to an open and honest culture.	

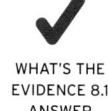

WHAT'S THE
EVIDENCE 8.1
ANSWER

WHAT'S THE EVIDENCE? 8.1

Bowles, L. (2016) Cocktail Conversations: listening to patients. *Nursing Times*, 112: online issue 2, 7–8 looks at an initiative in response to the Francis Inquiry, which places emphasis on listening to patients. This article focuses on a local initiative, which helped teams to provide high-quality care that reflects on, and learns from, people using and delivering the service.

- Read the article and reflect on your experiences of where you have been involved in receiving feedback from a patient on the care that they received.
- What action is taken if the feedback indicates dissatisfaction?

GO FURTHER

Review the following websites which support innovative approaches to improve services for patients.

NHS Improvement, available at: https://improvement.nhs.uk/improvement-hub/quality-improvement/

or the Academy of Fabulous (NHS) Stuff available at: http://fabnhsstuff.net/

There is also the report on the patient feedback challenge, which can be found here: www.opm.co.uk/wp-content/uploads/2014/02/PFC-Evaluation-Report-final1.pdf

WEBLINKS

NMC STANDARDS OF PROFICIENCY

The NMC regulates nurses and midwives and also serves to protect the public. One of the ways in which they do this is by setting and maintaining standards of education, training and conduct to ensure you're equipped with the skills and knowledge you need to practise now and in the future.

The NMC has developed new standards of proficiency for registered nurses (2018a) and the Education Framework: Standards for Education and Training (2018b).

The standards of proficiency are the minimum standards that you as a nursing student will need to meet in order to be considered capable of safe and effective practice by the NMC. Your education institution will also need to ensure that your programme is well-designed and effective to prepare you to meet these proficiencies in order to gain NMC registration.

The outcome-focused standards of proficiency presented in Table 8.2 are structured under seven headings. Each of these describes key components of the roles, responsibilities and accountabilities of registered nurses. While there is some overlap between the seven headings, it is hoped this approach will provide clarity to the public and the existing nursing and health professional workforce about the core knowledge, skills and competencies that they can expect of every registered nurse in the future.

Table 8.2 NMC Standards of Proficiency

At the point of registration, a registered nurse will:

1. Be an accountable professional

- be responsible and accountable for their actions
- act in the best interests of people, put them first, and provide nursing care that is person-centred, safe and compassionate
- solve problems and make sound decisions about care for people based on evidence and knowledge.

2. Promote health

- take a lead in helping people to improve and maintain their mental, behavioural, cognitive and physical health and wellbeing
- support and enable people at all stages of their lives to make informed choices about how to manage and improve their current health, and prevent ill health.

3. Assess needs and plan care

- assess the health and circumstances of people to inform the need for nursing intervention, care and support
- take into account the personal situation, characteristics, preferences and wishes of people, their families and carers
- accept that patients and families become experts in their own care and ensure they have the resources at their disposal to assist them to make informed decisions and that plans for intervention, care and support are tailored to their individual needs and preferences.

4. Provide and evaluate care

- take the lead in providing and supervising the delivery of nursing interventions, care and support to people of all ages and in any setting
- ensure that delivery of all aspects of care is compassionate and safe
- work in partnership with people, families and carers to evaluate whether the goals of care have been met in line with their wishes and preferences.

5. Lead nursing care and work in teams

- provide nursing leadership by demonstrating best practice and be accountable for delegating care appropriately to others, including lay carers
- play an active and equal role in multidisciplinary teams of professionals, collaborating and communicating effectively with colleagues, and with people and families to help them to manage their own care.

6. Improve safety and quality of care

- make a key contribution to continually improving the quality of care and treatment given, and improving people's experience of care
- be able to assess any risks to patient safety or experience, and take appropriate action to manage those, putting the best interests, needs and preferences of people first
- understand how to manage risks across organisations and settings.

7. Coordinate care

- engage with a variety of healthcare and other agencies and professionals, in order to support the delivery of complex care pathways and packages of care.

THE IMPORTANCE OF THE NMC CODE

As previously discussed in this chapter, the patient experience is a recognised indicator of the quality of care and the NMC supports this and recommends that nurses should:

- put the interests of people using or needing nursing or midwifery services first
- make their care and safety your main concern
- make sure their dignity is preserved and their needs are recognised, assessed and responded to

- deliver or advise on treatment utilising best evidence available and best practice
- reflect and act on any feedback you receive to improve your practice
- make sure that patient and public safety is protected
- raise concerns immediately whenever you come across situations that put patients or public safety at risk
- uphold the reputation of your profession at all times
- display a personal commitment to the standards of practice and behaviour set out in the *Code*.

ACTIVITY 8.2: CRITICAL THINKING – NMC STANDARDS

Reflect on your present practice and discuss with your mentor/supervisor how you can:

- deliver high-quality essential care to all persons in your care
- seek out every opportunity to promote health and prevent illness
- use leadership skills to supervise and manage others and contribute to planning, designing, delivering and improving future services.

The revised NMC *Code of professional standards for nurses and midwives* came into force on 31 March 2015, and reflects the changes in contemporary healthcare and society. It places patients and service users at the centre of practice with the objective of protecting the public and places emphasis on compassionate care, team work, record keeping, delegation and trust, accountability, raising concerns and co-operating with investigations and audits.

The Francis Inquiry (Francis, 2013), which publicised the failings in the care provided at Mid Staffordshire NHS Foundation Trust, made recommendations for change which included: putting patients first, culture change, fundamental standards of behaviour and openness, transparency and candour.

The *Code* is structured around four themes:

- Prioritise people
- Practise effectively
- Preserve safety
- Promote professionalism and trust.

The *Code* was developed in collaboration with the public, nurses and midwives, employers, educators and others who care about high-quality nursing care and should be used by nurses and midwives to underpin and guide their practice as a means of joining or maintaining their position on the NMC register and in defining their professionalism.

The *Code* presents the professional standards that nurses and midwives must maintain in order to enable re-registration to practice within the UK. It includes core standards of conduct, performance and ethics and is considered integral to quality improvement and the provision of safe, effective care. It also acts as a guide to reflecting on practice, professional approach and philosophy. It can be used by employers to support staff in maintaining standards as part of high-quality care provision. Your nurse lecturers will also use the *Code* to help you understand what it means to be a registered nurse.

The revised *Code* (2015) builds on the existing foundation of good nursing and midwifery practice but has also taken cognizance of the failings highlighted within the Francis Inquiry. The revised Code, therefore, contains six new requirements, which did not feature in the previous Code:

- Fundamentals of care
- Duty of candour
- Social media use
- Raising concerns
- Delegation and accountability
- Professional duty to assist in an emergency.

FUNDAMENTALS OF CARE

The *Code* (2015: 4) states that:

> The fundamentals of care include, but are not limited to, nutrition, hydration, bladder and bowel care, physical handling and making sure that those receiving care are kept in clean and hygienic conditions. It includes making sure that those receiving care have adequate access to nutrition and hydration, and making sure that you provide help to those who are not able to feed themselves or drink fluid unaided.

DUTY OF CANDOUR

The *Code* states that:

> The professional duty of candour is about openness and honesty when things go wrong and paragraph 14 (p.11) requires nurses and midwives 'to be open and candid with all service users about all aspects of care and treatment, including when any mistakes or harm have taken place'.

SOCIAL MEDIA USE

The *Code* emphasises that social media must be used responsibly, respecting others' right to privacy and upholding the reputation of the profession. Separate guidance has also been produced by the NMC in regard to the use of social media (www.nmc-uk.org/guidance).

RAISING CONCERNS

The *Code* highlights the responsibility of nurses and midwives to raise concerns about patient safety and to act on concerns raised to them. Your university may also provide you with specific advice in relation to this. The NMC has produced specific information about raising concerns, which can be accessed via the NMC website (www.nmc-uk.org/raisingconcerns).The Public Interest Disclosure Act enables nurses, midwives and students to make protected disclosures to the NMC and other organisations, protecting them from retaliation or victimisation when they raise concerns.

DELEGATION AND ACCOUNTABILITY

The *Code*, Paragraph 11 (p.10) requires nurses and midwives to be accountable for their decisions to delegate tasks and duties to other people, ensuring that delegated tasks and duties are within the other person's scope of competence, that they are appropriately supervised and supported and that the task is completed to the required standard.

PROFESSIONAL DUTY TO ASSIST IN AN EMERGENCY

The *Code*, Paragraph 15 (p.12) reintroduces the duty to offer help in an emergency, within the limits of knowledge and competency, and to arrange access to and the prompt provision of emergency care, wherever possible, while having regard to personal safety, the safety of others and the availability of other options for providing care.

REVALIDATION

Revalidation, which replaces post-registration education and practice (PREP) requirements, came into effect in April 2016 and is the new process that all nurses and midwives must follow in order to maintain their registration and eligibility to practise. Revalidation will encourage you to reflect on the role of the *Code* in your practice and allow you to demonstrate that you have embraced the standards within it. The process of revalidation occurs every three years in order to allow renewal of registration. The NMC has established a microsite for all the information you need to guide you through the revalidation process. Please explore this useful link, which will allow you to familiarise yourself and provide you with all the necessary information required for your future progression, following initial registration: revalidation.nmc.org.uk. Additional standards, guidance and circulars are also available via the NMC website (www.nmc.org.uk).

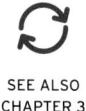

SEE ALSO
CHAPTER 3

ACTIVITY 8.3: CRITICAL THINKING

Think about your practice learning experiences so far.

Taking the NMC (2015) Code into consideration, write down any examples where you witnessed the four broad themes implemented in the delivery of care:

- Prioritising people
- Practising effectively
- Preserving safety
- Promoting professionalism and trust.

How did this impact on the care delivered?

CASE STUDY 8.1: AJIT

Ajit is 73 years old and until recently lived with his son and daughter-in-law. He has led an active life and enjoys reading, playing chess and spending time with his grandchildren. However, Ajit has been diagnosed with Alzheimer's Disease, which has progressed and he now requires long-term care.

Ajit tends to wander and this is a real concern for his family. How can you help to alleviate the family's concerns in relation to Ajit's care and safety?

CASE STUDY 8.1
ANSWER

CRITICAL THINKING STOP POINT 8.1 ANSWER

SEE ALSO CHAPTER 4

CRITICAL THINKING STOP POINT 8.1

SAFEGUARDING

Safeguarding adults is about protecting those at risk of harm (vulnerable adults) from suffering abuse or neglect. Safeguarding has been discussed earlier on in this chapter. Nurses have an important role to play in ensuring that patients receive the care or treatment that he/she needs as this is an integral aspect of safeguarding.

Referring to the case study, how would you help to ensure that Ajit receives the care or treatment that he needs?

CHAPTER SUMMARY

- In order to become a safe and effective practitioner who is fit for practice and purpose at the point of registration, your practice should be underpinned by fundamental nursing, professional, legal and ethical standards.
- Key to the provision of safe and effective care is the ability to assess, plan, implement and evaluate care delivery and to manage the challenges that face patients.
- The essential skills and knowledge required to nurse adults is complex, but through your active participation and application in both theory and practice and through robust support mechanisms, from your university and practice learning environments, you should be prepared appropriately for registration.
- The standards for pre-registration nurse education (NMC, 2018a) identify the knowledge, skills and attitudes that a graduate nurse needs to demonstrate at the point of registration.
- NMC Standards place patients and service users at the centre of practice with the objective of protecting the public, and places emphasis on compassionate care, team work, record keeping, delegation and trust, accountability, raising concerns and co-operating with investigations and audits.

GO FURTHER

CASE STUDY: CARE

Go to https://study.sagepub.com/essentialadultnursing for a further case study related to this chapter. If you are using the interactive ebook, simply click on the book icon in the margin to go straight to the resource.

Books

- Delves-Yates, C. (Ed.) 2018) *Essentials of Nursing Practice* (2nd edn.). London: Sage.
- Peate, I. (2017) *Fundamentals of Care: A Textbook for Health and Social Care Assistants*. London: John Wiley & Sons.

Journal Articles

FURTHER READING: JOURNAL ARTICLES

Go to https://study.sagepub.com/essentialadultnursing for further free online journal articles related to this chapter. If you are using the interactive ebook, simply click on the book icon in the margin to go straight to the resource.

- Dewar B. and Christley Y. (2013) A critical analysis of compassion in practice. *Nursing Standard*, 28(10): 46–50.
  In this article the authors explore the importance of a coherent vision and the need to anchor the compassion in practice policy in values that are important to healthcare staff.

- Valizadeh L., Zamanzadeh V., Dewar B., Rahmani A. and Ghafouriford M. (2016) Nurse's perceptions of organisational barriers to delivering compassionate care: a qualitative study. *Nursing Ethics* Online: https://doi.org/10.1177/0969733016660881?.
  A discussion on workload and organisational barriers to compassionate care delivery.

Weblinks

FURTHER READING: WEBLINKS

Go to https://study.sagepub.com/essentialadultnursing for further weblinks related to this chapter. If you are using the interactive ebook, simply click on the book icon in the margin to go straight to the resource.

- Care Inspectorate www.careinspectorate.com
  The Care Inspectorate (Scotland) website offers a wealth of information on service regulation and provides access to inspection reports.
- Care and Social Services Inspectorate www.cssiw.org.uk
  The Care and Social Services Inspectorate (Wales) website offers a wealth of information on service regulation and provides access to inspection reports.
- Care Quality Commission www.cqc.org.uk
  The Care Quality Commission (England) website offers a wealth of information on service regulation and provides access to inspection reports.
- National Institute for Health and Care Excellence (NICE) www.nice.org.uk/guidance
  The National Institute for Health and Care Excellence (NICE) provides access to quality standards in health, social care and public health.
- Regulation and Quality Improvement Authority www.rqia.org.uk
  The Regulation and Quality Improvement Authority (Northern Ireland) website offers a wealth of information on service regulation and provides access to inspection reports.
- Scottish Intercollegiate Guidelines Network (SIGN) www.sign.ac.uk
  The Scottish Intercollegiate Guidelines Network website provides access to national clinical guidelines containing recommendations for effective practice based on current evidence.

ACE YOUR ASSESSMENT

ONLINE QUIZZES

Revise what you have learned by visiting https://study.sagepub.com/essentialadultnursing

- Test yourself with multiple-choice and short-answer questions
- Do the chapter activities in the book and check your answers online

REFERENCES

Bowles. L. (2016) Cocktail conversations: Listening to patients. *Nursing Times*, 112, online issue 2: 7–8.

Care Quality Commission (2013) *Raising Standards, Putting People First*. Available at: www.cqc.org.uk/sites/default/files/documents/20130503_cqc_strategy_2013_final_cm_tagged.pdf (accessed 23/02/18).

Care Quality Commission (2015) *Fundamental Standards*. Available at: www.cqc.org.uk/content/fundamental-standards (accessed 23/02/18).

Department of Health (2012) *NHS Constitution for England*. Available at: www.gov.uk/government/publications/the-nhs-constitution-for-england (accessed 23/02/18).

Department of Health and NHS Commissioning Board (2012) *Compassion in Practice, Nursing, Midwifery and Care Staff, Our Vision and Strategy*. Available at: www.england.nhs.uk/wp-content/uploads/2012/12/compassion-in-practice.pdf (accessed 23/02/18).

Department of Health and NHS Commissioning Board (2016) *Leading Change, Adding Value*. Available at: www.england.nhs.uk/wp-content/uploads/2016/05/nursing-framework.pdf (accessed 23/02/18).

Department of Health, Social Services and Public Safety (DHSSPS) (2006) *The Quality Standards for Health and Social Care*. Available at: www.health-ni.gov.uk/articles/quality-standards-health-and-social-care (accessed 23/02/18).

Department of Health, Social Services and Public Safety (2011) *Quality 2020: A 10-year strategy to protect and improve quality in health and social care in Northern Ireland*. Available at: www.health-ni.gov.uk/topics/safety-and-quality-standards/quality-2020 (accessed 23/02/18).

Department of Health, Social Services and Public Safety (2011) *Transforming Your Care*. Available at: www.transformingyourcare.hscni.net/wp-content/uploads/2012/10/Transforming-Your-Care-Review-of-HSC-in-NI.pdf (accessed 23/02/18).

Francis, R (2013) *The Mid Staffordshire NHS Foundation Trust Public Inquiry: The Francis Report (2013)*. Available at: www.midstaffspublicinquiry.com/report (accessed 23/02/18).

Healthcare Improvement Scotland (2011) *Healthcare Quality Standard: Assuring person centred, safe and effective care: Clinical governance and risk management*. Edinburgh: Healthcare Improvement Scotland.

Institute of Medicine (2001) *Dimensions of Quality Care*. Available at: www.ihi.org/resources/Pages/ImprovementStories/AcrosstheChasmSixAimsforChangingtheHealthCareSystem.aspx (accessed 23/02/18).

NHS England (2014) *Five Year Forward View*. Available at: www.england.nhs.uk/wp-content/uploads/2014/10/5yfv-web.pdf (accessed 23/02/18).

Nursing and Midwifery Council (2015) *The Code: Professional Standards of Practice and Behaviour for Nurses and Midwives*. London: NMC.

Nursing and Midwifery Council (2018a) *Standards of Proficency for Registered Nurses*. London: NMC.

Nursing and Midwifery Council (2018b) *Educational Framework: Standards for education and training*. London: NMC.

Royal College of Nursing (RCN) (2018) *Principles of nursing practice*. Available at: https://www.rcn.org.uk/professional-development/principles-of-nursing-practice (accessed 26/08/18).

Scottish Government (2010) *The Healthcare Quality Strategy for NHS Scotland*. Edinburgh: Scottish Government.

Scottish Government (2016) *National Clinical Strategy for Scotland*. Edinburgh: The Scottish Government.

Welsh Government (2010) *Doing Well, Doing Better. Standards for health services in Wales*. Available at: www.wales.nhs.uk/sites3/Documents/919/ENGLISH%20WEB%20VERSION.pdf (accessed 23/02/18).

Welsh Government (2011) *Together for Health: A five year vision for the NHS in Wales* Available at: www.wales.nhs.uk/sitesplus/documents/829/togetherforhealth.pdf (accessed 23/02/18).

Welsh Government (2012) *Achieving Excellence. The quality delivery plan for the NHS in Wales*. Available at: www.wales.nhs.uk/sitesplus/documents/862/0812-Item14b-AchievingExcellence-TheQualityDeliveryPlanforNHSinWales2012-16.pdf (accessed 23/02/18).

Welsh Government (2012) *Working Differently – Working Together*. Available at: www.1000livesplus.wales.nhs.uk/sitesplus/documents/1011/Workign%20Together%20Workin%20Different%20Workforce%20Framework.pdf (accessed 23/02/18).

ASSESSMENT OF THE ADULT WITH ACUTE NEEDS

9

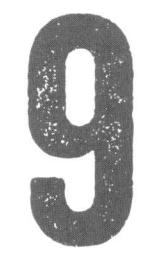

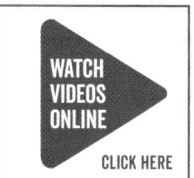

WATCH VIDEOS ONLINE CLICK HERE

JACQUELINE CHANG AND LAURA BELTON

THIS CHAPTER COVERS

- Why do you need to assess your patient?
- How to assess your patient
- Structuring your assessment
- Commonly used tools to aid nursing assessment and diagnosis

- What happens after the assessment?
- Preparation for placement.

> "
>
> 'You put the interests of people using or needing nursing or midwifery services first. You make their care and safety your main concern and make sure that their dignity is preserved and their needs are recognised, assessed and responded to.'
>
> **(NMC, 2015)**
>
> "

INTRODUCTION

This chapter highlights the importance of assessment in adult nursing, which as the NMC above makes clear is an essential part of your duty of care. We will also invite you to consider the skills and tools you will bring to the assessment role.

Assessment by a nurse happens throughout the patient's journey. Some assessments are formal; some are informal, often conducted when attending to personal care. As a nurse you will be collecting lots of information from a patient through conversations, questioning and visual observations. This chapter focuses on the formal assessments you will be learning when in practice and will carry out when you are qualified. It is important to recognise that many of the observations you undertake will be carried out informally, but must be recorded formally in order to justify the nursing care delivered.

WHY DO YOU NEED TO ASSESS YOUR PATIENT?

The nursing process is a cyclical process that informs nursing care. It was first introduced in 1967 by Yura and Walsh with four stages and has been adapted and developed over the years. There are now five stages to the nursing process (Figure 9.1). The assessment stage is vital as without it the other stages cannot happen and care cannot be delivered that is appropriate for that patient.

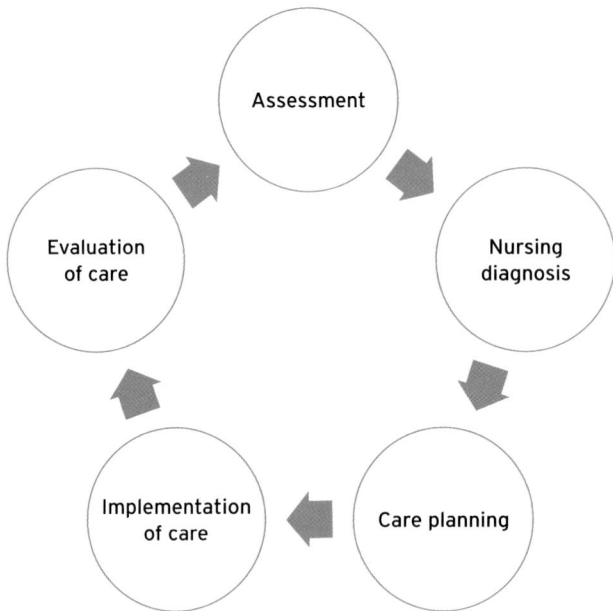

Figure 9.1 The stages of the nursing process

In order to provide patient-centred, individualised, beneficent care the patient must have a holistic assessment. Nursing assessment is the collection and organisation of information about a patient. While a full history is taken it is different from a medical assessment as it does not focus solely on the physical problem, but looks at the patient holistically, including psychosocial elements.

A patient is assessed by almost all members of the multidisciplinary healthcare team and the assessments highlight specific issues for those specific teams. The nursing assessment allows the nurse to identify the needs of the patient, and provide a nursing diagnosis from which the nurse can plan and deliver care based on the individual's assessment result. It is different from other assessments as, rather than focusing on the disease progression and treatment interventions, it focuses on the patient's needs at that time. As stated earlier, assessment is an essential stage of the nursing process.

Assessment also plays a part of the nurse's role in patient advocacy. As the nurse, you are the health-care professional who sees the patient the most and with your nursing team you provide 24-hour care. Due to this you are key to noticing, recording and relaying any changes in a patient's condition (Considine and Currey, 2015). As the nurse, you will act as a conduit between the patient and the medical team plus the wider multidisciplinary team (MDT) and as the patient's advocate, you are responsible for relaying pertinent information to relevant people.

Assessment is an essential element of the nurse's role and is highlighted throughout The *Code* (NMC, 2015).

ACTIVITY 9.1: CRITICAL THINKING

Considering the NMC Code (2015), which specific areas illustrate the importance of the nursing assessment for patient care?

Think back to Chapter 3 and consider the professional values that can be linked with assessment.

ACTIVITY 9.1
ANSWER

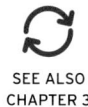

SEE ALSO
CHAPTER 3

In the NMC Standards of Proficiency for Registered Nurses (2018), Outcome statement 3 – Assessing needs and planning care – makes explicit the skills required at the point of registration by the Registered Nurse. *'Registered nurses assess and review the mental, physical, cognitive, behavioural, social and spiritual health needs of people, using this information to identify their requirements for nursing intervention, care and support.'* The importance of working in partnership with the patient to develop care plans that are patient centred is emphasised. By performing a holistic assessment, you will be able to treat your patient as an individual and avoid making assumptions. By listening to your patient and understanding their needs and preferences and what they are concerned about, you will be able to work in partnership with your patient to deliver person-centred care. It also ensures that you respond to your patient's needs be they physical, psychological or social (NMC, 2015). In short, it enables you to deliver values-based practice and, where necessary, to be their advocate. So let us consider how.

HOW TO ASSESS YOUR PATIENT

In order to assess a patient fully, you will need to obtain information about their current condition and their past medical history as well as their social situation and psychological status. You should aim to gather as much information as you can, and verbal information regarding their health status and medical history should be combined with all the medical records that you can find. It can be challenging to obtain information from a patient, particularly when they are acutely unwell, and you may find that a truly holistic assessment may have to take place over a few face-to-face interactions with a new patient. Depending upon the situation, it might be more important to perform a physical assessment rather than obtain a thorough nursing history. All information should be sought from, in the first instance, the patient themselves, but if they are unable to answer the questions then a family

SEE ALSO
CHAPTER 4

member or someone who knows them well would be an appropriate source. Consideration needs to be given here to the 'at risk' patient and the patient who lacks capacity, which is discussed in Chapter 4.

There are different types of physical nursing assessments: a mini assessment, which is a quick assessment of a patient's deteriorating health; an in-depth comprehensive assessment, which looks holistically at a patient; a focused assessment, which looks at a specific issue to allow for further interventions; and an ongoing assessment, which continues throughout the patient's care journey. This chapter will now consider all of these forms of assessment.

STRUCTURING YOUR ASSESSMENT

As already discussed, one of the challenges with performing an assessment is that you need to get a lot of personal information from a stranger as quickly as possible. There are different ways to manage communication in nursing and when assessing a deteriorating patient, it is not usually possible to plan out the assessment and deliver it as you may like. However, it is important to manage the communication and one way of doing this is by following the Calgary-Cambridge Guide to the Medical Interview (Silverman et al., 2013). Although designed with doctors in mind, it is a useful way of planning an assessment as the format is easy to implement as a five-stage assessment technique. It can be used in both acute and non-urgent situations using a series of steps.

THE CALGARY-CAMBRIDGE CONSULTATION GUIDE

The Calgary-Cambridge consultation guide was developed by Kurtz and Silverman in 1996 (Silverman et al. 2013). It can be applied to most clinical settings as it provides an easy-to-use structure that complements nursing's traditional holistic assessment approach (Munson and Willcox, 2007).

The guide consists of five tasks, which run as a sequence throughout the consultation, with two areas running parallel relating to structuring the consultation and developing a relationship with the client.

Task 1 – Initiating the session

Task 1 looks at establishing a rapport with the client. Munson and Willcox (2007) have suggested that the initial 90 seconds are paramount in creating a good foundation, as this is the time the client decides whether they like and trust you. This section also identifies the reason for the consultation.

ACTIVITY 9.2
ANSWER

ACTIVITY 9.2: CRITICAL THINKING

Think about how you would build rapport with a client. What communication skills would you use? Read Carl's case study (see Case Study 9.1); how would you build a rapport with him?

Task 2 – Gathering information

The second task in the Calgary-Cambridge guide looks at developing the client's story, what ideas they have about their condition and how they cope with their symptoms. Epstein et al. (2008) identified that an accurate history can provide 80% or more of the information required for a diagnosis; therefore, history taking is an essential part of the consultation process. The mnemonic PQRST (Zator Estes, 2014), which we will explore later, is useful in gathering information about symptoms.

Task 3 – Explanation and planning

Task 3 emphasises the need for a shared approach between the client and the practitioner; the client needs to be involved in the decision making which promotes the client taking responsibility for their own condition.

This section focuses on building a partnership that helps to keep the client informed and allows the practitioner to know what the client understands about their condition.

Task 4 – Physical examination

Nurses utilise a range of assessment tools to help guide a physical examination and to record any results and plan the care to be delivered. We will look at some of these later in this chapter.

Task 5 – Closing the session

This gives the patient the final chance to ask any questions and allows the practitioner to close the session. It is vital to make sure that your patient understands what the next stage of their care is and that they know what to expect from the care. You also need to highlight to your patient anything that they should be concerned about, known as **red flags**, and most importantly, when and how to call for you. This is referred to as '**safety netting**'.

ACTIVITY 9.3
ANSWER

ACTIVITY 9.3: REFLECTION

Think about how often you safety net with your patients and list three reasons explaining why it is important.

Are there any particular clinical settings where you think safety netting is done well? Can you give any examples?

Nursing has developed its own tools to structure the assessment process and we will look at these next.

HISTORY TAKING – A HOLISTIC NURSING ASSESSMENT

There are various classic models that help nurses structure an assessment of a patient. The most commonly used one is the **Activities of Living** (AL) by Roper et al., which was first published in 1979. It has been updated over the years by the authors but the structure has remained unchanged. This model is popular due to the clear way it works through the patient's physical, social and psychological health needs. The ALs are particularly useful because they assess how the patient is at that point as well as how they are usually, and help to see if there have been any changes. A thorough AL assessment looks at the 12 activities (see Table 9.1), the factors that influence them (biological, social, economic, environmental and psychological) and the dependence or independent levels of the patient for each AL.

Each clinical area you work in will have its own documentation to be used for patient assessment. However, most will be based around a functional model such as the Activities of Living (Roper et al., 2000) or Gordon's Functional Health Patterns Framework (Gordon, 1994). Both these frameworks work through the body systems and, when completed, give a holistic view of the patient (see Table 9.1).

Table 9.1   A comparison of different holistic assessment models

Roper, Logan & Tierney's Activities of Living (2000)	Gordon's Functional Health Patterns (1994)
Maintaining a safe environment	Health perception and health management
Communication	Nutritional-metabolic
Breathing	Elimination
Eating and drinking	Activity and exercise
Elimination	Sleep and rest
Washing and dressing	Cognition and perception
Controlling temperature	Self-perception and self-concept
Mobilisation	Roles and relationships
Working and playing	Sexuality and reproduction
Expressing sexuality	Coping and stress tolerance
Sleeping	Values and belief
Death and dying	

An important element of the functional systems assessment is to ask the patient and family what has changed with each of the activities. It is essential to know what is a new issue and what is a chronic issue.

Effective listening is an essential element of assessment as outlined in the earlier activity regarding communication. You need to be able to listen for clues when talking with your patient to be able to perform an effective assessment. In order to do that, open-ended questions are a useful communication technique to utilise.

COMMONLY USED TOOLS TO AID YOUR NURSING ASSESSMENT AND DIAGNOSIS

To aid the holistic assessment discussed earlier in this chapter nurses use a range of assessment tools. Some tools assess a very specific element of a person's health, for example, a pain assessment tool. Some are more generic and help to give an overall picture of a person's health status, an early warning score, for example. The specific, focused tools that look at particular problems will be discussed in the relevant chapters of this book. This chapter will look at some of the major common generic assessment tools and explain how to apply them to practice.

ACTIVITY 9.4: CRITICAL THINKING

Why do nurses need generic and specific risk assessment tools?

✔
ACTIVITY 9.4
ANSWER

COMMONLY USED GENERIC ASSESSMENT TOOLS

ABCDE

The ABCDE approach to assessment is a systematic method of assessing the acutely unwell patient and often forms the basis of a mini assessment. It is a quick and effective method of assessing a patient and identifying urgent care needs and is also commonly known as the Primary Survey.

The guidelines from the Resuscitation Council (2018) instruct that on approach to the patient they should always be asked 'how they are' to assess for a response. If the person is unresponsive and not breathing then cardiopulmonary resuscitation (CPR) would need to be commenced while calling for emergency help.

Airway – is the patient's airway clear? Are they talking/breathing? Is the breathing noisy? Is there an obstruction?

Breathing – do they look like they are struggling to breathe? In what way? Are there any signs of respiratory distress? Look, listen and feel for any abnormalities. Measure respiratory rate and pulse oximetry.

Circulation – are you able to palpate a pulse? Are they cold or clammy? Are they pale? Are they bleeding? Measure pulse, blood pressure and capillary refill time (CRT).

Disability – are there signs of a head injury or a loss of consciousness? Have they had any medications that can cause a lack of consciousness? Assess their pupils. What is their blood sugar? What is their AVPU or Glasgow Coma Scale score?

Exposure – are there signs of hypothermia, bleeding, infection, rash or swelling?

Depending on where you are working you may look further into the causes of an anomaly of the ABCDE assessment as part of your role and perform further investigations. Alternatively, if you identify an issue from the ABCDE assessment your management would be to alert other healthcare professionals to escalate the patient's care.

The Resuscitation Council (2018) states that the ABCDE approach to all deteriorating or critically ill patients is the same. The underlying principles are:

1. Use the Airway, Breathing, Circulation, Disability, Exposure (ABCDE) approach to assess and treat the patient
2. Do a complete initial assessment and reassess regularly
3. Treat life-threatening problems before moving to the next part of the assessment
4. Assess the effects of treatment
5. Recognise when you will need extra help. Call for appropriate help early
6. Use all members of the team. This enables interventions (e.g. assessment, attaching monitors, intravenous access) to be undertaken simultaneously
7. Communicate effectively – use the Situation, Background, Assessment, Recommendation (SBAR) or Reason, Story, Vital signs, Plan (RSVP) approach

8.   The aim of the initial treatment is to keep the patient alive, and achieve some clinical improvement. This will buy time for further treatment and making a diagnosis

9.   Remember – it can take a few minutes for treatments to work, so wait a short while before reassessing the patient after an intervention.

ACTIVITY 9.5
ANSWER

ACTIVITY 9.5: CRITICAL THINKING

What further investigations would you perform should you find an anomaly during the primary survey?

The Primary Survey is often thought to be limited to certain clinical areas such as A&E and ITU as its purpose is to identify and correct life-threatening conditions (Gumm, 2007). However, Considine and Currey (2015) argue that to utilise this tool in all areas would help to identify life-threatening conditions in all patients who may appear stable but are starting to deteriorate. Their argument is that if all nurses assessed all patients using the Primary Survey then acute deterioration may be detected earlier.

A common way deteriorating patients are detected in general wards is through the use of an Early Warning Score, which is also referred to as a track and trigger tool.

The National Early Warning Score (NEWS)

The Royal College of Physicians (RCP) led the development of a National Early Warning Score (NEWS) to improve the care of the acutely ill patient. It should be noted that some areas use a Modified Early Warning Score (MEWS) and it is always vital to check what tool the clinical area you are working in is using.

The RCP (2012) recognised that many hospitals used their own Early Warning Score system to assess patients and felt that having a standardised scoring system would be beneficial. The NEWS is based on a simple scoring system in which a score is allocated to physiological measurements already undertaken when patients present to, or are being monitored in, hospital. Six simple physiological parameters form the basis of the scoring system, which are:

1.   Respiratory rate
2.   Oxygen saturations
3.   Temperature
4.   Systolic blood pressure
5.   Pulse rate
6.   Level of consciousness.

The RCP (2012, p.x) advises that 'A score is allocated to each parameter as they are measured, with the magnitude of the score reflecting how extremely the parameter varies from the norm. The score is then aggregated. The score is uplifted for people requiring oxygen. It is important to emphasize that these parameters are already routinely measured in hospitals and recorded on the clinical chart.'

It should be noted that the NEWS is not appropriate for children, pregnant women or people with chronic obstructive pulmonary disease as their results might not be accurate (RCP, 2012). See the most up-to-date NEWS 2 (2017) below (Table 9.2).

Table 9.2   National Early Warning Score (NEWS) 2

NEWS key	0 1 2 3	FULL NAME			
		DATE OF BIRTH		DATE OF ADMISSION	

		Score	
	DATE / TIME		DATE / TIME
A+B Respirations Breaths/min	≥25 / 21–24 / 18–20 / 15–17 / 12–14 / 9–11 / ≤8	3 / 2 / / / / 1 / 3	≥25 / 21–24 / 18–20 / 15–17 / 12–14 / 9–11 / ≤8
A+B SpO₂ Scale 1 Oxygen saturation (%)	≥96 / 94–95 / 92–93 / ≤91	/ 1 / 2 / 3	≥96 / 94–95 / 92–93 / ≤91
SpO₂ Scale 2† Oxygen saturation (%) Use Scale 2 if target range is 88–92%, eg in hypercapnic respiratory failure. †ONLY use Scale 2 under the direction of a qualified clinician	≥97 on O₂ / 95–96 on O₂ / 93–94 on O₂ / ≥93 on air / 88–92 / 86–87 / 84–85 / ≤83%	3 / 2 / 1 / / / 1 / 2 / 3	≥97 on O₂ / 95–96 on O₂ / 93–94 on O₂ / ≥93 on air / 88–92 / 86–87 / 84–85 / ≤83%
Air or oxygen?	A=Air / O₂ L/min / Device	/ 2 /	A=Air / O₂ L/min / Device
C Blood pressure mmHg Score uses systolic BP only	≥220 / 201–219 / 181–200 / 161–180 / 141–160 / 121–140 / 111–120 / 101–110 / 91–100 / 81–90 / 71–80 / 61–70 / 51–60 / ≤50	3 / ... / 1 / 2 / ... / 3	≥220 / 201–219 / 181–200 / 161–180 / 141–160 / 121–140 / 111–120 / 101–110 / 91–100 / 81–90 / 71–80 / 61–70 / 51–60 / ≤50
C Pulse Beats/min	≥131 / 121–130 / 111–120 / 101–110 / 91–100 / 81–90 / 71–80 / 61–70 / 51–60 / 41–50 / 31–40 / ≤30	3 / 2 / 1 / ... / 1 / 3	≥131 / 121–130 / 111–120 / 101–110 / 91–100 / 81–90 / 71–80 / 61–70 / 51–60 / 41–50 / 31–40 / ≤30
D Consciousness Score for NEW onset of confusion (no score if chronic)	Alert / Confusion / V / P / U	3	Alert / Confusion / V / P / U
E Temperature °C	≥39.1° / 38.1–39.0° / 37.1–38.0° / 36.1–37.0° / 35.1–36.0° / ≤35.0°	2 / 1 / / / 1 / 3	≥39.1° / 38.1–39.0° / 37.1–38.0° / 36.1–37.0° / 35.1–36.0° / ≤35.0°
NEWS TOTAL			TOTAL
	Monitoring frequency / Escalation of care Y/N / Initials		Monitoring / Escalation / Initials

National Early Warning Score 2 (NEWS2) © Royal College of Physicians 2017

Source: National Early Warning Score (NEWS) 2: Standardising the assessment of acute-illness severity in the NHS. Updated report of a working party. London: RCP, 2017. Reproduced with permission of the Royal College of Physicians.

As the NEWS is standardised it allows the assessment of acute illness severity when patients present acutely to hospital and also when being assessed in primary care settings and the ambulance services. The RCP recommends that the NEWS is used to monitor all patients in hospitals, tracking their clinical condition and alerting the clinical team to any clinical deterioration which would trigger a timely clinical response.

The RCP (2012) recommends that the score should be determined from seven parameters, which includes the six stated above plus one weighted score for supplemental oxygen being delivered by mask or nasal cannula.

There are three trigger levels for clinical alert: low, medium and high. A low score would be a NEWS result of 1–4, a medium score would be 5–6. A high score is 7 or more. Patients would score an extra 2 points for using oxygen. If there is an extreme variation in an individual physiological parameter, that would be classified as a 'red' score.

The score would highlight the level of urgency of the clinical response required, such as a low score requiring a registered nurse who would decide how often clinical assessment is required or if the clinical care of the patient needs to be escalated. A medium score would prompt assessment urgently by a skilled clinician competent in acute illness and a high score would require urgent emergency assessment by a clinical or outreach team, and the patient would usually require transferring to a higher dependency clinical area.

Sprinks (2013) noted that four out of five NHS Trusts have adopted or plan to adopt the NEWS since its launch in 2012, but a poll of 13 NHS Trusts showed a mixed reaction with one specifically saying that they would not replace their own system which was in place due to the cost and time it took to develop their own assessment.

CRITICAL
THINKING
STOP POINT 9.1
ANSWER

CRITICAL THINKING STOP POINT 9.1

Consider the nurse's role in identifying the deteriorating patient. What are the benefits of using a standardised NEWS across the NHS?

CASE STUDY 9.1: CARL

You have been asked by a GP to assess a patient in the community. The patient's daughter has called asking the GP to visit her father who has been increasingly short of breath for the past three days. The GP asks you to visit and when you speak to the GP you request a copy of the patient's medication. This does not arrive before you visit but the GP does tell you that the patient is known to have COPD and is on oxygen at home.

When you visit in the early afternoon, Carl's daughter answers the door and explains that Carl cannot come to the door and that he is not able to talk in sentences. He is using his oxygen via nasal cannula. He is sitting in his pyjamas downstairs in a riser/recliner chair with some dirty plates with leftover food on the table next to him.

- Consider what observations you need to take and how you will record them?
- What medical history do you need to obtain from Carl and from his daughter? Which history-taking model would you consider using?
- Which other agencies will you need to contact?

PQRST - Provocation/Palliation, Quality/Quantity, Region/Radiation, Severity, Timing

The PQRST model is mainly used to assess pain but can also be used to assess any presentation.

Provocation and palliation – what makes it better or worse? Consider different positions, analgesia and mobilisation.

Quality/Quantity – what kind of pain is it (e.g. stabbing, sharp, dull, constant)?

Region and radiation – where is the pain? Where are the symptoms? Does any pain radiate?

Severity – could use a pain scale here, such as 1–10, or 1–5, or 1–3.

Timing – when is it better or worse, for example better after eating or in the morning? How long have you had the symptoms?

ACTIVITY 9.6: REFLECTION

What kind of patients have you looked after where a PQRST assessment would have been appropriate?

ACTIVITY 9.6
ANSWER

Once your assessment of a deteriorating patient is complete, it is essential to escalate the situation appropriately. You must now pass on the information to the relevant members of the multidisciplinary team (MDT) in order to provide the care required.

SBAR - Situation, background, assessment, recommendation

SBAR is a communication tool that helps health workers structure their handovers. It was first used in the military and now is used widely in healthcare throughout the world. The handovers may be to other nurses or to any member of the healthcare team, often doctors. The handover may be face to face, over the telephone or in written form, for example, email or fax. The tool ensures the required information is given in an organised, thorough and effective manner. Its purpose is to prevent information being omitted by some healthcare professionals during handover. Its intention was to standardise handovers to ensure patient safety specifically in situations where an escalation of care is required.

Situation – state who you are, where you are calling from, the patient's name and main problem

Background – any clinical information that may be helpful related to the current situation – age, admission reason, test results, medical history

Assessment – vital signs, ABCDE, current problem and its pattern

Recommendation – what do you need? When do you need it?

Having looked at some commonly used generic assessment tools, this chapter will now focus on some of the available assessment tools which focus on specific symptoms.

As stated earlier in this chapter there are many assessment tools that look at specific physical symptoms. The nurse performs these assessments on the patient and the results are used to diagnose and treat. However, every patient admitted should have the following assessments:

NEWS, MUST, Waterlow, BMI, urinalysis and, where appropriate, VIP, FRAT and pain assessment. These will be discussed in this section.

ACTIVITY 9.7
ANSWER

ACTIVITY 9.7: REFLECTION

Think of assessments you have observed and performed during your placements. What tools did you use or see used and what was the rationale for using the ones chosen?

As this is a personal reflection and everybody's experience has been different, an answer guide has not been supplied.

COMMONLY USED SPECIFIC ASSESSMENT TOOLS

Malnutrition Universal Screening Tool (MUST)

SEE ALSO
CHAPTER 35

This is a common assessment tool used to assess a person to determine if they require nutritional support. It is a clear, easy-to-follow risk assessment tool. The full MUST toolkit is available at www.bapen.org.uk.

The Malnutrition Universal Screening Tool (MUST) score is described by the Malnutrition Advisory Group (2003) as a five-step screening tool to identify adults who are malnourished, at risk of malnutrition or obese. It was designed for use in a variety of care settings by all care workers. The score has been identified as a simple, quick tool that can be used easily by nurses when carrying out an initial assessment in the community and hospital setting. It identifies clients who may need minimal input, such as nutritional advice, or more complex cases who may need more specialist input.

The MUST score has five steps:

- Step 1: To measure height and weight to obtain a BMI score using the height and weight chart
- Step 2: Note percentage unplanned weight loss and score using tables
- Step 3: Establish acute disease effect and score
- Step 4: Add scores from steps 1, 2 and 3 together to obtain overall risk of malnutrition
- Step 5: Use management guidelines and/or local policy to develop care plan.

The score can also be calculated using alternative measurements such as ulna length and knee height if necessary.

The Malnutrition Advisory Group (2003) developed the MUST score as it was recognised that around 5% of the general population have a BMI of below 20 kg/m, meaning they are underweight. It was identified that around 15–40% of people admitted to hospital who are living with chronic conditions or living in residential care are more likely to be underweight. The implications of this would mean an extra cost to the NHS as these patients will usually have a longer hospital admission.

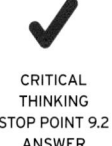

CRITICAL
THINKING
STOP POINT 9.2
ANSWER

CRITICAL THINKING STOP POINT 9.2

Think about restrictions to using the MUST score as part of your assessment. What do you do once you have obtained the results?

Waterlow Assessment

The Waterlow score was devised in 1985 by Judy Waterlow for use by her students while she was working as a clinical nurse teacher. Although designed in the hospital setting it is widely used by healthcare professionals in a variety of healthcare settings including A&E and nursing/residential homes. Waterlow (2005) advised that it is a simplistic tool which is to be used alongside professional judgement to determine the risk status of the client.

The Waterlow assessment tool is a scoring system that was designed to provide guidance on nursing care and the types of preventative aids associated with the three levels of risk status, wound assessment and dressings. It is essential to remember that when this assessment tool is used in the primary care setting, this is a vastly different environment to the one in which the score was developed.

NICE guidelines (2014) for the prevention and management of pressure ulcers recommend that nurses should be aware that all patients are potentially at risk of developing a pressure ulcer and require an assessment of pressure ulcer risk. The risk assessment should look at clients receiving NHS care in all settings including emergency departments, primary and secondary care. It also recommends that a valid score such as the Waterlow score be used to support clinical judgement when assessing pressure ulcer risk.

The Waterlow score looks at several different aspects. These are:

- build/weight for height
- continence
- skin type, visual risk areas
- mobility
- sex/age
- appetite
- special risks such as tissue malnutrition, neurological deficit, major surgery/trauma and medication.

The client is scored against each category and the higher the sum of scores the higher their risk rate, e.g. 10+ At risk, 15+ High risk and 20+ Very high risk.

The client's score indicates if and what further care is required, such as whether a pressure-relieving mattress should be used or whether nutritional supplements are advised.

Body Mass Index (BMI)

The Body Mass Index is a tool used to assess whether a person is of a healthy weight, is underweight or is overweight and to what degree. It measures a person's height against their weight and gives a score. BMI charts are available on www.bapen.org.uk as the BMI score is an essential element of the MUST assessment.

Falls Risk Assessment tool (FRAT)

A falls risk assessment is a common tool utilised in the clinical environment. Falls are common-place in patients aged over 65 and cost the NHS over £2 billion a year (Tian et al., 2013). Assessing a person's risk of falling allows precautions to be put in place, thereby protecting vulnerable patients.

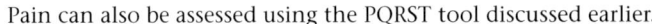

WHAT'S THE EVIDENCE? 9.1

Matarese, M., Ivziku, D., Bartolozzi, F., Piredda, M. and De Marinis, M.G. (2015) 'Systematic review of fall risk screening tools for older patients in acute hospitals', *Journal of Advanced Nursing*, 71 (6), pp. 1198-1209.

Falls are the most reported adverse incidents among older hospitalised adults. Several tools are used to detect fall risk in acute hospitals, but many of them have not been validated in older inpatients. Selecting the most accurate tool for older inpatients is challenging in clinical nursing practice.

A few risk screening tools have been tested exclusively with older inpatients in prospective validation studies in acute care settings. The Hendrich fall risk Model II and the St. Thomas Risk Assessment Tool in Falling elderly inpatients (STRATIFY) are the most tested fall risk screening tools with older hospitalised adults. The predictive accuracy is not satisfactory for any of the screening tools.

Pain

If someone is in pain it can be indicative of an undiagnosed clinical condition and, therefore, a thorough pain assessment is important. There are various methods of assessing pain, which mainly involve the patient giving a verbal pain score and depending on the local policy that may be a score out of 3, 5 or 10. Nurses also assess a patient's facial expressions and any involuntary groaning in order to decide if they are in pain at that point. This is particularly important for the unconscious patient as they have no other way of expressing the pain and they need the nurse to observe their involuntary actions. In order for the assessment and, therefore, treatment to be effective, the location and type of pain must be assessed.

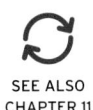

**SEE ALSO
CHAPTER 11**

Pain can also be assessed using the PQRST tool discussed earlier.

Venous Thromboembolism score (VTE)

In 2010 the Department of Health released guidelines stating that all patients should be assessed for level of mobility. Any patients with reduced mobility and all surgical patients should be considered at risk of developing a thromboembolism. There are various risk factors to developing a thromboembolism and the VTE assessment highlights who is at risk via a checklist-style form and whether or not the patient requires prophylactic medication and interventions such as anti-embolic stockings.

Visual Infusion Phlebitis score (VIP)

Any patient with a venous cannula in situ should have a VIP score to ensure the line is patent and that complications from the cannula are not occurring. The VIP score should be performed at least daily.

Alert, responds to vocal stimuli, pain stimuli or unresponsive to all stimuli (AVPU)

This tool assesses a patient's alertness and responses to certain stimuli and gives a score. The lower the score, the lower the cognitive responses. Pupil reaction to light should also be assessed.

Glasgow Coma Scale (GCS)

This is a tool used to assess a person's level of consciousness. There are three elements to assess and each are scored and then added together. The total score gives the GCS.

SEE ALSO
CHAPTER 27

CASE STUDY 9.2: JAMES

A 24-year-old man with Down's Syndrome is admitted to your medical assessment unit via his GP due to abdominal pain and a history of vomiting a green fluid. His temperature is 37.8°C. His heart rate is 92 bpm. His respiration rate is 22 rpm. His oxygen saturations are 98% on air. His blood pressure is 94/55 mmHg. He states his pain is acute, stabbing and scores it as 4 out of 5.

- What is his NEWS score?
- What questions do you want to ask him?
- What is your nursing plan?
- How will you assess his capacity?

Following your assessments, you bleep the doctor. What are you going to tell them? How are you going to structure your handover?

CASE STUDY 9.3: ALICE

You visit Alice, a 72-year-old woman, at home. She lives with her son and his family. She has had diarrhoea and vomiting for three days.

She is confused and dehydrated. She feels dizzy and faint and is struggling to speak properly or to walk independently.

Her vital signs are: Temperature 38.4°C. Pulse 102 bpm. Respiration rate 21 rpm.

- What assessments are you going to do?
- What is her NEWS score?
- What further investigations do you want to perform?
- What is the nursing diagnosis?
- What is the nursing plan?
- Who are you going to refer to and what are you going to tell them?

Assessment tools are designed to be understandable, reliable and repeatable in order to ensure all patients receive the same required care without the result being affected by the person performing the assessment. This makes them safe and effective. The following activity will help you to critique an assessment tool to assess its validity and reliability.

ACTIVITY 9.8
ANSWER

ACTIVITY 9.8: CRITICAL THINKING

Thinking of the assessment tools you have used in practice, identify two positive and two negative qualities of each tool. Find some evidence to support your thoughts. Consider any difficulties you had collecting the information you needed and any problems interpreting the information you did get. Did you need to ask any extra questions that weren't on the form? Did the result you got match what you thought before you did the assessment?

As this is a personal reflection and everybody's experience has been different, an answer guide has not been supplied.

WHAT HAPPENS AFTER THE ASSESSMENT?

Once the assessments have been performed and the nurse has made a diagnosis, care needs to be planned and implemented. Based on an ABCDE assessment, the following are common interventions:

- Airway
  - Maintain patency
- Breathing
  - Oxygen therapy and positioning
- Circulation
  - IV access, blood tests and IV fluids
- Disability
  - Monitor AVPU/GCS, pupils and blood sugar
  - Pain control measures
- Exposure
  - Monitor temperature
  - Complete NEWS chart, continuously monitor and use SBAR to escalate.

When an adult patient is unwell it is essential that, as the nurse looking after them, you notice deterioration. This is done through an ongoing assessment. Every time you interact with a patient you should be assessing them. When providing personal hygiene, you can assess psychological status, hydration, nutritional status and look for signs of pressure sores. When helping a patient to mobilise, assess them for pain which they have not mentioned to you or a weakness that has not been noted before. When helping with elimination look for signs of dehydration, infection, constipation or obstruction. When undertaking regular vital signs, note a change in the trend and consider the causes for this. When having a conversation check for signs of confusion or increased drowsiness. The signs that nurses pick up when delivering patient care is part of the ongoing assessment which is then interpreted and documented and escalated. Sepsis is known as the silent killer (NICE, 2017) and is largely on the increase because it may not be identified at the early stages when the nurses are delivering essential care. Through ongoing assessment and reviewing of the patient, a deteriorating adult can be escalated early and have their death prevented.

PREPARATION FOR PRACTICE PLACEMENTS 9.1

Now that you have read about the purpose and value of assessment tools and the variety of tools available, it is important to utilise that knowledge and understanding when in clinical placement.

While this chapter has highlighted commonly used assessment tools, some clinical areas modify the tools to suit their particular services so it is important to check what assessment tools they use. As mentioned earlier in this chapter, some pain scores are out of 10, some out of 5 and some are out of 3. You must know what you need to ask your patient in order to provide an assessment that is comparable to and repeatable by other members of the team. Another example is the difference between the NEWS and the MEWS and you must know which one you are using.

Documentation is often discussed with student nurses but the importance of it cannot be overstated. Assessments must be clearly and accurately completed. They must be dated and include the correct time. They must be signed by the person completing the assessment. Actions taken as a result of the assessment should also be documented, as the care plan for that patient may need to be altered depending on the result of the assessment.

CHAPTER SUMMARY

This chapter has:

- Highlighted the important role a nurse's assessment plays in ensuring the safe delivery of care for an acutely unwell adult
- Provided examples of models which are used to structure a patient assessment
- Given examples of commonly used assessment tools which aid a nursing diagnosis
- Outlined examples of key interventions to research further in subsequent chapters
- Explained the importance of the nurse performing ongoing assessments on their patients and escalating when warning signs are triggered
- Advised you on how to best prepare for assessing patients on your clinical placements.

GO FURTHER

Go to https://study.sagepub.com/essentialadultnursing for a further case study related to this chapter. If you are using the interactive ebook, simply click on the book icon in the margin to go straight to the resource.

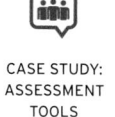

CASE STUDY: ASSESSMENT TOOLS

Books

- Dougherty, L., Lister, S., West-Oram, A. (2015) *The Royal Marsden Manual of Clinical Nursing Procedures* (9th ed). Chichester: Wiley and Sons Ltd.
  An excellent book for students which describes the use of a range of tools.
- Howatson-Jones, L., Standing, M., Roberts, S. (2015) *Patient Assessment and Care Planning in Nursing* (2nd ed). London: Sage/Learning Matters.
  A good introduction to nursing assessment, diagnosis and principles of care planning.

- Peat, I. and Dutton, H. (2013) *Acute Nursing Care: Recognising and Responding to Medical Emergencies*. Oxford: Routledge.
  An overview of assessing and managing acutely ill and deteriorating patients.

Journal Articles

FURTHER READING: JOURNAL ARTICLES

Go to https://study.sagepub.com/essentialadultnursing for further free online journal articles related to this chapter. If you are using the interactive ebook, simply click on the book icon in the margin to go straight to the resource.

- Fawcett, T. and Rhynas, S. (2012) Taking a patient history: the role of the nurse. *Nursing Standard*, 26 (24): 41-46.
  This article will help you understand the complexity and processes involved in history taking.
- Mayo, P. (2017) Undertaking an accurate and comprehensive assessment of the acutely ill adult. *Nursing Standard*, 32 (8): 53-63.
  A good summary of the approach to assessing acutely ill adults.
- Smith, D. and Bowden, T. (2017) Using the ABCDE approach to assess the deteriorating patient. *Nursing Standard*, 32 (14): 51-63.
  The article will help you develop your skills in assessing the deteriorating patient using the ABCDE approach.

Weblinks

FURTHER READING: WEBLINKS

Go to https://study.sagepub.com/essentialadultnursing for further weblinks related to this chapter. If you are using the interactive ebook, simply click on the book icon in the margin to go straight to the resource.

- https://tfinews.ocbmedia.com/
  Online training resource to learn about the use of the National Early Warning Score (NEWS)
- www.resus.org.uk
  Website of the Resuscitation Council (UK) which includes resuscitation guidelines and resources such as using the ABCDE approach
- www.gp-training.net/training/communication_skills/calgary/calgary.pdf
  An in-depth version of the Calgary-Cambridge Guide to the Medical Interview

ONLINE QUIZZES

ACE YOUR ASSESSMENT

Revise what you have learned by visiting https://study.sagepub.com/essentialadultnursing

- Test yourself with multiple-choice and short-answer questions
- Do the chapter activities in the book and check your answers online

REFERENCES

Considine, J. and Currey, J. (2015) Ensuring a proactive, evidence-based, patient safety approach to patient assessment. *Journal of Clinical Nursing*, 24(1–2): 300–7.

Epstein, O., Perkin, G., Cookson, J., Watt, I., Rakhit, R., Robins, A. and Hornett, G. (2008) *Clinical Examination*. The Netherlands: Elsevier.

Gordon, M. (1994) *Nursing Diagnosis: Process and Application*. St Louis, MO: Mosby.

Gumm, K. (2007) Emergency Department Trauma Management. In Curtis, K., Ramsden, C. and Friendship, J. (eds) *Emergency and Trauma Nursing*. Sydney: Mosby, pp.706–32.

Munson, E. and Willcox, A. (2007) Applying the Calgary-Cambridge model. *Practice Nursing*, 18 (9): 464–8.

National Institute for Health and Care Excellence (2014) *Pressure ulcers: prevention and management*. Available at: www.nice.org.uk/guidance/cg179/chapter/1-Recommendations

National Institute for Health and Care Excellence (2017) *Sepsis: recognition, diagnosis and early management*. Available at: www.nice.org.uk/guidance/ng51

NMC (2015) *The Code: Professional Standards of Practice and Behaviour for Nurses and Midwives*. Available at: www.nmc.org.uk/standards/code/read-the-code-online/

NMC (2018) *Future nurse: Standards of proficiency for registered nurses* [online]. Available at: www.nmc.org.uk/standards/standards-for-nurses/standards-of-proficiency-for-registered-nurses/

Resuscitation Council (UK) (2018) *The ABCDE approach* [online]. Available at: https://www.resus.org.uk/resuscitation-guidelines/abcde-approach/

Roper, N., Logan, W. and Tierney, A. (2000) *The Roper-Logan-Tierney Model of Nursing: Based on activities of living*. Edinburgh: Churchill Livingstone

Royal College of Physicians (2012) *National Early Warning Score (NEWS) Standardising the Assessment of Acute-illness Severity in the NHS*. Available at: www.rcplondon.ac.uk/projects/outputs/national-early-warning-score-news

Silverman, J.K., Kurtz, S. and Draper, J. (2013) *Skills for Communicating with Patients* (3rd ed). Oxford: Radcliffe Publishing.

Sprinks, J. (2013) Swift take-up of standardised early warning system across NHS trusts. *The Nursing Standard*, 27 (21): 7.

BAPEN (2003) The MUST Explanatory Booklet: A Guide to the 'Malnutrition Universal Screening Tool' (MUST) for Adults (2003). Available at: www.bapen.org.uk/pdfs/must/must_explan.pdf (Accessed 29th August 2018).

The Waterlow Score (2005). Available at: www.judywaterlow.co.uk/waterlow_score.htm

Tian, Y., Thompson, J., Buck, D. and Sonola, L. (2013) *Exploring the System-wide Costs of Falls in Older People in Torbay*. London: The Kings Fund.

Yura, H. and Walsh, M. (1967) *The Nursing Process: Assessing, planning, implementing, evaluating*. Norwalk, CT: Appleton Century Crofts.

Zator Estes, M.E. (2014) *Health Assessment and Physical Examination* (5th edn). Clifton Park, NY: Cengage Learning.

PREPARING ADULTS FOR SURGERY, PERI- AND POST-OPERATIVE SURGICAL CARE

10

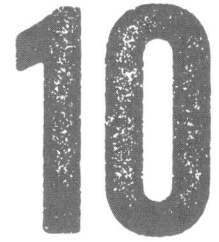

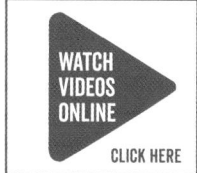

LUCIE LLEWELLYN AND LEE PENG LUI

THIS CHAPTER COVERS

- The different stages of the patient journey through surgical care from pre-assessment through to the post-operative ward
- The role of the nurse during each of these stages
- Care of the patient during their surgical journey

- Principles of anaesthesia, surgical a sepsis and post-anaesthetic care
- Assessment and management of the risks associated with the peri-operative environment.

> " "I knew that my operation and recovery would be physically demanding, but didn't realise how psychologically draining it would be for both myself and my family, especially when things didn't quite go to plan and I couldn't always get the answers I needed"
>
> **Allen, patient** "

INTRODUCTION

As seen in Allen's quote above the peri-operative journey is not only a physically demanding one, but is also psychologically stressful and it is, therefore, important that you have the necessary knowledge to provide effective care and support not only to your patient, but also to their family and carers. It is important to have a good understanding of the different stages in the patient journey through the surgical process, from pre-assessment once the patient has been informed that they require a surgical procedure, through to the time they return to the ward following surgery. Within this chapter you will learn more about the different stages of the peri-operative journey that the patient goes through and what the role of the nurse is at each stage, along with the roles played by other members of the multidisciplinary team. It is important to remember that surgical procedures are not without risk, and patient safety is paramount at each stage of the journey; however, it is also important to ensure that patient dignity is not compromised

WHAT IS SURGERY?

To put it into context there were approximately 7.2 million primary surgical procedures performed in the National Health Service in 2010/2011 (Health Episode Statistics (HES) data), and almost 6.7 million of these were elective cases that included both therapeutic and diagnostic interventions. Surgical procedures are either performed as an elective or an emergency.

An elective surgical procedure is planned, with time factored in for patient preparation (both physical and psychological) and a date set for the procedure to take place. This can either be as an inpatient, with the patient staying in the hospital overnight, or as day surgery when the patient will go home on the same day as they have their procedure. An emergency surgical procedure is unplanned and is essential for a patient's survival. As an emergency procedure is unplanned, there is limited time for patient preparation and this can place increased physical and psychological demands on the patient which will need addressing following surgery.

There are a number of reasons for patients to undergo a surgical procedure, and the expected outcome will vary according to why they needed that particular procedure. There are five different categories of surgical procedures:

- Curative: performed to restore health through the removal of diseased or damaged tissue, potentially using radical methods, e.g. cholecystectomy (removal of diseased gall bladder)
- Conservative: performed to improve health and preserve function through the removal of diseased or damaged tissue, using non-radical methods, e.g. lumpectomy (removal of localised breast cancer)
- Palliative: performed for relief of adverse symptoms to improve quality of life when curative or conservative procedures are not feasible, e.g. pleurodesis to relieve pain in mesothelioma patients (closes pleural space to reduce painful pleural fluid accumulation)
- Diagnostic: performed to confirm or determine a diagnosis, e.g. tissue biopsy
- Transplant: performed to replace a malfunctioning organ, e.g. heart transplant for heart failure caused by cardiomyopathy.

THE OPERATING DEPARTMENT TEAM

The operating department team consists of anaesthetists, surgeons, operating department practitioners and registered nurses, team leaders/matrons, theatre managers, theatre support workers/healthcare assistants/associate practitioners/nursing associates, surgical care practitioner, surgical first assistant, and physician's assistant (anaesthesia).

── GO FURTHER ──

The Association of Perioperative Practice provides a summary of the job roles and duties of personnel working in the operating department which you may wish to explore further www.afpp.org.uk/adverts/ redirect/184/635

WEBLINKS

Visit www.rcseng.ac.uk/ for further information on the Surgical Care Practitioner role.
Visit www.nmc.org.uk/standards/nursing-associates/ for the Nursing Associate role.

THE WHO SURGICAL SAFETY CHECKLIST

When the patient arrives in theatre, the WHO Surgical Safety Checklist (WHO, 2009) is completed, initially in the anaesthetic room, and then in the operating theatre before surgery commences and then again at the end of the procedure. A final risk assessment is carried out in the post-anaesthetic care unit when the nurse uses pre-determined criteria to ascertain if the patient is safe to be discharged and where they should be discharged to.

The aim of the checklist is to improve communication within the multidisciplinary team in theatres and enhance patient safety to prevent Never Events from occurring. There are three phases in the WHO checklist:

1. Sign In – this is carried out by the anaesthetist and the anaesthetic nurse/operating department practitioner (ODP) to verify with the patient:

    *   their identity
    *   their consent for surgery, the actual surgical procedure and site
    *   surgical marking to identify side, right or left (if applicable).

    In addition to this the anaesthetist and the anaesthetic nurse/ODP will also review:

    –   whether the anaesthetic machine, equipment and medication checks are completed
    –   if the pulse oximeter is attached to the patient and is functioning
    –   if the patient has any known allergies or is at risk of a difficult airway, aspiration or blood loss exceeding 500mls.

2. Time Out – this is carried out after induction of anaesthesia, but before surgical incision with the entire team present. A nominated coordinator, any healthcare professional in the operating team, will be responsible for initiating the 'Time Out' and completing the actual checklist. Each team member will introduce him/herself by name and role. The team will:

    *   confirm the correct operation, correct site, and correct position for the correct patient
    *   review anticipated surgical critical events, anaesthetic concerns, confirmation of instrument sterility and discuss any equipment issues or concerns
    *   review and confirm that the surgical site infection bundle and VTE prophylaxis have been undertaken
    *   confirm essential imaging is displayed as appropriate.

3. Sign Out – the last phase that is carried out after the surgery, before the patient or any team member leaves the operating room. The nominated coordinator will verify with the whole team:

    *   the operation is recorded
    *   the surgical counts are complete and correct
    *   the correct labelling of surgical specimens
    *   issues with equipment are identified and addressed
    *   if there are concerns for post-operative recovery.

ACTIVITY 10.1: CRITICAL THINKING

- What are the barriers to the implementation of the WHO Surgical Safety Checklist?
- How could these barriers be managed/removed to ensure successful implementation of the WHO Surgical Safety Checklist?

PRE-ASSESSMENT

The first phase of the patient's peri-operative journey once they have found out that they require a surgical procedure is pre-assessment. This is a process that has a number of different facets that should take into consideration not only the physical and psychological needs of the patient, but also their social needs. By doing this the patient should have a clearer understanding of what is going to happen to them and reduce their potential anxieties, as well as being as fit as possible for their procedure (NHS Modernisation Agency, 2003). It also allows for identification of any essential resources that will be needed for both the procedure and for discharge, as well as reducing the number of cancelled surgical operations for avoidable reasons.

Pre-assessment encompasses not only assessment and history taking in relation to physical, psychological and social factors, as well as identification of specialist requirements during admission and on discharge, but also patient education and information giving.

According to the AAGBI (2013) the pre-assessment nurse can achieve this through the use of a screening questionnaire to identify any health problems and make appropriate referrals to either an anaesthetist or surgeon as required. Information that should be gathered from patient assessment and history taking should cover:

- presenting complaint and symptoms
- diagnosis (if relevant)
- past medical history
- previous surgical history
- anaesthetic history
- medications
- allergies
- family history
- social and psychological history
- activities of daily living
- systems review.

(Walsgrove, 2011)

In addition to gathering this information a pre-assessment nurse with specialist training will also carry out a physical examination and a range of pre-operative tests. Historically, patients have had too many tests performed on them prior to surgery and according to the latest NICE (2016) guidelines on 'Routine preoperative tests for elective surgery', consideration should be given to the selection of tests in relation to the grade of surgery the patient is having, as well as their ASA score (see Table 10.1), which is a simple scale used by anaesthetists that describes the patient's fitness to have an anaesthetic. By following this guidance patients should have the minimal number of tests needed, which will not only minimise their discomfort, but is also seen to be a more appropriate use of hospital resources. The different tests that a patient may have are in Table 10.2.

Table 10.1 ASA Physical status classification system

ASA Physical status classification	Definition
ASA 1	A normal healthy patient
ASA 2	A patient with mild systemic disease
ASA 3	A patient with severe systemic disease
ASA 4	A patient with severe systemic disease that is a constant threat to life
ASA 5	A moribund patient who is not expected to survive without the operation
ASA 6	A declared brain-dead patient whose organs are being removed for donor purposes

(American Society of Anesthesiologists, 2014)

Table 10.2 Pre-operative tests dependent on grade of surgery and ASA physical status classification (NICE, 2016)

- Pregnancy test
- Sickle cell disease or sickle cell trait test
- HbA1c test
- Urine test
- Chest x-ray
- Electrocardiogram
- Blood tests

The aim of educating patients and giving them information, both verbal and written, is to reduce their fears and anxieties, and ensure that they have received all of the necessary information to enable them to be prepared for their surgical procedure. Patients need to be informed on how long they should fast for:

- 6 hours solid food
- 2 hours clear fluids.

It is important that patients adhere to these times; if they do not fast for long enough then there is the risk of aspiration during induction of anaesthesia. If they fast for too long then this can have a negative impact of dehydration, electrolyte imbalance and nutritional intake. Information regarding medications management is also important as patients are not always clear which of their regular medications they should continue as stopping these medications would be detrimental to the patient in terms of symptom control, for instance steroids, antihypertensives, anticonvulsants. Patients also need information as to which medications should be discontinued in the lead up to their surgery due to negative interactions with anaesthetic agents or potential to cause surgical complications such as bleeding, e.g. aspirin, monoamine oxidase inhibitors (MAOIs), as well as herbal medications such as St John's Wort.

Patient education is important in relation to what to expect following their surgical procedure, both in the immediate post-operative period and in terms of their needs following discharge from hospital, as this can also help to reduce the anxiety and fear associated with surgical procedures and ensure patients have the right systems in place to support them when they go home.

Pre-assessment is also key in determining whether patients are suitable to be selected to have their surgical procedure via day surgery. There is an increasing number of patients who are having their surgical procedure as a day case, which will allow them to go home on the same day as their procedure and recover at home. This is seen as not only beneficial for the patient, but is also beneficial to the hospital as it will have a positive impact on the utilisation of resources. The pre-assessment nurse plays a vital role in this as their assessment will identify whether a patient is suitable to be operated on as a day case, and effective patient selection will ensure that major and minor risks are reduced, in relation to patient outcomes.

ADMISSION AND PRE-OPERATIVE PREPARATION

Patients are either admitted in advance of their surgical procedure or on the day of surgery, which is why it is important that they receive clear instructions and pre-operative information such as fasting times to ensure that they are adequately prepared. Regardless of when the patient is admitted they will be seen by the anaesthetist, where additional assessment will take place to ensure that the patient is fit for anaesthesia and to identify any potential problems, such as a difficult airway. The patient will also be seen by the surgeon who will be operating on them, to confirm or acquire informed consent, to clarify any last questions from the patient and to mark the operation site with an indelible pen (WHO, 2009).

The role of the ward nurse at this time is to help the patient to prepare for their procedure and to provide additional support as required. The ward nurse will need to ensure that the patient has followed pre-operative instructions such as fasting times, skin preparation, hair removal (if appropriate), VTE assessment has been completed and the patient is wearing their anti-embolism stockings. In addition, the ward nurse will need to ensure the pre-operative checklist has been completed before the patient leaves the ward for theatre.

The pre-operative checklist is used to confirm the patient's identity and confirm that informed consent has been given. It also provides a baseline set of observations, which are used to guide care of the patient throughout the peri-operative journey, and are important when it comes to discharging the patient back to the ward, which will be discussed later within this chapter. The checklist also ensures that all necessary preparations have been carried out and all relevant information goes to theatre with the patient. Once the call is received from theatre that they are ready for the patient the ward nurse should make one last check to clarify that the pre-operative checklist is completed and then escort the patient to theatre, either by walking them down to the theatre suite if the patient is able to mobilise or accompanying the patient if they are being transferred by theatre porters. However the patient makes their way to theatre it is important that they keep warm, so as not to lose heat prior to surgery, which can delay the start of surgery (NICE, 2016).

INFECTION CONTROL

The operating department is a self-contained unit with restricted entry to authorised personnel only. Traffic patterns are established in the operating department to define movement of personnel to minimise the risk of infection. It is defined by transition, unrestricted, semi-restricted and restricted zones. Clinical waste and contaminated items should not travel down the same corridor as clean and sterile items (move from clean to dirty). The design of the operating department should accommodate the day-to-day workload, staff and patient numbers. In the operating room, movement and number of personnel and opening of theatre doors should be kept to a minimum. The doors of the operating room must be kept closed at all times to maintain positive air pressure in the room. You should observe the **sterile field** and sterile trolley when moving around to prevent contaminating the field.

Temperature and humidity in the operating room is important to maintain infection control. Daily checks on temperature, humidity and ventilation prior to the start of the operating list should be done to ensure they are within the recommended range and that the air flow system is working.

PATIENT SAFETY

Patient safety should be at the heart of all healthcare systems. Protecting patients from avoidable harm via risk assessment and management is an integral part of peri-operative nursing. According to WHO (2017), 234 million surgical procedures are undertaken worldwide yearly and 50% of complications associated with surgery are avoidable. Hence it is important that you are able to identify hazards and risks, and undertake measures to reduce or eliminate these risks within the peri-operative environment (NMC, 2015). Risk reduction can enhance patient and staff safety and outcomes, improve quality, and decrease healthcare costs. We need to develop a culture whereby risk assessment and management is everyone's business. Transparency, candour and open culture should be encouraged so that incidents are reported and lessons are learnt (Francis, 2013).

Human Factors in healthcare is defined as 'enhancing clinical performance through an understanding of the effects of teamwork, tasks, equipment, workspace, culture and organisation on human behaviour and abilities and application of that knowledge in clinical settings' (NHS England, 2012). By understanding Human Factors, we can better understand how individuals' behaviour and the interactions among work systems affect human performance, and how to minimise errors. NHS England (2012) recommends incorporating Human Factors principles in risk assessment and management as well as in root cause analysis. The Royal College of Nursing Human Factors Model shows how actions or omissions can impact performance and practice, and the factors that influence care (www.rcn.org.uk/clinical-topics/patient-safety-and-human-factors).

GENERAL ANAESTHESIA

The word 'anaesthesia' comes from the Greek word meaning without sensation. General anaesthesia (GA) is a medically induced coma through the use of a combination of anaesthetic agents in the 'Triad of Anaesthesia' (Figure 10.1). These drugs bring about a state of unconsciousness, pain relief and muscle relaxation, in a reversible manner, in order for surgery to be performed (Simpson and Popat, 2003).

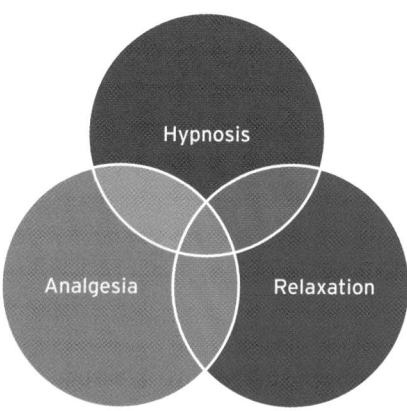

Figure 10.1 Triad of anaesthesia

The process of general anaesthesia consists of induction (from consciousness to unconsciousness), maintenance (surgery to be performed) and reversal (unconsciousness to consciousness). General anaesthesia is induced by either intravenous anaesthetic drugs or inhalational volatile agents (Table 10.3). Intravenous anaesthetics produce rapid induction and maintain the patient for a few minutes until maintenance anaesthesia takes over. Inhaled anaesthetics are known to trigger **malignant hyperthermia** (anaesthetic emergency), so they are contraindicated in those with known, or a family history of malignant hyperthermia.

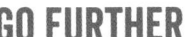

GO FURTHER

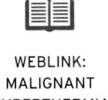

WEBLINK: MALIGNANT HYPERTHERMIA

The Association of Anaesthetists of Great Britain and Ireland offers guidelines and publications on various topics, one of which you might wish to explore further is Malignant Hyperthermia at www.aagbi.org.

Table 10.3 Some examples of intravenous anaesthetics and inhaled anaesthetics

Intravenous anaesthetics	Inhaled anaesthetics
Benzodiazepine, e.g. midazolam	Nitrous oxide
Barbiturates, e.g. thiopental	Halothane
Non-barbiturates, e.g. propofol, etomidate	Isoflurane
Dissociative anaesthesia, e.g. ketamine	Sevoflurane
	Desflurane

The other part of the triad is analgesia, which is not only important to relieve pain but also to reduce the autonomic response to surgery and too much use of anaesthetics (Simpson and Popat, 2003). Opiate analgesics are natural or synthetic drugs that act on the opioid receptors which are found throughout the central and peripheral nervous systems and other organs to block the transmission of pain, produce sedation and euphoria. However, opioids also have many unwanted side effects, such as respiratory depression, nausea and vomiting, constipation and bowel atony, and addiction.

Here are some examples of opioids that you may come across in theatres:

- Fentanyl
- Alfentanil
- Morphine
- Pethidine
- Diamorphine
- Oxycodone
- Remifentanil.

Relaxation or immobility is achieved by neuromuscular blocking drugs (Table 10.4). These drugs work by blocking the transmission of acetylcholine on the nicotinic receptors at the **neuromuscular junction** where the motor neuron excites the skeletal muscle fibres (Aitkenhead et al., 2013).

There are two types of muscle relaxants: non-depolarising and depolarising neuromuscular blocking drugs. Non-depolarising muscle relaxants compete with acetylcholine at the nicotinic receptor sites on the motor end plate to prevent transmission and depolarisation. As the action is competitive, the onset of action is slower compared to depolarising muscle relaxant. Depolarising muscle relaxant mimics the action of acetylcholine by attaching itself to the receptor sites and the motor end plate stays depolarised for several minutes as repolarisation is inhibited. The initial depolarisation causes muscle twitches and fasciculations. As the onset is very rapid, depolarising muscle relaxant is commonly used in **rapid sequence induction**.

Non-depolarising muscle relaxants can be reversed by an anticholinesterase drug (neostigmine). However, depolarising muscle relaxant is not reversible but is hydrolysed by a naturally occurring enzyme known as plasma cholinesterase. In the presence of atypical plasma cholinesterase, the duration of action of depolarising muscle relaxant becomes prolonged (Gwinnutt and Gwinnutt, 2012).

Table 10.4 Neuromuscular blocking agents

Non-depolarising muscle relaxants	Depolarising muscle relaxants
Short acting (commonly used in day surgery) - Mivacurium	Suxamethonium (succinylcholine)
Intermediate acting - Atracurium - Vecuronium - Rocuronium	
Long acting (commonly used in ITU) - Pancuronium - Cisatracurium	

AIRWAY MANAGEMENT

Airway management is central to the entire field of anaesthesia. The aims are to maintain airway patency, provide adequate oxygenation and ventilation, and prevent and protect the patient from aspiration and regurgitation (Simpson and Popat, 2003). The basic methods of airway management include bag face mask ventilation, laryngeal mask airway and endotracheal intubation.

Face masks come in various types and sizes (Figure 10.2), and should fit snuggly around the mouth and nose to provide a tight gas seal. Most of the face masks are clear nowadays to allow for observation of air misting (indicating patent airway) and presence of vomitus (in the event of regurgitation). During induction, face mask is used to pre-oxygenate the patient prior to insertion of laryngeal mask airway or endotracheal intubation. Sometimes, the anaesthetic assistant will assist by holding the face mask on the patient's face gently while the anaesthetist administers intravenous anaesthetics to the patient. A face mask may be employed during short non-invasive procedures whereby the anaesthetist will hold the face mask with one hand and with the other hand ventilate the patient with the breathing bag. Appropriate airway adjuncts (Figure 10.3) such as an oropharyngeal or nasopharyngeal airway may be inserted to facilitate bagging of the patient. However, holding the face mask can be tiring; in this case the laryngeal mask airway is an advantage.

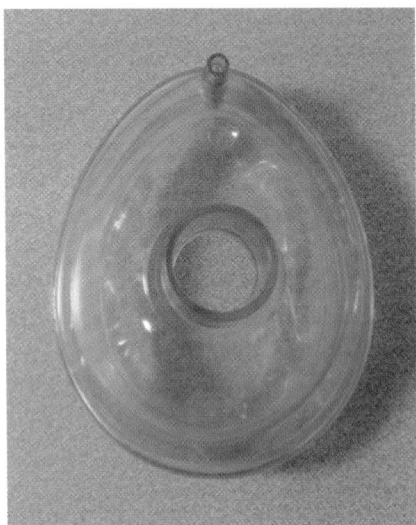

Figure 10.2   Face mask

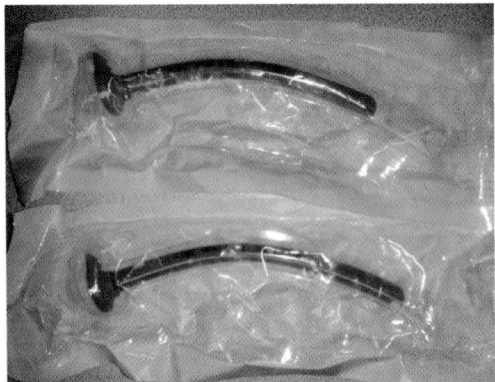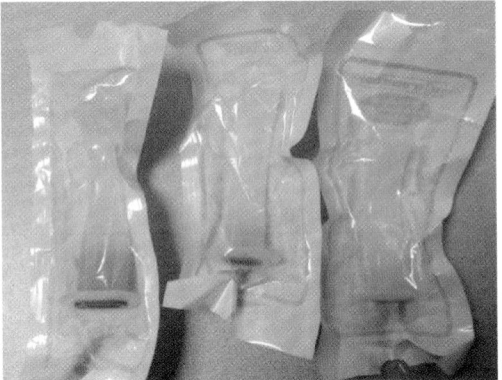

Figure 10.3   Airway adjuncts – nasopharyngeal airways (left) and oropharyngeal or 'Guedel' airways (right)

Laryngeal mask airway (LMA) or supraglottic airway devices (SADs) are now routinely used to deliver oxygen and gases to the patient during surgery (Figure 10.4). It is non-invasive and can be inserted immediately following induction. The LMA comes in many types and sizes, with the appropriate size chosen according to the weight of the patient. The anaesthetic practitioner will assist the anaesthetist with the insertion of the LMA by lowering the patient's mandible and opening the mouth, while the anaesthetist inserts the LMA along the floor of the hard palate and into the pharynx. The cuff of the LMA is deflated during insertion and inflated after insertion. The cuff will lie posterior to the larynx, thus it does not protect the airway from gastric contents aspiration and is indicated in patients who are not at risk.

If the patient is at high risk of regurgitation, endotracheal tubes (Figure 10.5) should be used because once the cuff of the tracheal tube is inflated it forms an airtight seal in the trachea preventing aspiration. It is also indicated in certain types of surgery, e.g. head and neck operations, laparotomy/laparoscopy, cardiothoracic surgery; when intubation is difficult; intermittent positive pressure ventilation is required; or when the patient is very ill. The anaesthetic assistant will check that the airway and intubating equipment are working and available prior to the patient arriving in the anaesthetic room. At intubation, the patient's head will be placed in the 'sniffing the morning air' position and tracheal intubation is performed with the aid of a laryngoscope (Figure 10.6), after the patient has been given an appropriate muscle relaxant. Attempts to intubate when the patient is not adequately relaxed may risk laryngospasm, thereby making intubation more difficult. Other intubating equipment, such as introducers and bougies, might be utilised when it is difficult to visualise the vocal cords. The tracheal tube can be railroaded via the bougie into the trachea. The Magill forceps (Figure 10.7) are useful to remove anything that might be obstructing the airway or guide the passage of the tracheal tube into the larynx or nasogastric tube into the oesophagus (Simpson and Popat, 2002).

CASE STUDY 10.1: GRACE

Grace is a 65-year-old woman who has been admitted to theatre for a hysteroscopy procedure under general anaesthesia. She is fit and healthy. When checking the patient in the anaesthetic room, Grace informed you that her last meal and drink was 4 hours ago.

ACTIVITY 10.2: CRITICAL THINKING

Referring to the above case study, what do you think will be the most appropriate airway management for the patient? Explain why.

ACTIVITY 10.2
ANSWER

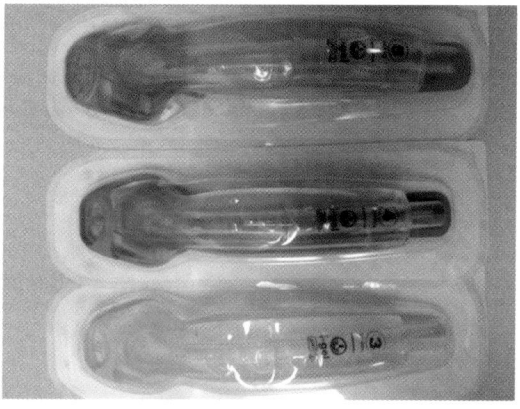

Figure 10.4   Different types of supraglottic airway devices/laryngeal mask airway (Sizes 3 to 5 i-Gels)

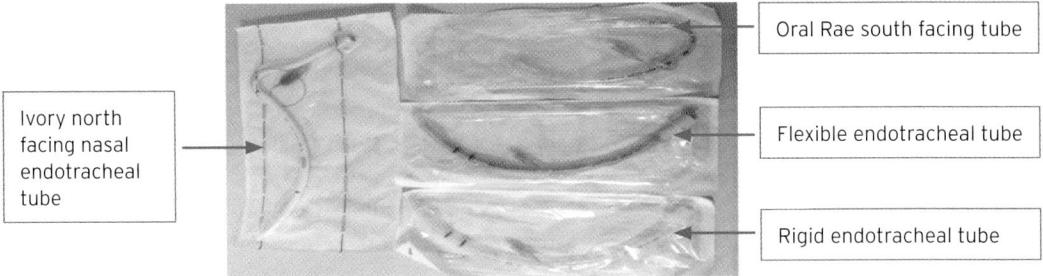

Ivory north facing nasal endotracheal tube

Oral Rae south facing tube

Flexible endotracheal tube

Rigid endotracheal tube

Figure 10.5 Tracheal tubes

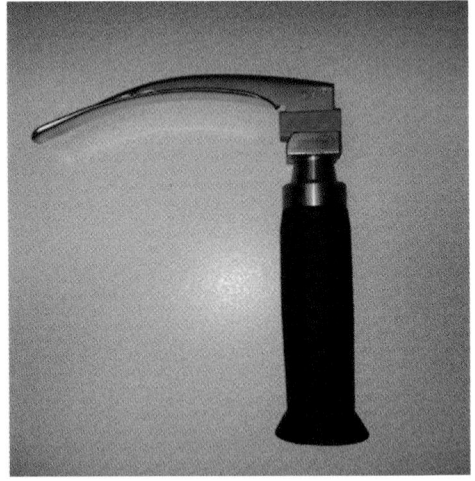

Figure 10.6 Laryngoscope and blade

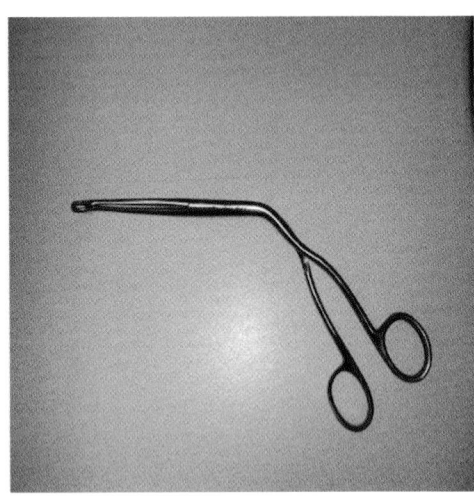

Figure 10.7 Magill forceps

REGIONAL ANAESTHESIA

SEE ALSO
CHAPTER 27

Before moving onto this section, it is recommended that you review the anatomy and physiology of the central nervous system and spinal meninges first.

Regional anaesthesia is the injection of a local anaesthetic drug (e.g. lignocaine, bupivacaine, levobupivacaine) into a 'region' of the body that is operated on to block pain or sensation, and to provide post-operative pain relief (see Table 10.5).

Table 10.5 Regional anaesthesia

Peripheral Nerve Blocks	Central Neuraxial Blocks
Cervical plexus block	Spinal block
Brachial plexus block	Epidural block
Femoral block	Combined spinal-epidural blocks
Ankle block	
Bier's block	

We will examine two of the most common blocks that you might encounter when on placement – spinal and epidural blocks. Spinal anaesthesia is a single injection of local anaesthetic (0.5% Marcain Heavy) into the subarachnoid space containing the cerebral spinal fluid (Cobbold and Money, 2010). It may be indicated for use when patients are unsuitable for general anaesthesia (i.e. those who have not fasted or are at risk of regurgitation). Spinal blocks provide a total loss of sensation for up to three hours and are commonly used in surgery below the umbilicus: such as lower limb surgery (total knee replacement/total hip replacement), urology (trans urethral resection of prostate (TURP) or cystoscopy), gynaecology, perineum procedures and obstetrics. The site of spinal injection depends on the surgery to be performed but is normally inserted between the region of second lumbar and first sacral vertebrae to avoid the spinal cord and fused sacral vertebrae (Fischer and Pinnock, 2004). The anaesthetic practitioner will assist the patient in to the lateral or sitting position with the body curled up to open the spaces between the lumbar spinous processes. Spinal anaesthesia can cause hypotension due to vasodilatation from blockade of sympathetic nerve fibres (Simpson and Popat, 2002). Consequently, it is essential that the patient has intravenous cannula sited prior to the procedure, so that in the event of hypotension vasoconstrictor/vasopressor drugs and intravenous fluids may be administered. Other possible complications of spinal anaesthesia include post-dural puncture headaches due to leakage of cerebral spinal fluid; urinary retention as a result of sympathetic nerve fibres blockade; nausea and vomiting secondary to hypotension; local anaesthetic toxicity or allergic reaction; respiratory distress if the block becomes too high; and infection (Simpson and Popat, 2002).

Epidural anaesthesia is the injection of local anaesthetic drugs (e.g. 0.25% bupivacaine) into the epidural space, which is the area between the dura mater and the vertebral wall (Fischer and Pinnock, 2004). Similar to spinal anaesthesia, epidural anaesthesia is indicated in abdominal or lower extremities surgery. In addition to general anaesthesia, epidural anaesthesia is used in thoracic and upper abdominal surgery, as well as providing post-operative pain relief, and control of chronic and labour pain. Like spinal anaesthesia, the patient may lie on the lateral side or in the sitting position. The complications of epidural anaesthesia are broadly similar to spinal block; in addition there are risks of catheter displacement, accidental injection into the epidural veins, and epidural a haematoma and abscess.

GO FURTHER

The Association of Anaesthetists of Great Britain and Ireland has guidelines on 'Best practice in the management of epidural analgesia in the hospital setting' (AAGBI, 2010). Please visit www.aagbi.org.

WEBLINK: EPIDURAL ANALGESIA

PRINCIPLES OF SURGICAL ASEPSIS

Asepsis is the absence of pathogenic micro-organisms that can cause infection (Phillips, 2013). There are two types of asepsis – medical and surgical asepsis. Medical asepsis is the exclusion of all microbes associated with communicable disease and is referred to as a clean technique. Surgical asepsis refers to the absence of all micro-organisms within any type of invasive procedure and is sterile. Aseptic technique includes steps taken to minimise the number of microorganisms in the environment and on equipment, with an aim to reduce the risk of contamination. Sterile technique involves all the processes of asepsis to create a sterile field. It is important to observe the sterile field and keep a distance from it to avoid contamination of the field.

Surgical site infection (SSI) is a type of healthcare-associated infection (HCAI) in which a surgical incision site becomes infected after a surgical procedure (NICE, 2013). SSI accounts for 16% of all healthcare-associated infections and can cause significant morbidity and mortality in surgical patients (NICE, 2013). Hence preventing SSI is the primary goal of the surgical team. The peri-operative practitioner has a responsibility to adhere to the principles of asepsis to maintain sterility within the operating field, and to eradicate both pathogenic and non-pathogenic micro-organisms in order to prevent contamination of the surgical wound.

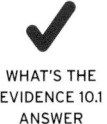

WHAT'S THE
EVIDENCE 10.1
ANSWER

WHAT'S THE EVIDENCE? 10.1

NICE offers guidance on surgical site infection www.nice.org.uk/guidance/CG74/

- What is the SSI Bundle of Care?
- What is the purpose of pre-operative showering?
- When is hair removal done? What should be used for hair removal? Why?
- When is antibiotic prophylaxis given? Why?
- Why is maintaining patient homeostasis important?

Table 10.6 Principles of surgical asepsis

Principles	Rationale
Sterile items are used within the sterile field	Unsterile items contaminate the sterile field
A sterile person is scrubbed, gowned and gloved	Can only touch sterile items when wearing sterile gowns and gloves
A sterile person must keep their hands in front of them at or above waist level	Gowns are only considered sterile in front from the chest to above waist level
Only the top of a sterile draped table is sterile at table level	Below table level is considered unsterile
An unsterile person should not reach across the sterile field	Micro-organisms from the unsterile person might accidentally be transferred onto the sterile field
A sterile person must face the sterile field and not turn their back or side to a sterile field	The sterility of objects which are out of view is questionable
Do not prepare the sterile field in advance	The degree of contamination is proportionate to the length of time
A sterile person must not touch unsterile items and an unsterile person must not touch sterile items	To avoid contamination
Keep movement within and around the sterile field to a minimum	To avoid contamination of sterile items or personnel
Check the sterile items for expiry dates and that the package is intact	To ensure sterility of the items

SURGICAL HAND ANTISEPSIS

The surgical hand antisepsis is an extension of handwashing and is also known as the antiseptic surgical scrub or antiseptic hand rub which is performed prior to putting on sterile surgical gown and gloves for a surgical procedure (AfPP, 2014). The purpose of the surgical hand antisepsis is to reduce the number of resident and transient flora, to suppress the growth of micro-organisms, to keep the population of micro-organisms to a minimum, and to reduce the microbial contamination of the patient's wound (AfPP, 2014; Phillips, 2013). Prior to carrying out the surgical hand antisepsis, the scrub personnel should wear the appropriate theatre attire, cap and face mask. A face mask is worn as it helps to contain micro-organisms from being expelled from the mouth and nose and it offers the wearer protection from splashes of blood and body fluids. When wearing a face mask, it should cover the nose and mouth, fitting snugly around the contour of the face and tied securely at the back. Avoid touching the filter part of the face mask once it is applied to prevent contamination of the hands. When removing the face mask, handle it by the tapes and discard it into an appropriate waste bin (Phillips, 2013).

WHAT'S THE EVIDENCE? 10.2

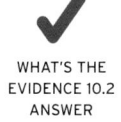

WHAT'S THE EVIDENCE 10.2 ANSWER

There have been numerous studies suggesting that the use of face masks has limited effect on surgical wound infections; however, the evidence in the literature is conflicting and not conclusive. Kelkar et al. (2013) carried out a study to a) check the efficacy of face masks in reducing bacteria dispersal in ophthalmic operating theatres and b) compare the fabric and 'two-ply' disposable face masks. Thirty staff were recruited from a multi-specialty hospital. Samples were taken prior to wearing the face mask, at 30mins, 60mins, 90mins, 120mins and 150mins. The authors found that the use of face masks during ophthalmic surgery statistically reduced the number of bacteria organisms falling on to the operative site and that the 'two-ply' disposable face mask performed slightly better than the fabric ones. However, regardless of the material of the face mask, results showed that after 30mins the bacterial count started to rise and after 120mins the bacterial counts had increased to pre-wear level.

- How long do you think you should wear the face mask for?

The wearing of jewellery is discouraged as this can be a source of microbial colonisation on the skin that could potentially be transmitted to the patient, and can also cause glove perforations (Association of Surgical Technologists, 2017). NICE (2013) recommends the removal of hand jewellery, artificial nails and nail polish before carrying out hand decontamination to reduce the risk of transferring micro-organisms during the surgical procedure.

A preliminary hand wash should be done prior to the surgical hand antisepsis (AfPP, 2017). A nail pick from the brush pack is used to remove debris from underneath the nails. In the past, the brush is used to 'scrub' the hands, hence the name 'scrubbing'. However, scrubbing using brush on hands (except nails) is not recommended as it can expose the dermis layer to infection. The hands should be rubbed vigorously for approximately two to five minutes, always keeping the hands above the elbow to prevent water from flowing down from the elbow (dirty) to fingertips (clean). Evidence comparing the duration of surgical hand antisepsis seems to suggest that the longer the duration of scrub the lower the count of colony forming units on the hands. However, the evidence should be interpreted carefully as findings are inconsistent (Tanner et al, 2016).

GOWNING AND GLOVING TECHNIQUES

Sterile surgical gowns and gloves are worn to prevent micro-organisms from being transferred from clothing and hands to the patients during surgical procedures, and they also offer protection to the surgical personnel from contamination (Phillips 2013). After surgical hand antisepsis, the hands and arms are thoroughly dried before donning sterile surgical gown and gloves. The scrub person will don the sterile surgical gown first. The sterile surgical gowns are folded inside out to facilitate the scrub person picking up and donning the gown without contaminating the outside of the gown. The gown should be considered contaminated and be discarded if the scrub person has touched the outside of the gown while donning it. Next, sterile gloves are worn using either closed or open gloving techniques. Closed gloving technique is preferred to prevent contamination of hands and the open gloving technique is practised when changing a contaminated glove during surgery or for procedures not requiring sterile gowns (Phillips, 2013).

Once gowned and gloved, the scrubbed person should keep the hands between the chest to the waistline level as this is the zone of sterility (Figure 10.8).

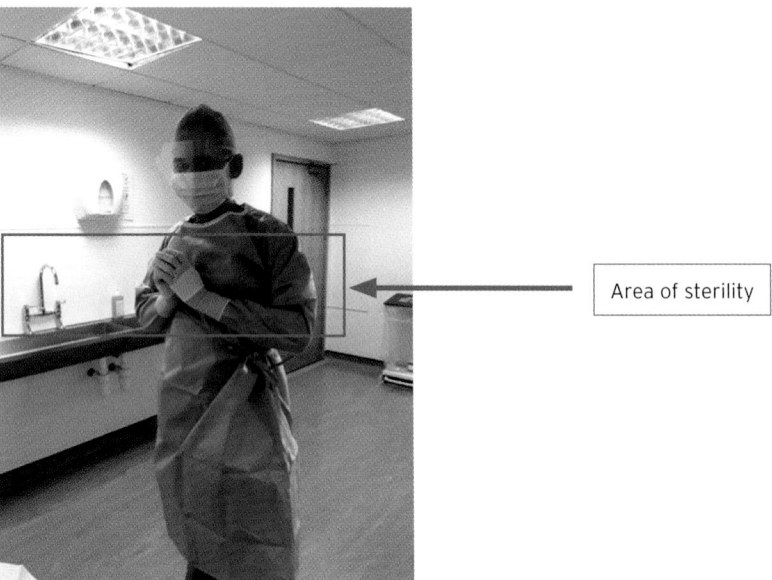

Area of sterility

Figure 10.8   Gowned and gloved, with the zone of sterility

CARE OF PATIENT DURING SURGERY

Patient positioning is important during surgery as anaesthetised and unconscious patients cannot communicate discomfort to staff, and poorly executed patient positioning can cause injuries to both the patient and staff. In order to position the patient safely and correctly, the surgical team should have a briefing beforehand so that the team know the position required for the surgery, and the type of equipment and positioning aids required. The team should also have good knowledge of anatomy and physiology and the physiologic effects of the position on the patient. Knowledge of the table mechanism is also essential. A moving and handling risk assessment should be carried out prior to executing any patient transfer and positioning to minimise any injuries.

There are four common surgical positions: supine, prone, lateral and lithotomy with variations such as Trendelenburg, Fowler's, jacknife and beach chair position. Positioning injuries can be caused by physical forces (pressure, shear and friction) and operating room conditions (moisture, room temperature, negativity) (Rothrock, 2015). Nerve injury, ocular injury, muscle and ligament strains, and skin pressure sores are some of the positioning injuries. To prevent positioning injuries and pressure sores, bony prominences and pressure points should be padded with gel pads. Care should be taken not to drag or pull the patient during positioning as this can create shear and friction.

Maintaining normothermia in the peri-operative patient is important to prevent inadvertent hypothermia as it has been shown that hypothermia can lead to increased post-operative complications.

GO FURTHER

Read NICE clinical guideline (CG65) *Hypothermia: prevention and management in adults having surgery* (www.nice.org.uk/guidance/cg65)

WEBLINK:
HYPOTHERMIA

CASE STUDY 10.2: KAREN

Karen, who is 35 years old, is admitted to theatre for laparoscopic appendicectomy under general anaesthesia. Her pre-operative temperature was 35°C and, on arrival to theatres, she said she 'felt extremely cold'. The plan is to position the patient in the supine position for surgery and to provide active warming.

ACTIVITY 10.3: CRITICAL THINKING

Looking at the case study and NICE clinical guidelines (CG65), how would you assist and support in the care of the patient to prevent a) inadvertent peri-operative hypothermia and b) positioning-related injuries?

ACTIVITY 10.3
ANSWER

POST-ANAESTHETIC CARE

The role of the nurse within the post-anaesthetic care unit (PACU) is predominantly to ensure that the patient is recovered safely using anaesthesia and surgery. This is done through careful assessment and management of the patient using a systematic approach to care following an ABCDE format, with an individualised plan for each patient.

Following surgery and anaesthesia, patients need to recover from the potentially hazardous effects of their anaesthetic within the PACU until their own protective reflexes return (AAGBI, 2013).

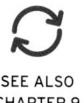

SEE ALSO
CHAPTER 9

One-to-one nursing care is required until the patient is able to maintain their own airway, their respiratory and cardiovascular systems are stable and the patient is able to communicate (RCoA, 2018). The patient is assessed, monitored and receives holistic care until they are ready to be discharged to the ward. Prior to the patient being transferred to the PACU, the nurse must carefully conduct a series of checks to make sure that they have all the necessary equipment (Table 10.7) and that it is functioning, ready for when the patient arrives, due to the potential hazards the patient may face during emergence from anaesthesia.

Table 10.7   Equipment required

- Cardiac monitor and leads, BP cuff, SpO_2 probe
- Drip stand
- Vomit bowl and tissues
- High flow suction unit, Yankauer suction catheter
- Oxygen point
- Bag-valve-mask
- Airway adjuncts – oropharyngeal and nasopharyngeal
- Gloves, aprons, alcohol gel

When the patient first arrives in the PACU their airway is always the first priority of care and the PACU nurse should position themselves at the head of the bed, in order to assess and manage the airway as required and attach oxygen, while receiving the handover from the anaesthetist and scrub practitioner. The anaesthetist must formally hand over the care of their patient to the PACU nurse (AAGBI, 2013), with an effective handover being seen as vital to maintain consistent continuity of care (Chadwick and Norman, 2012). While the PACU nurse is receiving handover, monitoring leads are attached to the patient and individualised alarm limits should be set that are +/– 20% of the patient's baseline observations. An initial set of observations should be taken (Table 10.8) following a systematic approach, and then documented.

Throughout this initial period care should be taken to ensure patient comfort and safety, as well as ensuring that infection control is adhered to. It is important to remember that, even though your patient is unconscious, hearing is the first sense to return, so it is essential that you communicate what you are doing with your patient, and if they wear a hearing aid that it is reinserted as soon as is practicable.

ACTIVITY 10.4
ANSWER

> # ACTIVITY 10.4: REFLECTION
>
> What information do you think the anaesthetist and scrub practitioner should hand over in relation to the care of the patient during anaesthesia and surgery?

OBSERVATIONS AND MONITORING

Following surgery and anaesthesia all patients should be monitored until they have fully recovered from the anaesthetic (AAGBI, 2013). This is done through visual observation of the patient, which is supplemented by vital signs, with pulse oximetry, non-invasive blood pressure monitoring and ECG as the minimum standard (AAGBI, 2013). On admission you should complete and document an initial set of observations (Table 10.8), as these will allow you to plan and manage care throughout the time your patient is in the PACU, and they should be compared to the pre-operative baseline.

Table 10.8   Initial observations on arrival in PACU

- Respiratory rate
- Oxygen saturations
- Heart rate
- Blood pressure
- Temperature
- AVPU or GCS
- Wound
- Drains (if appropriate)
- Invasive lines
- Urinary catheter (if appropriate)
- Pressure areas

ACTIVITY 10.5

Before reading further think what should be assessed/managed within an ABCDE structure for your patient in the PACU.

AIRWAY: ASSESSMENT AND MANAGEMENT

The patient's airway is the first priority of care as the protective reflexes – cough, gag and swallow – that would normally protect the airway from obstruction can be impaired due to the anaesthetic. On assessing the patient's airway a look, listen, feel approach should be used to assess for airway patency (Table 10.9) and identify potential airway obstructions (Box 10.1).

Table 10.9   Look, Listen, Feel approach to airway assessment

	Observation	Normal	Indication of airway obstruction
Look	Respiratory rate, depth and pattern	12-20rpm, regular depth and pattern	Tachypnoea, shallow breaths or irregular pattern
	Oxygen saturations	94-98% on O_2 88-92% on O_2 (COPD)	<94% on O_2 <88% on O_2 for COPD patients
	Patient colour	Normal	Pale, blue (cyanosed)
	Accessory muscles	Not used	Use of accessory muscles, e.g. scalene, sternocleidomastoid
	Mask misting	Mask misting present	Limited or no mask misting
	Level of consciousness	Conscious	Unconscious, semi-conscious

(Continued)

Table 10.9 (Continued)

	Observation	Normal	Indication of airway obstruction
Listen	Noise of breathing	Quiet	Snoring
			Gurgle
			Wheeze
			Crowing/stridor
			Silence
Feel	Movement of air (nose/mouth)	Air felt	No air felt

BOX 10.1: CAUSE OF AIRWAY OBSTRUCTION

- Tongue
- Foreign body, e.g. loose tooth, surgical pack
- Secretions
- Blood
- Laryngeal spasm
- Aspiration
- Tracheal haematoma
- Laryngeal oedema

If an obstruction is identified it is important that airway management is commenced straight away. Specific management of the airway will depend on the cause of the obstruction; however, there are three general stages of management that should be followed for all obstructions (Table 10.10) and you should only move on through the stages if the obstruction is not resolved. What is important though is that help is sought early, as a partial obstruction is easier to manage and if left untreated can soon become a complete obstruction and is harder to manage.

Table 10.10

Stage 1:
Simple airway manoeuvres: jaw thrust, head tilt, chin lift
Oxygen
Suction
Patient positioning
Airway adjuncts: oropharyngeal, nasopharyngeal

Stage 2:
Get help
Bag-valve-mask

Stage 3:
Intubation: prepare drugs, intubation equipment, assist anaesthetist

BREATHING: ASSESSMENT AND MANAGEMENT

The next step once the airway is secure is to move on to breathing. Potential respiratory problems that can occur in the PACU are hypoxia and hypoventilation. These are caused by residual paralysis from the muscle relaxants given in theatre, respiratory depression caused by overdose of opioid analgesia, pain from the surgery and atelectasis (lung collapse) due to ventilation and patient position during surgery.

Assessment of breathing mirrors the airway assessment as you will again need to adopt the look, listen, feel approach as set out in Table 10.9. As with airway assessment, respiratory rate is an important component of the assessment, and a patient who is **bradypnoeic** is at risk of both **hypoxia** and **hypercapnia**. It is also important to look at how your patient is breathing as the use of accessory muscles will indicate that the patient is working hard to breathe and if left untreated will tire quickly, leading to further compromise. It is important to note that when listening you will need to use a stethoscope to listen for the sounds of breathing, unlike the airway which you can hear with the naked ear. It is important that a systematic approach is adopted to performing chest auscultation to ensure that all fields of the lungs are listened to, and as chest auscultation is a specialist skill it is advised that you seek support to do this until competent. Other assessment skills that can be used to assess breathing through feel are palpation, **percussion** and **tactile fremitus**, all of which require practice and are not expected of the student nurse.

General management of respiratory problems will include titration of supplemental oxygen to maintain saturations of 94–98% for most patients following surgery and 88–92% for patients with COPD (O'Driscoll et al., 2017), as well as ensuring the patient is positioned to facilitate good lung expansion, i.e. sitting up if possible, and encouraging deep breathing and coughing. Specific management will depend on the underlying cause of the respiratory problem. If the patient is experiencing hypoventilation due to residual paralysis, then they will require reversal of the muscle relaxant, along with the use of bag-valve-mask to aid ventilation until the respiratory muscles are functioning appropriately. If hypoventilation is caused by the patient being unable to take deep breaths due to pain, then adequate analgesia is required to allow them to breathe without experiencing discomfort. However, if the patient is experiencing hypoventilation due to respiratory depression caused by opioid overdose, then naloxone will need to be given and alternative analgesia prescribed. If the patient is experiencing respiratory problems and these do not resolve with intervention, it is important that help is sought from the anaesthetist to prevent further deterioration.

CIRCULATION: ASSESSMENT AND MANAGEMENT

As previously mentioned, all patients on arrival to the PACU should be attached to a cardiac monitor and as such will have real-time cardiovascular monitoring that will include heart rate and rhythm, as well as blood pressure. In addition to monitoring, it also important to actually feel the patient's pulse to ascertain depth, which along with colour, warmth and measurement of the patient's capillary refill time, will give an indication as to how well perfused they are. Other assessments and monitoring that may be required will depend on the nature of the surgery that the patient has had or their underlying condition and these include ECG, central venous pressure monitoring and invasive blood pressure monitoring.

The cardiovascular system can be affected by a number of factors relating to the surgery and anaesthesia (see Table 10.11). Potential cardiovascular complications following surgery include hypotension, hypertension, bradycardia, arrhythmias such as atrial fibrillation or heart block and myocardial infarction.

Table 10.11

Anaesthetic drugs: volatile agents, reversal agents, opioids

Regional anaesthesia

Pain

Fluid loss: insensible loss during surgery, blood loss, dehydration

Management will depend on the cause of the cardiovascular compromise and should follow trends, not a lone blood pressure or heart rate reading. The most common cardiovascular problem following surgery is hypotension, which is either due to fluid loss (bleeding or clear fluid loss) or the vasodilatory effects of anaesthetic drugs or regional analgesia. Management is primarily fluid replacement with an intravenous crystalloid solution such as Hartmann's solution, and if the patient is actively bleeding and their haemoglobin is reduced the decision may be made to give blood instead. Fluids should be titrated in response to a change in cardiovascular observations and care should be taken not to over-load the patient. In addition to fluid replacement it is also important to consider the underlying cause of the hypotension and treat this accordingly.

Fluid balance monitoring is important within the assessment and management of circulation, and care should be taken to accurately document both fluid intake (e.g. oral, intravenous) and fluid output (e.g. urine, surgical drains, NG aspirate, vomiting) so that an accurate overall balance can be seen.

DISABILITY: ASSESSMENT AND MANAGEMENT

Neurological assessment of the patient while in the PACU can initially be carried out using the AVPU system. However, for some patients it will be more appropriate to perform a GCS assessment. Regardless of which assessment is performed it is important to monitor the patient's conscious level following surgery and document this on the observation chart to assess for deterioration.

Capillary blood glucose (CBG) measurements should be carried out regularly for all diabetic patients and if they are on a variable rate intravenous insulin infusion (VRIII) then this should be titrated accordingly. It is important that diabetic patients return to their usual treatment regimen as soon as possible following surgery, and that patients commence oral hydration and nutrition when able to.

Pain is a common problem following surgery and it is important that a comprehensive assessment is carried out to correctly identify the cause of pain to ensure the correct management is provided. This is important as not all pain experienced in the PACU is related to the surgical site (see Box 10.2).

SEE ALSO
CHAPTER 9

BOX 10.2: NON-SURGICAL CAUSES OF PAIN

- Sore throat from airway (endotracheal tube or laryngeal mask airway)
- Headache
- Poor positioning during surgery – back pain, joint pain, pressure on peripheral nerves, over-stretched ligaments
- Full bladder
- Tight bandages/dressings/plaster casts
- Myocardial infarction

Pain assessment should take into consideration the patient's self-report, physiological and behavioural signs and a simple to use pain scoring tool. Once assessed, pain should be managed using a multi-modal approach that incorporates both pharmacological and non-pharmacological interventions in order to reduce gaps in analgesia, reduce the amount of analgesia used and minimise the side effects of the analgesic drugs given. For most patients their pain will be quite severe and opioid analgesia such as morphine will be the initial drug of choice, which can either be given intravenously as boluses or via patient controlled analgesia (PCA). Other analgesia that may be given in the PACU include paracetamol, non-steriodal anti-inflammatory drugs (NSAIDs) and opioids, as well as local anaesthetic infusions via an epidural or a local block infusion. It is important that pain is assessed regularly so that the appropriate analgesia can be given.

It is also important to utilise non-pharmacological interventions as well, as this will help to treat pain, in particular the emotional component, and can include distraction, positioning and massage.

Post-operative nausea and vomiting (PONV) is a common complication following surgery that can affect 20–30% of all patients. Of these, up to 80% are at high risk for PONV (Pierre and Whelan, 2013) so identification of at risk individuals is important so that prophylactic treatment can be given during anaesthesia. Once in the PACU it is important to assess for PONV on a regular basis so that anti-emetic medication can be given in a timely manner.

As with pain management, the management of PONV also utilises a multi-modal approach as the different anti-emetics available – ondansetron, cyclizine, prochloperazine, metaclopramide – work on different receptor sites. The use of non-pharmacological management complements the use of anti-emetics through simple nursing care (see Box 10.3).

BOX 10.3: NURSING CARE FOR PONV

- Ensure adequate hydration - IV fluids
- Correction of hypotension
- Slow introduction of oral fluids - as appropriate
- Encouragement of slow, smooth movements
- Comfort measures - e.g. offer tissues, water to rinse mouth, wash face

Both pain and PONV if left untreated can lead to physiological and psychological problems that can impact on the patient's recovery, both in the short and long term, and can be avoided through careful assessment and management. They can also potentially cause a delay to the patient being discharged back to the ward.

EXPOSURE: ASSESSMENT AND MANAGEMENT

Temperature monitoring is important as patients are at risk of inadvertent hypothermia as a result of anaesthesia and surgery, and temperature should be monitored alongside the other vital signs. On admission to the PACU it is not uncommon to find a patient with a temperature below 36°C, and as such will need warming with either additional blankets or forced air warmers, in order to warm the patient prior to discharge. Patients with a temperature below 36°C are at increased risk of bleeding and other complications such as reduced level of consciousness.

A full top-to-toe assessment should be done in order to assess wound sites, pressure areas and skin condition, all of which should be documented within the patient's notes. It is important to regularly assess wound sites for bleeding, particularly if these are not easily seen. It is also important to monitor the perfusion of distal digits if the patient has a limb in plaster, as there is the risk of limb ischaemia due to venous occlusion.

DISCHARGE CRITERIA

In order for the patient to be discharged to the ward they will need to be assessed against criteria to determine if they are ready to be discharged, but also to determine where they need to be discharged to. According to the AAGBI (2013) and the RCoA (2018), every PACU should have a well-defined discharge criteria which patients should be assessed against to ensure that they are not put at risk by being discharged too soon or to the wrong clinical area.

According to the AAGBI (2013) the criteria in Box 10.4 should be met. However, if there is concern about the patient, or if there have been issues during surgery, then the patient may also need to be reviewed by the anaesthetist or the surgeon prior to discharge.

BOX 10.4: DISCHARGE CRITERIA

- Patient is fully conscious
- Able to maintain a clear airway and has regained their protective reflexes
- Breathing and oxygenation satisfactory
- Cardiovascular system is stable, no persistent bleeding
- Blood pressure and heart rate should approximate to normal pre-operative values
- Adequate peripheral perfusion
- Pain and PONV should be adequately controlled and suitable analgesia and anti-emetics prescribed
- Temperature within acceptable limits
- Oxygen, if required, should be prescribed
- IV cannula – patent, flushed and intravenous fluid prescribed if appropriate
- All surgical drains and catheters should be checked
- All documentation completed and medical notes present.

(AAGBI, 2013)

Once the patient has been assessed as fit for discharge, then the ward should be contacted to arrange transfer.

POST-OPERATIVE CARE – WARD

On returning to the ward following surgery it is important that the patient is settled and re-orientated to their environment. This is particularly important if the patient was admitted on the day of surgery, or has changed ward, as they will not be familiar with their environment. Explanations should be in language the patient understands and it is important that this is regularly reinforced as patients can experience a degree of amnesia and forget what they were told due to the effects of the drugs administered during anaesthesia.

Once the patient is back on the ward they may still need to be connected to a cardiac monitor, but this will depend on the patient's condition and the type of surgery. However, all patients will need to have their observations monitored and the frequency of observations are dictated by local policy and the patient's condition (see Box 10.5).

BOX 10.5: FREQUENCY OF OBSERVATIONS

- 15 minutes for first hour, or until observations stabilise
- Hourly for four hours
- Then four hourly
- N.B. frequency of observations increases if condition deteriorates/NEWS total increases.

In addition to the usual vital signs, additional monitoring and assessment in relation to the surgery will include fluid balance, pain, PONV, IV cannula, wound sites and wound drains. It is also important that your patient is reconnected to supplemental oxygen as per their prescription to maintain their oxygen saturations, as well as ensuring that all medications are administered in a timely manner.

Once your patient is settled on the ward it is important to ensure that they commence oral hydration and subsequently nutrition in a timely manner, being mindful that this is not rushed and that this may not be possible if they need to remain nil by mouth post-surgery. This is especially important for the diabetic patient, who will need to recommence their usual diabetic regimen as soon as possible.

Not only will you be caring for your patient at this time, but as a ward nurse you will also be caring for the patient's family who may be on the ward at the time the patient returns and could have been waiting anxiously for some time for news of their loved one. It is important that both the patient and their family are aware of when to call for help, and that the patient has access to their call bell. It is also important that they are aware of the change in patient:nurse ratio on the ward, as this would have been 1:1 or 1:2 in the PACU, and will more than likely be a much bigger ratio on the ward.

CHAPTER SUMMARY

This chapter has provided an overview of the different stages of the patient journey and the care of the patient during their peri-operative journey.

- A thorough pre-operative assessment will reduce surgical and anaesthetic risk to the patient and enhance patient peri-operative experience
- Patient safety is maintained via risk assessment and management
- WHO Surgical Safety Checklist to prevent Never Events

- General and regional anaesthesia. Airway assessment and management is important to identify and select the most appropriate method of securing the patient's airway during surgery. It is also imperative that the peri-operative nurse has sound knowledge and understanding of anaesthetic drugs and their effects on the patient.
- Post-operative care of the patient should follow a systematic approach of 'Look, listen, feel'.

GO FURTHER

CASE STUDY: FUNDAMENTAL CARE

Go to https://study.sagepub.com/essentialadultnursing for a further case study related to this chapter. If you are using the interactive ebook, simply click on the book icon in the margin to go straight to the resource.

Books

- Miller, R.D. and Pardo, M.C. (2011) *Basics of Anaesthesia* (6th ed.). Philadelphia: Elsevier Saunders. Comprehensive textbook that covers key issues in the care of the patient undergoing anaesthesia.
- Odom-Forren, J. (2017) *Drain's PeriAnaesthesia Nursing: A Critical Care Approach* (7th ed.). St Louis, Missouri: Elsevier. Comprehensive textbook that covers key issues in the care of the post-anaesthetic patient.
- Rothrock, J.C. (2015) *Care of the Patient in Surgery* (15th ed.). USA: Elsevier. Essential read that covers principles of peri-operative practice and detailed description of surgical procedures.

Journal articles

FURTHER READING: JOURNAL ARTICLES

Go to https://study.sagepub.com/essentialadultnursing for further free online journal articles related to this chapter. If you are using the interactive ebook, simply click on the book icon in the margin to go straight to the resource.

- Garrett, J.H. (2016) Effective perioperative communication to enhance patient care. *AORN*, 104: 112-117.
  Article on various communication tools to improve communication in peri-operative settings.
- Adedeji, R., Oragui, E., Khan, W. and Maruthainar, N. (2010) The importance of correct patient positioning in theatres and implications of mal-positioning. *Journal of Perioperative Practice*, 20(4): 143-147. This article looks at the risks of patient positioning and how to minimise these risks.
- Malley, A., Kenner, C., Kim, T. and Blakeney, B. (2015) The role of the nurse and the preoperative assessment in patient transitions. *AORN*, 102(2): 181.e1-181.e9. Informative article that discusses a study on the role of the nurse within pre-operative assessment and their contribution to transitions in care within the peri-operative environment

Weblinks

FURTHER READING: WEBLINKS

Go to https://study.sagepub.com/essentialadultnursing for further weblinks related to this chapter. If you are using the interactive ebook, simply click on the book icon in the margin to go straight to the resource.

- The Association of Anaesthetists of Great Britain and Ireland: www.aagbi.org
  Useful website with publications and guidelines relating to anaesthesia and post-anaesthetic care.
- British Association of Day Surgery: https://daysurgeryuk.net/en/home/
  Useful website about day and short stay surgery for patients, relatives, carers and healthcare professionals.

- National Institute for Heath and Care Excellence NICE (2016) *Hypothermia: Prevention and management in adults having surgery*: www.nice.org.uk/guidance/cg65
  Guideline on preventing inadvertent peri-operative hypothermia.

ACE YOUR ASSESSMENT

ONLINE
QUIZZES

Revise what you have learned by visiting https://study.sagepub.com/essentialadultnursing

- Test yourself with multiple-choice and short-answer questions
- Do the chapter activities in the book and check your answers online

REFERENCES

Aitkenhead, A.R., Moppett, I.K. and Thompson, J.P. (2013) *Smith and Aitkenhead's Textbook of Anaesthesia* (6th ed.). London: Churchill Livingstone Elsevier.

American Society of Anesthesiologists (ASA) (2014) *ASA Physical Status Classification System.* Available at: www.asahq.org/resources/clinical-information/asa-physical-status-classification-system (accessed 14/02/18).

Association of Surgical Technologists (AST) (2017) *AST guidelines for best practices for wearing jewelry* [Online]. Available at: www.ast.org/uploadedFiles/Main_Site/Content/About_Us/Standard%20 Wearing%20Jewelry.pdf (accessed 20/12/17).

Chadwick, S. and Norman, A. (2012) Handover of responsibility for patients in the post-anaesthetic care unit (PACU). In Colvin J. and Peden, C. (eds) *Raising the Standard: A Compendium of Audit Recipes for Continuous Quality Improvement in Anaesthesia* (3rd ed.). London: Royal College of Anaesthetists, pp.130–1.

Cobbold, A. and Money, T. (2010) Regional anaesthesia : back to basics. *Journal of Perioperative Practice,* 20 (8): 288–93.

Fischer, H and Pinnock, C (2004) *Fundamentals of Regional Anaesthesia.* Cambridge: Cambridge University Press.

Francis (2013) *Report of the Mid Staffordshire NHS Foundation Trust Public Inquiry.* Available at: www. gov.uk/government/publications/report-of-the-mid-staffordshire-nhs-foundation-trust-public-inquiry (accessed 20/12/17).

Gwinnutt, C. and Gwinnutt, M. (2012) *Clinical Anaesthesia : Lecture Notes* (4th ed.). Chichester: Wiley-Blackwell.

Kelkar, U. S., Gogate, B., Kurpad, S., Gogate, P. and Deshpande, M. (2013) 'How effective are face masks in operation theatre? A time frame analysis and recommendations', *International Journal of Infection Control,* 9 (1): 1–6.

Miller, R.D. and Pardo, M.C. (2011) *Basics of Anaesthesia* (6th ed.). Philadelphia: Elsevier Saunders.

National Institute for Health and Care Excellence (NICE) (2013) *Surgical Site Infection. NICE quality standard 49.* Available at: www.nice.org.uk/guidance/qs49 (accessed 16/03/17).

National Institute for Health and Care Excellence (2016) *Routine Preoperative Tests for Elective Surgery. NICE guideline NG45.* Available at: www.nice.org.uk/guidance/ng45 (accessed 22/06/17).

National Patient Safety Agency (NPSA) (2007) *Healthcare risk assessment made easy* [Online]. Available at: www.nrls.npsa.nhs.uk/resources/?entryid45=59825&q=0%C2%ACrisk%C2%AC&p=3 (accessed on 15/03/17)

NHS England (2012) *Human Factors in Healthcare: A Concordat from the National Quality Board.* Available at: www.england.nhs.uk/wp-content/uploads/2013/11/nqb-hum-fact-concord.pdf (accessed 15/03/17).

NHS Modernisation Agency (2003) *National Good Practice Guidance on Pre-operative Assessment for Inpatient Surgery* [online]. Available at: http://www.hello.nhs.uk/documents/Preoperative%20 assessment%20guidance%20for%20inpatient.pdf (accessed 15/03/17)

Nursing and Midwifery Council (NMC) (2015) *The Code* [online]. Available at: www.nmc.org.uk/standards/code/ (accessed 15/03/17).

O'Driscoll, B.R., Howard, L.S., Earis, J. and Mak, V. (2017) British Thoracic Society Guideline for oxygen use in adults in healthcare and emergency settings. Thorax, 72 i1–ii90

Phillips, N. (2013) *Berry & Kohn's Operating Room Technique* (12th ed.). Missouri: Elsevier Mosby.

Pierre, S. and Whelan, R. (2013) Nausea and vomiting after surgery. *British Journal of Anaesthesia,* 13(1): 28–32.

Rothrock, J.C. (2015) *Care of the Patient in Surgery* (15th ed.). USA: Elsevier.

Royal College of Anaesthetists (2018) *Guidelines for the Provision of Anaesthesia Services (GPAS). Guidance on the provision of anaesthesia services for post-operative care 2018.* (Chapter 4). Available at: https://www.rcoa.ac.uk/gpas2018 (Accessed 7/10/2018)

Simpson, P. and Popat, M. (2002) *Understanding Anaesthesia* (4th ed.). Oxford: Butterworth-Heinemann

Tanner, J., Dumville, J.C., Norman, G. and Fortnam, M. (2016) *Surgical hand antisepsis to reduce surgical site infection.* Cochrane Database of Systematic Reviews [online]. Available at: http://cochranelibrary-wiley.com/doi/10.1002/14651858.CD004288.pub3/abstract;jsessionid=5A81ECF5 E577790ADDC3E88DCFCCD389.f02t04

The Association for Perioperative Practice (AfPP) (2014) *A Guide to Surgical Hand Antisepsis* [online]. Available at: https://www.afpp.org.uk/filegrab/surgical-hand-antisepsis-poster-final.pdf?ref=1908

The Association for Perioperative Practice (AfPP) (2017) *A Guide to Surgical Hand Antisepsis* [online]. Available at: https://www.afpp.org.uk/filegrab/1surgical-hand-antisepsis-poster-final-27.07.17. pdf?ref=2142

The Association of Anaesthetists of Great Britain and Ireland (AAGBI) (2010) *Management of Severe Local Anaesthetic Toxicity.* Available at: www.aagbi.org/sites/default/files/la_toxicity_2010_0.pdf (accessed 15/03/17).

The Association of Anaesthetists of Great Britain and Ireland (AAGBI) (2013) *AAGBI Safety Guideline: Immediate post-anaesthesia recovery.* Available at: www.aagbi.org/sites/default/files/immediate_post-anaesthesia_recovery_2013.pdf (accessed 12/06/17).

Walsgrove, H. (2011) History taking. In Radford, M., Williamson, A. and Evans, C. (eds) *Preoperative Assessment and Perioperative Management.* Keswick: M and K Update, pp.33–53.

World Health Organization (WHO) (2009) *WHO Guidelines for Safe Surgery 2009: Safe surgery saves lives.* Available at: www.WHO.int/patientsafety/safesurgery/tools_resources/9789241598552/en/ (accessed 14/02/18).

World Health Organisation (2009) WHO Surgical Safety Checklist. Available at: http://www.who.int/patientsafety/topics/safe-surgery/checklist/en/. (accessed 7/10/2018)

World Health Organization (WHO) (2017) *Patient Safety.* Available at: www.who.int/topics/patient_safety/en/ (accessed 20/12/17).

PAIN ASSESSMENT AND MANAGEMENT

ANN KETTYLE

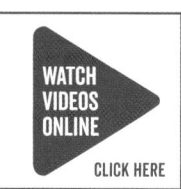

WATCH VIDEOS ONLINE

CLICK HERE

THIS CHAPTER COVERS

- The holistic assessment of pain
- Types of pain, their classification and potential causes
- Assessment of pain, non-verbal cues and tools (across all four fields of nursing)
- Pain assessment tools
- Biopsychosocial influences on pain
- The impact of cultural influences on pain assessment

- Management of pain
  - Management of acute pain
  - Management of persistent or cancer-related pain
- Impact of ineffective pain management.

REQUIRED KNOWLEDGE

- It will be helpful for you to have an understanding of the pathophysiology of pain before you start this chapter.

> " I was always in pain, it was my arthritis you see, and everyone kept telling me there was nothing they could do and that I should just keep taking the pain tablets. But they made me feel sick all the time and I didn't feel like eating. Then there was this new nurse at the GP's and she said that we should have a chat about it and see what we could do. She got me different medication and a review by the specialist doctor and now I am moving around a lot better and my appetite is back. "
>
> **Jeanette, patient**

> " As I get older I get more little niggles and it's always nice when someone listens to me and doesn't just hand me a tablet. "
>
> **Bill, patient**

INTRODUCTION

This chapter will provide information that will support you, as a nurse, in the assessment and management of pain to enhance patient recovery and quality of life. The routine assessment and management of pain is an essential skill required of all nurses (NMC 2018) and is an essential outcome for any patient. However, Wilson (2007) identified that a lack of nurses' knowledge has an impact on effective pain management.

All nurses should be familiar with McCaffrey's standard definition of pain: 'Pain is what the patient says it is' (Pasero and McCaffery, 2010). However, the problem with this definition is that it does not clearly identify that pain is not just a physical experience but also an emotional one endured by the individual. We will demonstrate throughout this chapter that, in order for you to better manage your patients' pain, it will be essential for you to recognise the emotional and psychological impact of the pain experience, as illustrated by the patient quotes above. This recognition and understanding will start with an accurate and relevant assessment of the pain your patient is describing.

We will also look at the differences between assessing and managing acute and chronic pain. Acute pain is often considered to be easier to manage as there is a foreseeable end to the pain event; however, you will learn throughout the chapter that it can be as complex and inadequately managed as chronic pain.

In 2015, the Faculty of Pain Medicine reported that approximately 14 million people in the UK live with chronic pain which affects their quality of life, at times prevents them from working, and impacts on their relationships with their families, significant others or carers. This chapter will demonstrate that nurses can, and sometimes do, disadvantage patients in their pain management. We will also look at how patients can sometimes disadvantage themselves in the management of their pain, as their own cultural and psychosocial influences can impact on their reception of the pain management measures suggested.

TYPES OF PAIN, THEIR CLASSIFICATION AND POTENTIAL CAUSES

There are two different types of pain:

Organic/Somatogenic pain – this is where there is a physical cause for the pain, e.g. injury/trauma, surgery or disease.

Psychogenic/Functional pain – this is where no physical reason can be found for the pain but the individual still experiences pain. This can be related to previously damaged tissue, which although healed can still generate pain, i.e. phantom limb pain.

Once you have identified the types of pain, you will then need to determine whether it is acute or chronic:

Acute pain is short term (less than 6 months) and is reversible if treated appropriately. It is usually of sudden onset and has a physical reason i.e. post-surgery or injury.

Chronic pain is pain that has lasted longer than 6 months and is related to an initial injury or disease, which has been treated, and is due to changes in the central nervous system. At this stage the pain may become the dominant disease (Pasero and McCaffery, 2010).

ACTIVITY 11.1: REFLECTIVE PRACTICE

ACTIVITY 11.1
ANSWER

- Take some time to reflect upon your own clinical practice.
- Can you identify examples of individuals with organic or psychogenic pain?
- Can you identify the pathophysiology of the pain process in those individuals?

Pain is classified according to its physiology, intensity, temporal characteristics, type of tissue affected and syndrome (these will be covered later in the chapter). Pain assessment must therefore be comprehensive and include:

- Classification of pain
- Pain physiology – nociceptive, neuropathic, inflammatory
- Intensity – mild, moderate, severe
- Time – acute or chronic
- Tissue involved – skin, muscles, viscera, joints, tendons, bones
- Syndrome/Disease – cancer, fibromyalgia, migraine, other.

ASSESSMENT OF PAIN, NON-VERBAL CUES AND TOOLS

Fayaz et al. (2015) identified that approximately one-third to one-half of the UK population are living with chronic pain while Gregory and McGowan (2016) report that 35% of inpatients experience severe pain with approximately 50% of medical patients reporting pain. It is unacceptable for patients to experience pain and for it not to be managed appropriately; effective pain management will ensure that the patient experiences increased comfort, higher levels of satisfaction with their care, less detrimental effects of the pain and improved outcome (Brennan et al., 2007).

The key to effective pain management is effective communication skills, accurate assessment using the most appropriate assessment tool and the knowledge and understanding to be able to select the most appropriate pain assessment tool(s) available to enable the appropriate **analgesic** to be administered.

When first considering pain it is essential to classify the type of pain being experienced, as this will allow you to identify appropriate interventions. Classification can be achieved by asking the patient some simple questions (see the box below).

ASSESSING TYPE OF PAIN

Quality	Is this pain new to you? How would you describe the pain, i.e. aching, sharp, burning, dull, etc.?
Impact	What impact does the pain have on you, i.e. does it affect sleep, activity, appetite? Does the pain stop you from doing anything?
Site	Where is the pain? Does it move or does the location of the pain change at all?
Severity	How bad is the pain? A numerical assessment score can be used to assist the patient to score the severity of the pain.

(Continued)

(Continued)

Time	When did the pain start - sudden/gradual? Was there a clear trigger for the pain? Is the pain constant or does it come and go? Is there any change or is it constant through the day?
Aggravating/ Alleviating factors	What makes the pain better/worse? When is the pain better and by how much? How long does the relief last for?
Past response	What have you done in the past to relieve the pain, was it through any medication (over the counter or prescribed), change of position or heat/cold? How effective was this? Did the medication cause you any problems (i.e. allergy); did you have to increase the dose or continue to take the medication?
Expectations	What do you think is causing the pain? What do you want us to do to help you? What do you think we should do to help with the pain? What do you hope that we will be able to achieve? What do you want to be able to do that the pain stops you from doing? What are you most afraid of? (This may uncover the fear of cancer or addiction to the medication.)

Once the pain assessment has been completed you will be able to undertake further observation of the site of the pain to identify any abnormal signs, i.e. swelling or redness. You should also ensure that a doctor, qualified nurse or nurse practitioner undertakes a full examination as soon as possible and prescribes analgesics; if any tests are ordered you should ensure that they are carried out and results fed back to them. It is essential that the prescribed analgesic is administered immediately and its efficacy evaluated within 20 minutes.

Once the description and characteristics of the pain experience are identified the continued assessment of pain can be undertaken through the use of a valid pain assessment tool and can be accurately documented and repeated by anyone using the same assessment tool. This is essential in monitoring the pain and the effect of any interventions.

The assessment of pain is a continuous process and by following a simple mnemonic you should always be able to cover and document the key aspects of the assessment and management of pain (see the box below).

MNEMONICS TO FACILITATE ASSESSMENT OF PAIN

ABCDE mnemonic:

Ask about pain regularly and **A**ssess pain systematically

Believe the patient and their family in their reports of pain

Choose appropriate pain control and **C**onsider the patient/family/setting

Deliver interventions

Evaluate efficacy of interventions and **E**mpower patients and their families/carers/significant others

PQRST mnemonic for chest or abdominal pain:

Palliative/**P**rovocative factors - What makes the pain worse?

Quality - Describe the pain

Radiation - Where is the pain? (May be more than one site)

Severity - Compare this pain to other pain previously experienced or the pain in the same location but at a previous time

Temporal factors/**T**ime - When does the pain start? How long does it last for? How often does the patient get the pain? What time of day is the pain better or worse?

REVIEW POTENTIAL OBSTACLES TO ACCURATE PAIN ASSESSMENT

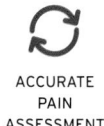

ACCURATE PAIN ASSESSMENT

ACTIVITY 11.2: REFLECTIVE PRACTICE

Reflect on the care of one or two patients where you identified that they might be in pain but they did not express this openly.

1. How did you know they were in pain?
2. Did you discuss this with them? If not, why not?
3. Why do you think the patient did not openly inform anyone that they were experiencing pain?
4. If you undertook a pain assessment, was it effective and did it support what you first thought?

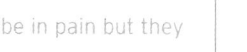

ACTIVITY 11.2 ANSWER

PAIN ASSESSMENT TOOLS

The first assessment tool is that of observation and even if there are communication barriers, non-verbal signs (cues) can indicate if someone is in pain. The patient may be showing obvious signs of distress such as crying or shouting or holding the painful area. But there are some less obvious, but discernable, signs that could be seen, for example, restlessness, becoming withdrawn, quiet or agitated, staying still, becoming pale or looking exhausted. You may also observe physical indicators of pain such as discolouration of the skin, pallor or neurological changes (such as reduced strength).

NON-VERBAL CUES/SIGNS

Observational assessment of pain should be accurately documented and there are tools to assist this, i.e. The Riley Infant Pain Scale and The PAINAD scale (Dipiro et al., 2017), which superseded the FLACC scale (Merkel et al., 1997). The Riley Infant Pain Scale reviews facial expression, sleep, movement, crying and touch using a Likert scale approach to rate the infant's movement in response to pain, but can be used for patients with a communication deficit. The PAINAD and FLACC scales were primarily developed for the elderly with cognitive impairment who demonstrate subtle changes in pain behaviour; however, due to their flexibility they may be appropriate for other patients with cognitive impairment. The PAINAD scale reviews breathing, vocalisation, facial expression, body language and consolability. The carer or nurse is required to score against the descriptors to identify whether pain is being experienced and to what level.

Peter and Watt-Watson (2002) state that the gold standard, and most valid, pain assessment is the patient's self-report of their pain and should include intensity of the pain, location and any associated anxiety or behaviour. However, lack of sleep, mood, and medications may affect the accuracy of the self-report. Furthermore, Watt-Watson et al. (2001) determined that nurses often distrust the patient's self-report of pain and often ignore or inaccurately document this report of pain or under-medicate even when self-reported pain scores are high. This is especially true in those experiencing chronic pain where understanding on the part of the healthcare provider results in increased patient satisfaction (Jenerette et al., 2015; Prem et al., 2011).

But what if the patient already has another condition and the related treatment is impacting on their perception of pain? They may be sedated or have depression, an anxiety disorder, a personality disorder or schizophrenia. This area of nursing is not researched sufficiently for assumptions to be made but you are advised to take due care when considering pain assessment for a patient with a known mental health condition. Furthermore, pain assessment must be completed along with measurement of vital signs as many medications in mental health nursing can cause serious physical illness; for example, in schizophrenia the use of antipsychotics increases the risk of **silent myocardial infarction.**

ACTIVITY 11.3
ANSWER

ACTIVITY 11.3: REFLECTIVE PRACTICE

Take some time to reflect on your own practice. Have you ever not believed a patient's self-report of pain? Ask yourself the following questions:

- Why did you not believe them?
- Did they show other signs of being in pain?
- How did you ascertain they really were in pain?

There is a vast range of pain assessment tools and they can be described as uni-dimensional or multi-dimensional. Uni-dimensional tools measure one aspect of the pain experience, i.e. intensity, and are quick and easy to use, whereas multi-dimensional tools acquire information about the quality of the pain as well as the intensity. These do, however, take longer to complete and require the patient to have good communication skills. To assess pain comprehensively you should use a combination of the two but may find that you are limited to the tools used in the practice area; however, this should not stop you from undertaking a full pain assessment in order to optimise care and outcome.

Table 11.1 Pain assessment tools

Uni-dimensional pain assessment tools	Multi-dimensional pain assessment tools
• Visual analogue scales or picture scales, i.e. Wong Baker, Riley Infant Pain Scale • Numerical rating or verbal descriptor scales, i.e. numeric pain intensity scale • Body diagrams	• McGill pain questionnaire (short and long) • Brief pain inventory (short and long) • Behavioural pain scales • Pain/comfort journals • Multi-dimensional pain inventory • Pain information and beliefs questionnaire • Pain and impairment relationship scale • Pain cognition questionnaire • Pain beliefs and perceptions inventory • Coping strategies questionnaire • Pain disability index

Uni-dimensional pain assessment tools	Multi-dimensional pain assessment tools
	• Hospital anxiety and depression questionnaire (HAD scale)
	• Neuropathic signs and symptoms, i.e. Leeds Assessment of Neuropathic Symptoms and Signs (Bennett, 2001)
	• Cognitively impaired/dementia pain scales, i.e. Abbey pain scale checklist for seniors with severe dementia (Royal College of Physicians et al., 2007).

ACTIVITY 11.4: REFLECTIVE PRACTICE

ACTIVITY 11.4
ANSWER

Reflect back on your own practice experience and the pain assessment tools you have used and consider:

1. Was the tool used the most appropriate?
2. Could you have used a different tool to obtain a more patient-centred assessment?

The above lists are not exhaustive and it is essential that the most appropriate assessment tool be used depending on the patient.

GO FURTHER

For pain assessment in those with a learning disability and dementia review the following articles:

• Beacroft, M. and Dodd, K. (2011) 'I Feel Pain' - audit of communication skills and understanding of pain and health needs with people with learning disabilities, *British Journal of Learning Disabilities*, 39 (2).
• Jones, S and Mitchell, G. (2015) Assessment of pain and alleviation of distress for people living with a dementia, *Mental Health Practice*, 18 (10), pp. 32-36.

Cognitive impairment is not limited to children as there are many adults who are unable to express their pain in a way that we understand, for example those with dementia or a learning disability. It is not that they do not experience pain, as is often thought, but that they have difficulty communicating their pain (Beacroft and Dodd, 2010). This impairment can mean that pain is underestimated and may ultimately lead to death if not appropriately managed. Many people assume that the parent of a child with a learning disability would know whether that child was experiencing pain. However, a study by Clarke et al. (2007) found that some parents did not identify that their child was in pain, at that time. Therefore, recognising the behavioural changes of an individual who is cognitively impaired is key to identifying whether they are experiencing pain, and there are tools to assist you, such as DisDAT (Regnard et al., 2007) or the Non-Communicating Adults Pain Checklist (NCAPC) (Meir et al., 2012). Pollard (2007) suggested that individual tools should be developed for each patient with a learning disability to ensure that pain is not overlooked in any hospital or care setting (Guidelines and Audit Implementation Network, 2010).

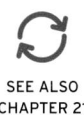

SEE ALSO
CHAPTER 21

Key factors for assessing pain in the older person are their communication skills, their reluctance to complain of pain (a cultural or social influence) and whether they have other conditions that may be impacting on the pain or their ability to communicate it.

BIOPSYCHOSOCIAL INFLUENCES ON PAIN

It is not only our cognitive ability that impacts on the assessment of pain but also our psychological, biological and social reaction to pain (the biopsychosocial perspective). The process of 'pain perception-cognitive awareness-appraisal-interpretation-pain behaviour' is fluidly influenced by the consequence of each stage but also limited by the cultural and social values of the individual. Linton and Shaw (2011) describe pain as a 'threat' that could provoke a flight/avoid/escape or fight response indicating that this response emphasises the link between pain, fear and anxiety and could result in increased anxiety or aggression (verbal or physical) on the part of the patient.

Everyone holds certain assumptions about how pain works and what it means to feel a certain stimulus and it is these beliefs that help us to process information more rapidly or automatically (Turk et al., 1999). However, our social setting also influences our beliefs/attitudes and our response to the pain, i.e. we may ignore pain if we are at work or we may take time off as pain means we need to rest (something we have learnt). Furthermore, our expectation of how long the pain should last will also have a link to our psychosocial wellbeing – if the pain lasts longer than expected, due to the condition or poor management by the healthcare professional, then we may have a negative attitude for future episodes of pain. When we process the pain we 'think' through the possible meaning and outcome; however, some individuals exaggerate what they are feeling, imagining the worst possible outcome, i.e. the pain is not going away, it will only get worse, it is so bad it must mean I have cancer. This over-exaggeration is called pain catastrophising and can have a negative impact on the outcome (Linton and Shaw, 2011).

ACTIVITY 11.5
ANSWER

ACTIVITY 11.5: REFLECTIVE PRACTICE

Consider your thoughts regarding the meaning of pain:

- Do you believe pain should be ignored?
- What does pain mean to you?

Summary of potential influences and possible outcomes

Table 11.2

Influences from service user, patient or healthcare professional	Influences from the process	Outcome

• Perception of illness
• Background beliefs about treatments, e.g. homeopathy, medicine, etc.
• Perception of the risks
• Individual personality
• Prejudices, e.g. attention-seeking behaviour
• Past experience
	• Is the process just looking at the biomedical side or also the emotional side?
	• Is the process giving the patient:
	  - Time
	  - Enough information in a way they can handle?
		• Is the patient benefiting:
		• Cognitively – are you taking into account or changing their beliefs about their illness, treatment, understanding and their fears?

Influences from service user, patient or healthcare professional	Influences from the process	Outcome
• Personal preferences and attitudes, i.e. you are the doctor so do what you need to, I want to be involved • Knowledge and information • Emotional state • Trust • Empathy • Environmental – are we in a place where we can discuss pain openly? • Abilities, i.e. vision, hearing, mobility • Concurrent medication and/or conditions	• Is the process person-centred and in partnership with them? • Is there a choice of treatment/interventions?	• Affectively – are you supporting and enhancing their emotional state and sense of satisfaction? • Behaviourally – are you supporting informed concordance to their treatment and the use of subsequent health and social care services?

THE IMPACT OF CULTURAL INFLUENCES ON PAIN ASSESSMENT

When assessing pain we should also consider cultural influences, not just of the patient but also of the nurse and doctor, which affect understanding of the meaning of pain and coping strategies. Some African cultures believe pain is the result of societal transgressions; some Nepalese believe back and joint pain to be a normal part of aging (Clark-Callister, 2003; Campbell and Edwards, 2012). Coping strategies also vary across cultures – the Japanese have a cultural emphasis on stoicism, some cultures ululate loudly to express their pain, while others release a quiet 'whee' sound. Whatever our attitude, society or culture and upbringing we all experience pain differently and so you must ensure that you ask those in your care what pain means to them and how they cope with it. The most important thing, however, is to believe the patient about their experience of pain.

ACTIVITY 11.6: REFLECTIVE PRACTICE

Think about a situation that you have encountered where analgesics were withheld or not given when the patient required it; can you identify the main obstacle to achieving **analgesia**?

ACTIVITY 11.6 ANSWER

MANAGEMENT OF PAIN

The management of pain depends on the pain classification; if pain is classified as acute then management will generally be through medication, which is time limited to the duration of the pain. Chronic pain, however, will normally encompass medication and adjunct therapies, such as physiotherapy and/or occupational therapy, and may never end. Pain is a warning signal and it should never be ignored, either by patients or by health professionals. However, as a nurse you should bear in mind that it is possible for patients to ignore their own pain. If the pain is chronic, patients may have become accustomed to it and no longer recognise it, or if, for example, someone is in an accident, they may be distracted by the accident itself and not recognise the pain they are in. This capacity to be distracted allows the 'attention' message to be interrupted (by distracting the patient) and, to some extent, alleviate the pain.

Whichever type of pain is experienced the initial, and most important, component of pain management is the patient closely followed by you, the nurse. Your experience and communication skills will enable you to support the patient in effectively managing their pain. You should start by asking them their preferences:

ACUTE PAIN

- What have you done in the past/been given to manage this type of pain? You may ask this of a carer or family member/parent.
- Would you like to try this action for this pain?

MANAGEMENT OF ACUTE PAIN

Acute or **nociceptive pain** occurs as a result of 'injury' to the body (trauma, **myocardial infarction** or surgery), infection (appendicitis, ear infection) or disease and can be divided into somatic or visceral pain. Somatic pain is localised and commonly described as pinprick, sharp or stabbing; the pain mechanism is activation of the delta fibre in the periphery and is associated with superficial injury (laceration or burn). In visceral pain the mechanism is activation of the C fibre and is commonly described as aching, pressure or difficult to localise. A third type of pain associated with acute pain is neuropathic pain, also a chronic pain, which is described as burning, pricking, tingling and is a result of a peripheral or central activation of the nerve fibres, e.g. post-traumatic neuralgia, limb amputation (phantom limb syndrome). Another form of acute pain is referred pain; this is where the nociceptors in the viscera are activated, which results in the perception of pain in a body surface. For example, myocardial pain in a heart attack is felt as pain in the inner aspect of the left arm, and pain in the tip of the shoulder usually comes from irritation of the central region of the diaphragm.

The medical management of acute pain is primarily medication and the National Institute for Health and Care Excellence (NICE) publishes guidelines on a regular basis, with other professional bodies, to assist you in managing pain effectively.

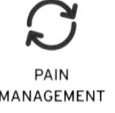

PAIN MANAGEMENT

Your intervention can reduce some of the complications associated with pain – remember, you must never ignore someone in pain. Pain is not normal or to be expected and while the patient is waiting for their analgesic there are some things that you can do to reduce the risks or to relieve the pain completely.

ACTIVITY 11.7: CRITICAL THINKING

Before we go on to discuss analgesics, consider how you might assist a patient in managing their pain.

Following a landmark report 'Pain after Surgery' (Royal College of Surgeons/College of Anaesthetists, 1990), which identified that pain management was inequitable, all major hospitals have been using an acute pain service (APS) and this can be accessed by community teams. The service consists of an anaesthetist, an acute pain clinical nurse specialist, a pharmacist, a physiotherapist and, at times, a clinical psychologist. However, the APS may not provide 24-hour cover or you may encounter someone in acute pain in a different setting so it is essential that you understand the pharmacological approaches to pain management.

Analgesics are available in a range of preparations to facilitate the effectiveness of the pain relief and to accommodate the patient's preference. The choice of route will affect the absorption rate of the medication and thus the time it takes for the drug to work.

Routes

- Oral
- Oral transmucosal absorption, either sublingual or buccal – administered orally and absorbed through the mucosa in the mouth
- Transdermal – the drug is administered through the skin, usually through an adhesive patch
- Rectal – a preferred route to oral administration if the patient is nauseous or vomiting, e.g. morphine or paracetamol
- Parenteral – the drug is administered as an injection or infusion.

ROUTES OF
ADMINISTRATION

A key consideration in analgesia is that each individual will absorb and respond to the analgesic drug in different ways and this can be seen by the variable requirements of each patient. However, there are some standard protocols to be followed to ensure that the patient receives effective pain control and the most efficient method is a **titrated** approach as this allows you to determine the least powerful drug to be administered to achieve the most effective pain relief.

Once you have completed a pain assessment and established that the patient requires analgesia and for which type of pain, you must administer the medication as quickly and safely as possible. If the patient has an appropriate preference for a type of analgesic this must be considered and the prescriber must discuss this with the patient to ensure that they receive optimum analgesia.

SEE ALSO
CHAPTER 13

The type of pain will also determine the intervention/analgesic (see Table 11.3 below and acute pain analgesics):

Table 11.3 Summary of types of acute pain and possible interventions

Type of pain	Examples	Intervention
Somatic pain	IV access	Cold packs
(localised pain)	Otitis media	Tactile stimulation
	Extensive abrasions	Paracetamol
	Stomatitis	Non-steroidal anti-inflammatory drugs (NSAIDs)
		Opioids
		Local anaesthetic
Visceral pain	Joint/muscle injury	NSAIDs
(generalised)	Colic and muscle spasm	Opioids
	Sickle cell crisis	Intraspinal local anaesthetic
	Appendicitis	Antispasmodic drugs
	Kidney stones	Paracetamol

It is essential that you monitor the patient after administration of any analgesic for signs of distress or any side effects, e.g. an **opioid** may cause respiratory depression and many analgesics cause nausea. Any side effects must be treated promptly to ensure the safety and comfort of the patient, for example administering naloxone in cases of respiratory depression caused by opioid administration. Reassessment of pain following analgesia is commonly overlooked and results in ineffective pain management and outcomes so it is essential that the pain level is reassessed, approximately 20 minutes after the analgesic has been administered, to ensure that it has been effective; if there is no relief then the patient must be reviewed by a doctor or nurse prescriber for the consideration of further or different analgesics (Bucknall et al., 2007). Pain relief must be administered regularly to achieve optimum comfort; however, if pain relief has initially been effective but the patient then complains of further pain you should review the patient to identify any other factors, reassess the pain and administer any other appropriate medication (e.g. an anti-emetic), as this may indicate a deterioration in their condition. At times **adjuvant** medication, a drug given to enhance the analgesic effect, should also be considered (see Table 11.4).

Table 11.4   Adjuvant therapy

Type of pain	Example drug
Muscle	Baclofen or diazepam
Gut spasm or colicky pain	Buscopan
Ischaemic pain, which tingles or shoots	Gabapentin
Ischaemic pain, which burns	Amitriptyline

However, if any of the above adjuvant medications are prescribed they must be taken as directed and never stopped without first discussing with a doctor.

MANAGEMENT OF PERSISTENT OR CANCER-RELATED PAIN

Persistent or cancer-related pain has the most detrimental, long-term impact on an individual and, therefore, its effective management can have a positive effect on the individual's quality of life. The World Health Organization (WHO) (1986) three-step 'ladder' is the 'gold standard' for managing this type of pain (see Figure 11.1).

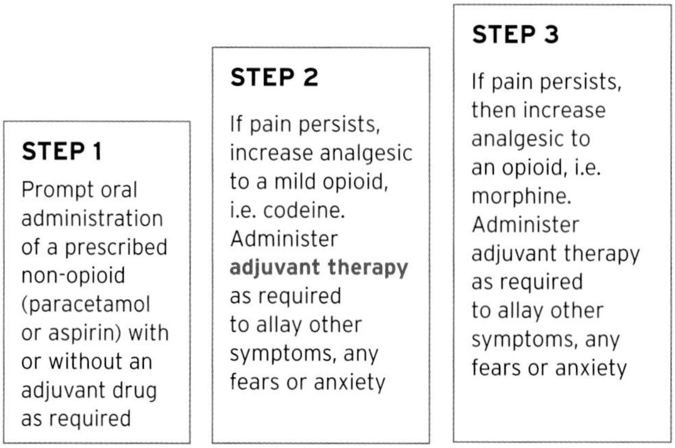

STEP 1
Prompt oral administration of a prescribed non-opioid (paracetamol or aspirin) with or without an adjuvant drug as required

STEP 2
If pain persists, increase analgesic to a mild opioid, i.e. codeine. Administer **adjuvant therapy** as required to allay other symptoms, any fears or anxiety

STEP 3
If pain persists, then increase analgesic to an opioid, i.e. morphine. Administer adjuvant therapy as required to allay other symptoms, any fears or anxiety

Figure 11.1   Pain-relief ladder (WHO, 1986)

However, to better understand the pain experience the pain management team may ask the patient to keep a diary of their pain experience, including what aggravates it, what relieves it and how often it occurs.

BIOPSYCHOSOCIAL APPROACH TO PAIN MANAGEMENT

If analgesia is not achieved then different approaches can be used, using the biopsychosocial approach, to establish an acceptable degree of comfort, minimise the impact to the patient and enhance their quality of life. By using the biopsychosocial approach you can improve the outcome of not only the pain intensity but also of the patient's mood, distress, sleep disruption, social functioning, active coping and medication use. However, too much support can make a patient feel useless or wanting more which can lead to greater disability and depression. The principal person in managing chronic pain is the patient and by supporting, and working with them to develop coping skills you will enhance their pain management.

It is important to identify and be aware of an individual's coping strategies so as to ascertain when they are no longer coping, and there are many tools available to assess these. Most coping strategy assessment tools cover illness focus and wellness focus by scoring the individual on the following:

- Ability to move/restriction of movement
- How often and when they need to rest
- How often and why they ask for assistance
- How much/little they exercise
- What they do to relax
- Whether they are able to perform tasks without difficulty (i.e. pace and persistence)
- Self-statements to manage pain
- Frequency of requesting social support.

These types of tools are usually called pain-coping inventories and most care environments will have access to one or more examples so you will be able to choose the most appropriate one for your patient.

ACTIVITY 11.8: REFLECTIVE PRACTICE

Take some time to reflect back on your clinical practice and identify one or more ways in which you observed a patient coping with their pain with/without any analgesic.

ACTIVITY 11.8
ANSWER

Coping strategies can be classified as active (internal) or passive (external) control; external control centres on what others can do to help an individual to manage their pain and is associated with greater pain, disability and depression whereas internal/active coping is associated with an enhanced outcome. However, the way that the patient focuses on their pain is just as crucial – if they are problem focused they will plan to deal with the pain and take action whereas if they are emotionally focused they try to alter their response to the pain and this results in ineffective pain management. However, the effect of any coping strategy will depend upon the individual, the pain itself, the emotions generated by the pain, the effectiveness of the distraction, access to healthcare interventions, social support and other resources available.

Your focus, when working with other healthcare professionals to help a patient manage their chronic pain, should be on changing thoughts, emotions and behaviours related to pain, helping them to cope with the reality of their condition, developing relaxation techniques, use of imagery/hypnosis/meditation, stress and anger management, and developing positive sleep behaviours.

An effective way of supporting the patient is through the use of **contextual cognitive behavioural therapy** (CCBT). A therapist will work with the patient to help them accept that their negative beliefs about their pain are accurate, assist them in developing realistic expectations of their condition and support them in the management of their pain (McCracken, 2005). CCBT also supports the individual to review and reset their goals/priorities, rather than focusing on their pain, and adjusting their lifestyle to achieve their goals, e.g. personal relationships. Furthermore, CCBT is recognised to be effective in reducing the pain experience, enhancing positive coping and reducing the behavioural expressions of pain and, with a multidisciplinary approach, the patient may be able to resume previously lost activities and have greater pain control (Guzmán et al., 2001).

PAIN
CLINICS

NEXT STEPS - THE PAIN CLINIC

The patient could also be referred to the pain clinic, where they can be assessed by a specialist multidisciplinary team who have a greater understanding of the pain process and management. The referral process can, however, be difficult and there needs to be greater education of healthcare staff as well as an increase in provision of specialist staff and pain clinics.

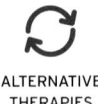

ALTERNATIVE
THERAPIES

It may be in part be due to the difficulty in accessing pain clinics that some people turn to alternative therapies. Some alternative therapies can be helpful and are offered on the NHS, e.g. aromatherapy in cancer care services; however, their use and efficacy is limited (Kwong et al., 2017). Other alternative therapies that may improve pain include: acupressure, physical manipulation, spinal cord stimulation and the use of **Entonox**, especially in cases of fracture.

ACTIVITY 11.9
ANSWER

ACTIVITY 11.9: CRITICAL REFLECTION

Reflect on an episode in practice where pain was effectively managed and consider:

- how the MDT was involved in the pain management;
- what was the evidence-based approach to the pain management used?

ANALGESIA

SYMPTOM CONTROL OF ANALGESIC SIDE EFFECTS

Many patients do not like taking analgesics due to the related side effects, i.e. drowsiness, nausea and vomiting; however, these can be managed while achieving optimal pain control and should be discussed with the patient prior to taking any action. It is essential that you always check for side effects in the computer-based formulary or the British National Formulary, which should be your best friend. However, it is essential that you know about common side effects so that you can intervene early. Visit the web link for common side effects of frequently used analgesics.

OPTIONS FOR MANAGING ANALGESIC-RELATED SIDE EFFECTS

Care should be taken when considering the management of side effects and you should always identify the exact cause of the side effect, to rule out other causes, and then consider the non-pharmacological approach first. The introduction of any further medication should only be considered after careful review of the patient's condition and history and after discussion with the patient/family/carer. For non-opioid analgesics the side effects can, at times, be managed by:

- reducing the dose of the analgesic, however it is important to titrate this to maintain pain control;
- changing the medication to a different one;
- changing the route of administration, i.e. from oral to transdermal route.

Other common side effects can be managed as follows:

- Constipation:
  - introducing a high-fibre diet
  - increasing fluid intake
  - increasing physical activity
  - ensuring that a mild laxative is also prescribed
  - enemas and suppositories if the above are ineffective.
- Nausea:
  - related to eating can be managed by prescription and administration of an anti-emetic, e.g. metoclopramide
  - related to movement or position (usually in the older patient) can be managed by one of the following:
    - anticholinergics
    - antihistamines
    - phenothiazines (e.g. prochlorperazine).
- Sedation can occur in up to 60% of patients and is more common in older adults. It can be managed by reviewing all of the patient's medication in order to minimise **polypharmacy** or where appropriate reduce the dose of, or change, the medication.
- Pruritus:
  - Anti-histamines – however, this should be done with caution in older adults as they also have side effects, i.e. dry mouth, constipation, blurred vision and confusion
  - A topical lotion.

The management of side effects in long- or short-term opioid therapy has been summarised on the web site; however, your immediate responsibility is to observe for respiratory depression and act immediately.

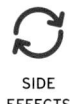

SIDE
EFFECTS

IMPACT OF INEFFECTIVE PAIN MANAGEMENT

Pain is thought to activate the stress response to injury; this in turn increases sympathetic nervous system activity, the release of catabolic hormones, impaired immune function and increased coagulation. We will now look at the physical impact to the patient.

If the sympathetic nervous system is activated, the heart rate, blood pressure and systemic vascular resistance is increased, which means that cardiac workload is increased and the heart needs more oxygen.

If demand exceeds delivery the heart can be 'injured' (myocardial ischaemia or infarction). If the patient already has a heart condition then this can make things even worse. If there are changes in local blood flow then the supply to the skin is decreased which impairs wound healing.

The pain-associated stress response can increase the rate of coagulation and this, along with reduced mobility due to pain, can increase the risk of thromboembolic complications, i.e. deep vein thrombosis (DVT) or pulmonary embolism (PE).

If the patient is experiencing severe pain in the upper abdomen or chest this can impair the depth of breathing and prevent the patient from being able to clear sputum or any excretions. The result could be less oxygen in the blood (hypoxaemia), lower respiratory tract infections and partial collapse or incomplete inflation of the lung (**atelectasis**).

The increased release of catabolic hormones can lead to increased protein breakdown, which can impair wound healing, and hyperglycaemia. This, along with immobility, can lead to muscle wasting, especially in the elderly; the end result is delayed healing and recovery.

The experience of ongoing (chronic) pain can often lead to depression due to individuals feeling restricted by their pain, having to make adjustments (sometimes detrimental) to their life in order to cope, feeling under pressure all of the time to carry on or because they are unable to maintain any physical activity (Goesling et al., 2013).

One of the most upsetting aspects of pain is the emotional distress that it causes, not only to the patient but also to family and friends; if pain is experienced then there is the perception that something is wrong and our welfare is threatened. This negative effect prompts common reactions to pain such as worry or fear of the unknown, anxiety, anger, frustration and depression. These negative responses to pain can impact on pain management, delay healing, heighten the pain experience or cause disability; therefore, we must also address the psychological wellbeing of the patient when we consider the management of pain. An individual's positive reaction to the pain experience (self-efficacy, personal control, expecting a positive outcome) can have a beneficial influence on the outcome. An example of this positive approach is that of needing to keep active when experiencing back pain rather than resting; in chronic back pain continuing to be active maintains movement, reduces risk of deterioration and reduces the disability experienced (Meng and Yue, 2015).

> I had experienced neuropathic pain from a neck injury, resulting in permanent head pain, for seven years before the surgeons could do anything about it. It left me feeling low and frustrated. However the most effective treatment I ever had was with a pain specialist nurse who actually listened to me and helped me to come to terms with the pain. He always asked me how the pain was affecting my life and listened to my answers; he helped me to develop ways to manage the pain and how I could still keep active, with some limitations.
>
> Anon

CHAPTER SUMMARY

On reading this chapter you will have developed your understanding of:

- The types of pain, their classification and potential causes
- Holistic assessment of pain, non-verbal cues and tools
- Pain assessment tools

- The biopsychosocial influences on pain
- The impact of cultural influences on pain assessment
- The management of pain including:
  - o   acute pain
  - o   persistent or cancer-related pain
- The impact of ineffective pain management.

——————— GO FURTHER ———————

Go to https://study.sagepub.com/essentialadultnursing for a further case study related to this chapter. If you are using the interactive ebook, simply click on the book icon in the margin to go straight to the resource.

CASE STUDY: HOSPITAL DISCHARGE

Books

- MacIntyre, P. and Schug, S. (2015) *Acute Pain Management: A Practical Guide* (4th ed.). Apple Academic Press Inc.: Oakville, Canada.
- Van Griensven, H., Strong, J. and Unruh, A (2013) *Pain* (2nd ed.). Edinburgh: Churchill Livingstone.
- Pasero, C. and McCaffery, M. (2010) *Pain Assessment and Pharmacologic Management*. Maryland Heights, MO: Mosby.

Journal Articles

Go to https://study.sagepub.com/essentialadultnursing for further free online journal articles related to this chapter. If you are using the interactive ebook, simply click on the book icon in the margin to go straight to the resource.

FURTHER READING: JOURNAL ARTICLES

- Urban-Kowalczyk, M., Pigońska, J. and Śmigielski, J. (2015) Pain perception in schizophrenia: Influence of neuropeptides, cognitive disorders, and negative symptoms. *Neuropsychiatric Disease and Treatment*, 11: 2023-31. http://doi.org/10.2147/NDT.S87666
- Potvin, S. and Marchand, S. (2008) Hypoalgesia in schizophrenia is independent of antipsychotic drugs: A systematic quantitative review of experimental studies. *Pain*, 138: 70-8. S0304-3959(07)00676-8 [pii]; doi: 10.1016/j.pain.2007.11.007 PMID: 18160219
- Al-Hashimi, M., Scott, S., Griffin-Teall, N. and Thompson, J. (2014) Influence of ethnicity on the perception and treatment of early post-operative pain. *British Journal of Pain*, 9 (3): 167-72. doi: 10.1177/2049463714559254

Weblinks

Go to https://study.sagepub.com/essentialadultnursing for further weblinks related to this chapter. If you are using the interactive ebook, simply click on the book icon in the margin to go straight to the resource.

FURTHER READING: WEBLINKS

- http://painconcern.org.uk/self-management-videos/breakingbarriers/self-management-vid/
- Pain Concern: http://painconcern.org.uk/
- National Institute for Health and Care Excellence (2012) Sickle Cell Disease: managing acute painful episodes in hospital. Available at: www.nice.org.uk/guidance/cg143
- National Institute for Health and Care Excellence (2017) Neuropathic pain in adults: pharmacological interventions in non-specialist settings. Available at: www.nice.org.uk/guidance/cg173
- National Institute for Health and Care Excellence (2016) Palliative care for adults: strong opioids for pain relief. Available at: www.nice.org.uk/guidance/cg140

- Scottish Intercollegiate Guidelines Network (SIGN) Management of Chronic Pain. Available at: https://www.sign.ac.uk/assets/sign136.pdf
- The British Pain Society: www.britishpainsociety.org/
  An excellent resource covering pain management across the lifespan and fields of nursing.

Commonly Used Guidelines

- Guidelines on acute pain management (ANZCA, 2013). Available at: www.anzca.edu.au/documents/ps41-2013-guidelines-on-acute-pain-management
- Practice guidelines for acute pain management in the perioperative setting (ASA, 2012). Available at: www.asahq.org/~/media/Sites/ASAHQ/Files/Public/Resources/standards-guidelines/practice-guide-lines-for-acute-pain-management-in-the-perioperative-setting.pdf
- Management of pain following acute stroke (University of Glasgow and NHS QIS, 2011). Available at: www.healthcareimprovementscotland.org/his/idoc.ashx?docid=5a14b14b-d75b-446e-ac03-86e15aa90ef2&version=-1
- Chest pain management. Available at: https://cks.nice.org.uk/chest-pain#!topicsummary
- Pharmacological management of cancer pain in adults. Available at: http://health.gov.ie/wp-content/uploads/2016/01/Pharma-Mgmt-Cancer-Pain.pdf
- Pain management for older people with learning difficulties and dementia (Joseph Rowntree Foundation, 2006). Available at: www.jrf.org.uk/report/pain-management-older-people-learning-diffi culties-and-dementia
- The College of Emergency Medicine: Management of pain in adults (2014). Available at: www.rcem.ac.uk/docs/College%20Guidelines/5w.%20Management%20of%20Pain%20in%20Adults%20(Revised%20December%202014).pdf

ONLINE QUIZZES

————— ACE YOUR ASSESSMENT —————

Revise what you have learned by visiting https://study.sagepub.com/essentialadultnursing

- Test yourself with multiple-choice and short-answer questions
- Do the chapter activities in the book and check your answers online

REFERENCES

Beacroft, M. and Dodd, K. (2010) 'I Feel Pain' – audit of communication skills and understanding of pain and health needs with people with learning disabilities. *British Journal of Learning Disabilities,* 39: 139–47. doi:10.1111/j.1468-3156.2010.00640.x

Brennan, F., Carr, D. and Cousins, M. (2007) Pain Management: a fundamental human right. *Anesthesia and analgesia,* 105 (1): 205–21. doi: 10.1213/01.ane.0000268145.52345.55

Bucknall, T., Manias, E. and Botti, M. (2007) Nurses' reassessment of postoperative pain after analgesic administration. *Clinical Journal of Pain,* 23(1): 1–7. Available at: www.ncbi.nlm.nih.gov/pubmed/17277638

Campbell, C.M. and Edwards, R.R. (2012) Ethnic differences in pain and pain management. *Pain Management,* 2(3): 219–30. http://doi.org/10.2217/pmt.12.7

Clark-Callister, L. (2003) Cultural influences on pain perceptions and behaviours. *Home Health Care Management & Practice.* 15 (3): 207–11. doi: 10.1177/1084822302250687

Clarke Z.J., Thompson A.R., Buchan L. and Combes H. (2007) Parents' experiences of pain and discomfort in people with learning disabilities. *British Journal of Learning Disabilities*, 36: 84–90.

The College of Emergency Medicine (2014) *Management of pain in adults*. Available at: www.rcem. ac.uk/docs/College%20Guidelines/5w.%20Management%20of%20Pain%20in%20Adults%20 (Revised%20December%202014).pdf

Dipiro, J.T., Talbert, R.L., Yee, G.C., Matzke, G.R., Wells, B.G. and Posey, L.M. (2017) *Pharmacotherapy: A Pathophysiologic Approach* (10th ed.). New York: McGraw-Hill

Faculty of Pain Medicine (2015) *Core Standards for Pain Management Services in the UK*. Available at: www.rcoa.ac.uk/system/files/FPM-CSPMS-UK2015.pdf

Fayaz, A., Croft, P., Langfrod, R.M., Donaldson, L.J. and Jones, G.T. (2016) Prevalence of chronic pain in the UK: a systematic review and meta-analysis of population studies, *BMJ Open*, 6 (6). Available at: http://bmjopen.bmj.com/content/6/6/e010364

Goesling, J., Clauw, D.J. and Hassett, A.L. (2013) Pain and depression: an integrative review of neurobiological and psychological factors. *Psychiatry Reports* (2013)15: 421. doi:10.1007/s11920-013-0421-0

Gregory, J. and McGowan, L. (2016) An examination of the prevalence of acute pain for hospitalised adult patients: a systematic review. *Journal of Clinical Nursing*, 25(5–6):583–98. doi: 10.1111/jocn.13094.

Guidelines and Audit Implementation Network, (2010) *Guidelines on Caring For People with a Learning Disability in General Hospital Settings*. Available at: https://rqia.org.uk/RQIA/files/81/81662c46-b7bb-43a5-9496-a7f2d919c2a3.pdf

Guzmán, J., Esmail, R., Karjalainen, K., Malmivaara, A., Irvin, E. and Bombardier, C. (2001) Multidisciplinary rehabilitation for chronic low back pain: systematic review. *BMJ*, 322: 1511–16.

Jenerette, C.M., Pierre-Louis, B.J., Mathie, N. and Girardeau, Y. (2015) Nurses' attitudes toward patients with sickle cell disease: a worksite comparison. *Pain Management Nursing*, 16(3): 173–81 http://dx.doi.org/10.1016/j.pmn.2014.06.007

Jones, S and Mitchell, G. (2015) Assessment of pain and alleviation of distress for people living with a dementia, Mental Health Practice, 18 (10), pp. 32–36.

Joseph Rowntree Foundation (2006) *Pain management for older people with learning difficulties and dementia*. Available at: www.jrf.org.uk/report/pain-management-older-people-learning-difficulties-and-dementia

Kwong, A., Ho, S., Wan, K., Ho, R. and Chow, K. (2017) Experiences of aromatherapy massage among adult female cancer patients: a qualitative study. *Journal of Clinical Nursing*. 26 (23–24): 4519–26 doi:10.1111/jocn.13784

Linton, S. and Shaw, W. (2011) Impact of psychological factors in the experience of pain. *Physical Therapy*, 91(5): 700–711. Available at: http://dx.doi.org/10.2522/ptj.20100330

McCracken, L. (2005) *Contextual Cognitive-behavioral Therapy for Chronic Pain*. Seattle: IASP Press.

Meir, L., Inger Strand, L. and Alice, K. (2012) A model for pain behavior in individuals with intellectual and developmental disabilities. *Research in Developmental Disabilities*, 33 (6): 1984–9. Available at: www.sciencedirect.com/science/article/pii/S0891422212001461

Meng, X.G. and Yue, S.W. (2015) Efficacy of aerobic exercise for treatment of chronic low back pain: a meta-analysis. American Journal of Physical Medical Rehabilitation, 94(5): 358–65. doi: 10.1097/PHM.0000000000000188. Available at: www.ncbi.nlm.nih.gov/pubmed/25299528

Merkel, S.I., Voepel-Lewis, T., Shayevitz, J.R. and Malviya, S. (1997) The FLACC: a behavioral scale for scoring postoperative pain in young children. *Pediatric Nursing*, 23(3): 293–7.

Nursing and Midwifery Council (NMC) (2018) *Standards of proficiency for registered nurses* [online]. Available at: www.nmc.org.uk/standards/standards-for-nurses/standards-of-proficiency-for-registered-nurses/

Peter, E. and Watt-Watson, J. (2002) Unrelieved pain: an ethical and epistemological analysis of distrust in patients. *Canadian Journal of Research*, 34 (2): 65–80.

Pollard, M. (2007) Is it pain? A framework for identifying pain in people with learning disabilities. *Learning Disability Practice*, 10 (6): 12–14. Available at: http://journals.rcni.com/doi/pdfplus/10.7748/ldp2007.07.10.6.12.c4271

Potvin, S. and Marchand, S. (2008) Hypoalgesia in schizophrenia is independent of antipsychotic drugs: a systematic quantitative review of experimental studies. *Pain*, 138: 70–78. S0304-3959(07)00676-8 [pii]; doi: 10.1016/j.pain.2007.11.007 PMID: 18160219

Prem, V., Karvannan, H., Chakravarthy, R.D., Jaykumar, S. and Kumar, S.P. (2011) Attitudes and beliefs about chronic pain among nurses – biomedical or behavioral? A cross-sectional survey. *Indian Journal of Palliative Care*, 17(3): 227–34. doi: 10.4103/0973-1075.92341

Regnard, C., Reynolds, J., Watson, B., Matthews, D., Gibson, L. and Clarke, C. (2007) Understanding distress in people with severe communication difficulties: developing and assessing the Disability Distress Assessment Tool (DisDAT), *Journal of Intellectual Disabilities Research*, 51: 277–92.

Royal College of Physicians, British Geriatrics Society, British Pain Society (2007) *The Assessment of Pain in Older People; National Guidelines. Concise guidance on good practice series, No 8.* London: RCP.

Royal College of Surgeons of England, College of Anaesthetists (1990) *Report of the Working Party on Pain after Surgery.* London.

Turk, D., Melzack, R., DeGood, D.E. and Shutty, M.S. (1999) Assessment of pain beliefs, coping, and self-efficacy. In Turk, D.C. and Melzack, R. (eds) *Handbook of Pain Assessment.* New York: Guilford, pp.320–45.

Watt-Watson, J., Stevens B., Garfinkel, P., Streiner, D. and Gallop, R. (2001) Relationship between nurses' pain knowledge and pain management outcomes for their postoperative cardiac patients. *Journal of Advanced Nursing*, 36(4): 535–45.

Wilson, B. (2007) Nurses' knowledge of pain. *Journal of Clinical Nursing*, 16: 1012–20. doi: 10.1111/j.1365-2702.2007.01692.x

World Health Organization (WHO) (2018) *WHO's cancer pain ladder for adults* [online]. Available at: www.who.int/cancer/palliative/painladder/en/

CLINICAL INVESTIGATIONS

12

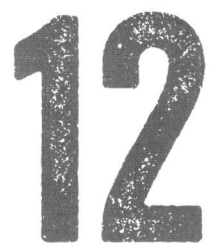

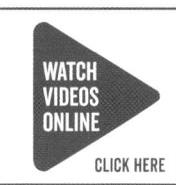

WATCH VIDEOS ONLINE

CLICK HERE

STEVE BEACH

THIS CHAPTER COVERS

- The clinical indication, patient preparation and care of the patient undergoing the following investigations.
  - Urinalysis
  - Bladder scanning
  - Capillary blood glucose
  - Venous blood tests
  - Electrocardiograph
  - Spirometry

  - Arterial blood gas
  - Arterial blood pressure
  - Central venous pressure
  - X-ray
  - Ultrasound
  - Computed tomography scans
  - Magnetic resonance imaging
  - Endoscopy.

My name is John and I am a nurse practitioner with a hospital at night team at a large teaching hospital. I use clinical investigations from blood glucose measurement and urinalysis to arterial blood gases and x-rays. These are valuable in assisting in making a differential diagnosis, monitoring disease process and reacting appropriately to treatments, such as settings for non-invasive ventilation and the rate for sliding scale insulin regimes.

However, it's important to remember that I should not rely on clinical investigations to make a diagnosis, but instead assist with constructing the most likely differential diagnosis.

As an autonomous practitioner, I am responsible for certain investigations from the ordering to the interpretation of the results. I have to ensure that the optimal information is available when requesting an investigation in order to give rationale for the request, especially if involving radiation. I also have the responsibility for interpreting certain results within my sphere of competence. I may then adjust treatment plans accordingly.

John, Hospital at Night Nurse Practitioner

My name is Jo and I am a 3rd year student nurse currently on placement on an acute medical ward. In my first two years, I assisted with and was exposed to a number of clinical investigations. At times I was not always fully aware of their diagnostic or therapeutic use. Now in my final year I am ensuring that I question the indication for all investigations I am involved in and am learning all the specific nursing care and preparation.

Jo, 3rd year student nurse

INTRODUCTION

Clinical investigations occur on a daily basis in all healthcare settings, both acute and community. They are requested, carried out and interpreted by a range of practitioners within the multidisciplinary team, both registered and unregistered. In the past decade, especially, the requesting and interpretation has been conducted by more advanced practice nurses and the performing of certain investigations such as venepuncture has been delegated to unregistered team members such as healthcare assistants and associate practitioners.

The term 'clinical investigation' refers to a range of procedures, invasive and non-invasive. These could be carried by the bedside or on the ward area, and include urinalysis, blood glucose measurement or arterial blood gas analysis. Others may see the patient being taken to another area of the hospital, such as x-ray, ultrasound or **CT scanning**.

Investigations in clinical practice have a variety of uses. The most important is, often, to confirm a possible diagnosis, such as x-ray to confirm a fracture or pneumonia, CT head to confirm cerebral haemorrhage or an ECG for ST elevation myocardial infarction. These can be carried out within minutes and the interpretation of results needs to be carried out and quickly in order to ensure the optimum outcome for the patient. However, practitioners must never underestimate the importance of the quality of the history taking and focused physical examination in order to construct their **differential diagnosis**. Clinical investigations often confirm the working hypothesis and account for only around 5% of the diagnosis.

In addition to confirming diagnosis, investigations can also assist in monitoring disease process in patients. For example, measuring the trend of inflammatory markers, such as white cell count and **C-reactive protein**, in order to assess the improvement in an infection being treated with intravenous antibiotics. They can also be useful in adjusting treatment, for example the ABG results can influence the settings of non-invasive ventilation in a high dependency clinical area.

This chapter will focus on a number of clinical investigations that you may encounter in clinical practice. It will consider the indications for carrying out an investigation, in addition to any preparation or care required for the patient before, during or after. As John has mentioned at the beginning of the chapter, the responsibility for these investigations may lie with advanced practice nurses in addition to medical practitioners.

The investigations you may be involved in undertaking as a nursing student include urinalysis, bladder scanning, capillary blood glucose measurement and the recording of electrocardiographs (ECG). You may also observe, assist or be involved in the preparation or care of patients undergoing many of the other investigations discussed. As Student Nurse Jo has mentioned, always consider the indication for the investigation and how this may impact on the care of your patients.

PREPARATION FOR PRACTICE PLACEMENTS 12.1

Before you start your placement, speak to the staff or visit that clinical area. Find out what clinical investigations are common to that practice area. Then you can research what these are, what conditions they assist to diagnose and any specific patient preparation or after care. You may also find it useful to speak to other nursing students who have already had a placement in that clinical area.

ACTIVITY 12.1: REFLECTIVE PRACTICE

Reflect on your clinical placements and consider what clinical investigations were carried out. Now, list the common ones and reflect on why they were undertaken.

URINALYSIS

This is a relatively cheap and quick investigation that is carried out in all areas of primary and secondary healthcare by a variety of healthcare staff. The procedure involves immersing a reagent stick into a clean urine sample (preferably mid-stream) and then waiting up to 120 seconds to read it. The change in colour of the differing sections may indicate the presence of glucose, ketones, nitrites, leukocytes, protein and blood (among others), which can be used in assisting with making a diagnosis. For example, in urinary tract infections, the presence of nitrites and leukocytes are usual, while in renal colic it is not uncommon to detect blood on the reagent stick. Glucose and ketones may also be detected in uncontrolled blood sugars such as in diabetes. Urinalysis is also useful in the monitoring for diseases such as the detection of proteinuria in pregnancy and **systemic lupus erythematosus (SLE)**. The practitioner carrying out the procedure must ensure they are wearing the correct **personal protective equipment (PPE)** and may have to assist some patients with hygiene post-procedure. It is imperative that the disposal of body fluids and correct hand hygiene are carried out as per local protocols.

SEE ALSO
CHAPTER 14

CRITICAL THINKING STOP POINT 12.1

Please take time to reflect on the need for PPE and good hand hygiene when correctly disposing of bodily fluids.

BLADDER SCANNING

This test is a bedside ultrasound procedure, used often by unregistered healthcare workers, to confirm the amount of urine present in the bladder. A healthy bladder can hold up to 300–400 ml in the day and up to 800 ml at night. Bladder scanning is indicated when there is a suspicion of urinary retention. Examples of when urinary retention may occur are in males who have an enlarged prostate gland, post-surgical procedure (especially those that are carried out with an epidural as the anaesthesia) and in severe constipation. The test is non-invasive, yet the practitioner must ensure that privacy and dignity is protected as the symphis pubis area must be visible. The ultrasound usually only shows the capacity of the bladder up to 999 ml: if it is higher than 999 ml then it will just indicate greater than this volume. Again, the operator may have to assist with hygiene post-procedure, as a lubricant would have been used. It is imperative that, if carried out by a healthcare assistant or other unregistered worker, the results are both documented and reported to a registered professional.

SEE ALSO
CHAPTER 29

CAPILLARY BLOOD GLUCOSE

This measures the amount of glucose (in mmol/L) present in the capillaries. The normal random blood glucose level for somebody who is not diabetic is between 4 and 8 mmol/L. It is a relatively quick and easy test to perform and is often carried out by unregistered healthcare workers or by carers or patients themselves. Patients who have been diagnosed with diabetes mellitus will usually have their own device at home and often have to titrate their dose of insulin depending on the result. If symptoms of hypoglycaemia are suspected, such as shaking, confusion or sweating, the capillary blood glucose should be measured immediately If the capillary blood glucose is less than 4 mmol/L, the patient should be given dextrose via a route appropriate for their condition. Other indications for this investigation are for those patients on long-term and high dose steroids, where hyperglycaemia may occur as a **type A adverse drug reaction**. Also, when an **ABCDE** approach is carried out on an acutely unwell patient, blood glucose should be measured to complete the Disability (D) assessment, as it may account for any loss or reduction in conscious level.

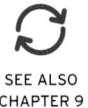

SEE ALSO
CHAPTER 9

The actual procedure varies depending on the device and so local protocol and training should always be followed. However, in the majority of devices the result is available within seconds. It is important that the fingertip utilised is cleaned prior to the test, but not with ethanol wipes as this may lead to an incorrect reading. Local protocols regarding correct use of PPE, the disposal of sharps and infection control should always be adhered to. As with any clinical test carried out by unregistered staff, the results should always be documented and reported to the registered nurse responsible for the care of that patient.

VENOUS BLOOD TESTS

There are multiple indications for venous blood tests and these are carried out daily in both primary and secondary healthcare settings. When the samples are delivered to the laboratory, results can often be available in the acute settings within 30 minutes to an hour, depending on the test. These procedures are often carried out by unregistered staff, such as phlebotomists and healthcare assistants, who would usually have extra training and be assessed on the appropriate competencies. The results can be interpreted to assist with a number of clinical purposes. Two of the most common purposes are to construct or deconstruct differential diagnoses and to monitor disease processes.

The procedure would involve a number of stages including the selection of a vein, the cleaning of the area and then the presentation of the needle device into the vein. It is imperative the correct bottles for the tests required are used, and that they are drawn in the correct order. This reduces the possibility of haemolysis (the breakdown of blood cells), which may lead to an incorrect result. Again, local policy on PPE, sharps and infection control must be adhered to. The practitioner must also ensure that positive patient identification occurs and that the correct patient details are entered onto the bottles. Table 12.1 shows normal ranges for common blood tests.

ACTIVITY 12.2: REFLECTIVE ACTIVITY

Venous blood tests are common procedures that you will witness on clinical placement. It is possible that a patient may feel dizzy or faint after these investigations. Reflect on why this may occur and how you would manage the situation.

> Taking venous blood samples are a common investigation that I request, carry out and interpret within my role. I have to ensure that I have a rationale for requesting such investigations as these can be painful and may cause bruising to the patient. There can also be a financial burden to the organisation when requesting unnecessary investigations. It is also vital that I interpret the results in a timely manner, in order for any abnormal result to be acted on if required and that any treatment plan is changed or amended.
>
> John, Hospital at Night Nurse Practitioner

Table 12.1 Common blood tests with normal values in adults

Blood Test	Normal Value
Haemoglobin (Hb)	130-170 grams per litre in men, 110-150 grams per litre in women
White cell count (WCC)	$3.7\text{-}9.5 \times 10^9$/L in men, $3.9\text{-}11.1 \times 10^9$/L in women
Platelets	$150\text{-}400 \times 10^9$/L
Sodium	133-146 mmol/L
Potassium	3.5-5.3 mmol/L
Urea	2.5-7.8 mmol/L
Creatinine	55-105 micromol/L
C-Reactive Protein (CRP)	Less than 10 mg/L

Electrocardiogram

An ECG or electrocardiogram (Figure 12.1) is a relatively quick and non-invasive procedure which is used to measure the rate and rhythm of the heart. It can also indicate when myocardial ischaemia and infarction may be present. There are multiple indications for this investigation. It is often carried out in the acute setting, where the patient has complained of symptoms such as **syncope**, chest pain or breathlessness and the result can assist in differentiating the correct diagnosis. The interpretation of this may need to be a rapid process, as in the cases of diagnosing an acute ST elevation myocardial infarction. The reduction of time to transport the patient to a cardiac catheter laboratory can be crucial for a positive outcome for the patient. The interpretation of this procedure is often done in the pre-hospital setting by paramedical staff or in hospital by either doctors or nurse practitioners. This investigation may also be utilised in the non-acute setting; for example, as a screening tool for patients in the pre-operative phase.

The procedure involves placing 10 leads attached to stickers onto the chest and limbs. The correct demographics should be entered into the ECG machine. The patient should be advised to keep still to ensure the most accurate tracing. This can be difficult for those patients in acute pain or who may be confused secondary to **hypoxia**. There can also be issues with the stickers remaining in place, for those patients who are sweaty or have a large amount of body hair. It is also important that the operator ensures privacy and dignity for the patient as it involves having their chest exposed. Figure 12.1 shows a normal ECG in relation to cardiac anatomy.

SEE ALSO
CHAPTER 25

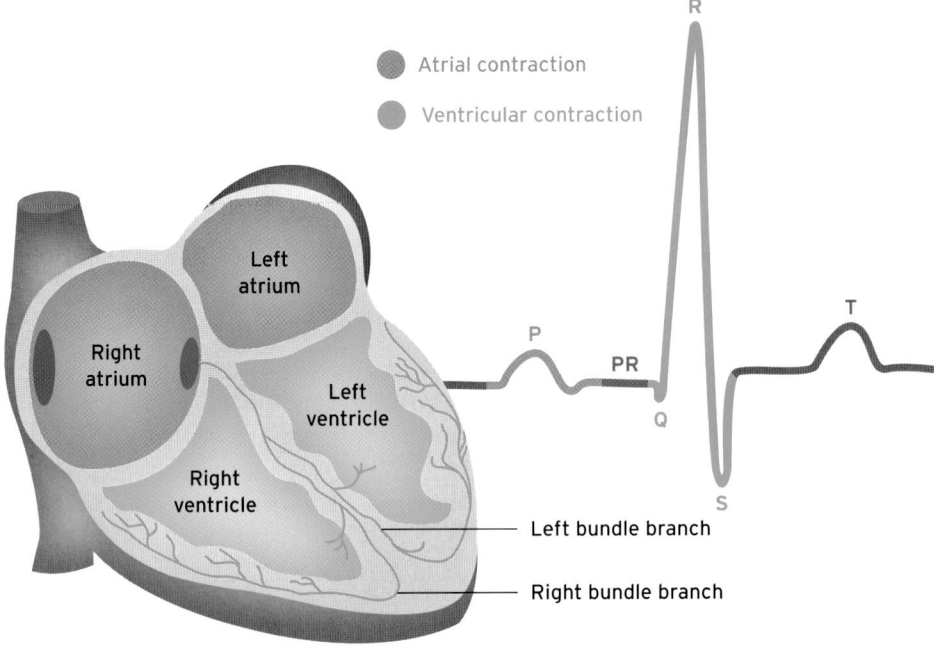

Figure 12.1

Source: Boore et al. (2016). Illustrated by Shaun Mercier, © SAGE Publications.

CRITICAL THINKING STOP 12.2

Consider a situation where you have had difficulties in attaching the electrodes to a patient's torso. What were the reasons for this? How did you manage the problem?

Table 12.2   Summary of professional groups who may perform investigations (with sufficient training)

Clinical Investigation	Professional Groups
Urinalysis	Healthcare assistants; registered nurses
Bladder scanning	Healthcare assistants; registered nurses
Capillary blood glucose	Healthcare assistants; paramedics and emergency medical technicians; registered nurses
Venous blood tests	Phlebotomists; healthcare assistants; registered nurses; medical practitioners
Electrocardiogram	Healthcare assistants; paramedics and emergency medical technicians; registered nurses; ECG technicians
Arterial blood gas	Medical practitioners; advanced practice nurses
Arterial blood pressure	Registered nurses; medical practitioners
Central venous pressure	Registered nurses; medical practitioners

Clinical Investigation	Professional Groups
X-ray	Radiographers
Ultrasound	Sonographers; Medical practitioners; Advanced practice nurses and paramedics; Midwives
Computed tomography scan	Radiographers
Magnetic resonance imaging	Radiographers
Endoscopy	Medical practitioners; Nurse endoscopists

SPIROMETERY

This investigation is a specialised respiratory procedure that is usually carried out by qualified pulmonary function technicians in acute hospitals or if in the community (predominantly GP surgeries) by specially trained practice nurses. Its function is to assist in the diagnosis of respiratory conditions, most commonly for COPD (chronic obstructive pulmonary disease). The investigation also assists in the monitoring of other respiratory conditions including asthma, idiopathic pulmonary fibrosis and cystic fibrosis. There is little preparation or after care required for this procedure. The test involves measuring two specific functions of the lung, the first being the FEV1, which is the forced expiratory volume in one second and the second being the FVC, forced vital capacity. This is the amount of air which can be forcibly exhaled from the lungs after taking the deepest breath possible. The technician will also calculate the ratio of these two measurements. This will give data to determine whether the patient may have a restrictive or obstructive lung function. If the FEV1/FVC ratio is 69% or less this can be indicative of restriction and, therefore, the possibility of COPD. The actual testing involves the patient blowing into a specialist device.

SEE ALSO
CHAPTER 24

ARTERIAL BLOOD GAS

Arterial blood gas or ABG is an invasive procedure, usually carried out from the radial artery using a heparinised syringe. The femoral or brachial arteries can also be used. The test is usually performed by doctors or nurse practitioners, and there are many indications. The result can give data regarding the oxygenation and acid-base balance of a patient. This can assist in differentiating if a hypoxic patient has either type 1 (hypoxia with normal/low CO_2 – see Table 12.3) respiratory failure or

Table 12.3 Example of an arterial blood gas result from a patient with type 1 respiratory failure

Parameter	Patient Result	Normal Values
pH	7.40	7.35-7.45
PaO_2	7.5 kPa	10.6-13.3 kPa
$PaCO_2$	4.0 kPa	4.7-6.0 kPa
Bicarbonate	24 mmol/L	22-28 mmol/L
Base Excess	+ 0.5	−2.0 – + 2.0

Table 12.4 Example of an arterial blood gas result from a patient with type 2 respiratory failure

Parameter	Patient Result	Normal Values
pH	7.26	7.35-7.45
PaO_2	7.0 kPa	10.6-13.3 kPa
$PaCO_2$	9.0 kPa	4.7-6.0 kPa
Bicarbonate	28 mmol/L	22-28 mmol/L
Base Excess	− 5.0	−2.0 − + 2.0

type 2 (hypoxia with a high CO_2 – See Table 12.4). This interpretation can assist with deciding on the most appropriate management. If this involves initiating NIPPV (**non-invasive positive pressure ventilation**), further results can assist in titrating the settings to the optimum. It is well documented that this procedure is very painful and so, if the patient requires multiple arterial punctures, an arterial line may be inserted in order to take multiple samples without the need to continually carry out venipuncture on the patient. Other indications include checking a potassium level quickly, as samples can be processed in a few minutes, rather than waiting for the laboratory result. In addition to oxygenation and acid-base balance, the ABG also measures lactate (which increases in the body in the presence of lactic acidosis when shock causes anaerobic cellular respiration). This can be an indicator of the mortality and morbidity of patients with septic shock or hypovolaemic shock from acute blood loss, i.e. gastrointestinal bleeding or trauma.

ACTIVITY 12.3: REFLECTIVE PRACTICE

Reflect on the psychological care and support you may need to give a patient undergoing this potentially painful procedure.

The procedure involves selecting the arterial site by feeling for a pulsation. The practitioner then cleans the area, as per local protocol, and inserts the needle of the heparinised syringe. If the puncture is successful, the syringe should fill itself due to the pressure of the artery: around 1ml is required. The practitioner should apply pressure to the area post-procedure until any bleeding has ceased. Local protocols regarding sharps, PPE and infection control should always be adhered to. A relative contraindication for this procedure is a raised INR level (indicating delayed clotting). The practitioner should always weigh up the benefits and risks if required to undertake this intervention.

This is a common and frequent investigation that I carry out when assessing acutely unwell adult patients. As it is a painful procedure, I must explain the rationale clearly to the patient in order to prepare them and gain informed consent. I always ascertain whether the patient is taking an anticoagulant medication, as I would need to consider the risk/benefit of the procedure. As this is an advanced role for nurses, I attended theory sessions regarding the procedure and was assessed for my competence prior to undertaking it independently.

John, Hospital at Night Nurse Practitioner

GO FURTHER

The website below will give you the opportunity to read more around the underpinning pathophysiology for ABGs. There is also a link to attempt some exam questions. www.oxfordmedicaleducation.com/abgs/abg-interpretation/

WEBLINK:
ABGS

CASE STUDY 12.1: BETTY

At this point in the chapter, many of the clinical investigations you may observe or carry out on clinical placement in the acute setting have been discussed. Take time now to consider the case study below.

Betty, an 84-year-old woman, is admitted to the Medical Assessment Unit via her GP, with a three-day history of increasing confusion, shortness of breath and urinary incontinence. Betty suffers from hypertension and takes a calcium channel blocker. She is a non-smoker and lives alone in a warden-controlled flat.

Assessment so far using the ABCDE approach:

A   Talking
B   Bilateral air entry, no added sounds. Respiratory rate 26 bpm. SpO$_2$ 93% on air.
C   Heart rate 122 irregular. Blood pressure 90/30mmHg. Capillary refill time 3 seconds.
D   Alert, but disorientated. Pupils equal and reacting to light.
E   Temperature 38.2°C, foul-smelling urine apparent.

Consider which clinical investigations may be requested on Betty's admission to assist with reaching a definitive diagnosis.

Give a rationale for each investigation.

CASE STUDY 12.1
ANSWER

SEE ALSO
CHAPTER 9

ARTERIAL BLOOD PRESSURE

Arterial blood pressure monitoring is a means of continually measuring the blood pressure of patients, who have or are at risk of having single and multi-organ failure, and are usually cared for in a high dependency or intensive care area. This reading is more accurate than the non-invasive blood pressure readings, usually carried out in less acute areas. The procedure involves the insertion of an arterial line, usually into a radial artery. This is a sterile procedure, which involves the infiltration of local anaesthetic, as it can be painful. You may be involved in assisting the medical practitioner. The transducer is then attached to the line and this is attached to the monitor, where the arterial waveform and arterial blood pressure reading is available. In most monitors these readings will be seen in red.

The other use of this arterial line is that you can take multiple blood gas samples, and so saves the patient from having multiple arterial punctures. This has been explored in the previous section.

CENTRAL VENOUS PRESSURE

As with arterial blood pressure monitoring, continuous monitoring of central venous pressure is also undertaken in high dependency patients. Central venous pressure, or CVP, is the measure of the amount of blood returning to the heart and the ability of the heart to pump blood back into the arterial system. As with the insertion of the arterial line, the CVP line is also inserted under sterile conditions. However, it is inserted into a central vein, usually the internal jugular vein via the subclavian approach. Again, you may be involved in assisting the medical practitioner. You should ensure the patient is lying flat. The line is then attached to a monitor and the measurement is continual. The measurement can be affected by cardiac failure, distributed shock and hypovolaemia, and so can give an indication regarding the fluid status of an individual. The normal values are 0–14 cm H_2O if measured at the sternum and 8–15 cm H_2O if measured at the midaxillary line. A lower value may indicate fluid depletion, while an increased number may indicate fluid overload.

X-RAYS

These investigations are common in both acute and community hospitals. This form of medical imaging uses electromagnetic radiation to highlight bone pathology, i.e. fractures on limb films, or air and consolidated matter on chest x-ray, to assist ruling in or out pneumonia (consolidation in the lung is usually due to bacterial infection) or pneumothorax (air in the pleural space). Although radiation is used, the majority of limb and chest x-rays utilise only a small amount, which is less than you would receive on a long haul flight. Abdominal and pelvis films require a larger dose of radiation, but again, have a high safety profile in single doses.

The requesting and operating of x-rays is governed by IR(ME)R 2000 (Ionising Radiation (Medical Exposure) Regulations) (DH, 2017). Those requesting, usually doctors or advanced nurses, must have undergone training and be present on a local register. Operators refer to qualified diagnostic radiographers. The images are interpreted at the time, usually by the practitioner who has requested the image. However, radiologists (doctors with a specialism in interpreting medical imaging) will write a report on each image within a few days; this is also now done by advanced practice radiographers.

As metal objects will show up as artefact on x-ray films, it is vital that patients are encouraged and assisted to undress into a gown or other light clothing prior to the investigation. It is also imperative that the operator and referrer confirm the pregnancy status of all females of childbearing age, as radiation may be harmful to the fetus.

WHAT'S THE EVIDENCE? 12.1

There is traditional thinking that all x-rays may harm the fetus of a pregnant patient. However, what is the evidence for this? What is the actual documented risk? Do all x-rays have the same risk?

ULTRASOUND

Ultrasonography is a non-invasive investigation using high frequency sound waves to create images of some parts inside the body. This is generally done by specially trained radiographers. However, many other professionals use ultrasound in their own specialist fields. For example, midwives and obstetricians use it to check on the growth of the fetus in pregnant patients while cardiac physiologists may carry out and interpret Echocardiograms (an ultrasound used to view the structure and function of the heart). More recently, in advanced trauma care, bedside ultrasound is often used as part of the primary survey of a trauma patient to rule out free fluid (bleeding) in the abdomen or cardiac tamponade (accumulation of fluid in the pericardial sac).

There is little specific preparation or after care for patients undergoing these procedures. However, some patients may need assistance in dressing and undressing, and some may need assistance with hygiene post procedure as a lubricant will be applied. As this investigation does not use radiation, it has a high safety profile.

COMPUTERISED TOMOGRAPHY SCANS

Computed tomography (CT) scans are investigations which use both x-rays and computers to create detailed images of the inside of the body. These are more specific and detailed than x-rays alone. However, they require a high intensity of radiation and are more expensive. Diagnostic radiographers have further post-registration training to perform these investigations. CT scans are usually interpreted by radiologists, yet some specialty doctors such as neurologists and neurosurgeons (specialists for the brain, spinal process and neurological system) will interpret them also. The scans have multiple indications for use. For example, in the case of a suspected stroke, the scan will differentiate between a haemorrhagic or ischaemic cause and so is vital when deciding whether to prescribe thrombolytic therapy (a powerful drug used to dissolve clots causing an ischaemic stroke). This investigation is also vital in the diagnosis of trauma patients, as it will show sites of internal damage and bleeding. Compared to MRI, which is discussed next, this investigation is quicker (a CT head can be performed in a few minutes) and more readily available out of hours in acute hospitals.

As with other medical imaging procedures previously discussed, the patient may need assistance with dressing and undressing. A peripheral cannula may also be required for some scans, as a dye or contrast may be injected intravenously, i.e. in a CTPA (pulmonary angiogram) the dye will highlight an obstruction such as pulmonary embolus. Prior to having contrast administered, allergies should be confirmed and renal function checked, as the contrast can have an adverse effect on the kidneys. If the patient is diabetic and taking metformin tablets, these should be stopped up to 48 hours post-administration of the dye. This is because the metformin is predominantly excreted by the kidneys and the contrast may cause a **nephropathy**. The renal function should be rechecked prior to recommencing the drug.

In addition to its diagnostic use, CT scanning is also useful in guiding further treatment, such as the location and shape of tumours prior to radiotherapy, and it also monitors disease, such as tumour growth.

MAGNETIC RESONANCE IMAGING

Magnetic resonance imaging (MRI) is probably the most complex form of medical imaging to date. It uses strong magnetic fields and radio waves to produce detailed images of the inside of the body. It is often more specific and sensitive than CT scanning, however, it has limitations: it is more costly, is rarely available out of routine hours and the investigations take longer. As the patient needs to remain still in a confined space for these periods, some become claustrophobic and their procedure has to be abandoned.

ACTIVITY 12.4: REFLECTIVE PRACTICE

Reflect on what it would be like as a patient to have an MRI scan. Remember, this investigation can take around 30 minutes. The area is enclosed and the patient must remain still.

- How do you think the patient is feeling?
- What strategies could you use to help to alleviate any fears?

There are many indications for MRI: it can be used to identify abnormalities in the brain, spinal cord, joints, heart and abdominal organs among others. The preparation for the patient is somewhat more vital than that of CT. A checklist must be completed prior to the procedure to identify if there is any metalwork in the patient's body from previous surgery and that all jewellery has been removed. As you can imagine, allowing a patient into a scan requiring strong magnetic forces with metalwork could be dangerous!

ENDOSCOPY

Endoscopic procedures look inside hollow organs and cavities of the body. The endoscope is a long, flexible tube, which encases a video-recording device. The three most common procedures are as follows; the first is the OGD (oesophagogastroduodenoscopy) where the scope is placed through the mouth and then views the oesophagus, stomach and duodenum. This investigation is often used for the diagnosis of gastric or duodenal ulcers or stomach cancer. Often the patient would have presented with a history of vomiting, epigastric pain or haematemesis (vomiting blood) to warrant a referral for this test. The second is a colonoscopy, where the scope is inserted through the anus, the rectum and then through the colon. This procedure can be used to confirm the diagnosis of inflammatory bowel diseases such as Crohn's disease and ulcerative colitis or diverticulosis. Patients referred for this investigation often have complained of rectal bleeding, mucous stools, and changes in bowel habit or abdominal pain. The third type of endoscopy is the bronchoscopy, where the scope is placed via a nasal passage into the lung, and may be used to diagnose diseases such as lung cancers. Patients referred for this intervention may have presented with a history of weight loss, breathlessness and haemoptysis (coughing up blood).

All of these procedures are usually carried out in acute hospitals by specially trained doctors or advanced nurses. They can be done routinely or as an emergency, for example to locate the bleeding point in acute gastrointestinal bleeding. The procedures are usually performed in a purpose-built endoscopy suite, although at times may be done in the operating theatre. In addition to their multiple diagnostic uses, endoscopic procedures also have therapeutic (treatment) indications. One example is the ERCP (endoscopic retrograde cholangiopancreatography), which is an endoscopic procedure to examine the pancreas and bile ducts, and gall stones can be removed.

The preparation and after care of patients undergoing these investigations resembles many of the activities required for surgical procedures. The patient will usually have to be nil by mouth for a number of hours pre-procedure to reduce the risk of vomiting during the procedure and to ensure that the stomach is visible. A peripheral cannula will often be inserted in order to administer sedation during the procedure, as usually the patient is sedated rather than fully anaesthetised. In the case of a colonoscopy, the patient will usually need to take a bowel preparation mixture in the day prior to the procedure, so that the rectum and colon are clear of faeces in order to obtain an adequate view. In cases where the patient has reduced mobility, they may need to be admitted into hospital for this preparation to ensure that assistance with hygiene and toileting can be given. As a sedative medication has been administered, it is imperative that vital signs and conscious level are monitored regularly during and after the procedure and that they are within normal limits for the patient prior to discharge. Post-procedure care should also involve ensuring that a patient has tolerated diet, fluids and has passed urine prior to safely discharging. Other post-investigation care may involve explaining any new medication that may have been prescribed. For example, a protein pump inhibitor such as omeprazole may be prescribed if a diagnosis of oesophagitis or gastritis has been made.

CASE STUDY 12.2: SUE

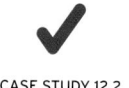

CASE STUDY 12.2
ANSWER

All the common clinical investigations have now been explored within this chapter. When considering the case study below, think back to any clinical placements you have been involved in within the primary care or community settings.

Sue is a 22-year-old office worker who presents to her GP practice with a three-day history of lower abdominal pain. She has no past medical history, but takes an oral contraceptive pill. She does not drink alcohol or smoke. She states she is sexually active and comments that her menstrual cycle is erratic.

Vital Signs: Temperature 37.2°C, heart rate 80 bpm, blood pressure 110/70mmHg, respiratory rate 17 rpm, SpO_2 99% on air.

Consider which investigations you would be able to do in this primary care setting for Sue in order to assist in reaching a diagnosis.

- Give a rationale for each investigation.
- Critically discuss the difficulties that may be faced in referring for or carrying out clinical investigations within the primary care or community setting.

CHAPTER SUMMARY

- Clinical investigations are varied, numerous and widely used in both primary and secondary care
- They often have a use in making differential diagnoses and some have a therapeutic use too
- They are carried out and interpreted by a range of registered healthcare professionals and unregistered support staff
- Clinical investigations have their limitations in practice in addition to their strengths.

GO FURTHER

Go to https://study.sagepub.com/essentialadultnursing for a further case study related to this chapter. If you are using the interactive ebook, simply click on the book icon in the margin to go straight to the resource.

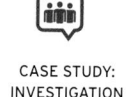

CASE STUDY:
INVESTIGATION

Books

- Haycock, A., Cohen, J., Saunders, B.P., Cotton, B.P. and Williams, C.B. (2014) *Cotton and Williams' Practical Gastrointestinal Endoscopy* (7th ed.). Chichester: Wiley-Blackwell.
  This book will assist with your understanding of the indications and procedure of gastrointestinal endoscopy.

- Higgins, C. (2013) *Understanding Laboratory Investigations. A Guide for Nurses, Midwives and Healthcare Professionals* (3rd ed.). Chichester: Wiley-Blackwell.
  This book will assist you in understanding the results of common blood tests that may be carried out in your clinical placement.
- Shoener, R.L. (2011) *RAD Notes: A Pocket Guide to Radiographic Procedures*. Philadelphia, PA: F.A. Davis Company.
  This book will assist with your understanding of the differing radiological procedures that you may observe in clinical practice.

Journal Articles

FURTHER READING: JOURNAL ARTICLES

Go to https://study.sagepub.com/essentialadultnursing for further free online journal articles related to this chapter. If you are using the interactive ebook, simply click on the book icon in the margin to go straight to the resource.

- Patout, M., Lamia, B., Lhuillier, E., Molano, L-C., Viacroze, C., Benhamou, D., Muir, J.F. and Cuvelier, A. (2015) A randomized controlled trial on the effect of needle gauge on the pain and anxiety experienced during Radial Arterial Puncture. *PLoS ONE*, 10(9): e0139432.
  This article discusses the evidence referred to in the chapter regarding the effect of pain and anxiety on the patient having an arterial blood gas sample taken.
- Rees, P.A., Moss, F. and Marsden, M. (2012) The use of guidelines to rationalise blood tests on emergency surgical patients. *International Journal of Surgery*, 10(8): S47.
  This article will assist you in discussing the financial and patient factors in the requesting and carrying out of unnecessary blood tests.
- Thompson, N., Murphy, M., Robinson, J. and Buckley, T. (2016) Improved nurse initiated X-ray practice through action research. *Journal of Medical Radiation Sciences*, 63(4): 203-8.
  This article will highlight the patient experience when nurses are requesting investigations that traditionally are requested by medical practitioners.

Weblinks

FURTHER READING: WEBLINKS

Go to https://study.sagepub.com/essentialadultnursing for further weblinks related to this chapter. If you are using the interactive ebook, simply click on the book icon in the margin to go straight to the resource.

- www.labtestsonline.org.uk/understanding/
  This website is an interactive tool to assist with your understanding of common laboratory investigations.
- www.radiologymasterclass.co.uk/
  This website is an interactive tool to assist with your understanding of common radiological procedures.
- www.youtube.com/watch?v=OmsNjUOvbSs
  This video brings to life the procedure of the upper gastrointestinal endoscopy, which is commonly seen on medical and surgical acute clinical placements.

ACE YOUR ASSESSMENT

ONLINE QUIZZES

Revise what you have learned by visiting https://study.sagepub.com/essentialadultnursing

- Test yourself with multiple-choice and short-answer questions
- Do the chapter activities in the book and check your answers online

REFERENCES

Department of Health (2017) *Ionising Radiation (Medical Exposure) Regulations 2000 (IRMER).* London: Department of Health.

Haycock, A. Cohen, J., Saunders, B.P., Cotton, B.P. and Williams, C.B. (2014) *Cotton and Williams' Practical Gastrointestinal Endoscopy* (7th ed.). Chichester: Wiley-Blackwell.

Higgins, C. (2013) *Understanding Laboratory Investigations. A Guide for Nurses, Midwives and Healthcare Professionals* (3rd ed.). Chichester: Wiley-Blackwell.

Shoener, R.L. (2011) *RAD Notes: A Pocket Guide to Radiographic Procedures.* Philadelphia, PA: F.A. Davis Company.

MEDICATION MANAGEMENT AND ADMINISTRATION

13

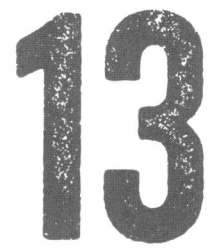

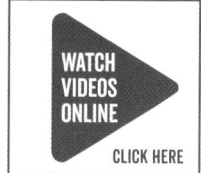
WATCH VIDEOS ONLINE
CLICK HERE

RONNIE MEECHAN-ROGERS AND KRIS PAGET

THIS CHAPTER COVERS

- The changing context of medicines management within the UK
- Medication management and relevant legislation
- The role of the nurse and multidisciplinary team in medication management
- Patient education and concordance
- An introduction to pharmacokinetics and pharmacodynamics.

> In my experience as a student, a topic that often causes disagreement is the use of covert administration, that is, the administration of any medical treatment in a disguised form. The complexity of this issue can often be underestimated. By disguising medication in food or drink, the patient is made to believe that they are not being given medication when in fact they are. As a nurse, we need to be sure that covert administration is always justified, for example, in order for it to occur, the patient should have been proven to lack capacity and it must be in their best interests. In a ward environment, I learnt the importance of discussing the options of covertly administering medication to a patient with the multidisciplinary team, in addition to relatives, carers and other advocates. Contacting a pharmacist for advice was essential in some of my patient cases as they were able to explain whether the medication would affect pharmacological properties and performance. It highlighted the importance of involving the multidisciplinary team in medicines management to provide holistic care.
>
> **Bethanie Howard, 3rd year student nurse**

Imagine if you will, an elderly patient, happily 'managing' their medication regime at home, in either a haphazard manner or coping with varying degrees of capability. The patient arrives in hospital as an 'elective or emergency' admission with medication which is promptly removed. Subsequently, the patient finds themselves submitted to a series of reasons why they cannot have the medications they are used to: 'computer it says no', 'not yet dearie', 'not until the Dr has seen you', 'we have run out', etc., etc. These answers frustrate patients, particularly at night and at the weekends and especially when they are in pain. Such measures are of course all for the benefit of the patient and are delivered by a series of disjointed 'safety' processes. Ideally a patient record could be electronically sourced, but probably neither succinctly or swiftly. Medication lists do not make allowances for the fact that a patient, expecting to make an early morning journey, will have quite wisely not taken a prescribed diuretic that morning. Have you ever tried to make a long journey, desperate for the lavatory with the urge being medication driven? It is unbearable – even unmanageable!

Patients can and do manage their medication successfully at home and could equally do this while in a hospital or care home which could reduce the number of drug errors in these areas. Hospitals are more likely to record 'missed doses' as a result of drugs not being available and staff not having the time to obtain further supplies from elsewhere, and care home residents can very easily be given medication intended for others as staff are unlikely to be fully trained or have the benefit of computer-driven record keeping. Competent patients can easily become disempowered and frustrated by hospital processes and nurses end up getting the blame for the system they have to implement. Undoubtedly, some patients will benefit from their medications being rationalised and even changed. However, in my experience this is rarely a smooth or effective process as pharmacy staff quite often check what a patient has brought with them on admission and simply order more of the same. It ought to be fine for doctors and nurses to 'take charge', but as a patient and a former medical professional, I feel there needs to be more accurate and timely processes in place. Alongside the extension of knowledge of medication, allowance must be made for a knowledgeable patient to continue their independence wherever possible. This can often be ascertained if a patient is able to attend a pre-admission session.

Yes, some patients do know too much and wish to be in control and may be a 'pain', and probably many more are quite happy with the established routines that they are submitted to. This I suppose is the circle that can never be squared!

Aprella Fitch, Patient

INTRODUCTION

The purpose of this chapter is to introduce you as an adult nursing student to medicines management or, as it's now more commonly called, **medicines optimisation**. During your pre-registration nursing programme you will gain knowledge and skills that relate to the administration of medicines and as Bethanie and Aprella point out above, it is important that you understand the many complexities involved in this aspect of your programme. It is important, therefore, that you recognise the importance of your role in relation to this aspect of nursing practice. This chapter will help you to understand and focus on the principles of safe medication optimisation, related specifically to nursing adults.

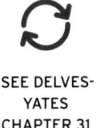

SEE DELVES-
YATES
CHAPTER 31

Medicines optimisation explores how patients and service users use medicines over time. It involves commencing different medicines while discontinuing others. Medicines optimisation explores and examines changes to behaviours, including non-medical therapies, in order to lessen the need for medicines. The overall aim is to improve safety and adherence to treatment, and reduce medicines waste.

Medicines optimisation ensures patients and service users get the precise choice of medication, when they need it most. By focusing on the experience of patients, service users and their families, the overall end goal for you and the health care team is to help:

- improve their outcomes;
- patients take their medicines correctly;
- avoid taking unnecessary medicines;
- reduce wastage of medicines and improve medicines safety.

Medicines optimisation differs from medicines management; primarily, it relates to outcomes and is individualised and patient centred rather than focusing on systems and processes. Ultimately, this approach is likely to ensure improved value from the investment in medications.

This chapter is underpinned by the National Institute for Health and Care Excellence (NICE) (2015) guidance on medicines optimisation and the Royal Pharmaceutical Society (RPS) (2013) good practice guidance for health care professionals. During your programme you will come into contact with a variety of systems and processes that are involved with medication administration; therefore, the chapter will cover prescriptions (including electronic systems), supplying, dispensing, administration, checking, disposal, licensing, PGDs, patients' own drugs, self-administration and controlled drugs.

The context of care that you will be exposed to as a nursing student will include both hospital and community settings and working with others such as doctors, non-medical prescribers and pharmacists. Therefore, it is important to understand your role as an adult nurse in relation to patient education and encouraging medication concordance. The chapter also aims to provide you with information on the principles of pharmacology including **pharmacokinetics** and **pharmacodynamics** in order that you can administer medications safely, and identify where you may need to liaise with medical staff and other prescribers to adjust medication regimes to ensure safe and effective medication optimisation. Remember, the administration of medicines and medicines optimisation forms a significant aspect of your everyday practice and is one of the most common nursing interventions carried out within clinical practice. When reflecting on the voices at the beginning of this chapter, hopefully you will see how important this is within your everyday practice.

THE CHANGING CONTEXT OF MEDICINES MANAGEMENT WITHIN THE UK

The context of health and social care for patients, service users, carers and their families has undergone a significant transformation over the past decade. With the introduction of new roles such as nursing associates, who will have a function in the administration of medicines (Health Education England, 2018), and increased delivery of healthcare within the community and primary care settings, it is important for you to understand the role of individuals who are involved with medications management as this is becoming more complex.

Patients, service users and their carers/families who access health and social care present with ever more complex needs. Nurses, nursing associates and associate practitioners, therefore, need a sound understanding of anatomy, physiology, pathophysiology, assessment skills and history-taking skills to ensure that multifaceted conditions can be managed safely and effectively.

As a nursing student it's essential that medicines management is not looked at in isolation and is fully integrated into the care and management of your patient. You will also be required to consider other elements of your education including professional issues, standards set by the professional regulator, legal and ethical considerations and policy that relates directly to health and social care.

In 2018 new standards for nursing education were published by the UK nursing regulator, the Nursing and Midwifery Council (NMC, 2018), with a greater emphasis on medicines management.

The Medicines and Healthcare products Regulatory Agency (MHRA) is an executive agency of the Department of Health. The MHRA's role is multifaceted and its responsibilities include ensuring that medicines, medical devices and blood components for transfusion meet applicable standards of safety, quality and efficacy, and helping to educate the public and healthcare professionals about the risks and benefits of medicines, medical devices and blood components, leading to safer and more effective use. The MHRA (2014) suggests that all health and social care practitioners are responsible for effective medicines management; the MHRA also articulates that for medicines management to be successful, medicines need to be cost effective, used for clinical outcomes and are aimed at achieving uppermost benefit, therefore reducing overall harm to patients, services users and their families.

From the standpoint of the MHRA, effective medications management requires health and social care staff (including nursing students) to work together collaboratively both within and across disciplines. This also includes effective working practices at an organisational level through to supportive supervision and administration policies. It's therefore essential that as a nursing student you are familiar with local policies and procedures and your level of competence at each stage of your educational programme.

The National Institute for Health and Care Excellence (2015) identifies several factors that influence effective medication optimisation. This includes changes to the demographics of the population of the United Kingdom, an increase in individuals living with a long-term condition, an ageing population and an increase in patients taking multiple medications (**polypharmacy**). All of these factors enhance the complexity of health outcomes for patients and, therefore, there is a risk that preventable and adverse events may result in unnecessary hospital admissions (Frontier Economics, 2014).

SEE ALSO
CHAPTER 2

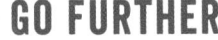

GO FURTHER

For more information regarding person-centred care in relation to medicines optimisation you can visit www.nice.org.uk/guidance/ng5/chapter/Person-centred-care

WEBLINK:
MEDICINES
OPTIMISATION

As you can now see, the context in which medicines management and optimisation operates has changed and so you now need to relate this to relevant legislation. The following section of this chapter intends to outline the historical trajectory of legislation and how this now relates to contemporary nursing practice.

MEDICATION MANAGEMENT AND RELEVANT LEGISLATION

As a nursing student it is important that you consider relevant legislation: some of this may be set in statute (law) or form part of guidance that is set by regulators, e.g. the NMC. Either way, this can be challenging for health and social care students to grasp. Legislation that governs medication management has been modernised, mainly to consolidate decades of UK legislation and to make this easier to understand.

There are two central pieces of legislation that you will be required to become familiar with. These are the Human Medicines Regulations (HMR) (2012) that has replaced the majority of the Medicines Act (1968), and the Misuse of Drugs Regulations (2001) which sits alongside the Misuse of Drugs Act (1971).

The Human Medicines Regulations (2012) consolidate the law of the United Kingdom concerning medicinal products for human use. The act is concerned mainly with administration, manufacturing and wholesale dealing, marketing authorisations of medicinal products, certification of homoeopathic medicinal products, traditional herbal registrations, **pharmacovigilance** and packaging and leaflets of medicinal products. The act is not limited to the above and also considers legislation around other factors. It's important to recognise that the act relates to all health and social care practitioners who are involved with medicines, whether they prescribe, dispense or administer and, therefore, relates to the wider multidisciplinary team.

There are three main classifications of medicines that are regulated by the HMR (section 30) and these will be discussed in turn.

1. A prescription only medicine (POM): Within this classification medicines must be accompanied with an authorised prescription. This must have been issued by a licensed practitioner. In most instances this will be a doctor, dentist, nurse prescriber or a pharmacist. It is important to consider that other professions such as physiotherapists, podiatrists and dietitians may be licensed to prescribe medication. Professions that are allied to medicines are often referred to as non-medical or supplemental prescribers.
2. A pharmacy medicine: This category relates to medicines that can only be supplied where there is a registered pharmacist. This can also include supermarkets where they have a designated pharmacy within the store. These do not generally require a prescription and are often related to over-the-counter medications.
3. A product that is subject to general sale: This category often relates to medication that can be purchased at your local shop. They are often limited in terms of their availability and size of the package.

Misuse of Drugs (1971 & 2001)

The Misuse of Drugs Act (1971) prohibits certain activities in relation to 'controlled drugs', in particular their manufacture, supply, and possession. The penalties applicable to offences involving the different drugs are graded broadly according to the harmfulness attributable to a drug when it is misused and for this purpose, the drugs are defined in the following three classes:

Class A includes: cocaine, diamorphine (heroin), dipipanone, lysergide (LSD), methadone and class B substances when prepared for injection.

Class B includes: oral amfetamines, barbiturates, cannabis, codeine and ketamine.

Class C includes: certain drugs related to the amfetamines, most benzodiazepines, tramadol, zopiclone, androgenic and anabolic steroids.

The Misuse of Drugs Regulations (2001) (and subsequent amendments) defines the classes of persons who are authorised to supply and possess controlled drugs (CDs) while acting in their professional capacities and lay down the conditions under which these activities may be carried out. In the regulations, drugs are divided into five schedules, each specifying the requirements governing such activities as import, export, production, supply, possession, prescribing and record keeping which apply to them.

Schedule 1 includes drugs such as lysergide, which is not used medicinally. Possession and supply are prohibited except in accordance with Home Office authority.

Schedule 2 includes drugs such as diamorphine (heroin) and morphine and are subject to the full controlled drug requirements relating to prescriptions, safe custody and the need to keep registers, etc. (unless exempted in Schedule 5).

Schedule 3 includes the barbiturates, buprenorphine, midazolam, temazepam and tramadol. They are subject to the special prescription requirements. Safe custody requirements do apply. Records in registers do not need to be kept (although there are requirements for the retention of invoices for two years).

Schedule 4 includes in Part I benzodiazepines (except temazepam and midazolam, which are in Schedule 3), and zopiclone, which are subject to minimal control. Part II includes androgenic and anabolic steroids. Controlled drug prescription requirements do not apply, and Schedule 4 Controlled Drugs are not subject to safe custody requirements.

Schedule 5 includes those preparations, which, because of their strength, are exempt from virtually all controlled drug requirements other than retention of invoices for two years.

Controlled Drugs

NICE (2016) has produced guidelines for healthcare staff who are involved with prescribing, dispensing and administering controlled substances. The guidelines recognise that, due to the risk of misuse and the potential risks of addiction, these medicines are subject to additional legislation. The legislation relates to the prescribing, storage, administration, record keeping and the destruction of medicines that fall within the schedules outlined earlier.

In most instances there is a requirement for two individuals to certify a controlled substance; one of these is usually a registered nurse. A register of the medication is recorded within a controlled drug register and a signature is required from both practitioners. All controlled drugs are requisitioned using a specific controlled drugs order book and are signed for and added to the register once they have been received within the clinical area. The controlled drugs cupboard has to be a separate cabinet that contains only controlled drugs and this has a unique key. In the event that a controlled drug needs to be destroyed, two practitioners also need to sign to evidence that this has happened.

Remember, it is important that as a student nurse that you work within the legal and ethical frameworks. These frameworks are there to protect you and the public from harm and, within your professional practice, prosecution. Legislation surrounding administration, storage and control of medicine needs to be considered within your own role and that of other healthcare professionals.

THE ROLE OF THE NURSE AND MULTIDISCIPLINARY TEAM IN MEDICATION MANAGEMENT

Prescribing

In 2012, the RPS produced a competency framework for all practitioners who are involved with prescribing. These guidelines have been updated with the backing of NICE and have been republished in 2016 for all regulators, e.g. the NMC and General Medical Council (GMC), professional bodies (e.g. RCN), and prescribing professions (e.g. medical practitioners, registered nurses who hold a prescribing qualification, dentists and pharmacists) (RPS, 2016).

The RPS (2016) recognises that when prescribed safely and used effectually, medicines can have positive health benefits for patients. Medicines are by far the most commonly used intervention to treat underlying conditions or pathology. **Polypharmacy** use to treat patients with medical conditions has increased, partly in response to patients having one or more underlying conditions, long-term conditions that can affect one or more body system or, as stated earlier in this chapter, an ageing population with multifaceted needs.

The RPS and RCN (2014), NICE (2015) and the DH (2016) all recognise that this added complexity of the management of patients requires professions involved with prescribing to enhance techniques that relate to successful medicines use and the manner by which these professions support patients.

Medical practitioners, dentists and veterinary surgeons are required to prescribe medicines upon completion of their undergraduate programmes. More recently, supplementary or independent prescribers are now able to prescribe medication within their sphere and scope of practice; usually this is after they have undertaken an approved education programme. The role of the registered nurse over the coming decade will evolve, and a broadening of additional prescribing responsibilities is likely as long as patient safety is protected and health outcomes for the public are beneficial.

Understanding the RPS (2016) prescribing framework will be beneficial on many levels. First, this will help you to identify prescribing errors or irregularities when administering medication to patients or providing information to patients about their medicines. Second, understanding the framework and recognising your limitations within your practice will support your education and preparedness to undertake this role in the future. Finally, you will have a greater understanding of why and how prescribers make decisions, assess the patient, consider the options, reach a shared decision, prescribe, and provide information to the patient and their family and the wider MDT.

While you may not be involved in prescribing of medicines during your education programme, this may be something that you are required to undertake from an agreed formulary once you are a qualified nurse. In line with the increasing demand for more nurses to become nurse prescribers, you will need to know about evidenced-based medicines management in order to prepare you for this role once qualified.

GO FURTHER

For more information on the prescribers' competency framework you can visit www.rpharms.com/resources/frameworks/prescribers-competency-framework

WEBLINK:
COMPETENCY
FRAMEWORK

Interpreting prescriptions

It is important to remember that within a hospital environment, nurses only have authority to administer medication under the supervision of a licenced prescriber, and in most instances this will be a doctor; however, this may also be a supplementary/independent nurse prescriber (RCN, 2014). As a student, you will need to be familiar with drug charts used within your clinical area at that time. You need to be aware that different NHS trusts and independent sector organisations may have different charts. While they will all contain similar information, the way that the information is presented may vary. It is also important to understand that while some areas may have a paper drug chart, others may be presented electronically. Different medication administration approaches will be discussed later within this chapter.

Each healthcare organisation will have its own policies and procedures that will govern the administration of medicines and medical products, e.g. blood products. You will need to be familiar with these and ensure that your practice is in accordance with these policies – they are there to protect you and the public!

ACTIVITY 13.1
ANSWER

ACTIVITY 13.1: REFLECTIVE PRACTICE

Having read the information regarding interpreting prescriptions, can you identify the different types of prescriptions, including paper and electronic, and identify the strengths and weaknesses of each of these in relation to your practice placement experiences?

The NMC (2015) published *The Code: Professional standards of practice and behaviour for nurses and midwives*. The *Code* outlines behaviours and standards that registered nurses must attain and reminds practitioners of their rights and responsibilities. As such, all nurses are accountable for their actions and omissions including medicines management.

The *Code* needs to be used alongside other regulatory advice. The RCN recognises the complexity of medication management and administration of medicines and states:

> The administration of medicines is an important aspect of the professional practice of persons whose names are on the Council's register. It is not solely a mechanistic task to be performed in strict compliance with the written prescription of a medical practitioner (can now also be an independent and supplementary prescriber). It requires thought and the exercise of professional judgement (RCN, 2017).

There are important aspects involved when administering medicines to individuals or groups of patients; these are often referred to as the rights (5 Rs) of medication (see below). You also need to consider other aspects, such as **pharmacokinetics, pharmacodynamics, pharmacotherapeutics** – the patient's response to medication, half-life, contraindications and other factors that will be explained in greater depth later in this chapter. When you deliberate all of these factors it is easy to see that the administration of medicines is not a mechanistic completion of a check list; professional judgement, clinical decision-making skills and interpreting the presentation of the patient are all essential (RCN, 2017).

When considering legislation surrounding the supply and possession of medication, doctors are approved to undertake these activities providing they are within their lawful practice (GMC, 2013). In most instances, a prescription must be made by a medical practitioner and the prescription must include the frequency of the administration, the route by which the drug will be administered and the dose to be given, and must be signed by the prescriber. If there is any ambiguity, then as a nurse you should challenge this with the prescriber.

Prior to administering the medication and following the 5Rs, always think allergy first. Always ask the patient if they think that they are allergic to any medication or substances, e.g. latex. There may be circumstances where the allergy has not been recorded on the patient's drug chart or that this is known but a prescribing error has occurred. This initial check is helpful in reducing the risk of adverse drug reactions or, in serious cases, anaphylaxis. NICE (2014) has published guidelines to assist staff to identify and manage drug allergies. The guidance outlines the assessment required and the steps that practitioners need to make; familiarise yourself with this in accordance with local policies and procedures.

ACTIVITY 13.2: REFLECTION

In a group, or as an individual, identify those practitioners who you have worked with who are prescribers and identity the context in which they are able to prescribe medicines.

ACTIVITY 13.2
ANSWER

Systems errors, medication errors and the effect that this can have on patient outcomes will be discussed in greater depth in the patient safety chapter.

The 5 rights relate to:

SEE ALSO
CHAPTER 5

- The right patient

While this may sound straightforward, one of the most common drug errors is that the wrong medication has been given to the wrong person. You will be required to check the patient's identity against their drug chart/prescription. This is more commonly being undertaken electronically using a bar code that is worn on the patient's wrist that will correspond with a matching bar code on the patient's prescription chart. In some areas you will also be required to authenticate the patient's date of birth. It would be a good idea at this stage to ask the patient if they have any known allergies.

- The right drug

You will need to identify the correct drug that is outlined within the prescription. If you are unfamiliar with this drug you can verify your understanding of this by using a reputable reference source. In most instances this is the British National Formulary (BNF). You will also have to demonstrate that you understand the therapeutic action of the medication (its use) and if this is appropriate to treat your patient's underlying condition. Other considerations during this stage will be any side effects that this may have and if this drug will interact with other drugs that are prescribed on the prescription chart.

- The right time

Medications are administered at various times of the day and night. Factors that necessitate how often a medication should be given can include the half-life of the drug, interaction of the drug with food molecules or higher levels of pH within the stomach in order to absorb substances across membranes. In order to ensure a medicine remains within its therapeutic index (when the drug remains effective without it becoming toxic or ineffective), it is important that the doses of the medication are delivered on time.

- The right dose

The correct dose for medication needs to be understood. This can be very complex, especially in critical care units, the operating department or within the emergency department. This is generally calculated by the prescriber in terms of body weight, which is usually measured in kilograms. Doses vary according to the age and the condition of the patient that you are treating. Your ability to calculate doses in the correct unit of measurement is essential.

- The right route

Medications are designed to be administered using a variety of methods. It is important that you are familiar with all of these as they will have an impact on the speed and proficiency of the absorption of the medicine. Administering medication via the wrong route of administration can have serious and life-threatening consequences. Ensure that you become familiar with the routes of administration of the drugs that you are giving to patients, and that you are able to identify how they affect factors such as absorption and distribution.

PREPARATION FOR PRACTICE PLACEMENT 13.1

As an individual, or as a group, identify each aspect of the 5 rights of drug administration and outline their importance to patient safety.

Medication administration approaches

There have been a number of technological advances that have influenced the process of medication administration within and outside of the NHS. Many healthcare organisations have electronic medication systems in place in an attempt to reduce adverse drug events, reduce the time that practitioners are involved with medication administration and reduce the overall cost and wastage of medicine procurement.

When undertaking your practice learning experiences, it is likely that you will be exposed to a variety of different administration approaches. It is important that as a nursing student you are familiar with each system used within your area and that you have undertaken mandatory training to ensure that you know how to work within the organisation's policies correctly, and that you ensure you base your practice in regard to medicines management around the NMC (2015) *Code*.

Patient Group Directives

NICE (2017) has updated its guidance on the use of patient group directives (PGD). It suggests that PGDs allow healthcare professionals to supply and administer specified medicines to predefined groups of patients, without a prescription. This guideline aims to ensure that patient group directives are used in line with legislation, so that patients have safe and speedy access to the medicines they need. The RCN (2006) in its guidance to nurses, identifies that the legislation (Statutory Instrument, 2000a) states that:

> Patient Group Direction means – in connection with the supply of a prescription only medicine … a written direction relating to the supply and administration of a description or class of prescription only medicine … or a written direction relating to the administration of a description or class of prescription only medicine, and which in the case of either is signed by a doctor … and by a pharmacist; and relates to the supply and administration, or to administration, to persons generally (subject to any exclusions which may be set out in the Direction).

The RCN (2006) goes on to say,

> In practice this means that a PGD, signed by a doctor and agreed by a pharmacist, can act as a direction to a nurse to supply and/or administer prescription-only medicines (POMs) to patients using their own assessment of patient need, without necessarily referring back to a doctor for an individual prescription.

The NMC *Standards for Medicines Management* (2007) and a further circular in 2009 (NMC, 2009) clarified the regulator's position on the role of the nursing student. Registered nurses and midwives cannot delegate the supply and/or administration of medicines under PGD. While you will be expected to understand PGDs and their use within practice you are not permitted to administer or supply medication via this directive until you graduate. It should be noted, however, that the standard and guidance on PGDs are likely to be superseded by the new pre-registration nursing standards published in 2018 by the NMC. At the time of writing, however, it is important that you understand PGDs and their use within practice but you are not permitted to administer or supply medication via this directive until you graduate.

PATIENT EDUCATION AND CONCORDANCE

NICE (2009) identifies that between 30 and 50% of individuals do not follow prescribed regimes for one reason or another. The traditional viewpoint identified patient compliance with prescribed medication as the basis of the problem. There is a wider acceptance now, with patients who have multiple pathologies and polypharmacy, that medicine-taking is a complex behaviour and influencing this involves partnership working between patients, providers of healthcare and healthcare systems.

A large proportion of the patients we look after are elderly and living with multiple long-term conditions and, as such, there is often a large regime of medications that they take daily. Throughout my experience of working in the acute and community settings, many patients often do not know what medications they are taking and what they are taking them for. The National Institute for Health and Care Excellence (NICE) (2009) states that providing patients with information is a method to increase their concordance to their medication regimes and, therefore, nurses are in the ideal position to provide this education to patients. In order to do this effectively, we have to know what we are talking about, and this can only be done through learning the indications for medications and how they work within the body. Having this knowledge means that we can interpret this information and then provide it in a manner that the patient understands, and to the detail that they would like.

Travis Norton, 3rd year student nurse

The NHS Constitution (Department of Health and Social Care, 2012) establishes the principles and values of the NHS in England. It sets out rights to which patients, public and staff are entitled, and pledges which the NHS is committed to achieve, together with responsibilities, which the public, patients and staff owe to one another to ensure that the NHS operates fairly and effectively. As such, the need for nursing staff to be equipped with the knowledge and skills necessary to educate the public about their medication regimes is inherently embedded within the rights for patients within the Constitution. The complexity of medications management and long-term conditions necessitates the need for the promotion of self-care models enabling patients to manage their conditions more effectively (Nicol, 2015).

Successive governments have highlighted the nurse's role as central to the success of patient education in terms of managing long-term conditions. When considering medications management and patient education, the NMC (2007) expects nursing practitioners to engage fully with the education of prescribed regimes, using plain language. Nurses need to educate patients about the use, side effects and contraindications of the medication, and what they should do if they feel unwell and are unable to take their medication. It is important to recognise that the education that is provided to patients about their medicines is given using an inter-professional approach; so, in essence, nurses, doctors and pharmacists will all be involved with this important role.

The term 'adherence' is now used to describe the extent to which patients' medicine-taking behaviour matches agreed recommendations from the prescriber. This understanding presumes an agreement between patient and prescriber. Attention is, therefore, required to the decision-making process between prescribers and patients (NICE, 2009). The problems that arise when patients are not fully involved are shown in Case Study 13.1.

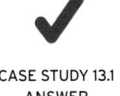

CASE STUDY 13.1
ANSWER

CASE STUDY 13.1: GEORGE WILSON

Mr George Wilson, a 75-year-old gentleman, has been admitted to hospital via A&E for investigations after a concerned neighbour became alerted to his condition. On admission he is breathless, and his ankles are swollen. He appears quiet, distressed and withdrawn. He was recently commenced on oral diuretics by his GP. George is usually active but informs you that he feels he cannot leave the house as he is frightened not to be close to the toilet. George stopped taking his diuretics a week ago as he was incontinent.

- What was the primary reason why George did not adhere to his medication regime?
- How could you ensure that George was able to take his medication safely with minimal disruption to his activities of daily living?

GO FURTHER

WEBLINK:
CONCORDANCE

For further reading regarding adherence and concordance visit www.nice.org.uk/guidance/cg76

GENERAL PRINCIPLES OF PHARMACOLOGY

You will no doubt as a nursing student have looked through the BNF with a certain amount of trepidation. The number of medicines that are prescribed for patients is growing; this is likely to increase with the introduction of personalised medicine and **genomics.** As a nursing student you will only be able to fully participate and contribute to the care of patients and service users if you understand how medicines work, what side effects they may cause and how illness can affect your patient's ability to absorb, distribute, metabolise and eliminate the drug. Pharmacology has many complicated aspects and terminology. Don't be frightened by these terms over your programme of education – you will become familiar with them. One such term – pharmacokinetics – relates to the science that explores and identifies the way the human body affects the drug, i.e. the factors that influence its absorption, distribution, metabolism and elimination.

ACTIVITY 13.3: CRITICAL THINKING

As an individual, or in a group, think about some experiences you have witnessed where patients may respond differently to the same drug and attempt to identify possible causes for this.

ACTIVITY 13.3
ANSWER

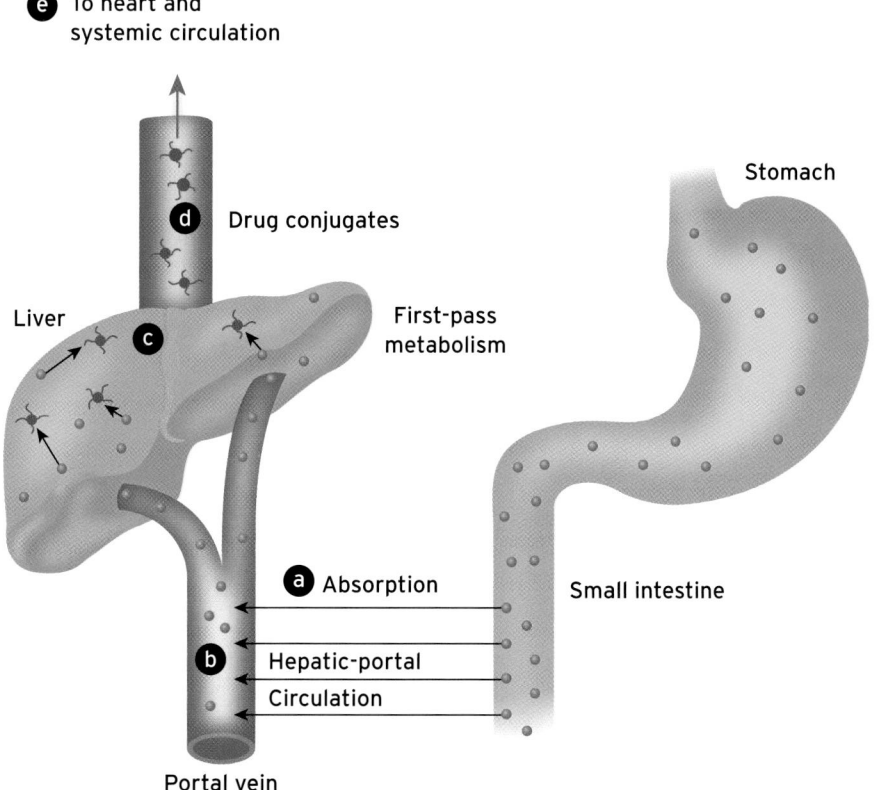

Figure 13.1 Hepatic first-pass metabolism

Available at: www.endoca.com/blog/cbd/how-cbd-metabolized/ accessed 1/5/17

Absorption

In the case of ingested or oral drugs (also referred to as **enteral**), these are drugs that are administered via the gastrointestinal system. In this instance the medication has to pass through the gastrointestinal (GI) wall in order to enter the plasma. Any substance that is absorbed via the GI wall will be transported to the liver via the **hepatic portal vein** prior to being delivered to the body's tissues and organs.

a – Drug absorbed from GI Tract.

b – Passes from the portal vein to the liver.

c – First Pass. The liver will re-package the drug and the concentration of a drug is reduced. This re-packaging can also produce metabolites that may also produce pharmacological effects, e.g. codeine has metabolites that are stronger than the parent drug itself – morphine.

d – Distributed around body.

e – Bioavailability. Drug available in circulation.

The majority of drugs are administrated orally, by mouth, and include liquids, tablets and capsules. The stomach contents and the speed of emptying have huge implications on the **absorption** of the drug and consequently the level of the drug in the blood, e.g. a drug taken with food will slow its passage into the small intestine where most drugs are absorbed to the portal system (see Figure 13.1). The prescription of some drugs will state with food, e.g. ritonavir (used to manage HIV-1), as the drug is better absorbed mixed with food matter (chyme). Some drugs can irritate the stomach causing pain or inflammation so taking them with food will reduce this effect, e.g. ibuprofen, a non-steroidal anti-inflammatory drug. Absorption is increased for some drugs when not in the presence of food and they should be taken at least an hour before a meal, e.g. flucloxacillin, an antibiotic. Drug presentation will also reflect its absorption rate, e.g. nifedipine MR (modified release), a short-acting drug that requires its action to be prolonged through its formulation that enables the timing and/or the rate of release of the drug substance to be controlled. Drug presentation must never be altered, e.g. dismantle a capsule or crush a tablet, unless indicated on the prescription, identified in your local policy or as advised by the pharmacist. This is important to remember when caring for patients with a nasogastric tube or fine feeding tube as a drug could expand in the tube and block it (e.g. ciprofloxin), or the patient could suffer from adverse effects of the unprotected drug, (e.g. enteric coated NSAID crushed will cause gastric irritation and possibly bleeding into the stomach).

Now that you have been introduced to the notion of absorption, let's consider some of the **parenteral** routes (which means to avoid the GI tract) of drug administration and how drugs are absorbed.

Buccal cavity administration is when the drug is placed between the cheek and gums OR in the cheek pouch. The inner cheeks have multiple fine capillaries that are able to absorb the drug quickly directly into the blood stream and miss passing through the digestive system. This is a useful method of administration if the patient is having issues swallowing or the effects of the drug would be decreased by passing through the stomach. Nicotine (smoking cessation) is an example of this method of administration; the person receives an almost immediate controlled dose of nicotine to divert them from smoking tobacco.

Sublingual administration is placing the drug under the patient's tongue. The area under the tongue has multiple fine capillaries that quickly absorb the drug, but importantly they are absorbed more rapidly by this method compared to buccal cavity administration. Nitroglycerin (GTN) spray or tablets are immediately administered prior to or during a painful angina cardiac attack using this method, ensuring a rapid response and improvement to the patient's condition. Some of the nursing considerations with this method of administration are raised in Activity 13.4 below.

ACTIVITY 13.4: CRITICAL THINKING

What advice do you need to give to patients who are using the sublingual route of medication administration? Identify what may happen if the patient swallows tablets intended for the sublingual route.

If a patient has open ulcers or mucositis, how would this affect the administration of sublingual or buccal routes of administration?

ACTIVITY 13.4
ANSWER

Drugs to administrate into the rectum will be packaged usually as suppositories, a jelly or an enema (liquid). A jelly or a pessary are more commonly used to administer a drug into the vagina. The heat of the rectum or vagina will encourage the pessary or suppository to dissolve and so the absorption of the drug. Once absorbed, the drug will have limited first pass but will immediately be distributed around the body. Drugs administered by the rectal and vaginal methods will only be effectively absorbed if the tissue is well perfused; it has a good blood supply. If there is any evidence of prolapse, e.g. collapse or protruding of any type of tissue through the vagina or the rectum, inform a practitioner immediately and do not administer the drug. Faeces will act as a barrier and limit the absorption surface area so it is important to establish your patient's bowel habits and routine before administering a drug by this method. Remember, the drug would need to be retained long enough for it to be absorbed; ensure your patient understands how the drug works or they may go to the toilet and expel it.

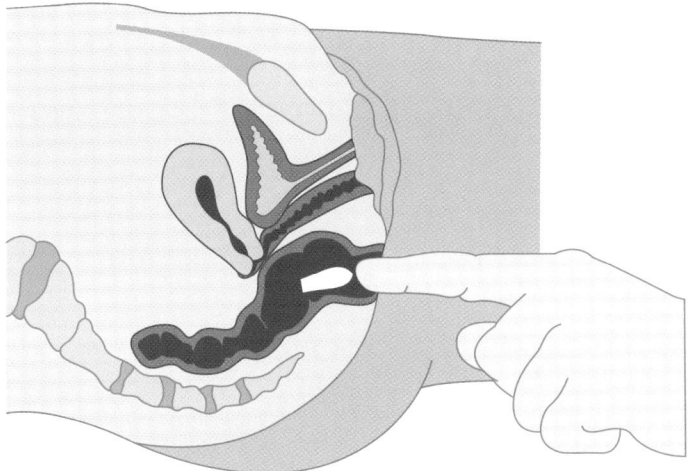

Figure 13.2 Rectal route of administration

Subcutaneous (SC) administration is by injecting the drug into the fatty layer between the dermis and muscle. Areas of the body ideal for this type of injection are the upper arms, thighs and lower abdomen. The drug can be administered by this method as a bolus, via a syringe driver, or an infusion of a low volume of fluid over a period of time via a pump. Insulin is administered using a subcutaneous method as if given orally the drug would be destroyed by the enzymes in the stomach.

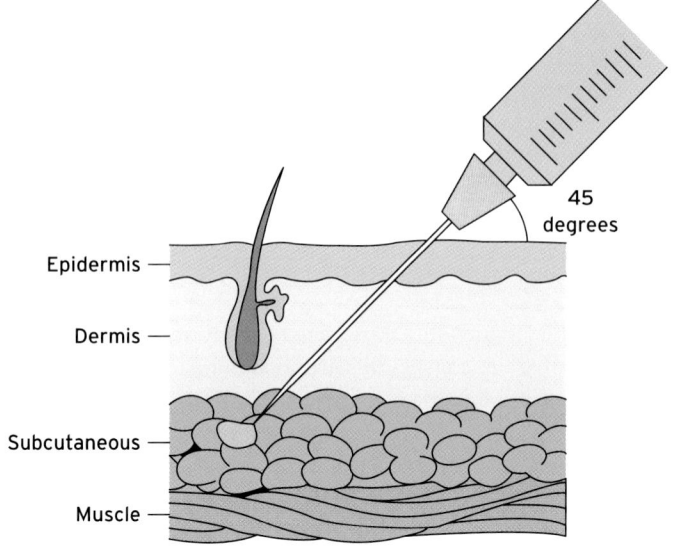

Figure 13.3 Subcutaneous route of administration

Intramuscular (IM) route is via injection of the drug directly into a muscle: the deltoid (upper arm shoulder), ventrogluteal (outer upper thigh), dorsogluteal (outer upper bottom) or the vastus lateralis (outer lower thigh). Intramuscular injections are rarely used as there are quicker methods to administer a drug, e.g. intravenous, and also less painful methods, i.e. subcutaneous.

Transdermal route involves layered patches that are adhered to the patient's skin and administer a drug consistently over a period of time: at the end of their life cycle they are removed and replaced with a new patch. They are very useful for the long-term administration of a drug ensuring stable therapeutic level, also patients like them as they are non-intrusive and reduce the amount of oral drugs.

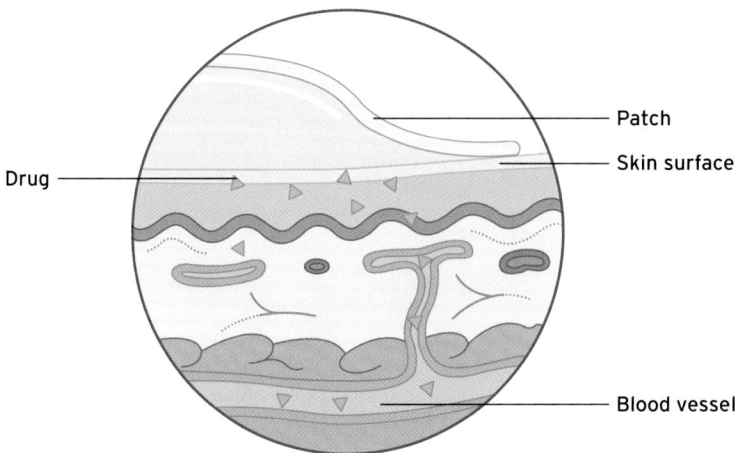

Figure 13.4 Transdermal route

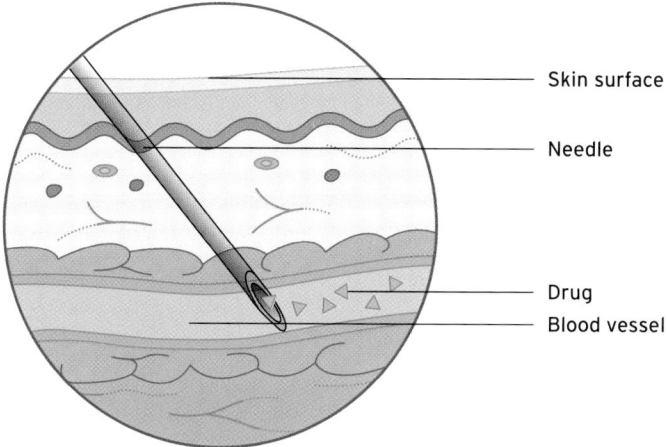

Figure 13. 5 Intravenous route

To ensure skin integrity the patient should be advised that the site is changed with each new patch, with the date and time indicated. Fentanyl patches are used to manage severe chronic pain.

Intravenous route involves injection or infusion directly into the vascular system and consequently it is immediately distributed around the body travelling to its point of action. It is important to recognise that, as the quickest method of drug administration, any adverse effects or allergic reactions will also develop very rapidly, requiring a speedy response.

Now that you have had an opportunity to explore how some drugs are administered and absorbed either via an **enteral** or **parenteral** route, let's investigate the next stage of pharmacokinetics – distribution.

Distribution

The rate or time a drug reaches its point of action depends on the rate and volume of blood and the solubility of the drug. The higher and larger the blood supply, the quicker the distribution. Solubility relates primarily to how drugs cross membranes within the human body. Remember, lipid-soluble drugs pass more effectively across cell membranes and the blood brain barrier than water-soluble drugs. Bound to large plasma proteins (**albumin**) in the blood, the drug is transported around the body to its point of action. The binding of the drug to the plasma protein does not initiate any therapeutic effect and only the unbound drug remains functional. Certain age groups including the very young and older adults can have significantly lower levels of albumin. This can result in more unbound drug being free to exert an effect, resulting in toxicity.

GO FURTHER

For more information on plasma protein binding visit www.nottingham.ac.uk/nmp/sonet/rlos/bioproc/plasma_proteins/page_five.html

WEBLINK:
PLASMA
PROTEIN

Metabolism

Following its action, the drug will be transported by the plasma proteins to the liver where it will be inactivated and be prepared to be removed from the body. The majority of drugs will be metabolised by oxidation and hydroxylation making them less fat soluble and more water soluble, and consequently easier to be eliminated via the kidney. Some drugs or their metabolites require removing in bile and emptied into the gastric intestinal system. Remember, while the liver is the organ responsible for **metabolism**, the kidneys, intestinal tract, skin and lungs also play a part in drug metabolism.

Elimination

The final phase of pharmacokinetics is **elimination**. Here, the drug is removed from the body. The majority of drugs will be eliminated in urine, bile, sweat, saliva and some in faeces. Renal and gastrointestinal diseases or conditions will impede normal removal of these waste products. The means by which the kidneys eliminate products is by active glomerular filtration. In this instance, drugs are secreted into the proximal convoluted tubule and are then pushed out into urine. Patients with acute kidney injury, renal failure or kidney diseases may have difficulties in excreting drugs; older adults particularly have a reduction in kidney function and, therefore, should be monitored closely to ensure toxins do not remain within the body.

CHAPTER SUMMARY

- There are a number of contextual changes and legal frameworks required for adult nurses to practise safely in relation to medicines management and optimisation
- The role of the nurse is expanding in relation to medicines management, including prescribing
- The routes of administration can affect the way in which drugs are absorbed
- Pharmacokinetics describes how drugs are absorbed, distributed, metabolised and excreted

GO FURTHER

CASE STUDY: ANTICOAGULANTS

Go to https://study.sagepub.com/essentialadultnursing for a further case study related to this chapter. If you are using the interactive ebook, simply click on the book icon in the margin to go straight to the resource.

Books

- Ashelford, S., Raynsford, J. and Taylor, V. (2016) *Pathophysiology and Pharmacology for Nursing Students.* London: Learning Matters/Sage.
- An integrated introduction to both the biology of disease and the therapeutic agents that are used to manage them, includes the relevant pharmacology of common disorders.
- Spires, A., O'Brien, M. and Andrews, K. (2011) *Introduction to Medicines Management in Nursing.* London: Learning Matters/Sage.
- Although aimed at first years this is a good book to help you revise the basics.
- Starkings, S. and Krause, L. (2018) *Passing Calculations Tests in Nursing.* London: Learning Matters/Sage.
- Designed to help you face calculations tests with confidence and pass first time!

Journal Articles

FURTHER READING: JOURNAL ARTICLES

Go to https://study.sagepub.com/essentialadultnursing for further free online journal articles related to this chapter. If you are using the interactive ebook, simply click on the book icon in the margin to go straight to the resource.

- Car, J., Shin Tan, W., Huang, Z., Sloot, P. and Franklin, B.D. (2017) eHealth in the future of medications management: personalisation, monitoring and adherence. *BMC Medicine*, 15:73.
- https://doi.org/10.1186/s12916-017-0838-0
- A paper that explores the role of eHealth in patients' medicines management journey to ensure adherence.
- Fylan, B., Armitage, G., Naylor, D. and Blenkinsopp, A. (2017) A qualitative study of patient involvement in medicines management after hospital discharge: an under-recognised source of systems resilience. *BMJ Quality and Safety*, Published Online First: 16 November 2017. doi: 10.1136/bmjqs-2017-006813.
- Looks at how resilience has a part to play in ensuring safety when patients are discharged home with medications.
- Wright, K. (2013) The role of nurses in medicine administration errors. *Nursing Standard*, 27 (44): 35–40.
- Provides a different way of looking at drug errors.

Weblinks

FURTHER READING: WEBLINKS

Go to https://study.sagepub.com/essentialadultnursing for further weblinks related to this chapter. If you are using the interactive ebook, simply click on the book icon in the margin to go straight to the resource.

- Genomics Education Programme
- www.genomicseducation.hee.nhs.uk/
- Provides a huge number of resources around genomics.
- Medicines Optimisation
- www.rcn.org.uk/clinical-topics/medicines-optimisation
- Explains what medicines optimisation is and provides a number of useful resources.
- Royal Pharmaceutical Society
- www.rpharms.com/
- An essential resource for all healthcare professionals whether you prescribe or not.

ACE YOUR ASSESSMENT

ONLINE QUIZZES

Revise what you have learned by visiting https://study.sagepub.com/essentialadultnursing

- Test yourself with multiple-choice and short-answer questions
- Do the chapter activities in the book and check your answers online

REFERENCES

Department of Health, Social Services and Public Safety (2016) *Northern Ireland Medicines Optimisation Quality Framework*. March 2016. Available at: https://www.health-ni.gov.uk/sites/default/files/consultations/dhssps/medicines-optimisation-quality-framework.pdf

Department of Health and Social Care (2012) *NHS Constitution for England*. Department of Health and Social Care.

Frontier Economics (2014) *Exploring the Costs of Unsafe Care in the NHS: A report prepared for the Department of Health*. Available at: www.frontier-economics.com/documents/2014/10/exploring-the-costs-of-unsafe-care-in-the-nhs-frontier-report-2-2-2-2.pdf

General Medical Council (2013) *Good Practice in Prescribing and Managing Medicines and Devices*. Available at: www.gmc-uk.org/Prescribing_guidance.pdf_59055247.pdf

Health Education England (2018) *Advisory Guidance. Administration of Medicines by Nursing Associates*. Available at: https://hee.nhs.uk/news-blogs-events/news/new-guidance-medicines-management-nursing-associates-published

Medicines Act (1968) Available at: www.legislation.gov.uk/ukpga/1968/67

Medicines and Healthcare products Regulatory Agency (MHRA) (2014) *Improving Medication Error Incident Reporting and Learning*. Available at: www.england.nhs.uk/wp-content/uploads/2014/03/psa-med-error.pdf

Misuse of Drugs Act (1971) Available at: www.legislation.gov.uk/ukpga/1971/38/contents

Misuse of Drugs Regulations (2001) www.legislation.gov.uk/uksi/2001/3998/contents/made

National Institute for Health and Care Excellence (2009) *Medicines Adherence: Involving patients in decisions about prescribed medicines and supporting adherence*. Available at: www.nice.org.uk/guidance/cg76

National Institute for Health and Care Excellence (2014) *Drug Allergy: Diagnosis and management*. Available at: www.nice.org.uk/guidance/cg183

National Institute for Health and Care Excellence (2015) *Medicines Optimisation: The safe and effective use of medicines to enable the best possible outcomes*. Available at: www.nice.org.uk/guidance/ng5

National Institute for Health and Care Excellence (2016) *Controlled Drugs: Safe use and management*. Available at: *www.nice.org.uk/guidance/ng46*

Nicol, J. (2015) *Nursing Adults with Long Term Conditions*. London: Sage.

Nursing and Midwifery Council (2007) *Standards for Medicines Management*. Available at: www.nmc.org.uk/standards/additional-standards/standards-for-medicines-management/

Nursing and Midwifery Council (2009) *Supply and/or administration of medicine by student nurses and student midwives in relation to Patient Group Directions (PGDs)* NMC Circular 05/2009. Available at: https://www.nmc.org.uk/globalassets/sitedocuments/circulars/2009circulars/nmc-circular-05_2009.pdf

Nursing and Midwifery Council (2015) *The Code. Professional standards of practice and behaviour for nurses and midwives*. Available at: www.nmc.org.uk/standards/code/

Royal College of Nursing (2006) *Patient Group Directions. Guidance and Information for nurses*. Available at: www.rcn.org.uk/professional-development/publications/pub-001370

Royal College of Nursing (2014) *Nurse Prescribing*. Available at: www.rcn.org.uk/get-help/rcn-advice/nurse-prescribing

Royal College of Nursing (2016) *Fact Sheet Nurse Prescribing in the UK*. Available at: www.rcn.org.uk/about-us/policy-briefings/pol-1512

Royal College of Nursing (2017) *Medicines Optimisation*. Available at: www.rcn.org.uk/clinical-topics/medicines-optimisation

Royal Pharmaceutical Society (2013) *Medicines Optimisation: Helping patients to make the most of medicines*. Available at: https://www.rpharms.com/Portals/0/RPS%20document%20library/Open%20access/Policy/helping-patients-make-the-most-of-their-medicines.pdf

Royal Pharmaceutical Society and Royal College of Nursing (2014) *Working together to help patients make the most of medicines*. Available at: www.rpharms.com/Portals/0/RPS%20document%20

library/Open%20access/Development/Workforce%20and%20Education/rps-make-the-most-of-medicines-web.pdf

Royal Pharmaceutical Society (2016) *A Competency Framework for All Prescribers*. Available at: www.rpharms.com/resources/frameworks/prescribers-competency-framework

The Human Medicines Regulations 2012. Available at: www.legislation.gov.uk/uksi/2012/1916/pdfs/uksi_20121916_en.pdf

INFECTION PREVENTION AND CONTROL

14

CLAIRE CHALMERS AND HEATHER GOURLAY

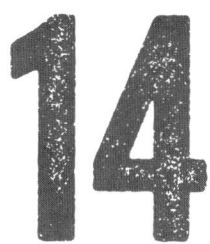

THIS CHAPTER COVERS

- Assessing the risk of infection
- Control measures to reduce the risk of infection
- Managing the infectious patient

- Monitoring infection prevention and control practices
- Promoting good infection prevention and control practice.

REQUIRED KNOWLEDGE

Before reading this chapter it will be helpful to:

- Revisit any previous education and training materials relating to infection prevention and control, including Chapter 24 (Infection Prevention and Control) and Chapter 18 (Assessing and Managing Risk) within the 1st year book *Essentials of Nursing Practice*
- Review your understanding of standard infection control precautions

- Revisit local policy relating to infection prevention and control
- Review *The Code – Professional standards of practice and behaviour for nurses and midwives* (NMC, 2015).

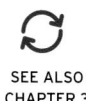 SEE ALSO CHAPTER 3

> ❝ I choose to get the flu jab to help keep me, my family and my community healthy. I encourage all my friends to consider getting it too, so we can stay healthy together as we age. ❞
>
> **David, Service User**

> ❝ If any nurse, even a director of nursing, sees a spill in a hospital then it is his or her responsibility to get it cleaned up. Infection control is everyone's business. ❞
>
> **Professor Paul Martin, UWS Depute Principal (and former Chief Nurse of Scotland)**

INTRODUCTION

Infection prevention and control is an integral component of high-quality health and social care practice. Understanding and appropriately implementing the principles of infection prevention and control will protect patients, health and social care workers, carers, visitors and the public at large. Assessing, responding to and minimising risk of infection is central to good infection prevention and control practice, as well as to the improvement of healthcare quality and public safety.

Yet despite the long-standing recognition that effective infection prevention and control is everyone's responsibility, the burden of healthcare-associated infection persists worldwide (WHO, 2011; CDC, 2016; ECDC, 2015; HPA, 2012; HPS, 2016) and non-compliance with standard precautions continues to be reported in the findings of healthcare research (Gammon et al., 2008; WHO, 2011; Perieeira et al., 2015; Colet et al., 2017). In turn, the range of interventions and approaches to support the prevention and control of infection continues to grow amidst health and social care systems that are becoming increasingly complex and challenging.

This chapter aims to enhance your knowledge of relevant microbiology, epidemiology and immunology (Table 14.1), and to develop your knowledge and skills in the prevention, control and management of infection, including your understanding of the importance of assessing infection risk.

ASSESSING THE RISK OF INFECTION

With advanced understanding in the fields of microbiology, epidemiology and immunology, our appreciation of the causes, spread and management of the micro-organisms capable of causing infection and/or infectious diseases continues to grow.

Table 14.1   Definitions of key fields aligned to infection prevention and control

Field	Definition
Microbiology	The study of micro-organisms or microbes – living things too small to see without the use of the microscope
Epidemiology	The study of patterns and causes of health-related issues, including disease, in populations
Immunology	The study of immune systems (or immunity)

Evidence base: Weir and Stewart (1997); Wilson (2000); WHO (2018)

Since the advent of germ theory, the invention of the microscope and the development of diagnostic techniques (such as culture media), progress in the science of microbiology has established the existence of thousands of different species of micro-organisms within the environment, including on and in the human body. There are four broad categories of micro-organisms, distinguishable by cell size, shape, colour, staining properties, respiration and reproduction (Inglis, 2007):

- Bacteria are single cell organisms of varying sizes between 0.3–14µm. There are three main shapes, determined by its cell wall: spherical/round (cocci); rods (bacilli) and spiral. The grouping of these individual-shaped cells (into bunches, chains and pairs) helps to further classify them. Bacteria with different cell wall structures and properties cause them to react differently to staining with Gram stain (and therefore be grouped on the basis of their staining characteristics as either Gram positive or Gram negative).

- Viruses range in size (30–400nm), the largest being as big as a small bacteria. Unlike bacteria which contain both DNA and RNA, viruses contain DNA *or* RNA (either single or double stranded, linear or circular). Viruses can be grouped into three main types based on their shape (cubic, helical and complex), and further defined by the structure and properties of their outer surface (enveloped or naked/non-enveloped). Lacking the ingredients to replicate and grow on their own, their outer structure and its properties are key determinants of its survival as well as its identification.
- Fungi range in size from microscopic to macroscopic, and can be grouped on the basis of their growth forms. The two main forms which exist are yeasts (small, round and unicellular) and moulds (strings which interlace and branch).
- Parasites include protozoa (complex single-celled microscopic organisms) and helminths (worms, which are multi-cellular organisms). Helminths can be subgrouped into nematodes (roundworms), cestodes (tapeworms) and trematodes (flukes), and while larvae may be only 100–200μm in size, adult worms can grow to become metres in length.

The relationships between micro-organisms and humans vary, but importantly, not all interactions lead to infection. From birth, into and throughout adulthood, colonisation (the presence of micro-organisms on the human body surface without harm) occurs. Colonising micro-organisms can be resident (found in certain areas of the body on a regular basis) and transient (present on the body for short periods of time). Made up mainly of bacteria (Grice and Segre, 2011), these establish what is described as the body's normal flora. The relationship between the micro-organisms of the normal flora and the human host can be referred to ecologically as commensalism, a class of relationship where one organism (the micro-organism) benefits (by securing a suitable habitat) from the other (the human) without affecting it. Common commensal bacteria found on the skin include *Staphylococcus epidermis*, *Staphylococcus aureus* and *Propionibacterium acnes* (Akst, 2014). Another perspective is to consider the relationship as symbiotic (or interdependent), where the micro-organism and human are mutually benefiting from each other – the micro-organism securing a suitable habitat, and the human securing protection from harmful micro-organisms by the presence of the micro-organisms which make up the normal flora.

CRITICAL THINKING STOP POINT 14.1

- Consider other areas of the human body (such as the respiratory and gastrointestinal tracts).
- What common commensals might be present in these areas?

In relationships where micro-organisms become harmful to the human host, the micro-organisms are described as parasitic (or pathogenic). Pathogens are micro-organisms which can be disease causing. Pathogens can also colonise parts of the body, in which case a colonised individual would be described as a carrier. A carrier is capable of spreading infection to others.

The ability of pathogens to cause disease is influenced by a range of interconnecting factors, which come together and result in infection. This range of factors is commonly known as the chain of infection (see Figure 14.1). For infection to occur, all six links of the chain of infection must occur together. Understanding the chain of infection and how breaking any one or more of the links can prevent infection is key to assessment of the risk of infection, and to good infection prevention and control practice.

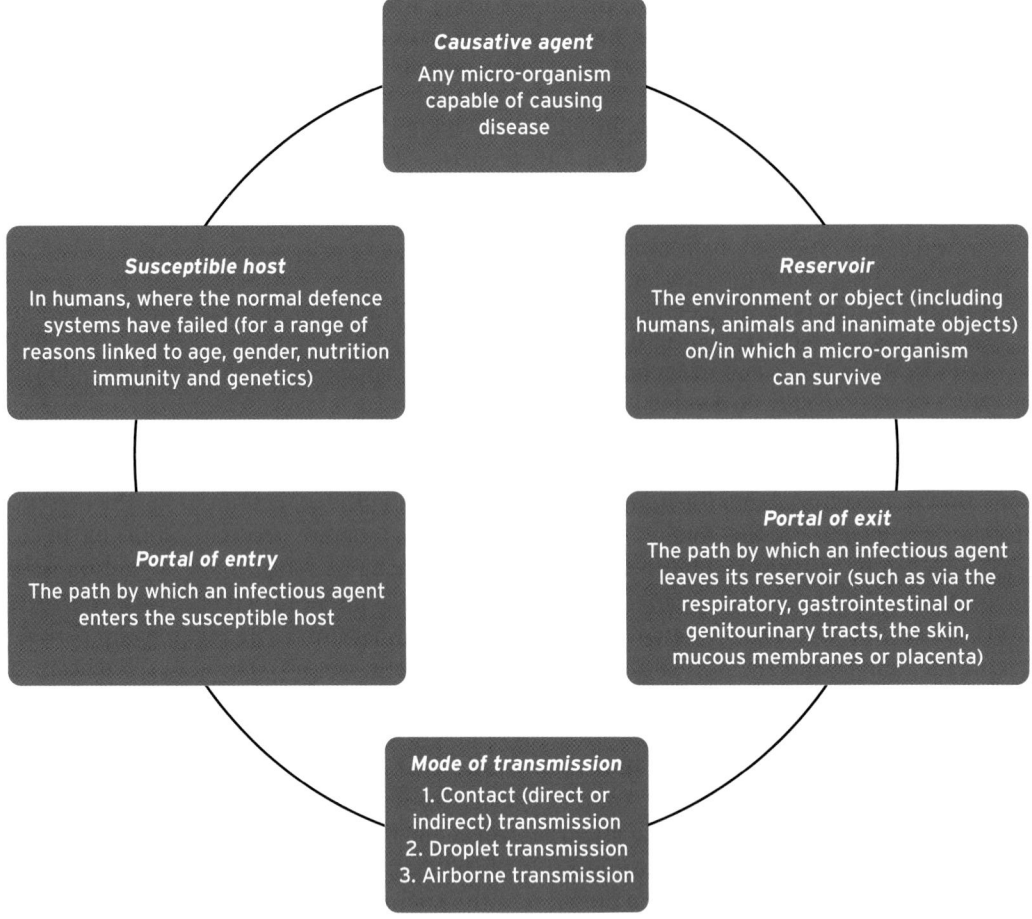

Figure 14.1   The chain of infection

ACTIVITY 14.1: REFLECTION

Reflect upon your role and responsibility in breaking the chain of infection

- Can you identify some common micro-organisms and how they are transmitted?
- Do you know what measures you can take to reduce the risk of transmission of infection?

Recognising the signs and symptoms of infection and infectious disease is another important aspect of infection prevention and control. The signs and symptoms of infection are wide ranging (see Table 14.2), but fever (or pyrexia) is considered one of the key features of infection. Fever is a high temperature, generally of 38+°C. Fever is sometimes the only sign of infection, and sometimes absent in infection (or related to other non-infectious conditions) – so assessment of temperature alone is not sufficient to facilitate a diagnosis of infection. Understanding the need for holistic assessment to support investigative procedures is central to identifying the microbial cause, securing a diagnosis and ensuring appropriate care/treatment.

Table 14.2 Signs and symptoms of infection

Localised infection:	
Generally described as infection that is limited to a specific area of the body. The signs and symptoms are those of acute inflammation, including inflammatory exudate.	• Redness • Swelling • Heat • Pain • Pus/foul-smelling discharge
Systemic infection:	
Generally described as infection that affects the bloodstream, with symptoms spread throughout the body.	• Fever • Aching and weakness • Chills (shivering) • Nausea and vomiting

Evidence base: Source: Inglis (2007)

CASE STUDY 14.1: WILLIAM

William is a 50-year-old gentleman, admitted to hospital for an open cholecystectomy. It was explained to William prior to his surgery that the surgeon would make a single cut in his abdomen, and take out his gallbladder. William stayed in hospital for three days following his surgery, and was advised that it would take around six to eight weeks to recover.

- What pre-operative, peri-operative and post-operative infection prevention and control practices might be implemented to prevent surgical site infection?

William was encouraged to get up and move around shortly after his surgery, and advised that once home, he should get back to his everyday activities as soon as he felt well enough to do so. He was advised to take things easy if he experienced pain, and to avoid any heavy lifting or straining for the first few weeks after his surgery.

- What advice might William be offered to minimise the risk of surgical site infection?

William returned home and was recovering well. He attended the GP surgery to have the sutures in his wounds removed after ten days.

- What assessment would the Practice Nurse carry out before undertaking William's suture removal?
- Describe the procedure of removal of sutures, including the elements of standard infection control precautions involved in the conduct of aseptic technique.

The Practice Nurse noticed that the wound dressing appeared to have been tampered with and on questioning William, he told the Practice Nurse the wound had become very itchy and he had lifted the corner of the dressing to scratch the itch. On removal of the wound dressing, the Practice Nurse suspected the wound was infected.

- What signs and symptoms might lead the Practice Nurse to suspect the wound infection?
- What might have caused the wound to become infected?
- How might the Practice Nurse manage this suspected wound infection?

To support holistic assessment, epidemiological enquiry as well as microbiological and non-microbiological investigations will be carried out. Assessment of a patient's general health and wellbeing, lifestyle activities and contacts will begin to establish some epidemiological clues about the cause of an infection. Non-microbiological investigations (such as neutrophil count) can assist in understanding the progression of infection, while microbiological investigations (such as microscopy) will be used to identify the micro-organism responsible for the infection. Specimen collection is an important role in the holistic assessment of infection.

SEE ALSO
CHAPTER 37

ACTIVITY 14.2: DECISION MAKING

You are on placement on a surgical ward, and your mentor asks you to collect a specimen of urine from a patient with an in-dwelling catheter, who is showing signs of infection.

- What signs and symptoms might the patient be showing?
- What steps would you take to collect the specimen of urine?
- How would you explain the procedure to the patient?

CONTROL MEASURES TO REDUCE THE RISK OF INFECTION

Control measures to reduce the risk of infection are embedded within an understanding of the chain of infection, and the actions that can be taken to break these individual links. It is now commonly accepted that the primary strategy for preventing and controlling infection is the application of standard infection control precautions (SICPs) (or standard precautions). The application of SICPs as part of care provision is determined by:

1. The level of interaction between the healthcare worker and the patient/client
2. The anticipated level of exposure to potential sources of infection – sources include blood and other body fluids, secretions and excretions (excluding sweat), non-intact skin and mucous membranes, and any item or equipment within the care environment which may become contaminated.

The underpinning principle of SICPs dictates there is a minimum standard of infection control precaution to be used in the care of all patients, on the basis that health and social care professionals are not always able to know the infection status of each and every patient/client at the outset of their care. On this basis, SICPs are intended for use by all health and social care staff in all health and social care settings at all times whether infection is known to be present or not. This approach aims to ensure the safety of patients/clients, staff and visitors to health and social care environments.

WHAT'S THE EVIDENCE? 14.1

The evolution of standard infection control precautions

General practice to support infection prevention and control has evolved and developed over many decades, and can be evidenced in the changes made to guidelines over the past 40 years. For example:

Updating of isolation precautions

Early infection control practices focused on the isolation of infected patients in separate facilities, the principle being to segregate infected patients from non-infected patients. Into the 20th century, these isolation practices shifted from facilities to environments, with cubicle systems of isolation within multiple bed areas of hospital wards being introduced. Within these environments, barrier nursing (a set of nursing procedures such as hand washing, gown use and equipment decontamination designed to prevent the transmission of infection) was introduced.

In 1983, the CDC *Guideline for Isolation Precautions in Hospitals* was published, with an increased focus on individual decision making. It encouraged and supported choice in the selection of isolation precautions for patients and in the precautions used by individuals in caring for patients on isolation precautions, based on the likelihood of exposure to infective material. This new approach focused decision making on precautions necessary to isolate the infection but not the patient. Within this guideline, the section entitled 'Blood Precautions' was updated and expanded to include patients with AIDS and body fluids other than blood. This new 'Blood and Body Fluid Precautions' guidance recommended blood and body fluid precautions when a patient was known or suspected to be infected with blood-borne pathogens.

The introduction of universal precautions

In 1987, the CDC *Recommendations for Prevention of HIV Transmissions in Health-Care Settings* advocated changing the term 'Blood and Body Precautions', to 'Universal Blood and Body Precautions' (or 'universal precautions'). This new approach acknowledged the fact that many patients with blood-borne infections were not recognisable, and recommended the application of blood and body fluid precautions consistently for all patients regardless of their known or suspected blood-borne infection status. Universal precautions extended the focus on gloves and gowns to include the use of masks and eye protection, the intention being to prevent parenteral, mucous membrane and non-intact skin exposure to blood-borne pathogens. At the same time, body substance isolation was introduced, with a focus on the isolation of all moist and potentially infectious body substances from all patients regardless of their presumed infection status. Glove use was encouraged before any anticipated and actual contact with moist body substances such as mucous membranes and non-intact skin.

The shift to standard infection control precautions

Since the above recommendations on universal precautions and body substance isolation, a range of policy updates and terminologies have been introduced as knowledge and understanding of disease transmission improves. Today, the term 'standard infection control precautions' (SICPs) (or standard precautions) is the most commonly used term to describe the group of precautions designed to prevent cross-transmission from recognised and unrecognised sources of infection. Combining the major features of universal precautions (designed to reduce the risk of transmission of blood-borne infection) and body substance isolation (designed to reduce the risk of transmission of infection from moist body substances), they are applied to all patients regardless of their infection status, based on the underpinning principle that all blood and body fluids (except sweat) may contain transmissible infectious agents.

Evidence base: Garner (1996); Siegel et al. (2007, updated 2017)

While additions and changes to the elements of standard infection control precautions arise from the newly emerging and re-emerging infectious diseases and their prevention and control, for now the elements of SICPs are generally considered as:

1. Patient placement
2. Hand hygiene
3. Respiratory hygiene and cough etiquette
4. Personal protective equipment (PPE)
5. Management of care equipment
6. Control of the environment
7. Safe management of linen
8. Management of blood and body fluid spillages
9. Safe disposal of waste (including sharps)
10. Occupational safety/exposure management.

Patient placement

Patient placement relates to the assessment of bed and patient spacing of those within health and social care environments, where the potential risk of transmission of infection may pose a risk to patients, healthcare workers and visitors. Assessment of this risk is important to ensure appropriate patient placement. In the context of standard infection control precautions, those admitted to inpatient environments displaying no signs of infection, and those with no known history of colonisation and/or infection with multi-drug resistant organisms (such as MRSA), will most likely be placed in a general environment.

General patient placement of immunocompromised patients is supported where robust implementation of standard infection control precautions are in place. In the absence of evidence to support single room (protective) isolation for most immunocompromised patients, Wigglesworth (2003) suggests that the use of a single room in such cases may heighten awareness of the need for rigorous implementation of standard precautions.

Patient placement for those with known or suspected infection and/or colonisation will be considered within the section on transmission-based precautions.

Hand hygiene

Hand hygiene is a general term that refers to any action of hand cleansing with the purpose of physically or mechanically removing dirt, organic material and/or micro-organisms from the hands, and involves the use of plain soap and water. Hand antisepsis aims to reduce/inhibit the growth of micro-organisms and can be undertaken by the application of an antiseptic handrub or by performing an antiseptic handwash. Hand antisepsis can be hygienic or surgical (see Table 14.3). Hand care is action taken to reduce the risk of damage or irritation to the skin of the hands (such as the application of hand cream).

Table 14.3 Approaches to hand antisepsis

Hygienic hand antisepsis	The treatment of hands with either an antiseptic handrub or antiseptic handwash to reduce the transient microbial flora without necessarily affecting the resident skin flora.
	• Hygienic handrub: Treatment of hands with an antiseptic handrub to reduce the transient flora without necessarily affecting the resident skin flora.
	• Hygienic handwash: Treatment of hands with an antiseptic handwash and water to reduce the transient flora without necessarily affecting the resident skin flora.

Surgical hand antisepsis	Antiseptic handwash or antiseptic handrub performed pre-operatively by the surgical team to eliminate transient flora and reduce resident skin flora.
	• Surgical handscrub(bing)/presurgical scrub refers to surgical hand preparation with antimicrobial soap and water.
	• Surgical handrub(bing) refers to surgical hand preparation with a waterless, alcohol-based handrub.

Evidence base: Source: WHO (2009a)

Hand hygiene is considered an important element of standard infection prevention and control practice, and one of the most effective methods of preventing the transmission of pathogens associated with healthcare (WHO, 2009a). To appreciate the purpose of different approaches to hand hygiene, it is necessary to understand the microbiology of the skin.

CRITICAL THINKING STOP POINT 14.2

- Revisit your understanding of the skin's normal flora, discussed earlier in this chapter, and describe the difference between resident and transient skin flora.
- Revisit your knowledge and understanding of hand hygiene. How would you describe the impact of the different types of hand hygiene on resident and transient flora of the hands?

Healthcare workers involved in both direct and indirect patient care must also be able to correctly perform hand hygiene at the right time. Prior to hand hygiene, healthcare workers should ensure their nails are short, with no nail varnish or false nails. Cuts or abrasions should be covered with a waterproof dressing, and no wrist watches, stoned rings, bracelets or bangles are worn (a plain wedding band can be worn). Care should be taken to ensure the area under any ring is washed and dried effectively. The WHO 'Five Moments for Hand Hygiene' (WHO, 2009b) define the key moments for hand hygiene as:

1. Before touching a patient
2. Before clean/aseptic procedures
3. After body fluid exposure risk
4. After touching a patient
5. After touching patient surroundings.

ACTIVITY 14.3: REFLECTION

Reflect on your responsibility to minimise the risk of infection through appropriate hand hygiene practices. Revisit the WHO 'Five Moments for Hand Hygiene', to ensure you understand the reasons why and when you should conduct hand hygiene during the delivery of patient care.

Respiratory hygiene and cough etiquette

The inclusion of respiratory and cough etiquette as a standard infection control precaution is relatively new, emerging from observations of limited control measures by patients, healthcare workers and visitors with respiratory symptoms during SARS outbreaks. The resulting transmission of SARS-CoV highlighted the need for infection control measures to minimise the risk of transmission of respiratory pathogens contained in large respiratory droplets and includes:

- covering the mouth/nose when coughing, sneezing and blowing the nose with disposable tissue, and disposing of used tissues promptly and appropriately;
- washing hands after contact with respiratory secretions and/or objects contaminated by such secretions;
- avoiding contact with the eyes/nose/mouth from contaminated hands;
- promoting good respiratory/cough hygiene practices in patients and visitors.

Personal protective equipment

Within health and social care settings, personal protective equipment (PPE) is specialised equipment or clothing (including gloves, aprons/gowns, eye and face protection, footwear and headwear) used to protect against contact with an infectious agent or body fluid that may contain an infectious agent. A range of legislation (see Table 14.4) combine to ensure healthcare employers provide PPE which affords adequate protection against the risks associated with planned tasks which might expose an employee to substances hazardous to their health. Healthcare workers have a responsibility to comply with this legislation, ensuring that suitable PPE is worn for the task being undertaken.

Table 14.4   Legislative underpinning of PPE

Legislation	Requirements of legislation
PPE at Work Regulations (1992)	Employers have duties regarding the provision and use of personal protective equipment (PPE) at work, where PPE is equipment that protects a user against health and/or safety risks in the workplace
Control of Substances Hazardous to Health Regulations (2002)	Employers are required to prevent and/or reduce workers' exposure to substances hazardous to their health
Health and Safety at Work Act (1974)	Employers are required, so far as is reasonably practicable, to ensure the health, safety and welfare of employees at work

Evidence base: HSE (2018)

In the healthcare setting, the intention of PPE is to create a barrier between potentially infectious material and the healthcare worker. The decision to select and use PPE must consider:

1. The type of exposure anticipated
2. The durability and appropriateness of the PPE for the task to be undertaken
3. The fit.

In selecting PPE, consider if touch, splashes or sprays, or large volumes of blood and/or body fluids are anticipated, and if the choice of equipment is sufficiently durable to withstanding the level of exposure and the category of precaution. Employers have a responsibility to provide PPE in a range of sizes suitable to the needs of the workforce – and employees have a responsibility to select the correct size to avoid risk of equipment failure and ultimately risk of exposure to infection.

STEP-BY-STEP CLINICAL SKILL 14.1

Personal protective equipment – selecting and using gloves

Before you start

Ensure all PPE is stored in a clean and dry area until required. Be aware of manufacturer's guidance on single and multiple use.

REMEMBER:

- The use of gloves does not replace the need for appropriate hand hygiene practices.
- Gloves should be removed and discarded between tasks to avoid risk of transmission of infection.

Care setting considerations:

The potential need to use PPE in a range of care settings is possible. Make sure you have a sufficient supply of appropriate PPE close to the point of use (and stored appropriately to avoid degradation), particularly when working in community settings, where access to supplies may be more limited.

Select the appropriate type of glove according to assessed risk (see Table 14.5):

Table 14.5   Assessment of procedure vs glove type

Assessment of procedure	Glove type
The procedure is assessed and determined to be a surgical procedure	Sterile latex/nitrile or neoprene surgical gloves are the glove type of choice
The procedure is assessed and determined to be a sterile or invasive procedure	Sterile latex/nitrile or neoprene gloves are the glove type of choice
The procedure is assessed and determined to be a non-sterile procedure, but with a risk of blood or body fluid contamination	Non-sterile latex/nitrile or neoprene gloves are the glove type of choice
The procedure is assessed and determined to be cleaning of equipment or the environment	Non-sterile latex/nitrile or neoprene gloves are the glove type of choice

Evidence base: WHO (2009a); HPS (2016)

Conducting a risk assessment of the likely exposure to the risk of infection ensures the requirement for personal protective equipment (PPE) is assessed.

- Gloves are not indicated where there is no potential exposure to blood or body fluids, or contaminated environment – unless as a contact precaution (where a patient has a known or suspected infection) (see Table 14.6).

Table 14.6   A risk assessment of the likely exposure to the risk of infection

Type of exposure	Examples	Risk of exposure to blood or body fluids/ contaminated environment/ contact precautions	Gloves required
Direct patient exposure	Taking vital signs (blood pressure, temperature and pulse); Administering injections; Carrying out personal hygiene (bathing/dressing).	NO	NO

(Continued)

(Continued)

Table 14.6 (Continued)

Type of exposure	Examples	Risk of exposure to blood or body fluids/ contaminated environment/ contact precautions	Gloves required
Indirect patient exposure	Administering oral medications; Distributing/ collecting patient meal trays; Bed making.	NO	NO

Source: WHO (2009a); HPS (2016)

CRITICAL THINKING STOP POINT 14.3

- List the types of PPE you have come across during your clinical placements.
- Document when they might be used and how.
- How compliant are you with the use of all types of personal protective equipment?
- Consider what action you could take if, following risk assessment, you identified the appropriate personal protective equipment was not available to you?

Management of care equipment and the care environment

The infection risk from care equipment and the care environment is dependent upon a number of factors including their level of contamination with blood and body fluids; the number and type of micro-organisms present; and the extent of contact between the equipment/environment and the patient (as a susceptible host). Appropriate classification and assessment of risk from care equipment and the care environment will ensure that risk of transmission of infection is reduced.

There are numerous ways to classify care equipment, the aim being to assist in understanding how best to safely use and decontaminate the items. One approach to classifying care equipment is to consider how often it can be used safely. This approach gives consideration to manufacturer's guidelines of usage. For example:

- ***Single use items of care equipment*** (such as needles and syringes) are those which can be used once on a single patient, before being placed in the appropriate waste stream for disposal. This type of equipment is not intended for reuse or reprocessing, even on the same patient.

- **Single patient use items of care equipment** are those which can be reused with the same patient. Reuse and reprocessing of this type of equipment are both dependent upon compliance with manufacturer's instructions and guidance.
- **Reusable items of care equipment** can be subdivided into those which are invasive (such as surgical instruments) and those which are non-invasive (such as bedpans, blood pressure cuffs, commodes and crutches). Both types of reusable care equipment are used once and then required to undergo an appropriate level of decontamination before reuse.

WHAT'S THE EVIDENCE? 14.2

The high risk practice of reusing single-use medical devices

In 2017, a white paper entitled 'Reuse of Single-Use Devices: Understanding Risks and Strategies for Decision-Making for Health Care Organizations' was commissioned by the Joint Commission International (Mansur, 2017), to address the concerning trend to reuse single-use medical devices.

The paper discusses and appraises the significant risk to the patient associated with such practices, highlighting how the reprocessing and reuse of such care equipment has the potential to compromise performance; result in inadequate decontamination outcomes; and render the manufacturer unliable for the product as a result of it not being used in accordance with their instructions.

The aim of the paper is to raise global awareness of the threat to patient safety, and to educate and support understanding of the risks associated with such practice.

The care environment, for the purposes of environmental decontamination, can be sub-divided into the 'public component' (the area not involved in patient care, such as lobbies and waiting areas, offices and corridors) and the 'patient component' (the area involved in patient care such as wards, clinical areas, treatment rooms and bathrooms). Ensuring appropriate and proportional environmental decontamination, the WHO (2009a) specifically defines the 'patient zone' as all inanimate surfaces touched directly or indirectly by the patient and by the healthcare worker involved in the patient's care (such as beds, bed rails, bed tables and bed linen). Touched surfaces have been further divided by level of hand contact: minimal hand contact surfaces (such as floors and ceilings) require less frequent decontamination than frequent hand contact surfaces (such as call buttons and door handles).

Decontamination

While recognising these different zones and surfaces may warrant different decontamination regimes, the overall aim is always to minimise the number of micro-organisms present while making the areas as unhospitable as possible to those most likely to cause infection. Decontamination is the process to remove pathogenic micro-organisms from objects so they are safe to handle, use, or discard, and can involve cleaning, disinfection and/or sterilisation. Before engaging in decontamination of care equipment and/or environments, assessment of the risk posed by the equipment or environment must be carried out, to determine the level of decontamination required – this will be influenced by how, where and with whom the equipment and environment has been used (see Table 14.7).

Table 14.7 Decontamination methods

Cleaning	The manual or mechanical removal of visible soil (e.g. organic and inorganic material) from objects/surfaces with water and detergents/enzymatic products. *An essential part of disinfection/sterilisation processes.*
Disinfection	The process to remove many or all pathogenic micro-organisms, except bacterial spores from objects/surfaces using liquid chemicals or wet pasteurisation.
Sterilisation	The process to eliminate all forms of microbial life, using physical or chemical methods (for example, using steam under pressure, dry heat, or liquid chemicals).

Evidence base: Rutala and Weber (2008, updated 2017)

Healthcare staff involved in the care of equipment and environment, including the management of linen, must understand the types of care equipment, categories of care environments and purposes of each decontamination method if they are to select and implement safe and effective decontamination practices.

ACTIVITY 14.4: REFLECTION

- Reflect on your knowledge and understanding of the methods of decontamination available.
- Have you witnessed or been involved in the decontamination of reusable care equipment and/ or the care environment during your clinical placements?
- Reflect on these experiences.

Safe disposal of waste (including sharps)

Effective management of *healthcare waste* requires an understanding and compliance with legislation relating to health and safety, infection control, the environment, transport and controlled drugs. To ensure that healthcare waste does not pose a risk of infection, waste is categorised (or streamed) to support appropriate segregation and disposal:

- Healthcare (including clinical) waste is waste produced as a result of healthcare activities, such as sharps and dressings.
- Special (or hazardous) waste is waste containing hazardous substances such as drugs or chemicals, and can be produced in clinical and non-clinical settings.
- 'Offensive waste' (or 'hygiene waste') is non-infectious waste that may cause offence due to the presence of healthcare-related waste items, body fluids or odour.
- Domestic/commercial waste is non-hazardous waste produced in domestic or commercial premises, as a result of the normal day-to-day use of the premises. This type of waste can be classified as recyclable (such as paper, cardboard, glass and plastic), or residual (not able to be recycled).

Most healthcare organisations will adopt a colour coding system of bags and containers to support the separation and disposal of the different kinds of waste produced. As producers of waste, healthcare workers must understand the local waste streams, to ensure waste is disposed of correctly. The management of sharps forms part of waste management strategies.

WHAT'S THE EVIDENCE? 14.3

The safe use of sharps – the findings and value of audit in reducing the risk of infection

Aziz et al. (2009) reported their findings from audit of sharps management in the University Hospital of South Manchester NHS Foundation Trust in July 2008. The audit focused on the observation of equipment, practice and awareness of sharps management, and involved visiting each ward area, outpatient department and operating theatre included in the audit, to:

- check the sharps containers in use;
- observe sharps management practice; and
- discuss and determine staff awareness of sharps management.

Findings from the audit observed all areas had equipment (such as sharps containers, needles and syringes) that met legislative requirements (BS 7320 and UN3291). While all areas had sufficient numbers of sharps containers, not all in use were correctly assembled, labelled or appropriately sited. Observation of staff practices found disposal of sharps at the point of use, with only 10% of areas making use of the temporary closure facility. In terms of staff awareness, the findings reported a good understanding of correct procedures for disposing of sharps and of managing a needlestick injury.

   The article highlights the value of audit as a valuable tool for monitoring sharps management; identifying deficits in practice; and facilitating measures to address these deficits (in this case through education and awareness raising). This shows how the use of audit can contribute to reducing the risk of infection.

Management of blood and body fluid spillages

Blood and body fluids are considered hazardous and must be dealt with immediately. The management of blood and body fluid spillages requires a combined understanding of a number of standard infection control precautions, including hand hygiene, the selection and use of personal protective equipment, and the ability to choose appropriate decontamination and waste management approaches.

ACTIVITY 14.5: REFLECTION

- Have you had to deal with a blood or body fluid spillage while on clinical placement?
- Reflect on your understanding of standard infection control precautions and how these might assist in managing the spillage safely.

Occupational safety

Occupational safety is underpinned by the Health and Safety at Work Act (1974), noted previously in the chapter when considering the issue of PPE. With this legislation comes a responsibility for healthcare providers to take all possible measures to minimise the risks of infection to its employers. Occupational health departments play a significant role in supporting employers to minimise infection risk, by offering a range of services to monitor and promote health and wellbeing. Specifically related to protection of healthcare workers from infection, these are screening and immunisation, education and training, and incident reporting.

Screening and immunisation

Screening and immunisation are two control measures available to healthcare workers to protect them, as employees, from the occupational risk from work-associated infectious diseases, including vaccine preventable infectious diseases.

- Screening involves the assessment of general health (including any conditions of the skin and/ or immunosuppressive disorders) and history of infectious diseases, as well as immunisation and immune status. Wider screening practices may be initiated under specific and defined conditions (such as during an outbreak or an epidemic), or if a healthcare worker has been exposed to a specific infectious agent which warrants ongoing monitoring.
- Immunisation aims to protect healthcare workers, their patients, their family and the wider community from the risks of infection. Healthcare workers may be offered Hepatitis B (for those identified as non-immune), influenza and chickenpox (varicella) immunisations.

Accepting relevant immunisations should be viewed by healthcare workers as taking reasonable precautions to protect themselves from infectious diseases, while acknowledging their duty of care towards their patients. Despite this, the uptake of some immunisations by healthcare workers is generally suboptimal, despite evidence to demonstrate effectiveness in reducing the risk of infection (PHE, 2016).

WHAT'S THE EVIDENCE? 14.4

How effective is flu vaccine?

The effectiveness of flu vaccine is dependent upon many factors, including the health and age of the person receiving it. To help ensure flu vaccine is effective, the World Health Organization makes use of its knowledge and understanding of influenza (including data on currently circulating strains of influenza). It makes recommendations to manufacturers of vaccines on the flu strains to include for the coming season. When the vaccine is well matched to circulating strains, evidence from the UK and USA shows it can be 50-70% effective (Andrews et al., 2014; Jackson et al., 2013).

Sometimes, a different strain of influenza emerges after vaccine production has started, and because of time required for manufacture, this cannot be included. This can impact on the effectiveness of the flu vaccine, making it less effective. Poorer matched vaccines still offer protection against circulating strains.

Why is there a need for flu vaccine for clinical staff?

The influenza vaccination is offered to frontline healthcare workers in the NHS with the aim of reducing the risk of staff contracting the virus and transmitting it to their patients and service users. For 2015/16, Public Health England (2016) reported the influenza vaccine uptake rate for frontline healthcare workers was 50.6% (compared with 54.9% in 2014/15).

Clinical evidence supports the need for flu vaccination among healthcare workers:

- *Frontline healthcare workers are more likely to be exposed to the influenza virus during the winter period* – evidence estimated that one in four healthcare workers became infected with influenza, this being a much higher incidence than that expected within the general population (Elder et al., 1996). *Healthcare workers who receive the flu vaccination can protect themselves against flu.*
- *Healthcare workers may transmit flu to patients* – evidence exists to show that in outbreak situations, transmission from healthcare workers to patients may have facilitated the spread of infection to patients, including neonates (Pachucki et al., 1989; Cunney et al., 2000; Horcajada et al., 2003). Further studies have shown the effects of healthcare worker flu vaccination programmes on patient mortality and morbidity (Potter et al., 1997; Carman et al., 2006; Hayward et al., 2006; Lemaitre et al., 2009; Hollymeyer et al., 2009). *Healthcare workers who receive the flu vaccination can protect their patients/clients against flu.*

Evidence base: PHE (2016)

ACTIVITY 14.6: REFLECTION

As a healthcare worker, have you been offered the influenza vaccination?

Reflect on your decision to accept or decline this vaccination, and how this impacts on your duty of care to your patients.

Education and training

To ensure patients are cared for by practitioners, knowledgeable and skilled in the principles of infection prevention and control, healthcare workers should be provided with relevant education and training, commensurate to their role, and intended to support their practice. This will generally begin at the point of induction to their role, and continue as part of an ongoing programme of continuous professional development. To facilitate engagement and compliance, some training may be mandatory, and others optional.

Training programmes designed to support good infection control practice should include content on procedures associated with the conduct of SICPs and Transmission-based precautions (TBPs). This should be supported by local national and international policy, guidance and regulation, all of which should be underpinned with research-based evidence. More formal education leading to an academic qualification may be supported for specific groups of staff specialising in infection prevention and control practice (such as the Infection Control Nurse or Doctor). This additional level of specialist knowledge and understanding helps to fulfil their role as subject expert, clinical leader, trainer and change agent.

Incident reporting

Incident reporting, including prompt reporting of any occupational exposure (such as sharps injury) is essential to ensue healthcare workers are provided with the correct support and advice, treatment and follow-up. Engagement in training should ensure healthcare workers are aware of the policy and procedure to manage any infection-related incident, so minimising the risk of transmission and long-term impact on health and wellbeing.

Compliance with SICPs

Compliance with SICPs is important to ensure safe and effective practice at all times, and to reduce the risk of infection. However, sub-optimal compliance with infection prevention and control precautions continues to be reported in the findings of research. With evidence that a significant proportion of healthcare-associated infection is preventable, this poor practice is considered a contributing factor to the current rates of healthcare-associated infection identified within healthcare settings across the globe.

WHAT'S THE EVIDENCE? 14.5

Poor or suboptimal compliance with standard infection control precautions

Back in 2008, Gammon and Morgan Samuel undertook a review of 37 international research-based papers, to explore the extent of compliance, factors influencing compliance and the strategies evaluated to alter this non-compliance. The review concluded that compliance with infection control precautions was internationally suboptimal, with healthcare workers selective in their application of recommended practice. The review also found compliance to improve with specific interventions, but noted how research did not indicate the duration or sustainability of the changes.

Almost ten years on, and despite a greater understanding of the global impact and burden of healthcare-associated infection (WHO, 2011), the issue of non-compliance with standard infection control precautions persist.

In 2014, Cioffi and Cioffi undertook a further review of existing literature in this area, and reported evidence of suboptimal infection prevention and control practices, but explained this further by evidencing a resistance to change and poor clinical judgement and/or decision making. The universal/global nature of this poor practice, they note, suggests it is engrained in an insensitive culture – one which does not recognise the need for change. This resistance to change, they propose, explains the limited success of behaviour change strategies to address the problem, and that healthcare workers are not ready for the decision making required to support good practice. They conclude the need for more effective strategies to address the current behaviour/practices, and suggest social psychology as a potential route.

Jackson et al.'s (2014) qualitative study found infection control practice deviated from policy, and commented on its contribution to the existing evidence base of non-compliant and harmful infection control practices within the healthcare environment. The study did acknowledge the multi-factorial and complex nature of behaviour and the implications of this in terms of understanding beyond knowledge deficit.

Highlighting the global nature of this issue, a cross-sectional study over two countries (Hong Kong and Brazil) by Pereira et al. (2015) evaluated, using a self-administered questionnaire, the differences in standard infection control precaution compliance among nurses from these two countries, while Colet et al. (2017) explored the same issue using a similar methodology (cross-sectional, self-reporting study) in baccalaureate nursing students in a Saudi university.

The study by Colet et al. (2017) brings us up to date with current practices, and so it is disappointing to read that they too identified issues of compliance, with lowest rates of compliance in handwashing – the cornerstone of standard infection control precautions. Again, the concept of fostering an appropriate culture to support compliance is postulated in the concluding remarks.

Evidence base: Gammon and Morgan-Samuel, 2008;
Cioffi and Cioffi, 2014; Jackson et al., 2014; Pereira et al., 2015; Colet et al., 2017

MANAGING THE INFECTIOUS PATIENT

At times, the use of standard infection control precautions may not be sufficient to prevent and control the risk of transmission of infection. Transmission-based precautions are an additional set of measures/precautions, used in conjunction with standard infection control precautions, and implemented when patients/clients are either suspected or known to be infected (or colonised) with a specific infectious agent.

In the same way that the term 'standard infection control precautions' has evolved over time, so too has the term 'transmission-based precautions'. A range of alternative terminologies such as isolation precautions, barrier nursing, enteric precautions, source isolation and protective isolation have been used and, today, transmission-based precautions are considered to incorporate all of the measures previously recommended under these terms.

CRITICAL THINKING STOP POINT 14.4

Review the terms previously associated with what is now known as transmission-based precautions, to help develop your understanding of the factors involved in transmission-based precautions.

The categorisation and application of transmission-based precautions is determined by the route of transmission of the infectious agent. As some micro-organisms/infectious diseases have multiple routes of transmission (for example, SARS), more than one transmission-based precaution might be employed.

Airborne transmission/precautions

Airborne precautions are used in addition to SICPs for patients with infections transmitted through either airborne droplet nuclei or small particles size (5μm or smaller). Generated when talking, coughing or sneezing, or during procedures involving the respiratory tract (such as suction, intubation or bronchoscopy), the micro-organisms are then carried airborne and dispersed over long distances. They may then be inhaled by susceptible individuals who have not had any direct contact with the original infection source.

Preventing and controlling the spread of infection of airborne conditions requires special air-handling and ventilation systems. Those requiring airborne precautions are placed in single rooms with negative air-pressure ventilation, ideally externally exhausted. Where recirculation is required, it should be subjected to high-efficiency particulate air (HEPA) filtration.

Only a small number of common infectious diseases are communicated via the airborne route:

Table 14.8 Common infectious diseases communicated via the airborne route

From the patient	From the environment
Mycobacterium tuberculosis	*Aspergillus* spp.
Measles virus	Anthrax spores
Varicella-zoster virus (chicken pox)	Legionella

Droplet transmission/precautions

Droplet precautions are used in addition to SICPs for patients with infections transmitted through large particle droplets (greater than 5μm), also generated during coughing, sneezing, or procedures involving the respiratory tract (such as suctioning). Large droplet nuclei do not stay suspended in the air for long, and so travel only short distances. Transmission requires close respiratory and/or mucous membrane contact (within one metre) between the infected source and the recipient/susceptible host.

Patients requiring droplet precautions should be placed in single room isolation, and where no single room is available, consideration should be given to the scope to adopt alternative placement options such as cohorting. Any decision to adopt cohorting (grouping of people, generally those already exposed to a patient known or suspected to have an infectious disease) requires healthcare workers to undertake a risk assessment of patient factors and symptoms, to determine risks of transmission/spread of infection. Where cohorting is to be utilised, patients should be separated from each other by at least one metre. Curtains can be drawn to create an additional barrier, and staff cohorting (the use of a dedicated team of healthcare staff to care for patients infected with a single infectious agent) may also be implemented to minimise the risk of movement (and therefore potential contamination) between those known to be infected and those not.

Common infectious diseases communicated via the droplet route include:

- Mumps
- Rubella
- *Bordetella pertussis* (whooping cough)
- Respiratory syncytial virus
- *Pseudomonas aeruginosa*
- Influenza virus
- Adenovirus
- Rhinovirus
- *Mycoplasma pneumoniae* (pneumonia)
- Coronavirus
- *Neisseria meningitidis* (meningitis).

CASE STUDY 14.2: DAVID

David is a 72-year-old man, retired from work for the past 12 years. He is active, playing golf with his friends three times a week, and travelling to Spain with his wife regularly. He suffers from high blood pressure, which is managed by medication, and he watches his diet and watches how much alcohol he drinks (especially during his trips abroad).

Each winter, since turning 65 years old, he has been invited by his GP to attend the local surgery for his annual flu vaccine. David chooses to accept this invite, recognising that as he gets older, it can be more difficult to fight off infection, and he might be more likely to get sick because his immune system works less well.

- What are the benefits of immunisation – to individuals like David, his family, and to the wider community?
- What other immunisations might David have been offered as an older adult over 65 years, and why?
- Find out what other age groups are immunised and when.
- Reflect your eligibility and professional responsibility as a healthcare worker to receive the annual influenza vaccination.

SEE ALSO
CHAPTER 3

Contact transmission/precautions

Contact precautions are used in addition to SICPs for patients with infections transmitted through direct or indirect contact with an infected patient or contaminated objects in the infected patient's immediate surroundings. A contaminated person or object is known as a fomite.

This route of transmission is considered the most common. Direct contact might involve skin-to-skin contact, while indirect contact may be via the hands of a healthcare worker or poorly decontaminated communal equipment or surgical instruments.

Comparable to patients requiring droplet precautions, those requiring contact precautions will ideally be placed in a single room, and where this is not available, cohorting will similarly be assessed. Common infectious diseases communicated via the contact route include:

- Scabies
- MRSA
- VRE
- *Clostridium difficile*
- *Staphylococcus aureus*
- Herpes simplex virus (HSV).

CRITICAL THINKING STOP POINT 14.5

- Choose an organism you have come across in clinical practice.
- Identify how it is spread (mode of transmission), and the methods of control.
- Consider if SICPs are sufficient, or if TBPs are required to prevent and control the risk of transmission to others.

WHAT'S THE EVIDENCE? 14.6

The impact of isolation

In 2003, an article by Madeo explored the psychological impact of isolation, highlighting the need to assess patients individually and to plan their care so as to minimise the risk of cross infection as well as safeguarding against negative psychological effects from being isolated.

Sprague et al. (2016) again explored the impact of isolation as a transmission-based precaution, in terms of financial and other costs. They presented evidence to suggest that patients may 'pay a price' as a result of being isolated, and explored the notion of alternative approaches to isolation to manage infectious diseases.

While not advocating isolation as a practice be abandoned, both suggest the issue of isolation warrants continued attention.

ACTIVITY 14.7: REFLECTION

Reflect on the use of isolation as a transmission-based precaution.

- How might you feel being placed in isolation?
- What information might you give to a patient being placed in isolation?

MONITORING INFECTION PREVENTION AND CONTROL PRACTICES

The impact of poor and suboptimal practice provides sufficient reason to monitor practice. Monitoring practice is a good way to better understand infection patterns and trends. By understanding these, consideration can be given to the need to promote and improve infection prevention and control practices, where necessary. This approach fits well with the concepts of risk management, clinical governance and quality. There are many ways to monitor infection prevention and control practices.

Surveillance

Surveillance can be defined as 'the ongoing systematic collection, analysis, and interpretation of health data essential to the planning, implementation, and evaluation of public health practice, closely integrated with the timely dissemination of these data to those who need to know' (CDC, 1988). In short, it is the continuous scrutiny of all aspects of occurrence and spread of infection that are pertinent to effective control. A variety of types of surveillance exists:

Mandatory surveillance of surgical site infection and healthcare-associated infection such as *Clostridium difficile* associated disease, *Staphylococcus aureus* bacteraemia and gram-negative bacteraemia or MRSA and E. coli. Healthcare-associated infection (HAI) surveillance involves the collection of data on healthcare-associated infections, analysis of results and feedback to clinical staff on issues such as incidence (numbers of new cases over a defined period) and prevalence (total numbers of cases during a specific period). As well as monitoring incidence and prevalence of infections, HAI surveillance provides early opportunity for early investigation of problems/outbreaks and implementation of targeted control measures. These interventions can then be evaluated for their impact. This is important given the current rates of HAI and the implications and costs of their management.

Alert organism and alert condition surveillance involves the surveillance of organisms and conditions of local interest and significance, often in areas where patients are at higher risk of infection from these organisms/conditions (see Table 14.9).

Table 14.9 Examples of alert organisms and alert conditions

Alert organisms	Alert conditions
Clostridium difficile	Cellulitis or other soft tissue or surgical site infections (more than expected)
	Diarrhoea and/or vomiting in patients with no other obvious sources - 2 or more cases in a clinical area
All Mycobacterium tuberculosis	Infections relating to invasive devices/procedures (more than expected)
Respiratory *Pseudomonas aeruginosa*	Post-operative pneumonia or respiratory infection (more than expected)

Evidence base: HPS (2014)

Audit

Audit is a cyclical process (see Figure 14.2), assessing service provision against a pre-existing standard. This assessment most often makes use of a pre-existing and standardised tool, generally mapped closely to the standard against which practice will be assessed. Audit involves four key elements, which end at the identification of the need for change.

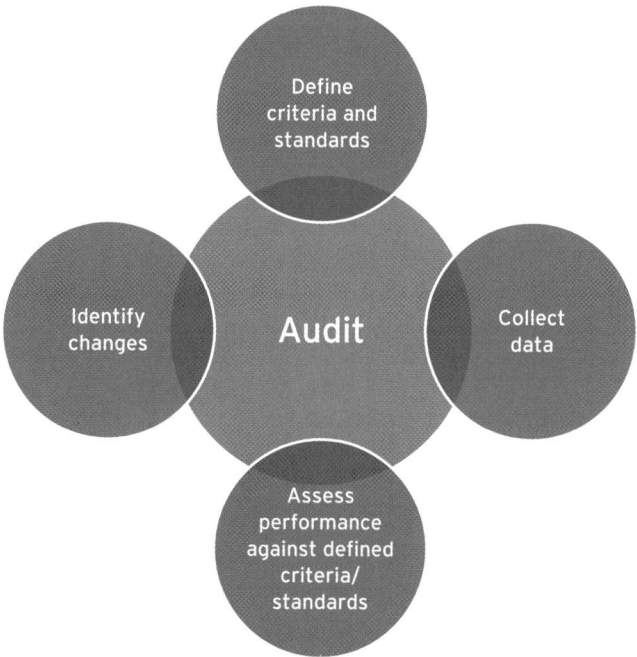

Figure 14.2 The audit cycle

Audit feedback and follow up (including the implementation of changes) enables practice changes/improvements to be made prior to re-audit. Audit generally makes use of a standardised audit tool to support the assessment of practice.

DECISION MAKING

- Discuss the concept of audit with your mentor when you are next on clinical placement.
- Find out if the placement area conducts audit of any practices - specifically infection prevention and control practices.

Look back exercises are long-standing monitoring exercises, which aim to identify, trace, recall, counsel and test those who may have been exposed to an infections (Damani, 2003). Look back exercises often involve the use of helplines to support contact, and press conferences/briefings to harness publicity. The decision to conduct a look back exercise is often decided at a high (but local) level, such as local authority or health service level.

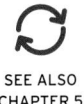

SEE ALSO
CHAPTER 5

Quality improvement/patient safety initiatives

While all monitoring aims to improve quality through the reduction in risk of transmission of infection, the advent of the quality agenda has seen a marked increase in the number and types of monitoring approaches which are underpinned with quality improvement methodology. Most of these initiatives can be described by standard abbreviations.

CRITICAL THINKING STOP POINT 14.6

Review the following list of abbreviations in the context of quality improvement and patient safety initiatives to monitor infection prevention and control practices. Explore their meaning and use through wider reading:

- Hazard Analysis and Critical Control Points (HACCP)
- Failure Modes and Effects Analysis (FMEA)
- Situation Background Assessment Recommendations (SBAR)
- Plan Do Study Act (PDSA)

Identify when and why these might be used in monitoring infection control practice within healthcare.

Research, evaluation and epidemiological studies are three further approaches to monitoring infection prevention and control practice. All provide a mechanism to better understand the appropriateness of current practice.

PROMOTING GOOD INFECTION PREVENTION AND CONTROL PRACTICE

Promoting good infection prevention and control practice is valuable, as this:

- facilitates patient safety/public protection – by limiting the risk of transmission of infection;
- improves awareness of, and compliance with contemporary infection control practices;
- supports quality/clinical governance issues, including the achievement of targets;
- limits media attention and/or the risk of litigation.

Promoting good infection prevention and control practice can operate at an individual, organisational, national or global/international level. Often, multi-factorial approaches are most successful and, for this reason, nations will adopt a global strategy, and this will then cascade down to local and at times individual levels.

Campaigning is an approach to promoting good infection prevention and control practices, and operates at local national and global levels. Working from the premise that something (often a behaviour) has to change (or awareness be raised), campaigns generally target a specific well-defined audience, and run for a dedicated period of time. Most campaigns will have a number of strategies with at least a communication strategy and an exit strategy. In recent years, there have been a number of notable campaigns linked to the promotion of good infection prevention and control practice.

- The World Health Organization (WHO) 'SAVE LIVES: Clean Your Hands' was a global campaign which called upon healthcare workers across the globe to wash their hands to prevent sepsis.
- The National Patient Safety Agency's (NPSA) 'cleanyourhands' campaign was a very high-profile campaign, again focused on hand hygiene practices of healthcare workers and patients – the organisation reports this campaign to have been hugely successful in changing hand hygiene behaviour and compliance levels.

Strategy and/or policy development is another approach to promote good infection prevention and control practices. Setting up a 'task force' or a 'think tank' at national level is a common approach to the development of national strategy. An example was the Scottish Government HAI Task Force, an overarching governmental body which coordinated (through consistency, leadership, expertise and rationalisation) the development and implementation of national strategy for reducing HAI.

CRITICAL THINKING STOP POINT 14.7

- Do you know of any current campaigns or task force/think tanks associated with infection prevention and control?
- Make use of social media and the internet to find a local, national or international campaign/ task force to explore.

Education is the final mechanism for promoting good practice. Education supports engagement with contemporary literature on a given topic, ensuring practices are research/ evidence based. The importance of evidence based infection prevention and control practice can be seen in enhanced patient outcomes, increased patient safety and improved quality of life.

CHAPTER SUMMARY

- There are numerous types of micro-organisms existing in a range of relationships with humans, not all of which are harmful. Disease-causing micro-organisms are known as pathogens
- The ability of pathogens to cause disease is affected by a range of factors, commonly described as the chain of infection. It is important to understand the chain of infection and the role you can play in preventing and controlling the transmission of infection
- Assessing the risk of infection is central to preventing and controlling the risk of transmission of infection
- Control measures to reduce the risk of infection include standard infection control precautions – measures used with all patients in all environments at all times to reduce the risk of infection
- In managing the infectious patient, standard infection control precautions are insufficient to minimise the risk of infection – and additional precautions, known as transmission-based precautions, are required in conjunction with standard infection control precautions
- Monitoring infection prevention and control practices is a good way to better understand infection patterns and trends
- Promoting good infection prevention and control practice enhances patient safety/public protection – by limiting the risk of transmission of infection.

CRITICAL REFLECTION

Holistic care

This chapter has outlined the importance of holistic assessment in the assessment of infection risk, and its prevention and control. Review the chapter and note down the factors which contribute to holistic assessment of a patient/client suspected of having or being at risk of infection. Think of the potential to care for patients and clients across the lifespan as well as across a range of health and social care settings. You may find it useful to list these and use this to reflect back on how you might utilise the different infection prevention and control approaches to reducing their risk of infection.

GO FURTHER

CASE STUDY: GASTROENTERITIS

Go to https://study.sagepub.com/essentialadultnursing for a further case study related to this chapter. If you are using the interactive ebook, simply click on the book icon in the margin to go straight to the resource.

Books

- Weston, D. (2013) *Fundamentals of Infection Prevention and Control: Theory and Practice*. Oxford: Wiley Blackwell.
- Weston, D., Burgess, A. and Roberts, S. (2017) *Infection Prevention and Control at a Glance*. Oxford: Wiley Blackwell.

Journal Articles

FURTHER READING: JOURNAL ARTICLES

Go to https://study.sagepub.com/essentialadultnursing for further free online journal articles related to this chapter. If you are using the interactive ebook, simply click on the book icon in the margin to go straight to the resource.

- Bouchoucha, S.L. and Moore, K.A. (2017) Infection prevention and control: Who is the judge, you or the guidelines? *Journal of Infection Prevention*. Available at: http://journals.sagepub.com/doi/pdf/10.1177/1757177417738332

  This article reports the findings of a qualitative study which explored the attitudes and behaviours of 29 registered nurses'/midwives' implementation of standard infection control precautions in a hospital in Australia. Data collected through interviews and focus groups was analysed using thematic analysis. The article focuses on the findings associated with one theme – 'staff judgement against guidelines', and discusses the deviation of staff from standard infection control precautions, despite the existence of mandatory guidelines.

- Weaving, P., Cox, F. and Milton, S. (2008) Infection prevention and control in the operating theatre: Reducing the risk of surgical site infections (SSIs). *Journal of Perioperative Practice*, 18 (5): 199-204. Available at: http://journals.sagepub.com/doi/pdf/10.1177/175045890801800503

  This article discusses how continuing advances in surgical techniques, asepsis, operating theatre protocols and ventilation systems are supporting patients to undergo both invasive and minimally invasive procedures with reduced risk.

- Gould, D. and Drey, N. (2013) Types of interventions used to improve hand hygiene compliance and prevent healthcare associated infection. *Journal of Infection Prevention*, 14(3): 88-93. Available at: http://journals.sagepub.com/doi/abs/10.1177/1757177413482608

  This review article highlights that hand hygiene is regarded as the most effective means of preventing healthcare associated infection, while highlighting the limited evidence of effectiveness. It considers the types of intervention used to promote hand hygiene and discusses their credibility, identifying factors which might influence the success of initiatives and interventions aimed at enhancing hand hygiene compliance.

Weblinks

FURTHER READING: WEBLINKS

Go to https://study.sagepub.com/essentialadultnursing for further weblinks related to this chapter. If you are using the interactive ebook, simply click on the book icon in the margin to go straight to the resource.

- www.who.int/infection-prevention/en/
  This site provides a global perspective on the topic of infection prevention and control
- www.hps.scot.nhs.uk/haiic/index.aspx
  The Health Protection Scotland website offers information on a range of topical infection prevention and control issues, and contains a dedicated HAI and infection control section, as well as hosting Scotland's national infection control manual.
- www.gov.uk/topic/health-protection/infectious-diseases
  This website is the health protection/infectious diseases site of Public Health England. It offers up-to-date information and guidance on a wide range of infectious diseases. It lists infectious diseases/conditions alphabetically, making information of specific conditions easy to find
- www.ips.uk.net/
  This site is the home of the Infection Prevention Society. Its aim is to inform, promote and sustain expert infection prevention policy and practice, and contains a wide range of information on the topic – including how to get involved directly.

ACE YOUR ASSESSMENT

ONLINE QUIZZES

Revise what you have learned by visiting https://study.sagepub.com/essentialadultnursing

- Test yourself with multiple-choice and short-answer questions
- Do the chapter activities in the book and check your answers online

REFERENCES

Akst, J. (2014) Microbes of the skin. *The Scientist*, June 13. Available at: https://www.the-scientist. com/?articles.view/articleNo/40228/title/Microboes-of-the-skin (Accessed 1st December 2017).

Andrews, N., McMenamin, J., Durnall, H., Ellis, J., Lackenby, A. and Robertson, C. (2014) Effectiveness of trivalent seasonal influenza vaccine in preventing laboratory-confirmed influenza in primary care in the United Kingdom: 2012/13 end of season results. *Euro Surveillance*, 19(27): 5–13.

Aziz, A.M., Ashton, H., Pagett, A., Mathieson, K., Jones, S. and Mullin, B. (2009) Sharps management in hospital: An audit of equipment, practices and awareness. *British Journal of Nursing*, 18(2): 92–7.

Carman, W.F., Elder, A.G., Wallace, L.A., McAuley, K., Walker, A., Murray, G.D. and Stott, D.J. (2006) Effects of influenza vaccination of healthcare workers on mortality of elderly people in long term care: a randomised control trial. *The Lancet* 2000, 355(9198): 93–7.

CDC (2016) *National and State Healthcare-Associated Infections Progress Report*. Available at: https//www.cdc.gov/hai/surveillance/progress-report/index.html (Accessed 1st December 2017).

CDC (2018) *Preventing Infections in Cancer Patients: protect: Know the Signs and Symptoms of Infection*. Atlanta, CDC. Available at: https://www.cdc.gov/cancer/preventinfections/symptoms.htm (Accessed 1st December 2017).

Cioffi, D. and Cioffi, J. (2014) Challenging suboptimal infection control. *Journal of Infection Control*, 2014, v11:i1 doi. Available at: http://www.ijic.info/article/view/13988/9515 (Accessed 20th December 2017).

Cogen, A.L., Nizet, V. and Gallo, R.L. (2009) Skin microbiota: A source of disease or defence? *British Journal of Dermatology*, 158(3): 442–55.

Cole, M. (2008) Compliance and infection control guidelines: A complex phenomenon. *British Journal of Nursing*, 17(11): 700–704.

Colet, P.C., Cruz, J.P., Alotaibi, K.A., Colet, M.K.A. and Islam, S.M.S. (2017) Compliance with standard precautions among baccalaureate nursing students in a Saudi university: A self-reported study. *Journal of Infection and Public Health*, 10(4):421–30.

Cunney, R.J., Bialachowski, A., Thornley, D., Smaill, F.M. and Pennie, R.A. (2000) An outbreak of influenza A in a neonatal intensive care unit. *Infection Control and Hospital Epidemiology*, 21: 449–54.

Damani, N.N. (2003) *Manual of Infection Control Procedures*. Cambridge: Cambridge University Press.

ECDC (2015) *Antimicrobial Resistance and Healthcare Associated Infection. Annual epidemiological report 2014*. Stockholm, ECDC. Available at: https://ecdc.europa.eu/sites/portal/files/media/en/publications/Publications/antimicrobial-resistance-annual-epidemiological-report.pdf (Accessed 20th December 2017).

Elder, A.G., O'Donnell, B., McCruden, E.A., Symington, I.S. and Carman, W.F. (1996) Incidence and recall of influenza in a cohort of Glasgow healthcare workers during the 1993–4 epidemic: Results of serum testing and questionnaire. *The British Medical Journal*, 313: 1241–42.

Gammon, J., Morgan-Samuel, H. and Gould, D.J. (2008) A review of the evidence for suboptimal compliance of healthcare practitioners to standard/ universal infection control precautions. *Journal of Clinical Nursing*, 17(2):157–67.

Garner, J.S. and the Hospital Infection Control Practices Advisory Committee (1996) Guideline for isolation precautions in hospitals. *Infection Control and Hospital Epidemiology*, 1996, Jan, 17(1): 53–80.

Grice, E.A. and Segre, J.A. (2011) The skin microbiome. *National Review of Microbiology*, 9(4): 244–53.

Hayward, A.V., Harling, R., Wetten, S. et al (2006), Effectiveness of an influenza vaccine programme for care home staff to prevent death, morbidity, and health service use among residents: Cluster randomised controlled trials. *The British Medical Journal* 2006; doi:10.1136/bmj.39010.581354.55.

Hollymeyer, H.G., Hayden, F., Poland, G. and Buchholz, U. (2009) Influenza vaccination of healthcare workers in hospitals – a review of studies on attitudes and predictors. *Vaccine*, 27:3935–44.

Horcajada, J.P., Pumarola, T., Martinez, J.A. et al. (2003), A nosocomial outbreak of influenza during a period without influenza epidemic activity. *European Respiratory Journal*, 21: 303–7.

HPA (2012) *Health care Associated Infection Operational Guidance and Standards for health Protection Units*. Available at: https://www.gov.uk/governemnt/uploads/system/uploads/attachment data/file/332051/HCAI Operationalguidancefinalemended 05July2012.pdf (Accessed 20th December 2017).

HPS (2014) *Local Infection Surveillance of Alert Organisms and Alert Conditions: IPCT actions to prevent and detect outbreaks and to minimise infections following healthcare*. HPS: Glasgow

HPS (2016) *Healthcare Associated Infection Annual Report* 2015. Available at: http://www.hps.scot.nhs.uk/haiic/sshaip/resourcedetail.aspx?id=1717 (Accessed 20th December 2017).

HSE (2018) *Health and Safety*. Available at: http//www.hse.gov.uk/legislation/hswa.html (Accessed 1st December 2017).

Inglis, T.J.J. (2007) *Microbiology and Infection* (3rd ed.). London: Churchill Livingstone.

Jackson, L., Jackson, M.L., Hallie Phillips, C., Benoit, J., Belongia, E.A. and Cole, D. (2013) Interim adjusted estimates of seasonal influenza vaccine effectiveness – United States. *MMWR*, 62(7):119–123.

Jackson, C., Lowton, K. and Griffiths, P. (2014) Infection prevention as a 'show': A qualitative study of nurses' infection prevention behaviours. *International Journal of Nursing Studies*, 51(3): 400–408.

Lemaitre, M., Meret, T., Rothan-Tondeur, M. et al (2009) Effect of influenza vaccination of nursing home staff on mortality of residents: a cluster randomised trial. *Journal of American Geriatric Society*, 57:1580–6.

Madeo, M. (2003) The psychological impact of isolation. *Nursing Times*, 18 February, 99(7):54.

Mansur, J.M. (2017) Reuse of Single-use Devices: Understanding risks and strategies for decision-making for healthcare organisations. A white paper by Joint Commission International. Available at: https://www.jointcommissioninternational.org/assets/3/7/JCI_White_Paper_Reuse_of_Single_Use_Devices2.pdf (Accessed 2nd December 2017).

NMC (2015) *The Code: Professional Standards of Practice and Behaviour for Nurses and Midwives*. London, NMC.

Pachucki, C.T., Pappas, S.A., Fuller, G.F. et al (1989) Influenza A among hospital personnel and patients. Implications for recognition, prevention and control. *Archives of Internal Medicine*, 149: 77–80.

Pereira, F.M., Lam, S.C., Chan, J.H., Malaguti-Toffano, S.E. and Gir, E. (2015) Difference in compliance with standard precautions by nursing staff in Brazil versus Hong Kong. *American Journal of Infection Control*, 43(7): 769–72.

PHE (2016) *Healthcare worker vaccination: Clinical evidence*. London: PHE.

Potter, J., Stott, D.J., Roberts, M.A. et al (1997) The influenza vaccination of healthcare workers in long-term care hospitals reduces the mortality of elderly patients. *Journal of Infectious Diseases*, 175: 1–6.

Rutala, W.A., Weber, D.J. and the Healthcare Infection Control Practices Advisory Committee (HICPAC) (2008, updated 2017) *Guideline for Disinfection and Sterilization in Healthcare Facilities, 2008*. Available from: https://www.cdc.gov/infectioncontrol/guidelines/disinfection/ (Accessed 2nd December 2017).

Siegel, J.D., Rhinehart, E., Jackson, M., Chiarello, L. and the Healthcare Infection Control Practices Advisory Committee (2007) *Guideline for Isolation Precautions: Preventing Transmission of Infectious Agents in Healthcare Settings*. Available at: https://www.cdc.gov/infectioncontrol/guidelines/isolation/index.html (Accessed 1st December 2017)

Sprague, E., Reynolds, S. and Brindley, P. (2016) Patient Isolation precautions: Are they worth it? *Canadian Respiratory Journal*, 2016. Available at: https://www.hindawi.com/journals/crj/2016/5352625/. (Accessed 2nd December 2017).

Weir, D.M. and Stewart, J (1997) *Immunology* (8th ed,). London: Churchill Livingstone.

WHO (2008) *Health Topics: Epidemiology*. Available at: http://www.who.int/topics/epide=miology/en/ (Accessed 1st December 2017).

WHO (2009a) *WHO guidelines on hand hygiene in health care. First global patient safety challenge. Clean care is safe care*. Geneva, WHO.

WHO (2009b) *Hand hygiene: Why, how and when?* Geneva, WHO. Available at: https://www.who.int/gpsc/5may/Hand_Hygiene_Why_How_and_When_Brochure.pdf

WHO (2011) Report on the Burden of Endemic Healthcare Associated Infection Worldwide: A systematic review of the literature. Available at: http://apps.who.int/iris/bitstream/10665/80135/1/9789241501507_eng.pdf?ua=1 (Accessed 1st December 2017).

Wigglesworth, N. (2003) The use of protective isolation. *Nursing Times*, 99(7): 26.

Wilson, J. (2000) *Clinical Microbiology. An Introduction for Healthcare Professionals* (8th ed.). Edinburgh: Balliere Tindall.

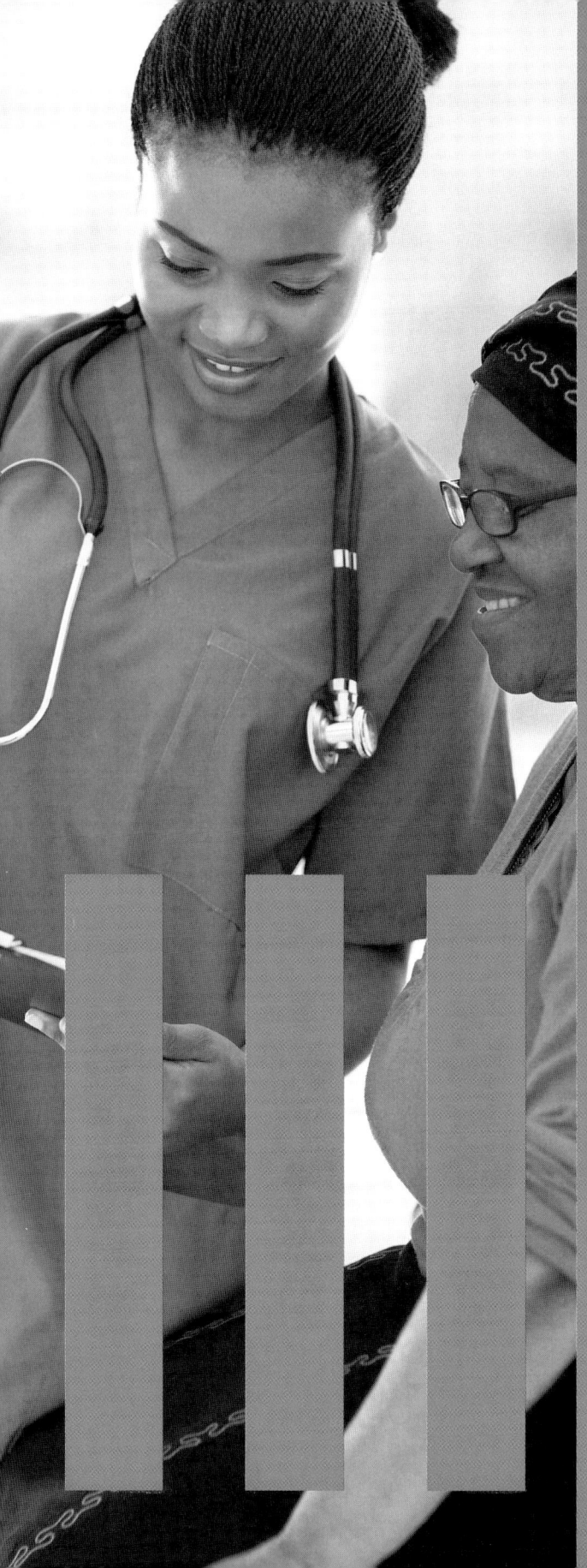

CARE OF THE CHILDBEARING WOMAN

15

LINDSAY GILLMAN

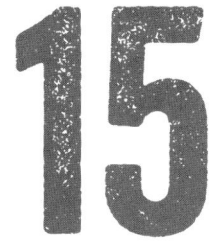

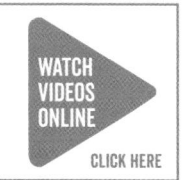

WATCH
VIDEOS
ONLINE

CLICK HERE

THIS CHAPTER COVERS

- Childbearing and the principles of care
- An overview of the normal physiological processes of pregnancy and birth
- The role of the adult nurse working with pregnant women during pregnancy and after childbirth
- Common emergencies in pregnancy and birth

- Safeguarding the mother and baby
- Perinatal mental health
- Guidance for providing appropriate support to mothers who are breastfeeding
- Medicines management during pregnancy and breastfeeding.

"

I really enjoyed going on my health visitor placement as it was one of the few opportunities that I had to learn about women's health. I found this really interesting, as pregnancy and childbirth related issues are encountered in many areas of adult nursing.

Amina, 3rd year student nurse

"

INTRODUCTION

As nurses, it is essential that we are aware of how pregnancy, childbirth and the postpartum period affects women's health in order to provide seamless care with other professionals within the multidisciplinary team, such as midwives, health visitors, GPs and obstetricians. The NMC Code requires that we must ensure that persons physical, social and psychological needs are assessed and responded to by promoting wellbeing, preventing ill health and meeting the changing health and care needs during all life stages (NMC, 2015). This chapter will increase your awareness of the life stage of pregnancy, childbirth and early motherhood so that you can provide appropriate care for women during this important life event.

CRITICAL THINKING STOP POINT 15.1

Before reading further, take a few minutes to think about what you currently understand by the term 'childbearing'.

THE PRINCIPLES OF CARE DURING CHILDBEARING

Childbearing is the term used to describe the continuum of pregnancy, from the process of conceiving, to birth and through to the postnatal period. Childbearing is a normal physiological process for most women and the aim of good care is to provide support during this time and to recognise when there may be pathological issues which require referral. In the United Kingdom, the primary care provider for most women is a midwife.

The principles of care as defined by the National Institute for Health and Care Excellence (2008) include that care should be provided by a small group of healthcare professionals with whom the woman feels comfortable, who can provide continuity of care. The purpose of this is to create a safe and trusting relationship and to ensure that individualised care can be provided. Continuity of care is particularly important for women who may need to discuss sensitive issues such as domestic violence, sexual abuse, psychiatric illness and recreational drug use, but it has known benefits for all women. If additional care is required by specialist teams, referral should be made through clear established pathways so that pregnant women who require additional care can receive it quickly. Referrals may be made to specialist midwives or nurses, social workers, health visitors, consultant obstetricians or other members of the health and social care team.

The core principle of care during childbearing is that the woman's autonomy is acknowledged and that their decisions are respected, even when this may conflict with the views of the healthcare professional. This principle is supported by the NMC Code (2015), the NHS Constitution (Department of Health 2015) and the Human Rights Act (1998). Although this will be a concept that you are familiar with, it is particularly important to remember this in the context of caring for a childbearing woman. Pregnancy is often emotive and there is the potential for the woman to be viewed as simply a means for carrying an unborn baby, and her rights violated in favour of those of the fetus. In the UK, the fetus does not have separate legal recognition in the common law of England and Wales, or under the European Convention, which means that women cannot be forced to accept treatment even if healthcare professionals consider it to be in an unborn child's best interest (Birthrights, 2013).

CRITICAL THINKING STOP POINT 15.2

- Why do you think we have emotional responses towards a fetus?
- In which situations do you think you might find it challenging to support a pregnant woman who declined recommended medical care or treatment?
- Why do you think you would feel challenged?
- Where could you get advice and support if you encountered this situation?

GO FURTHER

For more information on human rights in pregnancy visit the Birthrights website: www.birthrights.org.uk/

WEBLINK: HUMAN RIGHTS

THE NORMAL PHYSIOLOGICAL PROCESSES OF PREGNANCY AND BIRTH

The length (gestation period) of a human pregnancy is normally between 37 and 42 weeks, calculated from the first day of the woman's last menstrual period. The average gestation period is 40 weeks or 280 days. The term of gestation is divided into periods of approximately three months known as trimesters (see Table 15.1).

Table 15.1 Pregnancy trimester and corresponding gestation

Pregnancy trimester	Gestation in weeks
First	0–12
Second	13–27
Third	28–birth

Calculation of the expected date when the baby might be born (expected date of delivery or EDD) can be calculated by counting 40 weeks or 280 days from the first day of the last menstrual period (LMP). An easier way of doing this is to add nine months and 7 days to the date of the LMP. Remember that this is an estimated date of birth and women can be reassured that most babies are born within the two weeks either side of the calculated EDD.

CONCEPTION

Pregnancy starts with conception, which is usually defined as the implantation of the early embryo, known as the blastocyst, into the lining (endometrium) of the uterus. As the blastocyst embeds into the uterine lining, it develops specialised cells known as trophoblastic cells, which produce a hormone called human chorionic gonadotropin or hCG. One of the roles of hCG is to signal to the corpus luteum in the ovary to continue to produce the hormone progesterone. Progesterone plays an important role in pregnancy as it stimulates the growth of blood vessels that supply the endometrium and stimulates glands in the endometrium to secrete nutrients that nourish the early embryo; it also helps to maintain the endometrium throughout pregnancy. Pregnancy testing is based on the presence of hCG in the maternal urine or blood. The hormones of pregnancy, which include hCG, progesterone and oestrogen have additional effects on the woman's body that are often called the signs and symptoms of pregnancy. Signs and symptoms of pregnancy include amenorrhea, breast tenderness, nausea and vomiting and fatigue.

GO FURTHER

WEBLINK: PHYSIOLOGICAL PROCESSES

Visit the NHS Choices website to review your understanding of the physiological processes that occur in early pregnancy: www.nhs.uk/Conditions/pregnancy-and-baby/Pages/pregnancy-weeks-4-5-6-7-8.aspx

There is more information about the common symptoms that may occur in early pregnancy on the website.

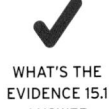

WHAT'S THE EVIDENCE 15.1 ANSWER

WHAT'S THE EVIDENCE? 15.1

Campbell et al. (2016) highlighted that nausea and vomiting in pregnancy may have a profound effect on women's health and their quality of life during pregnancy. These symptoms commonly experienced in pregnancy may also have a financial impact on the healthcare system.

The NICE (2008) guidelines recommend that women should be informed that most cases of nausea and vomiting in pregnancy will resolve spontaneously within 16 to 20 weeks and that nausea and vomiting are not usually associated with a poor pregnancy outcome.

The following interventions appear to be effective in reducing symptoms if a woman would like to consider treatment:

Non-pharmacological methods:

- ginger
- P6 (wrist) acupressure

Pharmacological methods:

- antihistamines

Information about all forms of self-help and non-pharmacological treatments should be made available for pregnant women who have nausea and vomiting.

Antenatal care for uncomplicated pregnancies, Clinical guideline [CG62]. Published date: March 2008. Last updated: January 2017. Available at: www.nice.org.uk/guidance/cg62/chapter/1-Guidance#management-of-common-symptoms-of-pregnancy

For additional resources, visit the website of the charity Pregnancy Sickness Support: www.pregnancysicknesssupport.org.uk/

ACTIVITY 15.1: REFLECTIVE PRACTICE

ACTIVITY 15.1
ANSWER

Visit healthtalk.org to hear some women's experiences of early pregnancy: www.healthtalk.org/peoples-experiences/pregnancy-children/pregnancy/symptoms-and-feelings-early-weeks

- What physical symptoms did the women experience?
- What emotions did the women discuss?

Reflect on the stories you have heard and consider how might you respond if a woman shared her experiences with you and asked for your advice?

PHYSIOLOGICAL ADAPTATION TO PREGNANCY

There are many physiological changes that occur in pregnancy that may produce signs or symptoms that would cause concern or be considered pathological in a non-pregnant woman. The hormones of pregnancy, particularly oestrogen and progesterone, enable the body systems to adapt to the various demands of pregnancy. It is important that, as nurses, we understand the causes of those symptoms and can recognise when referral to another practitioner may be required.

The cardiovascular system adapts to meet the changing maternal demands as the pregnancy progresses towards birth. An increase in maternal blood volume occurs by approximately 50% to meet the additional needs of the maternal and fetal systems via the utero-placental circulation. This is created by plasma expansion and results in hypervolaemia and physiological haemodilution. A low resistance environment is required to accommodate the increased blood volume without causing an increase in blood pressure. The increased levels of maternal progesterone cause a decrease in systemic vascular resistance. This often leads to a decrease in diastolic blood pressure in the first two trimesters, with a return to the non-pregnant level in the third trimester. The increase in blood volume raises maternal cardiac output by 35–50% due to a rise in heart rate and stroke volume. These changes enable the blood flow to the brain and coronary arteries to be kept stable in addition to increasing the blood flow to the uterus, liver, kidneys and breasts.

The metabolic rate rises during pregnancy; therefore, there is an increase in oxygen requirements. This is met by changes to the respiratory system, including an increase in minute and tidal volume and a small rise in the respiratory rate. Pregnancy also affects the urinary system with an increase in the glomerular filtration rate (GFR) by 40–50%, and an increase in urine production by up to 25%. Some substances including glucose, water-soluble vitamins and amino acids may be excreted in the urine. The gastrointestinal tract adapts during pregnancy under the effects of oestrogen, progesterone and relaxin. Progesterone affects the muscle tone of the tract and sphincters, causing symptoms such as indigestion and constipation. Indigestion in pregnancy is usually caused by reflux oesophagitis as the tone of the cardiac sphincter is reduced, while constipation is caused by both the reduced tone of the large intestine and increased sodium and water absorption in the colon.

During pregnancy, there are alterations in collagen formation and an increase in melanocytes, which results in changes to the elasticity and the pigmentation of the skin. Striae gravidarum, more commonly known as stretch marks, are caused by both hormonal and physical factors and may affect up to 90% of pregnant women. Chloasma, sometimes referred to as the 'butterfly mask' of pregnancy, is caused by increased pigmentation due a rise in melanin production. Another common feature that occurs during pregnancy is the linea nigra, which is a line of dark pigmentation seen on the abdomen in the midline, appearing from the second trimester. Changes to the skin caused by pigmentation usually fade in the postpartum period and often disappear completely. The changes in collagen fibres caused by the pregnancy hormones also cause laxity and increased mobility in the joints of the body. Softening of the pelvic joints and ligaments enables the pelvic cavity to enlarge during birth to accommodate the fetal head. Some women may experience pain in their pelvis during pregnancy due to the increased laxity and instability of the pelvic joints.

The maternal immune system adapts in a variety of ways during pregnancy to prevent rejection of the fetus and to provide some level of protection for it. The changes are complex and not completely understood; however, it is known that the woman becomes immunocompromised, although this does not seem to have an adverse effect on most pregnancies. The total white cell count increases in pregnancy, beginning in the first trimester and reaching a peak at approximately 30 weeks. This is mainly due to an increase in neutrophils providing an increased resistance to bacterial infection. Resistance to viral infections such as influenza, herpes and rubella may, however, be reduced.

CRITICAL THINKING STOP POINT 15.3

- What might be the consequence of physiological haemodilution in pregnancy on blood results such as haemoglobin (Hb) level?
- Why would it be important to have a pre-pregnant or early pregnancy blood pressure recorded?
- What physiological adaptations would you consider when interpreting a pregnant woman's blood pressure, pulse and respiratory rate?
- What information might you offer women who ask about having the flu vaccine in pregnancy?

THE PHYSIOLOGICAL PROCESSES OF BIRTH

Birth is a usually a normal physiological process that does not require medical intervention when it occurs spontaneously, at term in a healthy woman. However, for those who have not witnessed or experienced physiological birth, the way that birth is often represented as a medical emergency surrounded by high drama on television and in films is often considered the norm. Although the law in the United Kingdom makes it a criminal offence for anyone except a registered midwife or doctor to 'attend' a woman during childbirth except in an emergency, there are frequently situations where women give birth outside of their planned birth environment without a midwife or doctor present. As nurses, it is important that we understand how best to support a woman in these situations to ensure the safety of both mother and baby.

Oxytocin and adrenaline

Oxytocin is a hormone and neurotransmitter produced by the hypothalamus that influences the muscles of the uterus causing them to contract, and acts on the myoepithelial cells within the breast to enable breast milk to be expelled. Oxytocin is known as the 'love' hormone, as in addition to the action it has on muscles it also causes feelings of love, nurture and protection to be experienced. Oxytocin production and secretion is increased when we feel loved and cared for and can be stimulated by feelings of safety and security which can be created by a calm, dark, warm environment, soft voices and gentle touch. Oxytocin is also known as the 'shy' hormone as secretion can be halted by the presence of adrenaline, which is released as part of the 'flight or fight' response to threatening situations and fear. If you find yourself in a situation where a woman is in active labour outside of her planned birth environment, she is likely to be frightened about the outcome for her baby and anxious about maintaining her own privacy and dignity. Care provision that aims to reduce adrenaline secretion and facilitate oxytocin production is ideal for encouraging physiological birth. In practical terms this means that once you have called for assistance (in whichever way is most appropriate depending on your location), protecting the woman's privacy and creating an environment which is calm, warm and safe is the best thing that you can do.

Recognising the stages of labour

The stages of labour are referred to in numerical terms; the first, second and third stage, and define the processes that are occurring during labour and birth. It is often difficult to determine exactly when each stage begins and ends, with wide variations seen in terms of the length of each stage. There is much debate about how useful it is to categorise the process of labour in such a way; however, it is important that you know what to expect during physiological labour and birth, and what your role might be when attending a woman in an emergency.

1st stage of labour: This is the 'contractions' stage and is defined as when there are regular, painful contractions and progressive cervical dilatation from 4 cm (NICE, 2014). The regular uterine contractions cause the cervix to thin and open, to enable the passage of the fetus from the uterus to the vaginal canal. The length of time it takes for the cervix to fully open can be variable from a few minutes to many hours. As labour progresses the contractions generally become more intense, last longer and are closer together. When contractions are lasting between 50–60 seconds and occur every 2–3 minutes, labour is likely to be progressing towards the second stage. There are often other signs that accompany regular uterine contractions which may indicate that labour is progressing; these include low backache and/or discomfort felt deep in the pelvis, diarrhoea, the loss of the mucus plug from the cervix as it opens (sometimes referred to as a 'show') and spontaneous rupture of the fetal membranes (the 'waters breaking'). The fetal membranes contain amniotic fluid, which is usually straw coloured and has a slightly sweet smell.

2nd stage of labour: The second stage of labour is the 'pushing' stage and can be divided into two phases: passive and active. The passive phase begins from full dilatation of the cervix before or in the absence of involuntary maternal pushing with contractions. The active phase begins following full dilatation where there is active involuntary maternal pushing during contractions; the baby may or may not be visible (NICE, 2014). Just before active pushing commences women may feel the need to bear down as they experience rectal pressure, as though they need to open their bowels (many women do this as they push). Other signs include anal dilatation, a bulging perineum and the woman's vagina may start to open. With active pushing, the top of the baby's head may become visible, gradually stretching the vagina and perineum and the head will 'crown' (the largest part of the head will have moved through the vaginal opening). Once the head has been born (the baby's face will most probably be facing the mother's back), the baby's head will rotate to face the mother's thigh: this realigns the shoulders within the pelvis. With the next contraction, the shoulders and the rest of the baby are usually born. Sometimes, particularly with very rapid labours, the baby is born during one contraction. The baby will be attached to the placenta by the umbilical cord, which pulsates as the fetal blood within the utero-placental circulation continues to flow. Do not worry about clamping, tying or cutting the cord, it should be left untouched and intact.

3rd stage of labour: The third stage of labour is defined as the time between the birth of the baby to the birth of the placenta and membranes (NICE, 2014). The umbilical cord should be left intact and attached to the placenta, which is usually expelled from the uterus within an hour after the birth of the baby. Blood loss during this stage is variable, but is usually between 100 and 500mls.

ACTIVITY 15.2: REFLECTIVE PRACTICE

If a woman was in labour or giving birth unexpectedly, what you would do to support her in the different stages of labour while waiting for help to arrive?

What would be your key priorities during each stage?

CRITICAL THINKING STOP POINT 15.4

Visit the NHS Choices website and consider the options that are available to women when choosing where to give birth. www.nhs.uk/Conditions/pregnancy-and-baby/pages/where-can-i-give-birth.aspx

- What does the evidence suggest is the safest place to give birth?
- What are the reasons for this?

THE ROLE OF THE ADULT NURSE WORKING WITH PREGNANT WOMEN DURING PREGNANCY AND AFTER CHILDBIRTH

The role of the adult nurse in maternity care has changed significantly over the past few years, and nurses are now more likely to be included in aspects of care provision for pregnant women. The changing profile of childbearing women and the use of integrated care pathways mean that it is likely that you will provide care for pregnant or newly delivered women at some point in your role as a nurse.

One of the ways the profile of childbearing women has changed, is the age they are when they choose to start a family. The average maternal age at birth has increased by almost four years over the last four decades. The trend for women to delay childbearing until their 30s and 40s is reflected in the falling birth rates among the under 30s, and the rising birth rates at older ages (Haines, 2016). The number of births to women who are over 40 has increased in the last decade by 21.5% (NHS Digital, 2016).

In addition to being older, women may also be heavier; the UK has the highest prevalence of obesity of all the European countries with over 25% of women having a body mass index (BMI) of over 30 kg/m^2 (Devlieger et al., 2016). It is well documented that women who are obese and pregnant are at risk of complications during pregnancy and birth. Women may also have long-term medical conditions that may get worse during pregnancy, although some may also get better (this depends on both the condition and the health of individual). Advances in medical and obstetric management, in addition to progress in assisted reproductive technologies such as in-vitro fertilisation, has meant that many women who may not previously have been able to get pregnant, or carry a successful pregnancy to term due to a long-term condition, are now able to do so. These factors have the potential to create pathological features in what would otherwise be a physiological event. In some cases, there is the increased likelihood of a surgical birth (caesarean section), which carries with it the usual surgical risks. The rate at which babies are being born by caesarean section has increased significantly from 24.1% to 27.1% in the last decade, with a rate of almost 60% for women aged 45 and over (NHS Digital, 2016).

Being pregnant and older, overweight or having a long-term medical condition, known as co-morbidities, increases the risk of complications in pregnancy. This means that an integrated pathway approach to care should be initiated, with the inclusion of other healthcare professionals. This may include you in your role as a nurse in primary or community-based care, working on a medical or surgical ward, specialist care team or within a high dependency care area. Maternal morbidity and mortality may not be something you have thought about before, particularly in the context of working in the UK. Maternal deaths in high-income countries are rare events; however, many more women have severe pregnancy complications that can leave them with life-changing disabilities. The confidential inquiry into maternal death and morbidity in the UK and Ireland identified that in the two years between 2012 and 2014, tragically 200 women died during childbearing (pregnancy to one year after birth) – 81 women died from direct (obstetric) causes, and 119 from indirect (medical) causes. Following a review of the cases, the authors of the report concluded that 'the clear message remains the importance of coordinated multi-professional care covering the entire pathway before, during and after pregnancy' (Knight et al., 2016: 1).

This integrated approach to care has the potential to improve outcomes for women and babies by ensuring that they are seen by the right professional with the knowledge and skills to care for them, in the right place, at the right time (NHS England, 2013), which will include your knowledge and skills as an adult nurse.

CRITICAL THINKING STOP POINT 15.5

- In what circumstances could you be involved in providing care for a childbearing woman in your role as an adult nurse?
- What factors you would need to consider when providing care?
- Which other health or social care practitioners might be involved in the woman's care?

COMMON EMERGENCIES IN PREGNANCY AND BIRTH

There may be times when you need to support a woman who requires urgent care due to a pregnancy-related health issue. However, it is important to remember that childbearing women also experience medical emergencies such as a heart attack, stroke or pulmonary embolus. In all situations, the principles of emergency care remain the same: assessment and management of Airway, Breathing and Circulation.

Vaginal bleeding in pregnancy

Vaginal bleeding is relatively common in pregnancy, particularly in the first trimester, with approximately 25% of women experiencing some form of bleeding with or without abdominal cramping (Gubbin and Gould, 2016). Although it is a common occurrence, the severity of the situation depends on the cause, and the woman's haemodynamic state. Bleeding in the first trimester can be caused by a variety of factors; it may be a warning sign of a miscarriage, ectopic pregnancy or an unusual condition called a molar pregnancy. Bleeding accompanied by cramps felt in the lower abdomen may indicate that uterine contractions are occurring and the cervix may be dilating. Vaginal discharge that is blood streaked, or a light pink or brown in the absence of abdominal pain, is not usually a cause for concern. Women with any bleeding should be reviewed either by their GP or midwife in the first instance, or be referred directly to an Early Pregnancy Unit (EPU) for further assessment. Assessment usually includes an ultrasound scan (abdominally, trans-vaginally or both), blood tests for βhCG levels and a vaginal examination by speculum to view the cervix to see if it is opening (Royal College of Obstetricians & Gynaecologists, 2016).

The causes of bleeding in the second and third trimesters also include placenta praevia and placental abruption, which can both become emergency situations. Placenta praevia occurs when the placenta implants low down in the uterus close to or covering the cervix. Uterine contractions that lead to the cervix opening also cause the placenta to separate and bleeding occurs. Women are usually aware that they have placenta praevia, as it is diagnosed through routine ultrasound scans. If women who are known to have placenta praevia experience vaginal bleeding they should be reviewed urgently as this has the potential to become an obstetric emergency. Bleeding from placenta praevia is usually painless.

Placental abruption occurs when the placenta begins to detach from the uterine wall prematurely (before the birth of the baby). Placental abruption may cause bleeding and severe abdominal pain or there may not be any signs at all. Placental abruption should always be treated as an obstetric emergency. Significant bleeding in pregnancy is called an ante-partum haemorrhage.

Vaginal bleeding after birth

After birth, it is normal for vaginal bleeding which may be like a heavy menstrual period. Bleeding may continue for between two and six weeks, with the colour of the loss changing from bright red to a dark red-brown blood, followed by a pinkish and finally white discharge. If bleeding is very heavy and uncontrolled immediately after birth, this is called a postpartum haemorrhage and is always considered an obstetric emergency.

The cause of the blood loss from a postpartum haemorrhage needs to be established immediately so that the appropriate management can occur. The blood loss will either be from the uterine placental site or from trauma sustained during birth such as a tear in the cervix, vaginal wall or perineum. The placental site may bleed due to the uterus not contracting fully after the third stage of labour is complete, known as uterine atony. This may be due to exhaustion of the muscle fibres because of a very long or obstructed labour, or it may be due to retained fragments of placental tissue. Effective management of a postpartum haemorrhage includes various methods to ensure that the uterus is fully empty and contracted to control the bleeding.

Pre-eclampsia and eclampsia

There are different types of hypertension in pregnancy including chronic hypertension (high blood pressure before pregnancy), gestational hypertension (high blood pressure because of pregnancy) and pre-eclampsia (high blood pressure with proteinuria). The incidence of death from pre-eclampsia is now less than one per million women who give birth (Knight et al., 2016); however, the incidence of hypertension in pregnancy is a more common feature, affecting 10–15% of pregnant women (NHS Choices, 2015). Pre-eclampsia is diagnosed when there is new hypertension presenting after 20 weeks gestation with significant proteinuria. Eclampsia is a convulsive condition that is associated with pre-eclampsia and is considered an obstetric emergency. The symptoms of pre-eclampsia include:

- severe headache
- visual disturbances, blurred vision or seeing flashing lights
- severe pain just below the ribs
- vomiting
- sudden swelling of the face, hands or feet.

If women experience any symptoms of pre-eclampsia they should be advised to seek immediate medical advice (NICE, 2010a). Table 15.2 below shows the definitions of chronic and gestational hypertension, pre-eclampsia and severe pre-eclampsia.

Table 15.2 Definitions of chronic and gestational hypertension, pre-eclampsia and severe pre-eclampsia

Term	Definition	
Chronic hypertension	Hypertension that is present at the first antenatal visit or before 20 weeks gestation; or if the woman is taking anti-hypertensive medication when referred for maternity care	Mild hypertension: 140-149/90-99 mmHg
		Moderate hypertension: 150-159/100-109 mmHg
Gestational hypertension	New hypertension presenting after 20 weeks gestation without significant protein	Severe hypertension: ≥160/≥110 mmHg
Pre-eclampsia	New hypertension presenting after 20 weeks gestation with significant protein	
Severe pre-eclampsia	Severe hypertension and/or symptoms and/or biochemical and/or haematological impairment	

(Adapted from NICE, 2010a)

SAFEGUARDING THE MOTHER AND BABY

Some women will have complex social situations which have the potential to create additional vulnerabilities during pregnancy. These complex social factors may include poverty, homelessness, a history of drug or alcohol misuse, recent migrant or asylum seeker status, difficulty reading or speaking English, being aged under 20 years old, and experiencing domestic abuse. Access to care is particularly important for these women to ensure that the most appropriate care and support can be planned and provided. However, the evidence suggests that women with complex social situations may not initially seek antenatal care or attend follow-up appointments because of the perceived negative attitude of healthcare staff. A key principle of maternity care is that all women should be treated with kindness and dignity with respect for their views, values and beliefs. Women should be supported to make decisions about their care in partnership with healthcare professionals. This is particularly important for this vulnerable group of women, where early and sustained engagement with maternity care can have a positive effect on outcomes (NICE, 2010b).

Female genital mutilation (FGM) is another factor that may also cause a complex social situation if it is identified in an adult woman. This is because there may be the risk of FGM to her baby if it is a girl. FGM is illegal in the UK and there is a mandatory responsibility for safeguarding children under the age of 18 years who have had FGM, or are at risk of being subjected to it, under the Serious Crime Act (2015). When safeguarding requirements have been considered, women in this situation should be offered support that is sensitive and culturally appropriate.

If you become aware that a woman and her unborn child are vulnerable, the usual safeguarding procedures should be followed. It is important that any concerns about vulnerable women or babies are documented and shared appropriately. Many of the serious case reviews into the death or serious harm of a vulnerable individual have identified that professionals failed to share or record significant pieces of information (HM Government, 2015).

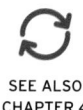

SEE ALSO
CHAPTER 4

PERINATAL MENTAL HEALTH

Most people are aware of what is often called the 'baby blues', which refers to a short period of low mood during the first week after birth. The cause of the 'baby blues' is thought to be the sudden hormonal and chemical changes that take place in a woman's body after birth. It is also likely to be influenced by disrupted sleep patterns and recovery from labour and birth.

Symptoms can include:

- feeling emotional and irrational
- crying for no apparent reason
- feeling irritable
- feeling depressed or anxious.

These symptoms are normal, usually only last for a few days and should resolve spontaneously. If symptoms continue for longer than a few days postnatally or occur during pregnancy, a more significant mental health issue may be developing. Women are vulnerable to developing mental health issues during pregnancy and the postnatal period just as they would be at any other time in their lives; however, pregnancy or childbirth may be the trigger for these to occur for the first time or for a previous condition to recur. The impact of a mental health issue in the perinatal period may be more significant for a woman as her ability to function and care for her family can be impaired.

The issues most commonly seen in the perinatal period and first year after birth include mild to moderate depression and anxiety, affecting between 12 and 20% of women. Postpartum psychosis is a serious and more rare condition affecting between 1 and 2 women per 1,000 and can occur in women without any previous mental health problems (NICE, 2016). Postpartum psychosis is recognised as a psychiatric emergency and signs may include mania, depression, confusion, delusions and hallucinations. In the 2015 confidential enquiry into maternal deaths, it was reported that 23% of the women who died, did so because of mental-health related issues with 1 in 7 of these deaths being caused by suicide (Knight et al., 2015). Although for most women, the symptoms that they experience may be not be so acute that they lead to this tragic outcome, it is important that the most appropriate support is sought as soon as women or members of their family express any concerns about their mental health.

It is important to remember that women who are concerned that they may have a mental health problem may be unwilling to discuss or disclose this during pregnancy or in the postnatal period. The reasons for this may include a perception of being perceived in a negative way, which may impact on the decisions made by health or social care professionals regarding the ability to care for a baby. It may be useful for you to use anxiety and depression identification questions to begin to discuss mental wellbeing with a woman when concerns about mental health have been expressed. The following depression identification questions should be asked at a woman's first antenatal visit and during the early postnatal period (NICE, 2016):

- During the past month, have you often been bothered by feeling down, depressed or hopeless?
- During the past month, have you often been bothered by having little interest or pleasure in doing things?

If a positive response is given to either question, the woman should be referred to her GP or mental health professional. Women should be referred to a specialist perinatal mental health service if they report:

- new thoughts of violent self-harm
- sudden onset or rapidly worsening mental symptoms
- persistent feelings of estrangement from their baby.

CRITICAL THINKING STOP POINT 15.6

Why do you think women may be reluctant to discuss their mental health concerns in the perinatal period?

What ethical and legal issues would you need to consider if you had concerns about a mother's mental health in the postnatal period?

SUPPORT FOR MOTHERS WHO ARE BREASTFEEDING

Breastfeeding is one of the most effective ways of ensuring that a baby gets the right nutrients and antibodies to be healthy, and because of this it is considered a high-impact public health intervention. There are many long-term benefits of breastfeeding for both the mother and baby, and recent research into epigenetics and the microbiome has identified that it may be even more important than previously thought. Breastmilk is a unique and dynamic substance that provides the baby with more than just food; it also contains hormones, anti-inflammatory factors, enzymes, immunoglobulins, white cells, viral fragments and transfer factors which help with absorption of the nutrients.

The first milk is called colostrum, which is creamy and yellow in colour, and contains anti-infective and anti-viral properties that are important for ensuring good gut health in the baby. Although the benefits of breastfeeding are widely known, not all women choose to breastfeed. Those who do may initiate breastfeeding after birth but may not continue for a variety of reasons. Many women may find breastfeeding more challenging than they expected before the birth of their baby, and often experience problems in the early days and weeks. Women should be advised to seek help from their midwife or health visitor if they are experiencing any problems with feeding or have concerns about the baby's health or weight gain. There are some key principles to consider when supporting a woman to breastfeed to ensure that the baby is positioned properly at the breast. The acronym CHIN is a useful way to remember them:

Close – the baby needs to be held close to the body; skin-to-skin contact is recommended

Head free – the baby's head should be free to move so that they can position themselves properly with their chin leading towards the nipple and their head tilted back

In line – the baby's body should be in line with their head so that their neck isn't twisted

Nose to nipple – the baby's nose should be in line with the nipple so that as they tilt their head backwards and lead with their chin towards the nipple, the nipple is drawn into their mouth at the correct angle

(Unicef UK, 2014)

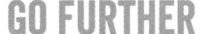

GO FURTHER

Look at the images of correct positioning and other useful information on the NHS Start4Life breastfeeding page: www.nhs.uk/start4life/breastfeeding#steps

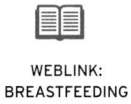

WEBLINK:
BREASTFEEDING

CRITICAL THINKING STOP POINT 15.7

- What are the factors that influence women's decisions about breastfeeding?
- What are some of the common breastfeeding problems?
- How can healthcare professionals best support breastfeeding mothers?

CONSIDERATIONS FOR MEDICINES MANAGEMENT DURING THE PERINATAL PERIOD

There may be times when you are required to administer medicines to a woman who is pregnant or in the postnatal period. There are some important points to remember to ensure safe medicines management for both the woman and the fetus or baby. Earlier in the chapter, the utero-placental circulation was introduced, and you learned that the maternal and fetal blood come into close contact during pregnancy to enable the transfer of gases, nutrients and waste products. The structure of the placenta offers some protection from unwanted substances crossing the maternal-fetal barrier; however, some substances including medicines can pass from the mother to the fetus. The main risk to the fetus is exposure to certain toxins in the medicines that can cause problems during development. If prescribed during the first trimester, medicines can produce congenital malformations (teratogenesis), with the greatest risk from the third to the eleventh week of pregnancy as this is when the embryonic structure and major organs are developing. During the second and third trimesters medicines can have toxic effects on fetal tissues, or affect fetal growth or development. Well-known examples of where medicines have caused damage to the developing fetus include the use of thalidomide to treat nausea in pregnancy during the 1960s, and more recently fetal exposure to valproate, used to control epilepsy during pregnancy.

During the postnatal period, there may be a risk of toxins from medicines transferring to the baby through breastmilk, therefore the benefits of taking medication when breastfeeding must be considered to outweigh the risks. Prescribers should be cautious about prescribing or recommending any medicines, alternative remedies or supplements during pregnancy and during breastfeeding. Women who are taking medication for a long-term condition should be advised to continue until treatment plans are reviewed by their GP, medical consultant or obstetrician. The British National Formulary contains information regarding prescribing in pregnancy and during breastfeeding and should be referred to for up-to-date prescribing and administration advice.

GO FURTHER

WEBLINKS

Valproate carries a high risk of developmental disorders and congenital malformations if taken in pregnancy. Visit the government webpage to read the leaflet explaining the risks and the advice for women: www.medicines.org.uk/emc/RMM.420.pdf

Read the NICE guidelines for prescribing in pregnancy: https://bnf.nice.org.uk/guidance/prescribing-in-pregnancy.html

---

CHAPTER SUMMARY

This chapter has explored the principles of maternity care and your role as an adult nurse within the multiprofessional team when providing care for childbearing women.

- Pregnancy and childbirth are normal physiological processes. The woman's body undergoes many physiological adaptations initiated by the pregnancy hormones.
- There may be some pregnancy or birth-related emergencies that you will encounter in your role as an adult nurse. In all situations, the principles of emergency care remain the same: assessment and management of Airway, Breathing and Circulation.
- During childbearing, some women may be particularly vulnerable because of complex social situations. The usual principles of safeguarding must be applied.
- Perinatal mental health is an important aspect of maternity care. Prompt recognition and intervention can ensure women and their families get the help and support they need.
- Breastfeeding is a high-impact public health intervention with health benefits for both mother and baby. Women may need support to initiate and continue breastfeeding, and specialist help should be sought if women are experiencing difficulties.
- If a fetus is exposed to certain medicines from the maternal system, there can be significant detrimental effects on growth and development. Always check whether medicines are safe to be taken during pregnancy or breastfeeding.

GO FURTHER

Go to https://study.sagepub.com/essentialadultnursing for a further case study related to this chapter. If you are using the interactive ebook, simply click on the book icon in the margin to go straight to the resource.

CASE STUDY: PERSON-CENTRED CARE

Books

- Rankin, J. (ed.) (2017) *Physiology in Childbearing with Anatomy and Related Biosciences* (4th ed.). London: Elsevier.
  This book provides detailed information on the physiological aspects of childbearing.
- Leap, N. and Hunter, B. (2016) *Supporting Women for Labour and Birth: A thoughtful guide.* Abingdon: Routledge.
  A book detailing the importance of thoughtful support during labour and birth through the stories of women and their midwives.
- Avery, G. (2016) Consent (Chapter 5) in *Law and Ethics in Nursing and Healthcare: An introduction* (2nd ed.). London: Sage.
  This chapter is a good source for revision of the ethical and legal framework in relation to the principle of consent, with some interesting cases relating to pregnancy and childbearing.

Journal Articles

Go to https://study.sagepub.com/essentialadultnursing for further free online journal articles related to this chapter. If you are using the interactive ebook, simply click on the book icon in the margin to go straight to the resource.

FURTHER READING: JOURNAL ARTICLES

- Soma-Pillay, P., Nelson-Piercy, C., Tolppanen, H. and Mebazza, A. (2016) Physiological changes in pregnancy. *Cardiovascular Journal of Africa*, 27 (2): 89–94. Available at: www.ncbi.nlm.nih.gov/pmc/articles/PMC4928162/pdf/cvja-27-89.pdf

- This article presents a detailed account of the physiological changes in pregnancy, highlighting the differences between normal physiology and pathology.
- Nair, M., Kurinczuk, J.J., Brocklehurst, P., Sellers, S., Lewis, G. and Knight, M. (2016) Factors associated with maternal death from direct pregnancy complications: A UK national case-control study. *British Journal of Obstetrics and Gynaecology*, 122: 653-62. Available at: www.ncbi.nlm.nih.gov/pmc/articles/PMC4674982/
  The pre-existing conditions (co-morbidities) that can cause significant complications in pregnancy are discussed in this article.
- Montgomery, A., Hannon, G., Muhammad, S., Das, S. and Hayes, K. (2017) Tubal ectopic pregnancies: Risk, diagnosis and management. *British Journal of Midwifery*, 25 (11): 700-5. Available at: https://doi.org/10.12968/bjom.2017.25.11.700
  This article presents a review of the risk factors and current management methods for ectopic pregnancy.

Weblinks

FURTHER READING: WEBLINKS

Go to https://study.sagepub.com/essentialadultnursing for further weblinks related to this chapter. If you are using the interactive ebook, simply click on the book icon in the margin to go straight to the resource.

- Resources for parents and professionals to help support breastfeeding are available on the Best Beginnings website.
  www.bestbeginnings.org.uk/from-bump-to-breastfeeding
- The Pandas foundation is a charity that supports families experiencing antenatal or postnatal illness. The website provides information, resources and support.
  www.pandasfoundation.org.uk/
- This is the website for *bumps*, a service that provides specific information about the use of medicines and other chemicals in pregnancy.
  www.medicinesinpregnancy.org/

ONLINE QUIZZES

ACE YOUR ASSESSMENT

Revise what you have learned by visiting https://study.sagepub.com/essentialadultnursing

- Test yourself with multiple-choice and short-answer questions
- Do the chapter activities in the book and check your answers online

REFERENCES

Birthrights (2013) *Consenting to Treatment*. Available at: www.birthrights.org.uk/library/factsheets/Consenting-to-Treatment.pdf (last accessed 6 May 2017).

Campbell, K., Rowe, H., Azzam, H. and Lane, C.A. (2016) The management of nausea and vomiting of pregnancy. *Journal of Obstetrics and Gynaecology Canada,* 38 (12): 1127–37

Department of Health (2015) *The NHS Constitution for England*. Available at: https:// www.gov.uk/government/publications/the-nhs-constitution-for-england/the-nhs-constitution-for-england (last accessed 6 May 2017).

Devlieger, R., Benhalima, K., Damm, P., Van Assche, A., Mathieu, C., Mahmood, T., Dunne, F. and Bogaerts A. (2016) Maternal obesity in Europe: where do we stand and how to move forward?

A scientific paper commissioned by the European Board and College of Obstetrics and Gynaecology (EBCOG). *European Journal of Obstetrics & Gynecology and Reproductive Biology,* 201: 203–8.

Gubbin, J. and Gould, D. (2016) Management of vaginal bleeding in early pregnancy in the emergency department. *European Journal of Obstetrics & Gynecology and Reproductive Biology,* 206: e155–e156.

Haines, N. (2016) Statistical bulletin: *Births by parents' characteristics in England and Wales: 2015.* Office for National Statistics. Available at: www.ons.gov.uk/ peoplepopulationandcommunity/birthsdeathsandmarriages/livebirths/bulletins/ birthsbyparentscharacteristicsinenglandandwales/2015 (last accessed 27 September 2017).

Her Majesty's Government (2015) *Information Sharing Advice for Practitioners Providing Safeguarding Services to Children, Young People, Parents and Carers.* Available at: www.gov.uk/government/ uploads/system/uploads/attachment_data/file/419628/Information_sharing_advice_safeguarding_ practitioners.pdf (last accessed 14 October 2017).

Human Rights Act 1998, C.42 Available at: www.legislation.gov.uk/ukpga/1998/42/pdfs/ ukpga_19980042_en.pdf (last accessed 6 May 2017).

Knight, M., Tuffnell, D., Kenyon, S., Shakespeare, J., Gray, R. and Kurinczuk, J.J. (2015) *Saving Lives, Improving Mothers' Care: Surveillance of Maternal Deaths in the UK 2011-13 and Lessons Learned to Inform Maternity Care from the UK and Ireland Confidential Enquiries into Maternal Deaths and Morbidity 2009–13.* Available at: www.npeu.ox.ac.uk (last accessed 14 October 2017).

Knight, M., Nair, M., Tuffnell, D., Kenyon, S., Shakespeare, J., Brocklehurst, P. and Kurinczuk, J.J. (2016) *Saving Lives, Improving Mothers' Care: Surveillance of Maternal Deaths in the UK 2012–14 and Lessons Learned to Inform Maternity Care from the UK and Ireland Confidential Enquiries into Maternal Deaths and Morbidity 2009–14.* Available at: www.npeu.ox.ac.uk (last accessed 14 October 2017).

National Institute for Health and Care Excellence (2008) *Principles of care in Antenatal care for uncomplicated pregnancies overview.* Available at: https://pathways.nice.org.uk/pathways/antenatal- care-for-uncomplicated-pregnancies#content=view-node%3Anodes-principles-of-care (last accessed 6 July 2017).

National Institute for Health and Care Excellence (2010a) *Hypertension in pregnancy: diagnosis and management.* Available at: www.nice.org.uk/guidance/cg107/chapter/1-Guidance#reducing-the- risk-of-hypertensive-disorders-in-pregnancy (last accessed 11 October 2017).

National Institute for Health and Care Excellence (2010b) *Pregnancy and complex social factors: a model for service provision for pregnant women with complex social factors* Available at: www.nice.org.uk/ guidance/cg110 (last accessed 11 October 2017).

National Institute for Health and Care Excellence (2014) *Intrapartum care for healthy women and babies.* Available at: www.nice.org.uk/guidance/cg190 (last accessed 24 January 2018).

National Institute for Health and Care Excellence (2016) *Antenatal and postnatal mental health.* Available at: www.nice.org.uk/guidance/qs115 (last accessed 11 October 2017).

NHS Choices (2015) *High blood pressure (hypertension) and pregnancy.* Available at: www.nhs.uk/ conditions/pregnancy-and-baby/pages/hypertension-blood-pressure-pregnant.aspx (last accessed 14 October 2017).

NHS Digital (2016) *Hospital Maternity Activity 2015–16.* Available at: www.content.digital.nhs. uk/catalogue/PUB22384/hosp-epis-stat-mat-summ-repo-2015-16-rep.pdf (last accessed 27 September 2017).

NHS England (2013) *How to ensure the right people, with the right skills, are in the right place at the right time: A guide to nursing, midwifery and care staffing capacity and capability.* National Quality Board. Available at: www.england.nhs.uk/wp-content/uploads/2013/11/nqb-how-to-guid.pdf (last accessed 9 October 2017).

Nursing and Midwifery Council (2015) *The Code: Professional standards of practice and behaviour for nurses and midwives.* Available at: www.nmc.org.uk/standards/code/ (last accessed 14 October 2017).

Royal College of Obstetricians and Gynaecologists (2016) *Bleeding and/or pain in early pregnancy.* Available at: www.rcog.org.uk/en/patients/patient-leaflets/bleeding-and-pain-in-early-pregnancy/ (last accessed 14 October 2017).

Serious Crime Act 2015, C.9. Available at: www.legislation.gov.uk/ukpga/2015/9/pdfs/ukpga_20150009_en.pdf (last accessed 14 October 2017).

Unicef BFI UK (2014) *Breastfeeding and Relationship Building Workbook.* London: Unicef UK.

CARE OF THE HIGHLY DEPENDENT AND CRITICALLY ILL ADULT

16

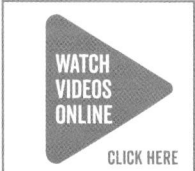

WATCH VIDEOS ONLINE

CLICK HERE

CAROLINE ADAM

THIS CHAPTER COVERS

- Understanding critical care
- Criteria required for admission to critical care
- How to provide person-centred, safe and holistic critical nursing care to patients and their families

- Nursing assessment and care management of the highly dependent and critically ill adult
- The transition of discharge and step down from critical care.

> I have suffered many psychological and physical issues during and after my time in the unit ... my mind created several 'memories', some of which I now know are clearly false and some are a distortion of an actual event. I would be lying in bed looking at the nurse's station and the nurse's faces would morph into animals ... the inability to properly communicate also cultivated a feeling of isolation. Hospital can be a lonely place if you're unable to communicate, particularly when under stress ...
>
> **Kevin, critical care patient, 2013**

> When I first walked into ACCU, I immediately noticed the change in atmosphere. There was a calmness; a change of light, monitors beeping and the suction sound of ventilators. I was nervous and I thought I was going to be out of my depth. Walking through the ITU and HDU units, I noticed there were fewer patients, one-to-one nursing, more space around the beds and lots of equipment. I believe my experience has honed my professional responsibilities, observation, communication, clinical and interpersonal skills as a student nurse. I took away with me invaluable knowledge and experience that will enhance my nursing practice in other clinical areas.
>
> **Cheryl, Part 1 student nurse, BSc adult nursing programme**

INTRODUCTION

Caring for highly dependent and critically ill adults is a challenging experience for all team members, including student nurses. The nature of the critical care environment and the dynamic pace can be overwhelming for all.

As previously noted by Cheryl (Part 1 student nurse), the thought of the specialist nature of this environment was initially daunting and anxiety provoking; she talks about the noises and being nervous while also acknowledging a feeling of calmness.

Suzanne, a highly experienced critical care nurse offers some reassuring words:

> "Intensive care is a complex but rewarding area to work within. For the student nurse/newly registered nurse, I believe it offers invaluable placement experiences providing opportunities to deliver fundamental, leading to advanced, nursing skills within a controlled and well-supported environment. The team look after each other, while ensuring every student's learning needs are addressed and at all times person-centred care is very evident."

Kevin (critical care patient) describes his feelings of isolation, particularly when unable to communicate verbally and when feeling stressed, as patients undoubtedly experience. Nurses working within this environment aim to provide quality care to highly dependent and critically ill adults. They need to be prepared to apply person-centred, evidence-based approaches, recognise and respond to the needs of acute illness while balancing the physical, psychological, and emotional needs of their patients. Nursing adults within a critical care environment will also require preparing the patient and their family for appropriate step-down and discharge.

These aspects of care are all considered throughout this chapter for you to gain an insight into high dependency and critical care. This will develop your knowledge, skills and help you to feel more prepared to work in this area.

The next section will outline the aim of critical care and acknowledge some of the challenges faced.

UNDERSTANDING CRITICAL CARE

The overall aim of critical care is to treat the underlying cause of the condition and support the body's organs until recovery can be optimised. Intensive care/therapy units (ICU/ITU) and high dependency units are often termed collectively as critical care. These are areas that look after patients who need a higher level of care than a general ward can provide, when extra monitoring and specialised supportive interventions are required (Scottish Intensive Care Society Audit Group [SICSAG], 2015). Patients are admitted for constant monitoring and support to keep body systems functioning when their conditions are serious and may be life-threatening. These areas have higher levels of staffing, specialist monitoring and advanced treatments and the staff are trained in caring for the most dependent and critically ill patients.

ICU beds are a very expensive and limited resource because they provide:

- specialised monitoring equipment
- medical expertise
- constant access to highly trained nurses (usually one nurse for each bed).

CHALLENGES FACING CRITICAL CARE IN THE 21ST CENTURY

- Ageing population: multi-disease and complexities of care
- Provision in a variety of settings:
    - inpatient
    - outpatient
    - home care
    - electronic ICU – allows critical care by remote monitoring
    - reduce costs and length of stay in acute settings
    - increasing use of technology
    - reducing readmission rates

Lengths of stay vary, depending on the extent of the illness or injury. Patients may be admitted either as a planned admission following major surgery or, depending on their past medical history, may develop complications because of surgery, or as an emergency admission following extensive surgery or an episode of acute illness or major trauma.

As patients recover and need less intensive care, they are sometimes transferred to a high dependency unit (HDU) before a general ward. Intensive care teams often continue to visit patients on the ward and some units offer 'follow-up' or 'outreach' services to provide additional support following a prolonged ICU stay.

ADMISSION TO CRITICAL CARE

Intensive care is often needed when one or more organ system has failed.

There are many different conditions and situations that can cause organ systems to fail. Some of the most common include:

- trauma – road traffic collision, falls, assaults and major burns
- an acute health condition – such as acute coronary syndrome, stroke, respiratory disorders, renal disorders, hepatic and gastrointestinal disorders
- acute infections – such as sepsis or pneumonia
- major surgery
- neurological disorders – haemorrhage, altered level of consciousness
- shock.

SEE ALSO
CHAPTER 4

SEE ALSO
CHAPTER 29

PREPARATION FOR PRACTICE PLACEMENTS 16.1

If you have been allocated a clinical placement in a high dependency or critical care environment, in order to help you prepare for this, you could research and find information related to this area.

(Continued)

(Continued)

Your university may automatically provide you with information prior to attending placement, i.e. learning profiles, when to contact the area, who to contact, placement learning outcomes, the university link allocated to this area. Find out from them if there is anything else you can do to help prepare you before placement commences.

Do you know of any other nursing students who have undertaken a similar placement experience that you can chat to?

Pre-placement: consider your learning needs, expectations and what you hope to achieve. Then when you start you may find it beneficial to reflect on your experiences, perceptions and provision of care and either discuss these with another student or your mentor or write these down as part of your learning portfolio.

Working within a critical care area requires good multidisciplinary teamworking and we will now explore who is involved in caring for critically ill adults.

TEAM ROLES WITHIN CRITICAL CARE

If you have had a clinical placement in a high dependency or critical care environment, you will have noticed that good professional working relationships and a team approach are central in providing direct patient care within this challenging environment.

Many healthcare professionals are involved in working collaboratively within a multidisciplinary team to ensure each patient is cared for holistically, with all their needs being addressed. There are various healthcare professionals involved:

- **Registered nurses and student nurses**: registered nurses caring for highly dependent and critically ill adults provide direct nursing care and routinely assess, plan, implement and evaluate individualised care. Nurses promote activities of living and assist with supporting these. Nursing staff always act as advocates for their patient, particularly at this time of vulnerability. A common role within critical care is educator of staff, patients and families.
- **Student nurses** are a crucial part of the team and learn about the complexities of caring for highly dependent and critically ill adults, while being actively involved with providing care, and at all times being supported and supervised.
- **Healthcare support workers** are valued team members who provide direct patient care under supervision of registered nurses. For some, their role also involves measuring patient observations and maintaining stock, equipment and supplies.
- **Nurse consultant, nurse manager, clinical nurse specialist**: Nurse consultants are experts and provide and promote evidence-based nursing care. They are involved in audits and conducting research to enhance patient outcomes. Nurse managers ensure quality person-centred nursing care is delivered; they manage staff, resources and budgets. Clinical nurse specialists provide education and direct patient care while collaborating with colleagues within the wider team.
- **Critical care doctors: consultant anaesthetists, intensivists and junior doctors**: patients admitted to critical care areas will be cared for during their stay by a team who have critical care experience.
- **Advanced critical care practitioners**: work with nursing and medical staff in enhancing direct patient care and outcomes; they practise advanced skills and are clinical educators.

- **Outreach/follow-up nurses**: provide support and follow-up for patients recently discharged from critical care, and educate clinical staff within hospital to care for highly dependent patients.

Wider team:

- **Physiotherapists**: assess and maintain patient muscle function and mobility; are involved in assessing, planning, implementing and evaluating movements and exercises.
- **Dieticians**: monitor and assess the dietary and calorific intake; encourage individualised care plans, which can include enteral feeding.
- **Pharmacists**: review patient medications, assess drug actions and interactions, maintain stock and assess and establish patients' *parenteral* needs.
- **Radiographers**: obtain patient x-rays on the unit.
- **Microbiologist/infection control team**: advise on infection control and prevention, also contribute to patient assessment and advise on appropriate treatments.
- **Administration and clerical staff**: maintain patient records and documentation along with receptionist and secretarial roles.
- **Specialist doctors**: surgeons, physicians, cardiologists, neurologists: referred to for specialist input and expertise.
- **Specialist nurses**: pain, stoma, tissue viability.
- **Speech and language team**: assess patients' swallowing ability and ability to communicate effectively; work with patient and team to develop techniques and strategies to improve.

CARING FOR EACH OTHER

Working within a specialised area can be very challenging and demanding and, over time, can have significant personal effects. Team members can be susceptible to burn out, which can be due to:

- caring for sick patients and supporting families every day
- ethical and moral conflicts associated with prolonging life; futility of treatments; withdrawing/ withholding/limiting treatments; pressures related to distribution and appropriate use of health-care resources; staffing workload/levels.

If you have been on placement in this environment you may have noticed that nurses are very aware of looking after each other. They are adept at supporting each other, debriefing thoroughly and encouraging strategies to reduce stress, anxiety and moral distress. This engenders a true sense of belonging, team spirit and caring.

ACTIVITY 16.1: CRITICAL THINKING

The multidisciplinary team (MDT) roles within critical care are many, as outlined previously within this chapter. Alongside your practical experiences up to now, discuss with your peers and /or mentor, the learning opportunities available for you within the wider team.

To gain an insight into the importance of teamworking (from another healthcare professional's perspective) you may wish to arrange to spend some time with them.

This next section will consider the admission criteria to critical care and provide an outline of the different levels of care.

CRITERIA REQUIRED FOR ADMISSION TO CRITICAL CARE

As patients become sicker and require more support and care, they will need more nursing input and monitoring. Normally, patients needing this higher level of care and support will be admitted to either a high dependency unit or intensive care.

Patients are admitted to critical care areas for advanced support and monitoring and during active treatment of an underlying clinical condition. The clinical condition that has resulted in the patient needing critical care should be identifiable, acute and potentially reversible. Admission for critical care is only appropriate if the patient can be reasonably expected to survive and receive sustained benefit in quality of life. An increasing requirement for organ support is not in itself a reason to admit a patient who is suffering their final illness, and who has no apparent expectation of recovery. If a patient has an advanced directive and stated or written a preference for or against intensive care, this must be taken into account.

DECISION TO ADMIT

Every patient's condition varies and, therefore, different interventions and support strategies are required. Patients may be at risk of clinical deterioration at any time due to damage to body systems, organs and cells, particularly when deterioration is left undetected and untreated.

Patients are admitted to a critical care area for a variety of reasons, planned or unplanned. Frequently, the ITU team will review the patient pre-admission taking cognisance of the overall benefits or limitations of admission to critical care, as it will not be in the best interests of all patients to be admitted. If patient transfer is to occur, then this should happen as soon as possible and families contacted and advised promptly.

There has been a change in the classification of high dependency and intensive care, which now focuses on the level of specific care required for patient needs.

LEVELS OF CARE DEPENDENCY

To be able to deliver safe, person-centred care to the highly dependent and critically ill adult it is essential that you understand the levels of care definitions, what level of acute care is required and the potential for the patient's clinical deterioration. Levels of care are numerically rated from 0 to 3. These levels are used to ensure accurate risk assessment, appropriate decision making and justification of the staffing skill mix in caring for the patient in the clinical environment (National Institute for Health and Care Excellence [NICE], 2007).

The level of care (see Table 16.1) is calculated daily from the scores based on support of five organ systems: respiratory, cardiovascular, renal, neurological and dermatological (Intensive Care Society, 2009).

Table 16.1 provides an explanation of the different levels and how they are determined.

Level 3	Level 2	Level 1	Level 0
Advanced respiratory support (connected to a ventilator via endotracheal tube or tracheostomy) OR Two or more organ systems are being supported (except basic respiratory and basic cardiac)	One organ supported	Epidural or/and general observations requiring more monitoring than can be provided on a general ward	A patient is assessed as level 0 if not assessed as level 1, 2 or 3 (e.g. no organ support and adequate monitoring could be provided on a general ward)

HOW TO PROVIDE PERSON-CENTRED, SAFE AND HOLISTIC CRITICAL NURSING CARE FOR PATIENTS AND THEIR FAMILIES

The main principle of the NHS is to provide high-quality care to all individuals, free at the point of need. High-quality care includes care that is safe, effective and results in as positive an experience possible for patients (Health Education England [HEE], 2013). Patient safety is an essential part of nursing care that aims to prevent avoidable errors and patient harm. Patient safety is a feature of a healthcare system and a set of tested ways for improving care. Staff can apply safety improvement methods to make systems of care more reliable (Royal College of Nursing [RCN], 2017). The RCN and Nursing and Midwifery Council's *Code* (2015) promote patient safety.

Working within healthcare there are many factors related to patient safety. One is termed 'human factors' – considering how people interact with each other and technology (Healthcare Improvement Scotland, 2012). 'Enhancing clinical performance through an understanding of the effects of teamwork, tasks, equipment, workspace, culture and organisation on human behaviour and abilities and application of that knowledge in a clinical setting' (Catchpole, 2010 as cited in Department of Health, 2012).

However, delivering healthcare can place individuals, teams and organisations under pressure. Staff must make difficult decisions in dynamic, often unpredictable circumstances. Decision making can be compromised, in such challenging situations, impacting on the quality of care and clinical outcomes, and potentially causing harm to the patient; poor performance also increases costs (HEE, 2013).

Therefore, to ensure safe, person-centred nursing care is provided, it is important to consider patient needs, while recognising and preventing clinical deterioration and delivering a holistic approach to nursing care. There are many other elements to be aware of: teamworking (already discussed), attitudes and good communication, which will be discussed next.

Good communication is important and we will consider the communication skills needed in this environment in more detail shortly. An effective communication system that is easy to understand and follows a standard approach is vital when communicating with colleagues, particularly when concerned about a patient's clinical deterioration. Patient safety is paramount and the focus should be on preventing adverse patient events by early recognition of deterioration and ensuring that this is communicated to relevant team members so minimising risk. Early recognition and treatment of the deteriorating patient can reduce the likelihood of adverse events and minimise the level of care required (Australian Commission on Safety and Quality in Health Care, 2010).

COMMUNICATION AND INTERPERSONAL SKILLS

The importance of effective communication and interpersonal skills for a nurse cannot be underestimated. These skills are particularly important in ICU as, during times of crisis, communication can often be misperceived.

Consider again Cheryl's quote at the beginning of this chapter. Cheryl felt that her experiences within a critical care environment helped to hone her interpersonal and communication skills, perhaps because having the ability to communicate well within this environment is so vitally important, if you are to provide safe and effective, person-centred care.

For nurses and healthcare professionals working within critical care this is one of the fundamental challenges to overcome. We are all different and react in various ways as a response to perceived stressors. The admission of a relative to critical care is an example of an intensely stressful situation, and you may witness reactions such as perceived anger, guilt or hysteria. It is part of the role of a nurse to find strategies to cope with these reactions.

ACTIVITY 16.2
ANSWER

ACTIVITY 16.2: REFLECTIVE PRACTICE

Consider a patient interaction that you have had where communication was perceived to be difficult. Why was this the case?

What could have made this more effective for you and the patient?

It is part of your role as a student nurse to ensure that your communication skills are effective and to develop the fundamental skills and strategies to enable positive patient and family interaction and satisfaction, patient safety and multidisciplinary team working. While caring for highly dependent and critically ill adults, observing non-verbal communication is vital as often patients are unable to communicate verbally, so reading non-verbal cues such as feelings, anxieties and pain is essential.

ACTIVITY 16.3
ANSWER

ACTIVITY 16.3: REFLECTIVE PRACTICE

•   Can you reflect upon a patient interaction when using your non-verbal cues was particularly useful?
•   What were the challenges involved and how did you overcome these?

Poor communication is one of the most common causes for dissatisfaction with health services. Communication issues can happen anywhere within the healthcare system. Transitions between care settings are particularly vulnerable. A key principle, therefore, is to reduce communication break-downs by making them more visible. Staff can then address omissions or misunderstandings before any harm comes to the patient (RCN, 2017).

Using your communication skills effectively is as important as your provision of physical care, support and technical skills. Caring for highly dependent and critically ill adults and their families, you will need to be aware, not only of the frightening experience for the patient of being critically ill and requiring specialist support, but also of the number and range of healthcare professionals involved in patient and family communications. These factors could affect how communication is interpreted, so it is important to address communication inconsistencies, ensuring that all communication is understood and the message received is clear.

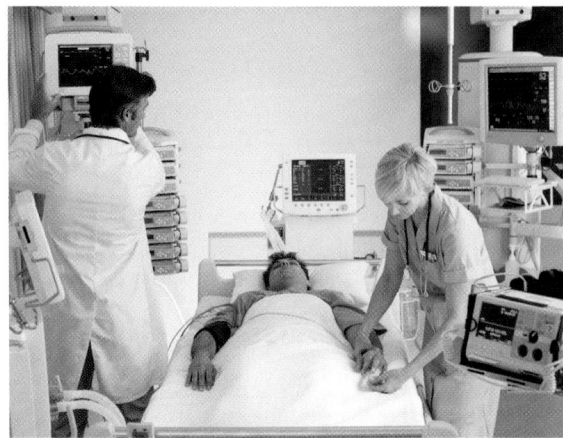

Figure 16.1
Source: iStock images

Every patient and their family is unique; no amount of tubes, wires, drugs and noisy monitoring equipment can ever conceal that the patient who is being cared for is an individual, with their own needs. Nurses learn the 'softer' skills of effective communication through experience and reflection; when caring for highly dependent and critically ill adults there must be an even balance between delivering technical and softer skills.

ACTIVITY 16.4: CRITICAL THINKING

ACTIVITY 16.4
ANSWER

- Have you had the opportunity to consider the high dependency/critical care environment from the patient's and family perspective?
- How could you make this transition easier for the patient and their family? What communication strategies and standards would you expect?

Please review the link below for further consideration of this: www.healthtalk.org/peoples-experiences/intensive-care/intensive-care-patients-experiences

Values-based, person-centred care is fundamental when delivering nursing care. The *Code* (NMC, 2015) states the importance of ensuring that these values are always part of our everyday nursing care. Person-centred care evolved from Tom Kitwood's work: he suggested that every person should be respected and valued and is a unique individual, and care should be delivered according to their values and beliefs. This approach is founded on individuality, respect, personal values and worth. Delivering person-centred care ensures that individual needs and wishes are being addressed, while providing dignity and compassion.

When caring for highly dependent and critically ill adults, person-centred care could potentially be influenced by several factors: use of complex technology and continual monitoring, along with disruption to normal physical, psychological, emotional and spiritual function.

ACTIVITY 16.5: REFLECTIVE PRACTICE

Can you identify barriers to the delivery of person-centred care to highly dependent and critically ill adults?

Now suggest strategies to overcome these.

This link is a film clip of an introduction to the environment of intensive care, and may help you to answer the above: https://vimeo.com/179850018

This article may help you to explore person-centredness:

Timmins, F. and Astin, F. (2009) Patient centred care: reality or rhetoric? *Nursing in Critical Care,* 14(5): 219–21.

We will now consider the physical, psychological, emotional and spiritual care needs of the individual requiring care and their families.

CONSIDERATION OF THE PHYSICAL, PSYCHOLOGICAL, EMOTIONAL AND SPIRITUAL ELEMENTS OF CARE

Physical needs

Nursing a highly dependent and critically ill adult requires delivery of individualised fundamental nursing care alongside more advanced technological support.

CONSIDERING THE PERSONAL CARE NEEDS OF THE PATIENT

- Maintaining good personal hygiene: cleanliness, prevention of infection, hair care, nail care
- Maintaining good oral hygiene, as patients may be nil by mouth/intubated: lip care, care of teeth/gums/tongue, prevention of infection and complications
- Preventing harm by maintaining skin integrity: assessment of skin, SSKIN bundle (Healthcare Improvement Scotland, 2011), frequent change of patient position, need for pressure redistributing and relieving equipment
- Maintaining good eye care: 'dry eye'/loss of blink reflex/impaired production of tears, care of aids: contact lenses, glasses
- Promotion of passive and active limb movements and exercises: limited mobility, loss of muscle tone and weakness, use of aids to encourage mobility, rehabilitation plans
- Nutrition and bowel care: nutritional needs must be assessed. ICU patients are often prone to bowel dysfunction, this therefore needs to be assessed and reviewed regularly.

Psychological needs

The importance of psychological and social support for patients and families in critical care cannot be underestimated. Providing person-centred care involves caring for the psychological needs of the individual and their family.

Within a critical care area sensory overload can be a major stressor for patients, and modifications should be made to reduce these as appropriate:

- Light – use of natural lighting, clear differentiation between day and night
- Noise – design of rooms/bed areas, background music, private areas away from the patient to facilitate discussions, designated time for rest periods
- Privacy – many healthcare professionals are involved in patient care and this can feel very intrusive for patients: facilitate a reduction in this where possible.

Delirium can often manifest in critically ill patients due to treatment interventions, which may include medications, sepsis and sleep deprivation, and as a result the patient may experience hallucinations and delusions. These may last for a few months post discharge and, of course, are extremely upsetting for the patient and family. **Post intensive care syndrome** is a recognised phenomenon and you will need to be aware of this when working in this environment; night-time is often the worst as the patient may experience flashbacks and be fearful of going to sleep. Talking about this can be helpful and, often while in hospital, the outreach/follow-up care team can help rationalise these experiences and help the patient to understand. A patient diary may further help the patient to reflect and accept that the hallucinations and delusions are imaginary. Sometimes, referral to a counsellor or psychologist may be required.

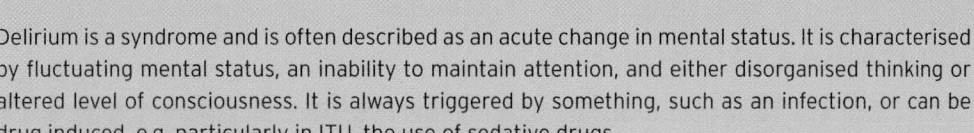

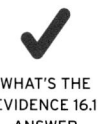

WHAT'S THE
EVIDENCE 16.1
ANSWER

Delirium in ITU

Delirium is a syndrome and is often described as an acute change in mental status. It is characterised by fluctuating mental status, an inability to maintain attention, and either disorganised thinking or altered level of consciousness. It is always triggered by something, such as an infection, or can be drug induced, e.g. particularly in ITU, the use of sedative drugs.

The incidence of delirium in the United Kingdom in ventilated critically ill patients is 55% to 69%; internationally the incidence varies from 20% to 50%.

What do you think may be some predisposing and risk factors that might trigger an episode of delirium and why?

Please access the website below and consider further ITU patients who develop a delirium and how you can support them.

www.icudelirium.co.uk

'Nursing a patient suffering from ICU-induced delirium can be challenging. Delirious patients are often in an acute confusional state, making it difficult to assess, reassure, orientate and care for them effectively. It is important that there is a regular assessment for delirium using an appropriate tool such as CAM-ICU. This will confirm the presence of hyper/hypoactive or mixed delirium. Pharmaceutical drugs are often used to help patients with hyperactive delirium to maintain their safety. However, early mobilisation, promoting good sleep, hygiene and minimising sensory stimulation are all key nursing interventions which have proven to reduce delirium. Watching a loved one in a state of delirium can be traumatic for families and friends. Therefore, an important aspect of the nursing role is to support families through this difficult time by explaining and reassuring them of the transitional nature of delirium.'

Audrey, senior charge nurse: adult critical care unit

It may be helpful to prepare the patient and family to expect psychological changes such as mood swings, changes in libido and relationships, depression and anxiety. While not all patients will experience these, for some it will be part of their journey to recovery and it is important that these factors are recognised, discussed and treated.

Emotional needs

Fear of the unknown and lack of understanding, for the patient and family, are two factors that must be addressed. Caring for emotional needs is just as important as caring for physical needs, and although providing practical nursing skills demands a lot of nurses' time, it is essential that interpersonal care must be prioritised. For nurses, the role of skilled communicator is vital in ensuring that the patient's and family's needs are addressed to ensure that information is relayed and understood. Being open and honest about progress, likely developments and making sure that all are involved in decision making is crucial to ensure lines of communication remain open.

The patient's stay in critical care has a significant effect on the family as a whole and you should encourage the family to discuss their experiences.

For the family who have endured the patient's journey it is common for them to experience:

- fear and anxiety
- uncertainty
- loss of control
- loss of family connection as a whole unit.

The family unit may be affected financially, due to inability to work, and lack of income may be a further stressor. The changes in relationship can be a major burden and may impede communication between patient and their family as they try to come to terms with all that has happened. This is an extremely difficult time for the family and support and guidance should be provided.

Family needs can include:

- reassurance
- support
- information which is honest and truthful
- to be near relatives
- to be comfortable

Care at the end of life must depend on the individual circumstances, with the focus on the comfort of the patient, then the needs of the family. The family will be involved in discussions and will be advised of what is going to happen, what to expect and often at this time will remain the patient's advocate. Nursing staff will provide continuous support and explanation but will also ensure that the family have privacy and time to themselves with their loved one.

Spiritual needs

Caring for the patient holistically involves looking after their spiritual needs and those of their family. Considering the values, beliefs, religious needs, traditions and culture of the individual should remain paramount to nursing staff when providing care. However, these needs can remain unfulfilled due to prioritising demands on urgency of treatment and providing practical nursing care. Taking the time to discuss spiritual needs and listening to what the patient's and family's wishes are will ensure their needs are met: reassurance, use of touch sensitively and involvement of family can help to demonstrate care and compassion.

For some individuals, their emotional and spiritual needs intensify when faced with a stay in ICU. Often there can be more outward signs of devotion displayed during times of serious illness. Spiritual needs are not only to be considered at end of life but these needs should be addressed throughout the patient's stay and appropriate support provided. Spiritual advisors can be a huge support and their presence may aid the patient and family at times of stress, distress, acute illness and end of life. The family may automatically contact their spiritual advisor if they have existing strong spiritual beliefs; however, nurses should always check the appropriateness to contact someone on their behalf.

It is important that any signs of clinical deterioration are immediately noted and interventions applied. We move on now to outline why and to discuss some general care management.

NURSING ASSESSMENT OF THE HIGHLY DEPENDENT AND CRITICALLY ILL ADULT

Nursing assessment and response to changes in the patient's condition

Generally, the signs of clinical deterioration are similar irrespective of the underlying condition. Normally, signs include changes related to respiratory, cardiovascular and neurological systems (Truhlar et al., 2015).

Early warning scoring systems are routinely used within acute hospital settings to identify patients at risk of deterioration and although there are currently many variations utilised within the UK, these are all fundamentally similar (NICE, 2007). One of the recommendations from the Department of Health (2000) suggested a tool be utilised in order to track and trigger physiological scores resulting from signs of patient deterioration.

A major part of the role of the nurse is the ability to: recognise, assess, communicate and effectively manage the sick and deteriorating patient, while working collaboratively within a team. To be able to know and understand when a patient is acutely unwell and then act accordingly are key skills required by all nurses but particularly those working in areas of acuity. Nurses need to learn to provide safe, effective patient assessment and respond to dynamic clinical changes appropriately. To work in this area, you will need to be equipped with the skills necessary to measure physiological parameters, make decisions using your clinical experience and judgement and, as we have already seen, communicate successfully to safeguard the continuity of person-centred care (Coulter Smith et al., 2014).

In order to detect and efficiently manage signs of patient deterioration, nurses must be competent in the use of a systematic, holistic approach to providing care. You will no doubt be familiar with the 'ABCDE' approach to assessment, which is widely utilised within clinical settings. It is recognised as a simple, systematic algorithm that focuses on patient safety and assessment (Resuscitation Council UK, 2015). When this algorithm is applied, and used in combination with additional patient data – vital signs, fluid and electrolyte balance, blood glucose and other relevant investigations – then definitive evidence of patient deterioration will become apparent and if necessary enables escalation to the next stage in care.

CARE MANAGEMENT OF THE HIGHLY DEPENDENT AND CRITICALLY ILL ADULT

General care management

Caring for patients who require intensive care requires complex and multifaceted nursing skills. Nurses provide round-the-clock care and monitoring, and there is a high ratio of nurses to patients – each person in ICU is usually assigned his or her own 'named' nurse; within HDU this is normally 1 nurse to 2 patients. This provides special expertise and the facilities for the support of vital functions and uses the skills of medical, nursing and other personnel experienced in the management of these problems.

Most units have facilities for treating severe, life-threatening illness. These commonly deal with respiratory failure, heart and circulatory failure, kidney failure, severe septicaemia (blood poisoning), and many others. Most units will transfer critically ill patients to specialist centres, for example, for head injuries, severe burns and for severe heart problems.

ICU nurses play a vital role in the patient's care, including the following:

- taking regular blood tests
- changing the patient's treatment in line with test results
- giving the patient the drugs and fluids that the doctors have prescribed
- recording the patient's blood pressure, heart rate and oxygen levels
- clearing fluid and mucus from the patient's chest using a suction tube
- turning the patient in his or her bed every few hours to prevent sores on the skin
- oral care: cleaning the patient's teeth and moistening the mouth
- personal care: washing the patient in bed
- changing the sheets
- eye care: putting drops in the patient's eyes to make it easier to blink.

GO FURTHER

**WEBLINK:
ICU**

You may find this a useful resource for further information: people talk about the nursing care they received while in ICU. www.healthtalk.org/peoples-experiences/intensive-care/intensive-care-patients-experiences/nursing-careicu#ixzz4ZnuMOWAI

Please review further information contained in the online resources at https://study.sagepub.com/essentialadultnursing website for more information related to respiratory, cardiovascular, neurological and renal conditions.

CASE STUDY 16.1: DAVID

David is a 40-year-old farm worker. He is single, lives alone and despite having some disability support needs he normally manages to work. His mother who is his next of kin lives several hours away. He arrived in A&E with an acute exacerbation of asthma and was only able to converse in short sentences and therefore unable to provide a full history. He has had a cough with productive sputum for the last week and has never been admitted to hospital previously. Acutely breathless, with a respiratory rate of 40 and oxygen saturation of 90%, with deteriorating arterial blood gases, it was quickly determined that he required intubation and ventilation. This required sedative drugs and no further information could be ascertained from the patient.

- How would you suggest collecting the necessary information to combine his care from the community and acute care?
- Describe supportive measures for the respiratory system and any interventions for acute asthma which may be required.

WHAT'S THE EVIDENCE? 16.2

Safeguarding adults

David has some disability support needs and as such the A&E staff may not be able to elicit a full history from him. He will naturally be anxious and scared. The staff may have concerns regarding safeguarding.

**SEE ALSO
CHAPTER 4**

Please refer to the NMC (2015) link for further information:
www.nmc.org.uk/standards/safeguarding

Cardiovascular Care
Please review further information contained within the online resources https://study.sagepub.com/essentialadultnursing

**SEE ALSO
CHAPTER 27**

Neurological Care
Please review further information contained within the online resources https://study.sagepub.com/essentialadultnursing

ACTIVITY 16.6: RESEARCH AND EVIDENCE-BASED PRACTICE

ACTIVITY 16.6
ANSWER

The following web link provides information on how to perform a GCS assessment. www.glasgowco mascale.org/whats-new

This is a good reminder of how to use GCS accurately to assess the neurological status of your patients.

CASE STUDY 16.2: KEN

Ken is an 18-year-old male. He recently attended A&E with altered consciousness. His friends have indicated that he may have drunk vodka and taken some 'E's'. While admitting Ken you realise that he seems confused, disorientated and is shouting. He suddenly deteriorates and no longer seems able to maintain his own airway. He is quickly intubated and ventilated. An urgent CT scan is performed and no abnormalities are detected.

His friends on further questioning reveal this is unusual behaviour for Ken. Normally he is fit and well, with no past medical history and does not abuse alcohol or drugs.

- How would you assess and manage the care of a patient with altered conscious level?
- What information would you provide his family?

RENAL CARE

Please review further information contained within the online resources https://study.sagepub.com/essentialadultnursing

---

CASE STUDY 16.3: MARGARET

Margaret is a 51-year-old woman, who lives with her two teenage children, Donna and Millie. Margaret recently separated from her husband and is finding it stressful working full time and looking after two teenage daughters. She is currently employed as a shop assistant. For the last week, Margaret has developed flu-like symptoms with a productive cough, and her two daughters phoned the GP when their mother was unable to get to the bathroom without help. Millie states that although unwell, her mum had been to work yesterday.

In A&E it is found Margaret has a respiratory rate of 31, her oxygen saturation is 88% and her chest x-ray shows pneumonia. The doctor explains to Donna and Millie that he is concerned that Margaret has respiratory sepsis and requires transfer to a critical care area for respiratory support and close monitoring.

(Continued)

(Continued)

- What further close monitoring may Margaret require?
- Describe supportive measures for the respiratory system and any interventions that may be required.

Later that day, Margaret's urine volumes are less than 10mls an hour and her kidney function is deteriorating. It is explained to her daughters that Margaret may be developing severe sepsis and may require renal support.

- What information would you give Margaret's daughters regarding sepsis and how this can affect other organs?

Click on the weblink below to find out more about SIGN 139 (Scottish Intercollegiate Guidelines Network) 'Care of deteriorating patients'.
www.sign.ac.uk

Following patient improvement from critical illness, continued care within an appropriate care area must be discussed, with recognition of individual needs, as stated below by Belinda in her quote (a critical care patient in 2010). This will now be explored.

THE TRANSITION OF DISCHARGE AND STEP-DOWN FROM CRITICAL CARE

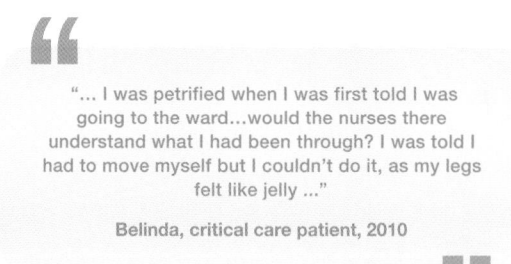

"... I was petrified when I was first told I was going to the ward...would the nurses there understand what I had been through? I was told I had to move myself but I couldn't do it, as my legs felt like jelly ..."

Belinda, critical care patient, 2010

TIMELY DISCHARGE AND APPROPRIATE STEP-DOWN FROM CRITICAL CARE

When a patient has been deemed as no longer requiring high dependency or critical care nursing and discharge is anticipated, this should be discussed with the patient and family promptly to help prepare and ease expectations of transition. The dependency level of the patient is considered along with their physiological data, results and physical capabilities. A detailed discussion should outline the differences in care provision: change in nurse-to-patient ratio, reduced level of monitoring and shared rooms. The patient will be encouraged to participate more in their own care and become less dependent in the days preceding transfer. Nurses need to consider individual patients' needs in response to updates about their condition and potential transfer or step-down from high dependency or critical care. For patients recovering from acute illness, rehabilitation should take account of their physical, psychological and emotional needs.

Normally, patients will have had a short clinical assessment carried out to ascertain their physical and non-physical risks; following this their rehabilitation needs will be considered and goals planned to achieve these. It is important that the patient (and their family if agreed) are involved in decision making and setting realistic rehabilitation goals to facilitate their recovery.

PREPARING PATIENT AND FAMILY FOR DISCHARGE AND STEP-DOWN

Many patients and families will require a lot of reassurance and support prior to step-down. Naturally, they will feel anxious about leaving the environment, the reduced level of nursing care, unfamiliar ward environment and generally getting better (NICE, 2009). Patients can feel particularly vulnerable and very wary about relocation to a general ward; they may have had a prolonged stay within a high dependency or critical care setting and will feel safe there. Nursing staff should promote the patient's step-down as a positive step in progression and recovery, while recognising that this may be an anxious time (as Belinda's quote suggests, at the start of this chapter).

CRITICAL THINKING STOP POINT 16.1

How might nurses reassure and support patients and their families during this anxious period?

To enhance recovery and aid a smooth transition from critical care to ward, discussions must be open and honest about the likely effects that will be encountered, with reassurance given that contact will remain between ward and critical care staff. It is difficult to predict individual patient experiences post-ICU but it is likely that most will encounter some psychological and physical challenges. Often it can take some time before a patient will return to the quality of life they had before their acute illness.

A structured clinical handover and treatment plan will be provided to the ward nursing and medical staff to ensure continuity of care. Ward staff will be advised of the patient's needs, abilities and limitations and will understand their recovery may be gradual. Patients and families should be reassured that it is natural to feel anxious about step-down but be encouraged that these feelings will lessen as the patient's condition continues to improve.

Recovery from critical illness can be straightforward and for many patients and their families this occurs without significant impact. However, recovery is individual and for some there can be many longer-term physical and psychological effects following an episode of critical illness (NICE, 2009).

Additional information identifying some of the potential effects is provided within the online resources at https://study.sagepub.com/essentialadultnursing

OUTREACH: IMPORTANCE OF SUPPORTING PATIENT, FAMILY AND STAFF

The aim of continuing to care for patients following discharge from critical care is to ensure that the patient, family and staff are managing this transition. This can be a challenging time as often the patient feels more vulnerable and, along with re-learning how to do some things physically, there will be a reduced level of nursing input, a different environment and team and routine to become familiar with. There will also be the challenges of managing their emotional, psychological, social and spiritual needs.

After discharge from the critical care area some patients may be followed up on a regular basis, by the critical care follow-up/outreach service to address any ongoing physical, nutritional, psychological and emotional needs.

Staff working with patients who have been transferred from critical care areas on general wards should be provided with education and training to recognise and understand their holistic needs. This should be the remit of the critical care follow-up/outreach team, combined with reducing the potential risks of patient readmission.

"Many patients post-ICU face complex and protracted recoveries. As yet there is no formal rehabilitation (rehab) programme to help these patients recover to their functional best. As a nurse who has worked with over 250 patients post-ICU I still find this deficit in rehab very frustrating. During my secondment as a critical care liaison nurse, I was able to provide support, advice and reassurance to patients and their families as they tried to negotiate the aftermath of critical illness. This proved to be extremely beneficial for patients and their loved ones – and to some extent I felt like I was providing them with a life line."

Audrey, senior charge nurse

ACTIVITY 16.7 ANSWER

ACTIVITY 16.7: CRITICAL THINKING

Now consider some of these potential longer-term effects following a lengthier stay within critical care.

Can you recognise the impact that these may have on the patient and their family and wider social circle?

PATIENT DIARIES

Diaries written during the period of a patient's stay within critical care have been used in many European countries since the 1990s in order to support patients and their families to understand and contextualise the ICU experience (Nydahl et al., 2014). Often, patients who are ventilated and sedated during critical illness do not remember, nor appreciate what happened to them throughout this time. Patient diaries are a valuable means of helping elicit understanding, by recording a second-person account of experiences, thoughts, progress and information. Normally, the diary is considered a positive method to help patients grasp the impact of their critical illness experience (Storli et al., 2008 as cited in Mallet et al., 2013).

"As nurses we have been very much aware of the mechanics of critical care and the importance of caring for patients and their relatives throughout their stay. It is only in recent years I have gained an understanding and more awareness of the patient's experience of critical care and the long-term effects for the patient. Supporting, encouraging and involving patients' relatives with patient diaries and post-critical care information, is instrumental in improving this experience for patients. We are becoming much more aware of the impact we have in our actions and how we can change, inform and educate staff and relatives to assist patients in their recovery post-critical care."

Janice, senior charge nurse

DISCHARGE PLANNING

Effective discharge planning from hospital to home is fundamental in ensuring that the patient's needs will be met and any ongoing care can be planned and continued seamlessly. Patients discharged home following an episode of acute illness, particularly high dependency or critical care, may be more likely to require additional support such as continuing rehabilitation – home adaptations and aids to help mobility, provision of home care and perhaps financial support (if the patient is unable to return to employment immediately). Effectively preparing for these factors will ensure that health and social care systems can work collaboratively to support individuals and their families.

Discharge planning is crucial and nurses are key team players in communicating effectively, applying local and national policies and guidance, and ensuring the provision of healthcare services addresses the needs of the patient and their family.

HEALTH PROMOTION

All nurses and healthcare providers must be cognisant of their role in promoting good health with patients and their families.

When caring for adults who have required high dependency and critical care, it may be appropriate to provide health promotion as part of their recovery plan. Suggestions and encouragement related to positive lifestyle changes include: nutrition, fluid intake, importance of physical activity and exercise, cessation of smoking, reduction in alcohol consumption, sleep and rest, employment and support groups. It is essential that advice is individualised to reflect person-centred care.

WHAT'S THE EVIDENCE? 16.3

Investigating risk factors for psychological morbidity three months after intensive care: a prospective cohort study.

Wade, D.M., Howell, D.C., Weinman, J.A., Hardy, R.J., Mythen, M.G., Brewin, C.R., Borja-Bolunda, S., Matejowsky, C.F. and Raine, R.A. (2012) *Critical Care*, 16: R192 BioMed Central

(Continued)

(Continued)

Wade et al. (2012) suggest that despite the growing numbers of post-ICU patients developing mental health issues, there are identifiable risk factors that could be reduced to prevent this increasing incidence.

Read this article and consider whether you agree with the authors.

What are the modifiable risk factors that could be influenced to make a positive outcome to post-ICU patients?

CHAPTER SUMMARY

- Caring for highly dependent and critically ill adults can be challenging and requires the underlying knowledge and understanding of the development of critical care, levels of care dependency, criteria for admission and team roles.
- Nurses must be familiar with care management of highly dependent and critically ill adults including major systems support and interventions required.
- Nurses have a key role to play in providing person-centred, safe and holistic nursing care.
- Planning for timely and appropriate transfers, step-down and discharges is vital to ensure a smooth and effective transition.

GO FURTHER

CASE STUDY: CRITICAL CARE

Go to https://study.sagepub.com/essentialadultnursing for a further case study related to this chapter. If you are using the interactive ebook, simply click on the book icon in the margin to go straight to the resource.

Books

- Delves-Yates, C. (ed.) (2018) *Essentials of Nursing Practice* (2nd edn.). London: SAGE.
  This book is a good resource to review nursing practice, the importance of communication and inter-personal skills and delivering effective care.
- Jevon, P. and Ewens, B. (2012) *Monitoring the Critically Ill Patient* (3rd ed.). Oxford: Wiley-Blackwell.
  This is a good starting point to enhance clinical knowledge and review many relevant aspects related to caring for a critically ill adult.
- Tait, D., James, J., Williams, C. and Barton, D. (2012) *Acute and Critical Care in Adult Nursing* (2nd ed.). London: SAGE.
  This book provides an overview of caring for acutely and critically ill adults.

Journal Articles

FURTHER READING: JOURNAL ARTICLES

Go to https://study.sagepub.com/essentialadultnursing for further free online journal articles related to this chapter. If you are using the interactive ebook, simply click on the book icon in the margin to go straight to the resource.

- Coulter Smith, M.A., Smith, P. and Crow, R. (2014) A critical review: A combined conceptual framework of severity of illness and clinical judgement for analysing diagnostic judgements in critical illness. *Journal of Clinical Nursing*, 23(5-6): 784-98.
  This review highlights some of the nursing skills required to care for critically ill patients.
- Teasdale, G. (2014) Forty years on: Updating the Glasgow Coma Scale. *Nursing Times*, 110(42): 12-16.
  A worthwhile resource to review assessment of individuals with an altered conscious level.
- The Intensive Care Society (2009) *Levels of Critical Care for Adult Patients* [Online] Available at: www.ics.ac.uk/EasySiteWeb/GatewayLink.aspx?alId=1159.
  This website is useful to find out more information related to defining levels of care for critically ill adults.

Weblinks

FURTHER READING: WEBLINKS

Go to https://study.sagepub.com/essentialadultnursing for further weblinks related to this chapter. If you are using the interactive ebook, simply click on the book icon in the margin to go straight to the resource.

- ICUsteps is a useful example of a charity support established by former intensive care patients, families and healthcare professionals to promote better support and rehabilitation following a critical illness. You may find this useful to browse: www.icusteps.org
- Resuscitation Council (UK) (2015) *Guidelines and Guidance: A Systematic Approach to the Acutely Ill patient (ABCDE Approach)*. [Online] Available at: www.resus.org.uk/resuscitation-guidelines/a-systematic-approach-to-the-acutely-ill-patient-abcde
  An important website to refresh the latest resuscitation guidelines and review the ABCDE systematic approach.
- Scottish Intensive Care Society (2015) *Audit of Critical Care in Scotland 2015, Reporting on 2014.* [Online] Available at: www.scottishintensivecaresociety.org.uk
  This is an interesting link to find out more about the Scottish Intensive Care Society.

ACE YOUR ASSESSMENT

ONLINE QUIZZES

Revise what you have learned by visiting https://study.sagepub.com/essentialadultnursing

- Test yourself with multiple-choice and short-answer questions
- Do the chapter activities in the book and check your answers online

REFERENCES

Australian Commission on Safety and Quality in Health Care (2010) *National Consensus Statement: Essential elements for recognising and responding to clinical deterioration.* Commonwealth of Australia: ACSQHC.

Coulter Smith, M.A., Smith, P. and Crow, R. (2014) A critical review: A combined conceptual framework of severity of illness and clinical judgement for analysing diagnostic judgements in critical illness. *Journal of Clinical Nursing*, 23(5–6): 784–98.

Department of Health (2000) *Comprehensive Critical Care: A review of adult critical care services.* London: The Stationery Office.

Department of Health (2012) *Human factors in Healthcare. NHS England. Clinical Human Factors Reference Group Interim Report.* Available at: www.england.nhs.uk/wp-content/uploads/2013/11/nqb-hum-fact-concord.pdf (accessed 12 June 2018).

Fazio, S., Pace, D., Flinner, J and Kallmyer, B. (2018) The Fundamentals of Person-Centered Care for Individuals with Dementia. *The Gerontologist*, 58(1). Available from : https://doi.org/10.1093/geront/gnx122

Healthcare Improvement Scotland (2011) *SSKIN Care Bundle*. Available at: www.healthcareimprovementscotland.org (accessed 12 June 2018).

Healthcare Improvement Scotland (2012) *Acute Adult Patient Safety Programme*. Available at: www.scottishpatientsafetyprogramme.scot.nhs.uk (accessed 12 June 2018).

Health Education England (2013) *Raising the Bar Shape of Caring: A Review of the Future Education and Training of Registered Nurses and Care Assistants*. Available at: www.hee.nhs.uk/our-work/shape-caring-review (accessed 12 June 2018).

Jevon, P., Ewens, B. and Pooni, J.S. (2012) *Monitoring the Critically Ill Patient* (3rd ed.). Oxford: Wiley-Blackwell Publishing.

Mallet, J., Albarran, J.W. and Richardson, A. (2013) *Critical Care Manual of Clinical Procedures and Competencies*. Oxford: Wiley-Blackwell Publishing.

National Institute for Health and Care Excellence [NICE] (2007) *Acutely Ill Adults in Hospital: Recognising and responding to deterioration. NICE Clinical Guideline 50*. London: NICE.

National Institute for Health and Care Excellence [NICE] (2009) *Rehabilitation after Critical Illness. NICE Clinical Guideline 83*. Manchester: NICE.

National Institute for Health and Care Excellence [NICE] (2014) *Head Injury: Triage, Assessment, Investigation and Early Management of Head Injury in Infants, Children, Young People and Adults*. London: NICE.

Nursing and Midwifery Council (2015) *The Code: Professional standards of practice and behaviour for nurses and midwives*. Available at: www.nmc.org.uk/standards/code/ (accessed 12 June 2018).

Nydahl, P., Knueck, D. and Egerod, I. (2014) Extent and application of ICU diaries in Germany in 2014. *British Association of Critical Care Nurses*, 20 (3): 155–62.

Resuscitation Council UK (2015) *Advanced Life Support*. London: Resuscitation Council (UK).

Royal College of Nursing (RCN) (2017) *Patient safety and human factors*. Available at: www.rcn.org.uk/clinical-topics/patient-safety-and-human-factors (accessed 12 June 2018).

Royal College of Physicians (2008) *The Use of Non-invasive Ventilation in the Management of Patients with Chronic Obstructive Pulmonary Disease Admitted to Hospital with Acute Type II Respiratory Failure*. London: RCP.

Scottish Intensive Care Society Audit Group (2015) *Quality Improvement Group. Minimum Standards and Quality Indicators for Critical Care in Scotland; Version 3.0*. Available at: www.sicsag.scot.nhs.uk/Quality/Quality_Indicators_2015.pdf

Scottish Intercollegiate Guidelines Network (2014) *SIGN 139: Care of Deteriorating Patients*. Available at: http://www.sign.ac.uk/assets/sign139.pdf (accessed 12 June 2018).

The Intensive Care Society (2009) *Levels of Critical Care for Adult Patients*. [Online] Available at: www.ics.ac.uk/EasySiteWeb/GatewayLink.aspx?alId=1159 (accessed 12 June 2018).

Truhlar, A., Deakin, C., Soar, J., Khalifa, G.E.A., Alfonzo, A., Bierens, J.J.L.M., Brattebo, G., Brugger, H., Dunning, J., Hunyadi-Anticevic, S., Koster, R.W., Lockey, D.J., Lott, C., Paal, P., Perkins, G.D., Sandroni, C., Thies, K.C., Zideman, D.A., Nolan, J.P. (2015) European Resuscitation Council Guidelines for Resuscitation 2005: Section 4. Adult Advanced Life Support. Resuscitation.10.10.16/j.resuscitation.2015.07017 pp.148–201

CARE OF THE FRAIL OLDER ADULT

17

MARGARET BROWN AND TRUDI MARSHALL

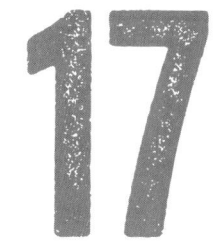

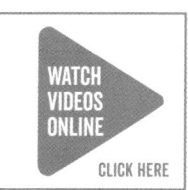

WATCH VIDEOS ONLINE

CLICK HERE

THIS CHAPTER COVERS

- An overview of frailty
- Recognition, screening and prevention of frailty
- Current models and frameworks for assessing frail older adults
- Evidence-informed interventions for the frail older person
- The needs of frail older adults in different environments
- Preparing to care for the person with frailty.

> " Frailty does not mean wrapping somebody in cotton wool. By talking to the person, and observing them as you converse, you will 'flesh out' the framework of the person you heard about at the handover. There is no need to be afraid to work with them, provided you have established a safe way to do so and if this means recruiting help, so be it. But so long as you remember they are a person, albeit perhaps with some limitations, you will get on fine. By adopting this approach, you may even hear some interesting stories into the bargain!
>
> **Gary, student nurse** "

INTRODUCTION

You will find it is common to hear the term 'frailty' being used to describe someone old and vulnerable but it is much more than this. While frailty can often be associated with ageing, it is not exclusively older people who become frail, yet it is a health state related to the ageing process. Frailty is likely to involve multiple systems of the body gradually losing the reserves that allow recovery and resilience (British Geriatric Society, 2014). It is now regarded as a medical 'syndrome', which is a collection of symptoms that result from disease processes. Frailty is not a single illness but the understanding we have of this is still evolving. Frailty also happens to an individual and each person is likely to be different, with varying backgrounds and health histories, together with their own multiple health concerns. However, despite the complexity of this condition, some of the causes of frailty are reversible.

Older frail people are vulnerable to the smallest changes in health and other circumstances and this can lead to rapid and serious decline, leading to hospital admission and even death. Therefore, frailty is recognised as a serious condition. Over the age of 65 years, 10% of people will have frailty, with 25–50% of people over 85 affected. As our population ages, the number of people with frailty is also likely to rise (British Geriatric Society, 2014).

All practitioners working in health and social care need to be aware of frailty, how to recognise and assess needs and how to reduce the impact on a person's life. As a student nurse working in community, hospital or care homes, you will be caring frequently for older people who are frail, in a wide range of settings, and it is important to have an understanding of this condition. This chapter will examine frailty in more detail by exploring recognition, assessment, management, care and prevention, in order to support you in your role.

While frailty can be portrayed negatively and can seem to be all about deteriorating health and wellbeing, as we heard in Gary's reminder people do not need to be wrapped in cotton wool. Therefore, this is also about people who will bring personal strength and resilience to their daily life with frailty. Hence, when we are examining frailty as a concept, we also need to examine the impact on the individual as they experience frailty.

So now we begin our examination of frailty by starting with a person. Mr Williams will be key to our understanding of frailty. His story will frame some of the issues.

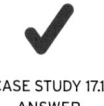

CASE STUDY 17.1
ANSWER

CASE STUDY 17.1: MR WILLIAMS

Mr Williams is 78 years old; he lost his wife 18 months ago following 52 years of marriage. He has a history of osteoarthritis, chronic obstructive pulmonary disease (COPD), hearing problems and has cataracts in both eyes. After his wife's death, he moved to a flat in a private housing complex near his daughter. This was a distance away from his old friends and the local church, but she is his only family and he felt this was for the best. Since he moved, he has tried to adapt and mixes with some of the people in the complex, occasionally looking after his young grandson.

What interventions to prevent frailty might be useful for Mr Williams at this time?

AN OVERVIEW OF FRAILTY

Here we need to understand frailty as a condition where the person fails to return to normal functioning after a period of illness, putting them at risk of negative outcomes including falls, delirium and functional deterioration in living skills (Clegg et al., 2013). Frail older people are essentially at higher risk of deterioration in their physical and mental health, even after a minor event such as an infection. They are also more likely to have multiple co-morbidities as well as functional, psychological and social needs. People 65 years and older use 66% of hospital bed days and about 25% of these are used by those over 80 years (HSJ/Serco, 2014). As older people are more likely to become frail they tend to account for the largest increase in acute hospital admissions, with the highest risk of acquired disability, cognitive decline and admission to residential care (Ellis et al., 2011). Therefore, as a student nurse, you will meet older frail people in most of your practice placements.

A limited ability to maintain homeostasis means even moderate life events can place the body under extreme stress. In addition, the person may have impaired physiological responses. The person may have a reduced recognition of hunger or thirst and wound healing is much slower. The frail older person is much more likely to have symptoms that can mimic dementia, as most acute health concerns they experience, such as infections, will include changes in their cognitive state.

SEE ALSO
CHAPTER 19

Biologically, indicators of frailty can manifest in muscle and weight loss, reduced walking speed, exhaustion and low energy expenditure. Psychologically, frailty can have an impact on older people, who may be unhappy when described this way. Society places value on independence and autonomy and frailty may be viewed as a series of losses. This can lead to a sense of helplessness and hopelessness, increasing the risk of depression. In turn, this can affect physical health and wellbeing. Loss of social contact, isolation and reduced finances can occur in old age, reducing opportunities and increasing loneliness. Body image may change for the person and the way others respond and refer to them. These can all affect how the frail older person copes with this transition, which may be experienced as a series of losses, with a limited future and more intervention and interference by others, together with a sense of being closer to death (Fillit and Butler, 2009).

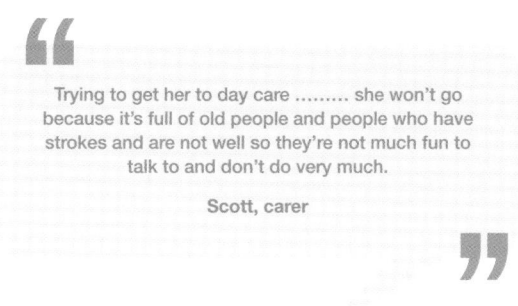

> Trying to get her to day care .... she won't go because it's full of old people and people who have strokes and are not well so they're not much fun to talk to and don't do very much.
>
> Scott, carer

As the idea of frailty brings with it negative connotations of dependency, this can also lead to a fear of being moved to a care setting. For older people who have caring responsibilities, such as a wife caring for a husband, they may realise that they are unable to continue being a support to others. Frailty can also place limitations on the person's other activities and interests. Being identified as frail can also lead to others treating the person differently and reducing opportunities to take part in activities in case the person falls or becomes unwell. This negative view of frailty should be examined and perhaps challenged, as this can lead to stigma, withdrawal and isolation, making prevention of further disability and support to maintain quality of life difficult. It is important to have an understanding of how it might feel to be older, yet still consider the experience of both healthy and frail older people. Try the visualisation activity below and check your own responses to ageing and frailty.

ACTIVITY 17.1
ANSWER

ACTIVITY 17.1: REFLECTIVE PRACTICE

Close your eyes and imagine you are 80 years old. Consider a life where you live independently, attend a range of activities including tai chi classes, swimming, a book club and are a volunteer at the local hospital. Your life is full of friends and family; you are still driving and are busy nearly every day. You have a few aches and pains and take colds like everyone else. Otherwise, you feel not too bad most of the time.

- Question 1

Now – eyes still closed – there is a mirror in front of you. How do you look? How do you feel about yourself now? How could you describe yourself?

Now consider a life where you had developed some common conditions associated with older age, you have cataracts so cannot drive or read, you have developed osteoarthritis too and so moving around has to be done more slowly and you have had a number of chest infections this winter. You are reluctant to leave the house in bad weather and have now given up your swimming and tai chi classes. You have lost weight and are not really sleeping well. Yet you are still the same person and hope to get back to life as you lived it.

- Question 2

Now think about how you look and feel. What would it be like to be described as frail?

WHAT'S THE EVIDENCE? 17.1

Read the research paper found on this link about the experience of frailty or find a recent paper that looks at this topic.

Skilbeck, J., Arthur, A. and Seymour, J. (2017) Making sense of frailty: An ethnographic study of the experience of older people living with complex health problems. http://onlinelibrary.wiley.com/doi/10.1111/opn.12172/full

Consider the findings of the research. Some of these might be similar to your own feelings during the activity. Are there any key differences that surprise you?

Providing psychological support is as important as physical care and this begins with developing relationships with the person and family. This will support them to understand the condition and develop strategies to manage daily life. The person may need support to address the grief and loss that can be generated by becoming frail and they may react with anger, distress or become depressed. Depression is generally under-recognised and under-treated in older age and there is a need for access to mental health services for older people. It is important to consider and discuss this in a positive way, as part of a holistic plan of care. The goal of care is not only to maximise function and treat ill health but also to enhance and maintain wellbeing and quality of life.

PATHWAY TO FRAILTY

Frailty does not have a sudden onset and can be a long journey for the person, yet this can give us a real opportunity to intervene at various parts of the pathway. Frailty begins with cells ageing and becoming damaged. When this damage can no longer be repaired or removed this leads to deteriorating body systems. As these accumulate over time, some people will reach the stage of frailty. Some older people will have better compensatory responses than others will and the body has some redundancy or reserve, where the damage is contained and does not show clinical symptoms. The evidence about how this happens and why it happens to some older people and not others is in the early stages and it needs much more work to make these links explicit (Rockwood et al., 2015). Current thinking is that frailty is the result of genetic, environmental, cellular and physiological factors that come together to result in multiple system frailty.

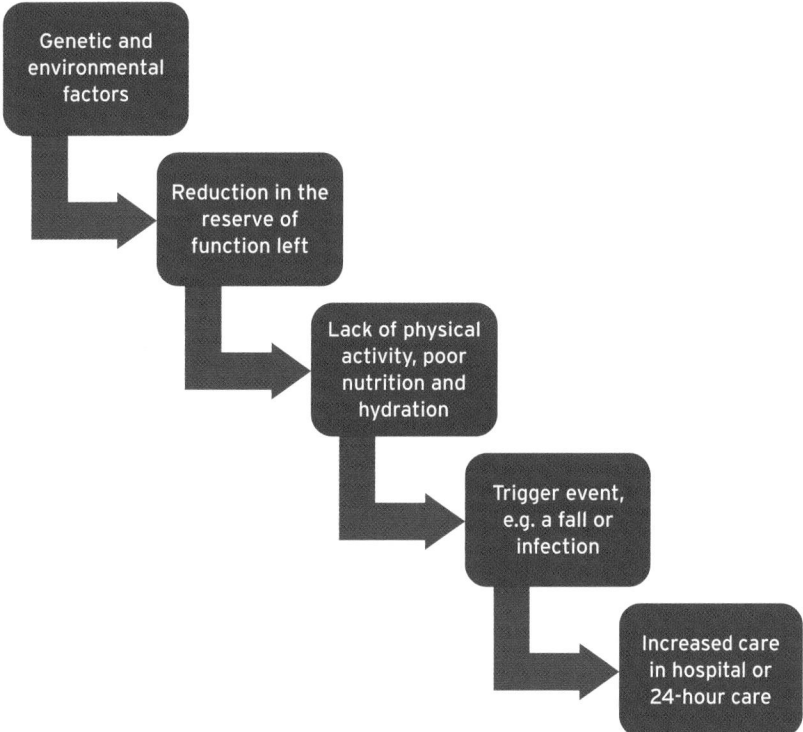

Figure 17.1 Frailty pathway

Figure 17.1 shows the most common pathway to frailty in older people; yet I am sure that you can see this could be different if appropriate interventions, care and treatment are available and implemented at the right time. While genetic factors cannot be changed, yet, most other lifestyle, environmental and health events could be prevented or ameliorated to some degree. It is important not to perceive frailty simply in terms of this inevitable pathway, rather a syndrome that has multiple causes, is complex and, therefore, requires a multifaceted approach that is continued and revised over time. An outcome- rather than disease-focused approach will be more useful for this complex condition.

RECOGNITION, SCREENING AND PREVENTION OF FRAILTY

Now we understand that frailty is a complex pathway, it is important to understand how to recognise and assess this condition. By recognising frailty as early as possible, we can improve long-term outcomes for older people. However, there is no widely recognised screening tool that can be used to identify frailty, particularly within a clinical setting. The case for screening older people for frailty is not proven and not only is there a lack of consistent assessment tools, there are also the challenges of making a correct diagnosis (British Geriatric Society, 2014).

Sternberg et al. (2011) undertook a systematic literature review to help identify an operational definition of frailty that could be used in clinical settings. They found that disability, reduced gait speed and impaired cognition were the most common characteristics identified in most frailty studies. However, there was no consensus and, in many cases, the characteristics could be altered depending on the intervention offered and the expected outcomes. Despite this lack of certainty, it is still important to identify tools and provide guidance in order to identify frailty. Identifying people who are frail early in the condition allows preventative interventions or restorative care.

Some frail older people present with a simple symptom that could be masking an underlying complex medical issue. These symptoms are often referred to as frailty syndromes (Table 17.1). These common syndromes mean that a frail older person could present to a service with one or more of these and you need to be alert to the more complex picture underlying them.

Table 17.1   Common frailty syndromes

Falls	Sudden collapse, report of 'legs gave way', or the person may be found lying on the floor.
Immobility	Sudden change in mobility, described as 'gone off legs'. May be found having been stuck in the toilet and not able to get up.
Incontinence	Change in continence. There may be new onset incontinence or a deterioration of urinary or faecal incontinence.
Delirium	Acute or suddenly worsening confusion. Low-level infection such as a urinary tract infection. Can be superimposed on dementia.
Adverse drug reactions/ polypharmacy	Increased susceptibility to effects and adverse effects of medicines. Taking a multiple range of medication, usually more than five different medications.
Dementia	A sudden deterioration in the person with dementia or deteriorating memory, thinking and understanding.
End of life	Increase in reports of pain and distress. Multiple morbidities are experienced and complicated by acute illness.

Adapted from the British Geriatric Society (2014)

CURRENT MODELS AND FRAMEWORKS FOR ASSESSING FRAIL OLDER ADULTS

Frailty is often framed in deficit models with a focus on what the person has lost or can no longer do. However, it is important to bear in mind that the frail older person will have strengths or assets that must be taken in to account in their assessment and care. Frailty is a process, not just an outcome, and in their journey through frailty many older people develop resilience and coping mechanisms to allow them to continue to be as independent as they can for as long as possible. If we only focus on deficits, this can lead to the person being increasingly dependent and speeds deterioration.

Reflecting a negative approach, there are two main models used to understand frailty: the phenotype model and the deficit model. The phenotype model was originally developed and validated by Fried et al. (2001). The phenotype model identifies frailty using specific characteristics of weight loss, reduced muscle strength, reduced gait speed, exhaustion and low energy expenditure. Using these variables the participants could determine those who were pre-frail, frail and robust. Those who were pre-frail reported one or two of these symptoms. Those who were frail had three or more of these symptoms. Robust older people had none of the above symptoms (Fried et al., 2001). This work is considered important because it suggests that there could be a set of observable characteristics that exist within individuals that could identify the risk of frailty.

The cumulative deficit model was derived from a large study of people with dementia. By examining the presence of a range of what were called 'deficits', including presence of a range of diseases and disabilities, an index of frailty was developed (Rockwood et al., 2005). In effect, the more 'deficits' the person had, the more likely they were to be frail. At a particular point, these deficits will reach a point where the person cannot survive. Although some did not obviously lead to illness or death, it was the accumulative impact that led to the increased risk of frailty and mortality. This is an important idea, that frailty is not linked to a single illness or event but is likely to be gradual and cumulative in the older person. Being able to grade frailty in this way can improve recognition and timely interventions to prevent deterioration or improve quality of life.

When we recognise that the person is at risk of frailty, the next step should be a holistic assessment. The complex overlapping problems frail older people experience necessitates assessment across multiple domains to develop a therapeutic plan for recovery and independence. This process is referred to as Comprehensive Geriatric Assessment (CGA) (British Geriatric Society, 2010). The CGA is a highly evolved form of ongoing care led by doctors, nurses and allied health professions (physiotherapy, occupational therapy, speech and language therapy, dietetics) who specialise in looking after older adults with frailty and work as a coordinated multidisciplinary team. This may be delivered in a specialist unit, ward or by a mobile team in other areas of medicine or surgical care or indeed in community settings. Table 17.2 indicates the key domains for assessment.

Table 17.2 Domains of the Comprehensive Geriatric Assessment

Medical	Severity of the presenting condition
	Other co-morbid conditions
	Review of medication
	Nutritional status
	List of identified problems
Mental health	Cognitive assessment
	Assessments of mood and emotional state
	Explore fears and anxieties
Functional capacity	Performance of activities of living
	Assessment of mobility, walking and balance
	Ability to move around
Social situation	Support available from others
	Financial circumstances and benefits
	Social networks and activities
Living environment	Housing or home environment
	Use of equipment
	Use of assistive technology
	Access to resources and support from the wider community

Adapted from the CGA (British Geriatric Society, 2010)

There is evidence that use of the CGA with frail older people improves clinical outcomes, reduces mortality and the need for long-term care and reduces the costs of health and social care. Several studies have been undertaken which identify that using the CGA with frail older people admitted to hospital means they are more likely to return home, less likely to experience functional or cognitive decline and have a lower in-hospital mortality rate (Ellis et al., 2011). Care for Older People in Hospital (Healthcare Improvement Scotland, 2015) highlights the importance of this assessment and states that older people presenting with frailty syndromes should have prompt access to a specialist team and a CGA where treatment is reviewed by the multidisciplinary team.

There is also a range of rating scales used in frailty research and clinical practice; these include the Edmonton Frail Scale (Rolfson et al., 2006) and the Groningen Frailty Indicator (Schuurmans et al., 2004). These use varied but similar indicators to record deficits, such as nutrition, functional independence, vision, hearing, mobility, polypharmacy and cognition. These measures are intended to identify people at various stages of frailty and can be useful in clinical practice. Specific measures of function and movement can also be helpful, such as the gait speed test (Studenski et al., 2011) used in community or hospital settings and the Timed Up and Go Test (TUG) (Shumway-Cook et al., 2000). These measures can be aligned with a CGA process, to identify risk and inform prevention and treatment plans.

SAFEGUARDING FRAIL OLDER PEOPLE

SEE ALSO
CHAPTER 3

Frail older people can be at risk in any care setting. Their vulnerability can expose them to suboptimal care and neglect, physical, emotional, financial, sexual and cultural abuse. It is the responsibility of all professionals and other practitioners to be aware and alert to the possibility of abuse and neglect occurring in any setting. Legislation is available throughout the UK to support and guide families and practitioners where there is any suspicion.

SEE ALSO
CHAPTER 4

However safeguarding is not only about abuse and neglect, but also about managing risk safely. As a student nurse, you will learn that this can range from reporting poor practice, to enabling older frail people to make decisions about their own life and recognising that risk cannot be avoided completely. You will find that communication, partnership and shared decision-making can allow the person to remain safe but respect their human rights.

EVIDENCE-INFORMED CARE FOR THE FRAIL OLDER PERSON

There are a number of interventions for the person living with frailty and it is important that these be offered in a timely and appropriate way. There are risks and benefits in all treatments and for the older person who is frail these need to be thoroughly evaluated and revisited. While a lack of treatment can result in rapid deterioration and distress, aggressive treatment approaches can have limited success, while causing pain and distress.

The primary consideration should be to provide relevant and realistic treatment and this begins with a comprehensive and multidisciplinary team approach. One of the risks is where treatments and protocols developed for adults with a single condition are applied to this complex group. Older frail people are generally not included in research into treatments or medications and this means that these are likely to have a different and sometimes unexpected impact, often with more adverse effects and less benefit. There are barriers to making decisions about treatment for frail older people in acute care, including the use of disease-focused rather than holistic models of care and poor communication about choices, risks and impact of treatment (Mallery and Moorhouse, 2011).

Acute illness can trigger treatment that may not be optimal for the frail older person and it is important to consider carefully the risks and benefits. Treatment may include medication, invasive investigations and surgery. There are risks and adverse outcomes for these interventions that could include an impact on function and memory, cause pain and discomfort and some may require time in hospital. The complexity of frailty should lead to discussions about quality of life, dignity and comfort and the management of symptoms when considering treatments (Mallery and Moorhouse, 2011).

PLANNING FOR CARE NEEDS

The frail older person and family members can only make plans for care now and in the future if they are informed about the current and future impact of the frailty syndrome. Greater understanding about these can help people make informed decisions about possible treatments and plans for future care needs. In particular, a greater understanding of the impact on wellbeing of complications of frailty, including pain, polypharmacy, falls, dementia and delirium can help avoid some of the distressing treatment delays or the use of inappropriate interventions. Part of your role will be taking part in empowering the person and family with timely and appropriate information leading to holistic and realistic health and treatment decisions, which can result in a better quality of life.

During a placement in a care of the elderly ward, a gentleman was admitted who, on first impressions, was comfortable in the ward area. Over the course of the next few days, however, it was increasingly clear that at times he was distressed in that environment and he would barely acknowledge staff. On noticing how different he was during a visit with his granddaughter, I approached her and she mentioned how talking about football always grounded him and allowed an avenue for other conversation. Later that same day, I put her advice to use and found that I could discuss aspects of his care, which he had previously not acknowledged before.

Gary, student

Prevention and management strategies for frailty have similar approaches and aims. The following interventions can be used for primary prevention: to maintain or improve the health status of the older person with frailty risk factors and for the person on the frailty journey.

Physical activity, good nutrition and hydration are key preventative strategies and may also slow or reverse some of the progress when the person is at risk of frailty. Maintaining optimum wellbeing after frailty is recognised and assessed means it is possible to improve health outcomes using a range of approaches.

Physical activity is considered the primary intervention for frailty and should target strength, endurance and balance rather than a single approach to being active. The advice is to engage in these at least three times a week for 30–45 minutes and do this for at least 5 months (World Health Organization, 2011). Improving gait, body strength and mobility can reduce the risk of falls and dependence on others for activities of living. Exercise can produce anti-oxidant and anti-inflammatory responses that can slow muscle wasting and increase the synthesis of protein; this can prevent or ameliorate the impact of frailty.

GO FURTHER

**WEBLINK:
NICE**

The National Institute for Health and Care Excellence (NICE) has developed guidance to try and support people to delay the development of frailty in addition to disability or dementia. You can access this at www.nice.org.uk/guidance/ng16.

HEALTH PROMOTION

Why not begin to think about these and begin with yourself.

Try to keep an activity diary for a week to see how well you are doing.

Divide the page into columns and check what your activity levels are and how your actions fit the multidimensional approach advocated to avoid frailty. In each column, note the type of exercise, i.e. brisk walking, swimming and the time taken.

Day of the week	Strength exercise	Endurance exercise	Balance exercise

Consider your own approach to wellbeing; were you able to achieve the standard set to prevent frailty? Remember, these activities should be a mix of all three types of exercise three days a week for at least 30-45 minutes on each occasion.

If you have achieved this, then very well done and you will be a great example to others. If you need to do more to achieve this, what plans do you need to have in place to work towards making your lifestyle frailty preventative?

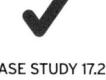

**CASE STUDY 17.2
ANSWER**

CASE STUDY 17.2: MR WILLIAMS

Remember Mr Williams. He was settling in well in his new home. He had made some friends and had enjoyed spending more time with his daughter and grandson. Then he fell in the shower, was bruised and had a real shock.

Afterwards he complained of more joint pain and became afraid of falls.

What interventions might benefit him at this point?

EATING AND DRINKING

**SEE ALSO
CHAPTER 37**

Poor nutritional status can be a contributing factor to frailty and can play a part in the interventions offered. Inadequate dietary intake has been linked with impaired immune response, risk of osteoporosis, increased risk of chronicity of diseases and peripheral artery disease. Additionally, the person can experience poor oral health, risk of skin breakdown, exhaustion, falls, increased dependence and, of course, frailty. The importance of adequate nutrition in the prevention of frailty is well established. It is suggested in a review of the available evidence that a good quality diet, high in micronutrients, such as vitamins C, D and E and folate, protein and antioxidant intake may lower the risk of frailty as there is an association between malnutrition (or the risk of malnutrition) and frailty (Lorenzo-López et al., 2017). This is not unexpected, as it is clear from the description and assessment of the frailty syndrome that weight loss is generally one of the key concerns.

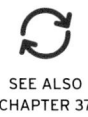

SEE ALSO
CHAPTER 37

MEDICATION AND FRAILTY

Polypharmacy, or the use of five or more medications by an individual, is a common concern for older people and particularly so for the person who is frail (Saum et al., 2017). Polypharmacy increases the risk of inappropriate prescribing, poor compliance and adverse reactions leading to falls, impairment of activities of living and hospitalisation. Age-related changes in renal, metabolic and gastrointestinal function affect how medication is absorbed and excreted and the higher number of medications taken can increase risk.

SEE ALSO
CHAPTER 13

Saum et al. (2017) suggest that while it is important to consider reducing the number of medicines frail older people are prescribed, it is vital that each person is managed as an individual.

Frailty is such a complex condition that pain and discomfort should be expected and recognition and management plans should be in place. It is vital that we remember that older people may not report pain unless specifically asked, and there is a range of assessment tools that should be routinely offered. In addition, plans to reduce infections, falls and delirium are key interventions. Ensuring the frail older person has a timely influenza and pneumococcal vaccination and recognising and treating any minor condition such as skin tears, coughs or dental caries can prevent more serious acute illness. These are more likely to be successful when family and other caregivers are involved in planning and care management. Effective, current and advance planning includes good assessment processes and involvement of the family and wider team. The provision of clear information and good advance planning can improve care outcomes and prevent unexpected episodes of acute ill health.

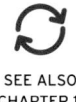

SEE ALSO
CHAPTER 11

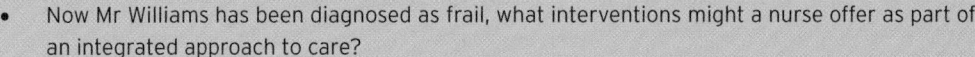

CASE STUDY 17.3: MR WILLIAMS

CASE STUDY 17.3
ANSWER

Here we meet Mr Williams again. It is six months later and despite being more active and working with his plan of care, he begins to complain of having no energy, poor appetite and has lost weight. Despite a thorough review by his GP, there is no single cause found and he is considered frail. At this, he became reluctant to go out and had no confidence in looking after his grandson.

- Now Mr Williams has been diagnosed as frail, what interventions might a nurse offer as part of an integrated approach to care?

Finally:
   Despite Mr William's journey through frailty bringing challenges, he has been supported to remain at home and encouraged to work with his family and the multidisciplinary team to maintain his wellbeing. Frailty can be a difficult experience but is not without hope.

PLACE OF CARE FOR FRAIL OLDER PEOPLE

Frail older people at home

Most older frail people would prefer to remain in their own home yet there are ongoing concerns about lack of responsive community care services, inappropriate admissions to hospital, lack of designated frailty units or teams and delayed discharge to a community setting (HSJ/Serco, 2014).

> My mother-in-law had a severe stroke 2 years ago that has left her with a right-sided weakness, poor mobility and difficulty both in swallowing and speaking. On discharge from hospital she received great care and support from an early supported discharge team, but once it was clear that her rehabilitation was not likely to progress and the team began withdrawing their expertise then things began to change. The number of visits she had from the care service were reduced and obviously the physiotherapist stopped coming. I am saying the care service visits were reduced but I think the maximum is what my mother-in-law gets, which is four visits a day. Thankfully, currently she has a small number of people who know her looking after her, so they all get in. They nearly always get to do what they have been tasked with doing and you can see my mother-in-law warming to most of them and looking forward to the visits.
>
> **Scott, carer**

Frailty needs a biopsychosocial approach and this should fit closely with an integrated care approach. Integration of health and social care services that work collaboratively with people and families can enable the person to be supported at home. Increasing opportunities for different types of services may improve the person's experience and care. The carer's and the frail older person's experience above could have been much improved, with a clear provision of what integrated care should be for the frail older person.

ACTIVITY 17.2 ANSWER

ACTIVITY 17.2: REFLECTIVE PRACTICE

Reflect on the experiences described in the film in the link below and how each person has adapted to their changing life at home.
   Consider:

1.   What adaptations are maintaining their independence?
2.   What factors might cause their move from their home to hospital or care setting?

www.youtube.com/watch?v=_pEMrqOANzA&feature=youtu.be

However, it must be borne in mind that frailty brings with it a susceptibility to developing acute illnesses and injuries. This means that it is likely that the person will be in need of hospital care at various points in the journey.

Frail older people in hospital

Cornwell (2012) noted that 27 reports and guidelines have been produced over the last 12 years about the care of older people in hospital, and that it was time to focus on solutions to the concerns raised. It is clear that these solutions should include high standards of practice by all staff and attention to the physical, psychological and social needs of the older person; in particular, caring for people as individuals and involving them in all decision-making. Three aspects of care in hospital have been identified as crucial to positive care outcomes: involving people, families and carers; providing access to specialist care; and minimising moves from setting to setting (HSJ/Serco, 2014).

Some of the adverse effects of hospitalisation are the reduction of independent functioning, increase in the use of medical interventions and mortality. Disability in activities of living is a common outcome including reduction in mobility, dressing, bathing and using the toilet. It is suggested that at least 30% of people 70 years and older in hospital will develop this increased disability (Covinsky et al., 2003). The lack of movement in hospital, poor diet offered and lack of support to maintain independence therefore play a dominant role in the outcomes of hospital care and further in the ability of the older person to return home. Oliver (2017) identifies that only a few days in bed can cause muscle weakness. Therefore, interventions to encourage mobility, a good diet and fluid intake and supportive care for activities of living framed within a frailty-focused and person-centred approach can improve outcomes.

SEE ALSO
CHAPTER 39

Innovations for the care of the frail older person includes specialised frailty units and frailty-focused teams. While these approaches appear to provide a very positive approach, it is unlikely that most hospitals can ensure that all patients who are frail will have the opportunity to be cared for by these units or teams. The rising numbers mean that frailty will be at the core of hospital care and, therefore, professionals should all be encouraged to learn how to make care and treatment approaches frailty focused. Families must be part of the team and are a rich source of both information and support for the team.

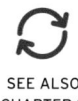

SEE ALSO
CHAPTER 2

> Talking with someone who knows your patient better than you ever will grants you a unique insight into that person's life, and can give you ways of grounding people – especially someone who is distressed in the ward environment – so that you can open a line of communication. It is essential to work in partnership with the person and those who know them so that you can provide optimal care, both medical and psychosocial. If you do identify a strategy to connect with them, ensure that this is passed to other staff!
>
> **Gary, student**

ACTIVITY 17.3: CRITICAL THINKING

ACTIVITY 17.3
ANSWER

Consider the benefits and risks for the older frail person who is cared for in a specialised frailty unit rather than a general medical ward. Identify up to three benefits and three risks that might occur.

Frail older people in care homes

The care home sector is part of the journey of many older people with frailty and should be seen as an important partner in the care experience. The media, professionals and the public can perceive care homes negatively and this may be the result of news stories, anecdotes or experiences. It may also be a result of our own fears of ageing and end of life. However, many care homes lead the way in integrating health and social care, and improvement in quality of care and a focus on quality of life is beginning to impact on the sector. One example of this is the work of My Home Life, which is a programme across the UK using an evidence-based approach to best practice. This programme is based on relationships and helping not only residents but also families and staff to work in a way that reinforces feelings of security, belonging, continuity, purpose, achievement and significance every day.

WEBLINK:
HOME LIFE

GO FURTHER

Access the My Home Life Page at http://myhomelife.org.uk/
You will find Best Practice themes identified and explore how these might apply to the older person who is frail.

PALLIATIVE CARE AND FRAILTY

SEE ALSO
CHAPTER 25

Frailty is a progressive condition and as the person becomes less able to cope with a range of factors related to multiple morbidity, they are overwhelmed. There is a need for a palliative care approach to be considered early and used to help the person live as well as possible. The uncertainty about when the person will reach the end of life makes support for family vital. The more structured approach of palliative care may allow for advanced planning, including an ongoing discussion of Do Not Resuscitate choices. Palliative care approaches for frailty may need some modification where they have been developed for traditional single disease processes, such as cancer. There needs to be a greater understanding of the interacting and competing illnesses and disabilities on the person's quality of life. Recognising that the person is reaching the end of the frailty journey is key and this can be recognised by an unrelenting decline in physical, psychological and cognitive function, unexplained weight loss and an increase in the frequency of acute illness with less recovery after each one (Moorhouse et al., 2015). Management of medications may include stopping any that may cause distressing symptoms and an increasing focus on the recognition, assessment and management of pain and discomfort. You will appreciate that the fragility of the body must be respected and comfort measures should be a priority. Not only family but also those who have provided care over long periods will need support and should be included in care activities where they wish to do so.

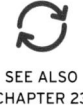

SEE ALSO
CHAPTER 23

So now, you are preparing to care for the person who is frail. Here is some practical advice from an experienced mentor who says:

Remember that people can have hearing and visual difficulties and you need to communicate clearly and make sure the person can see you and understand what you say. You must listen and give the person time to respond, the person may not understand what you say when they are very tired, frail and ill. Often the person is bedbound and a little contact like holding the person's hand can be very welcome. I would like a student to treat this person as a whole person and do not see them as a task. The frail person will have lots of things impacting upon their health, take this into consideration. The older generation may not complain and many don't want to be any trouble, so you need to check everything. Even if you are only in for a simple dressing you need to make sure that you look at everything. They may not complain but we need to pick it up.

Sheila, mentor

This advice to look at the whole person links to the biopsychosocial approach we have adopted in this chapter. You need to consider the complexity of the person's needs which may not be easy to identify, so good clinical and person-centred observation is essential. Good communication is enhanced by really understanding and learning about how the person is experiencing the world; this includes sensory challenges such as hearing and seeing as well as the impact of exhaustion and pain. A really important point is made about how some older people do not wish to be a 'burden' on the people caring for them, and their attempts to seem well can increase the risk of missing something important that can have considerable impact on health and quality of life. This careful, person-centred and holistic approach is also reflected in the student's words below.

> It can be very helpful to read through care plans and medical records, though this is not always practicable, therefore paying careful attention at handovers is essential to ensuring patient safety. Talk through any procedure and identify areas which enable participation. Especially in personal care, not only does this minimise any embarrassment for them, it also helps prevent institutionalisation, and maintains independence. If you don't understand, for example, cultural or religious implications, just ask. In my experience, this is preferable to people than basing actions on assumptions. A holistic approach, therefore, is necessary, since no two people are the same, even from the same culture. Just because something is or is not acceptable to one person, this doesn't hold true for all people.

Gary, student

CHAPTER SUMMARY

- Frailty is a complex syndrome mainly affecting older people and has multiple causes and effects.
- A multidisciplinary approach including the use of the Comprehensive Geriatric Assessment is more likely to produce successful outcomes.
- Person-centred and relationship-focused approaches are key to supporting the person living with frailty, family and supporters.
- Safeguarding the person living with frailty should also include risk enablement to allow choice and respect rights.
- Evidence-informed care approaches require a wide and comprehensive range of knowledge and skills for nurses.

GO FURTHER

Go to https://study.sagepub.com/essentialadultnursing for a further case study related to this chapter. If you are using the interactive ebook, simply click on the book icon in the margin to go straight to the resource.

CASE STUDY: FRAIL ADULT

Books

- Tetley, J., Cox, N., Kirsten, J. and Witham, G. (2018) *Nursing Older People at a Glance*. Oxford: Wiley, Blackwell. Chapter 23 focuses on frailty but is an excellent book on the older person.
- Theou, O. and Rockwood, K. (2015) (eds) *Frailty in Ageing: Biological, clinical and social implications*. Basel: Karger. This edited text covers all of the main concerns about frailty, ranging from biopsychosocial issues to care practice.

FURTHER
READING:
JOURNAL
ARTICLES

Journal Articles

Go to https://study.sagepub.com/essentialadultnursing for further free online journal articles related to this chapter. If you are using the interactive ebook, simply click on the book icon in the margin to go straight to the resource.

- Cornwall, J. (2012) The care of frail older people with complex needs: time for a revolution. London: The King's Fund. [Online] Available at: www.kingsfund.org.uk/publications/care-frail-older-people-complex-needs-time-revolution [Accessed 23rd March, 2017]
- Ebrahimi, Z., Wilhelmson, K., Eklund, K., Moore, C.D. and Jakobsson A. (2013) Health despite frailty: exploring influences on frail older adults' experiences of health. *Geriatric Nursing*, 34(4): 289–94. doi: 10.1016/j.gerinurse.2013.04.008. Epub 2013 May 10.
- Taube, E., Jakobsson, U., Midlöv, P. and Kristensson, J. (2016) Being in a bubble: the experience of loneliness among frail older people. *Journal of Advanced Nursing*, 72(3): 631–40.

FURTHER
READING:
WEBLINKS

Weblinks

Go to https://study.sagepub.com/essentialadultnursing for further weblinks related to this chapter. If you are using the interactive ebook, simply click on the book icon in the margin to go straight to the resource.

- Royal College of Nursing website that provides advice and resources to identify frailty in older patients and guidance on choosing helpful interventions.
www.rcn.org.uk/clinical-topics/older-people/frailty
- British Geriatric Society guidelines on the recognition and management of frailty in older people.
www.bgs.org.uk/index.php/fit-for-frailty

ONLINE
QUIZZES

ACE YOUR ASSESSMENT

Revise what you have learned by visiting https://study.sagepub.com/essentialadultnursing

- Test yourself with multiple-choice and short-answer questions
- Do the chapter activities in the book and check your answers online

REFERENCES

British Geriatric Society (2010) *Comprehensive assessment of the frail older patient.* [Online] Available at: www.bgs.org.uk/good-practice-guides/resources/goodpractice/gpgcgassessment [Accessed 10th January 2017]

British Geriatric Society (2014) *Fit for Frailty - Consensus best practice statement for the care of older people living with frailty in community and outpatient settings.* [Online] Available at: www.bgs.org.uk/index.php/fit-for-frailty [Accessed 19th January 2017].

Clegg, A., Young, J., Iliffe, S., Rikkert, M.O. and Rockwood, K. (2013) Frailty in elderly people. *Lancet,* 381: 752–62. [online] Available at: http://dx.doi.org/10.1016/S0140-6736(12)62167-9 [Accessed 10th January 2017].

Cornwell, J. (2012) *The care of frail older people with complex needs: time for a revolution.* London: The King's Fund. [Online] Available at https://www.kingsfund.org.uk/publications/care-frail-older-people-complex-needs-time-revolution [Accessed 23rd March 2017].

Covinsky, K.E., Palmer, R.M., Fortinsky, R.H., Counsell, S.R., Stewart, A.L., Kresevic, D., Burant, C.J. and Landefield, S.C. (2003). Loss of independence in activities of daily living in older adults hospitalized with medical illnesses: Increased vulnerability with age. *Journal of the American Geriatric Society*, 51(4): 451-8.

Ellis, G., Whitehead, M.A., Robinson, D., O'Neill, D. and Langhorne, P. (2011) Comprehensive geriatric assessment for older adults admitted to hospital: Meta-analysis of randomised controlled trials. *British Medical Journal*, 343 (7821): 469–73.

Fillit, H. and Butler, R.N. (2009) The frailty identity crisis. *Journal of the American Geriatrics Society*, 57(2): 348–52.

Fried, L.P., Tangen, C.M., Walston, J., Newman, A.B., Hirsch, C., Gottdiener, J., Seeman, T., Tracy, R., Kop, W.J., Burke, G. and McBurnie, M.A. (2001) Frailty in older adults, evidence for a phenotype. *The Journals of Gerontology series A: Biological Sciences and Medical Sciences*, 56(3): M146–M157.

Healthcare Improvement Scotland (2015) *Care for Older People in Hospital*. Edinburgh: NHS Scotland.

HSJ/Serco (2014) *Commission on Hospital Care for Frail Older People*. [Online] Available at: www.hsj. co.uk/frail-older-people/commission-on-hospital-care-for-frail-older-people-main-report/5076859. article [Accessed 12th October 2017].

Lorenzo-López, L., Maseda, A., de Labra, C., Regueiro-Folgueira, L., Rodríguez-Villamil, J.L. and Millán-Calenti, J.C. (2017) Nutritional determinants of frailty in older adults: A systematic review. *BMC geriatrics*, 17(1): 1–13.

Mallery, L.H. and Moorhouse, P. (2011) Respecting frailty. *Journal of Medical Ethics*, 37(2): 126–8.

Moorhouse, P., Koller, K., and Mallery, L. (2015) End of life care in frailty. In Theou, O. and Rockwood, K. (eds) *Frailty in Ageing: Biological, clinical and social implications*. Basel: Karger, pp. 195–209.

National Institute for Health and Care Excellence (2015) *Dementia, disability and frailty in later life - mid-life approaches to delay or prevent onset*. [Online] Available at: www.nice.org.uk/guidance/ng16. [Accessed 15th January 2017].

Oliver, D. (2017) Fighting pyjama paralysis in hospital wards. *British Medical Journal*, 357: p. j2096 doi: https://doi.org/10.1136/bmj.j2096.

Rockwood, K., Song, X., MacKnight, C., Bergman, H., Hogan, D.B., McDowell, I. and Mitnitski, A. (2005) A global clinical measure of fitness and frailty in elderly people. *Canadian Medical Association Journal*, 173(5): 489–95.

Rockwood, K., Mitnitski, A. and Howlett. S.E. (2015) Frailty: scaling from cellular deficit accumulation? In Theou, O. and Rockwood, K. (eds) *Frailty in Ageing: Biological, clinical and social implications*. Basel: Karger, pp. 15–32.

Rolfson, D.B., Majumdar, S.R., Tsuyuki, R.T., Tahir, A. and Rockwood, K. (2006) Validity and reliability of the Edmonton Frail Scale. *Age and Ageing*, 35(5): 526–9.

Saum, K.U., Schöttker, B., Meid, A.D., Holleczek, B., Haefeli, W.E., Hauer, K. and Brenner, H. (2017) Is polypharmacy associated with frailty in older people? Results from the ESTHER cohort study. *Journal of the American Geriatrics Society*, 65(2): e27–e32.

Schuurmans, H., Steverink, N., Lindenberg, S., Frieswijk, N. and Slaets, J.P. (2004) Old or frail: what tells us more? *The Journals of Gerontology Series A: Biological Sciences and Medical Sciences*, 59(9): M962–M965.

Shumway-Cook, A., Brauer, S. and Woollacott, M. (2000) Predicting the probability for falls in community-dwelling older adults using the timed up & go test. *Physical Therapy*, 80(9): 896–903.

Skilbeck, J., Arthur, A. and Seymour, J. (2017) Making sense of frailty: An ethnographic study of the experience of older people living with complex health problems. *International Journal of Older People Nursing*, 00:1:1-11. https://doi.org/10.1111/opn.12172

Sternberg, S.A., Schwartz, A.W., Karunananthan, S., Bergman, H. and Mark Clarfield, A. (2011) The identification of frailty: a systematic literature review. *Journal of the American Geriatrics Society*, 59(11): 2129–38.

Studenski, S., Perera, S., Patel, K., Rosano, C., Faulkner, K., Inzitari, M., Brach, J., Chandler, J., Cawthon, P., Connor, E.B. and Nevitt, M., (2011) Gait speed and survival in older adults. *Journal of the American Medical Society*, 305(1): 50–8.

World Health Organization (2011) Information sheet: *Global recommendations on physical activity for health 65 years and above*. [Online] Available at: www.who.int/dietphysicalactivity/publications/recommendations65yearsold/en/ [Accessed 24th March 2017].

CARE OF THE ADULT WITH LONG-TERM CONDITIONS

18

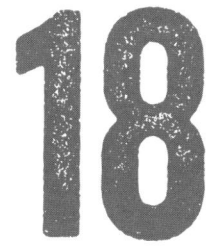

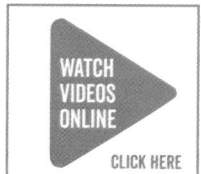
WATCH VIDEOS ONLINE
CLICK HERE

JANETTE BARRIE, SHEILA STEEL AND DIANE LOUGHLIN

THIS CHAPTER COVERS

- The main challenges of living with a long-term condition including the impact of social, economic and environmental factors

- Contemporary models of care to support people living with long-term conditions
- Self-management
- Anticipatory Care Planning.

" I feel frustrated through lack of understanding, I know I am telling the truth but people don't know and react differently and don't believe you're really ill, they don't take the time to listen.

Patient with advanced cardiac failure "

" I just want my life back, I used to run a successful business and now I struggle to make a cup of tea!

Patient living with arthritis "

INTRODUCTION

This chapter covers the care and experience of adults living with long-term conditions. The chapter will explore the main challenges for people and will consider some of these challenges in more depth. It will consider models of care to support people to live well and achieve their own personal outcomes. It will also explore the cultural change necessary to shift from a reactive model of care to an anticipatory approach which supports self-management with the patient and their family at the centre.

ACTIVITY 18.1
ANSWER

ACTIVITY 18.1

Write down what you think the term 'long-term condition' means.

Long-term conditions are conditions where there is no known medical cure and as such can only be managed or controlled. These conditions include: diabetes, asthma, chronic obstructive pulmonary disease and epilepsy (WHO, 2011). We live in diverse communities and during your community placements you will have the privilege of caring for people within their own homes, many of whom will have one or more long-term condition. You will note the incidence of long-term conditions is higher in the low socioeconomic groups and the effects of living with long-term conditions can severely impact upon mental health and quality of life (Tuzun et al., 2015). **Always remember when caring for people in their own homes, you are a guest and enter with the patient's permission.**

The number of people living with a long-term condition is quite staggering. More than 17.5 million adults in the UK alone live with one or more long-term condition, which equates to almost 28% of the entire adult population. This problem is not restricted to the UK; it is a problem experienced in most Western countries and a large part of Asian and African countries too. Conditions such as cardiovascular disease, cancer, chronic respiratory disease and diabetes are responsible for 63% of all deaths worldwide, which is 36 million of 57 million global deaths, with 80% of these deaths occurring in low- and middle-income countries (WHO, 2011). Interestingly, WHO suggests that if the major risk factors for many long-term conditions such as smoking, obesity, lack of exercise were eliminated, many long-term conditions would be prevented. This highlights the connection between long-term conditions, poverty and lifestyle with early death and we need to understand these risk factors in more detail if we are to influence the later effects (Lynch and Davey Smith, 2005).

ACTIVITY 18.2: REFLECTIVE PRACTICE

Reflecting on your current or previous clinical area:

- How many of the patients in your the care have a long-term condition?
- How many of those patients were admitted with a disorder other than their long-term condition?
- How many of those patients would you consider to be classed in a lower socioeconomic group?
- Do you think any of the patients related their lifestyle with their long-term condition?

THE MAIN CHALLENGES OF LIVING WITH A LONG-TERM CONDITION

There is no doubt the population is ageing. Traditional healthcare services have been designed to respond to acute illness and acute problems; however, because of advances in medicine, pharmacology and social support, people are living longer. With this increase in life expectancy there is the potential for:

- an increased prevalence of age-related long-term conditions
- multi-morbidity
- polypharmacy.

It is thought that 60% of people over the age of 65 years have multiple conditions (Tinetti et al., 2012). The term multi-morbidity is used when the person has two or more chronic conditions (Salisbury et al., 2014). As a nurse you will have detailed knowledge of a number of long-term conditions to enable you to carry out a person-centred assessment. At times, undertaking such an assessment can be quite difficult as multi-morbidity is commonly found in the lower socioeconomic groups where patients may not fully understand their condition due to poor health literacy. Some patients may have complex care plans and multiple medications. When the patient is taking multiple medications, this is known as polypharmacy. In order for the patient to live well with their long-term condition and to take their medication safely, as nurses we have a responsibility to make sure our patients understand their condition(s) and the plan of care.

POLYPHARMACY

Effective management of long-term conditions usually depends upon the use of medication. For those with multi-morbidity, this can result in the use of multiple medicines, which is thought to add further complexity to the person's condition. The more medicines a person takes, the more likely they are to experience an adverse drug reaction (Zhang et al., 2009).

Polypharmacy is defined as when the patient is taking five or more medications simultaneously (Kaufman et al., 2002), and it is thought that due to the ageing population and increased prevalence of long-term conditions, the older population are at greater risk of polypharmacy and the impact this can have on quality of life (Tseng et al., 2016).

Polypharmacy is also thought to be a reason for people not to take their medication. Other reasons include:

- poor health literacy
- low literacy and numeracy skills
- cultural factors
- inadequate social support
- and other conditions such as depression (Williams et al., 2008).

It is estimated that approximately 50% of people with long-term conditions do not take their medication (National Prescribing Centre, 2007). So, as nurses, what can we do to support people in taking their medications? If we consider the reasons why people don't take their medication then perhaps we can use interventions to offer support.

"I don't like the colour pink so I stopped taking my pink tablets. I knew they helped my heart but I didn't realise I'd end up in hospital if I stopped taking them."

Patient

"I've got that much medication, if I take them then they come back up quicker than they go down, I'm just sick, violently sick and I bring up the rest of the medication and that's not doing me any good."

Patient

ACTIVITY 18.3
ANSWER

ACTIVITY 18.3

Circle what you think the correct answer is to the following questions relating to polypharmacy in the UK.

1	The percentage of hospital admissions that are implicated in adverse reactions to medications	2.5%	4.5%	6.5%
2	Polypharmacy 'at risk' relates to what number of medications that are received regularly either daily or weekly?	10-12	13-15	>15

In a study of 256 residents from 55 care homes what do you think were the approximate numbers of:

3	Administration errors, i.e. wrong drug or dose	40	50	60
4	Medication not given	110	115	120
5	The percentage of an unnecessary drug being prescribed	25%	30%	35%

Source: https://www.kingsfund.org.uk/publications/polypharmacy-and-medicines-optimisation

Education, medication reminders and behaviour change are thought to improve concordance (Williams et al., 2008). If someone doesn't understand their condition(s), they may not understand why it is important to take a specific prescribed medication. Therefore, as a nurse you must teach your patients about their conditions and why a specific medication has been prescribed. Ultimately, it is the person's choice to take the medication or not; however, if they have all the information presented to them in an understandable format and we use a health literacy technique such as 'Teach-Back' to make sure they understand, then the choice they make will be an informed one.

TEACH-BACK

Teach-back is a useful technique to establish if our patients understand information and instruction. After receiving information or education about their condition, patients are asked to explain back in their own words what they have just heard in order to demonstrate their understanding of the information given or the clinical skill they must undertake to manage their condition, e.g. the use of an inhaler or self-administration of insulin. If the patient is unable to explain or describe the technique then the nurse should re-educate the patient perhaps using different words until the patient can demonstrate understanding. Teach-back has been shown to be a useful technique for patient education and supporting self-management (Dantic, 2014). Remember, when giving the patient information, it is our responsibility to make sure they understand before we can consider the interaction or consultation truly complete.

GO FURTHER

For more information and to view some helpful video clips, check out www.teachbacktraining.org/

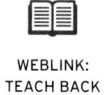

WEBLINK:
TEACH BACK

With the correct knowledge, skills, confidence and support, people can live quite well despite having many long-term conditions. As their health and care needs become more complex, the services to support them may increase, which results in many different people, agencies and disciplines being involved. To make sure care is delivered safely, efficiently and effectively there are a number of evidence-based nursing models and service models of care to help.

MODELS OF CARE TO SUPPORT PEOPLE WITH LONG-TERM CONDITIONS

To meet the health and care needs of people with long-term conditions there is a need for practical, proactive and supportive approaches to care. Forward thinking and planning ahead must be regarded as 'the norm' to embed quality, efficiency and safe practice. In order for this to happen, it is essential that a proactive, collaborative culture is adopted to meet the changing and often challenging health and care needs of individuals within an ageing society (Allen and Glasby, 2013).

Throughout the UK, there is a move towards formal integration between health and social care. Northern Ireland's Health and Social Care services have been formally integrated for a number of years and much progress has been made to do likewise within Scotland, England and Wales.

The integration of Health and Social Care facilitates a more inter-connected approach to care which results in a seamless service for the patient and their family. However, it is also thought to improve the efficiency of services financially challenged in today's economic situation.

Our approach to care is important. Models of care are required to optimise the experience and confidence of patients and to ensure the right thing is done at the right time for the right patient. Evidence-based models of care ensure a consistent approach, the best use of resources and the best possible outcome for the patient.

SUPPORT THROUGH ILLNESS TRAJECTORIES

There are many different long-term conditions as mentioned earlier in this chapter. In the past, diagnoses of certain conditions such as AIDS or cancer were considered terminal; however, with advances in science and pharmacology, conditions such as these are now considered long-term conditions, meaning the patient can live for many years despite having the condition. However, many of these conditions will have different stages resulting in the patient requiring different levels of support at different times.

The term health trajectory is described as the pattern of health and illness over time and is a result of biological, social, behavioural, environmental, economic and political factors as well as genetics. By understanding these factors and disease processes, it allows us to anticipate when people are at greater risk and helps us identify who and when people will require intervention and support on the trajectory facilitating a more person-centred approach to care (Henly et al., 2011).

Table 18.1 McCorkle and Pasacreta (2001) describe eight phases of the chronic illness trajectory:

	Phase	Definition
1.	Initial or pre-trajectory	Where no signs or symptoms are present
2.	Trajectory onset	The first signs and symptoms appear. This includes the diagnostic phase
3.	Crises	A potentially life-threatening situation occurs (e.g. may require emergency care)
4.	Acute	Symptoms require control with a prescribed regimen
5.	Stable	Symptoms are managed and controlled
6.	Unstable	Symptoms become uncontrollable by the previously adopted regimen
7.	Downward	Mental and physical status deteriorates
8.	Dying	Death is preceded by a period of days, weeks or hours

Patients will require different support and interventions along the trajectory according to their condition. We can use this framework to support person-centred anticipatory care by identifying where the patient is within this trajectory and ensure the most appropriate plan of care has been negotiated with the patient and their family.

The experience of patients can vary depending on the condition they have, e.g. those with cancer will have a different trajectory to those with heart failure or general frailty, with each having different periods of stability, intermittent crises, changing needs and end of life care support (Margereson, 2010).

The traditional approach to healthcare tends to be a disease-orientated approach which can often result in the patient experiencing fragmented care that leads to incomplete and ineffective interventions (Onder et al., 2015). Nurses are key to facilitating joined-up care using coordinating approaches such as care/case management, e.g. motor neurone disease and multiple sclerosis. However, it is when patients have multiple conditions and complex health and social care needs that care coordination or care management works best and will be discussed in more detail later in this chapter.

In response to the increasing number of people living with long-term conditions, different models of care have been explored with the aim of optimising patient experience and outcome, while ensuring the most efficient use of resources. The chronic care model, originally developed during the late 1990s in the USA, has been adapted by many countries throughout the world. It is described as a theoretical framework, which creates the right environment to empower people to be in control of their own long-term conditions. The model facilitates the opportunity for people to actively participate in defining their own care and outcomes by connecting them to the right people and the right support. There are six elements to the model, which if considered collectively, ensures a person-centred and collaborative approach to care (Wagner, 1998). The six elements are described below:

1. The healthcare system design
   - Making sure the way we deliver healthcare supports people with long-term conditions to reach their goals.
2. Self-management support
   - Where the focus is on the individual with the long-term condition recognising their central role in the management of their own condition.
3. Decision support
   - Routinely using robust evidence to inform clinical decision-making ensuring safe, effective and efficient person-centred care.

4. Delivery system design
   - Delivering integrated services to ensure continuity and seamless care.
5. Clinical information systems
   - Having electronic systems which support the care of people with long-term conditions ensuring communication of vital information and outcomes.
6. Community resources
   - Connecting all available and appropriate community resources and assets to support people with long-term conditions to live well.

The chronic care model has evolved over the years to reflect the strategic direction of healthcare, which is to embed care for people with long-term conditions within a primary care environment and in line with other initiatives such as patient safety, care coordination and cultural competency (Carrier, 2009) and, of course, integrated health and social care services.

GO FURTHER

Check out the chronic care model at www.improvingchroniccare.org/index.php?p=1:_Models&s=363
   Look at the elements and consider how this may transfer to your own primary care system.

WEBLINK:
CHRONIC
CARE

Another theoretical framework to support person-centred care for people with long-term conditions is the House of Care (Coulter et al., 2013). At the heart of this approach is person-centred conversations and collaborative care planning. Within this approach, people are encouraged to be actively involved in shaping their own care and local services have been redesigned to support this. This provides more time for the person to participate in their care planning process where the healthcare professional takes into account the strengths and assets the person has already acquired when living with their long-term condition(s). By identifying the person's goals and exploring care and support options through this collaborative discussion, care and support priorities can be identified with the plan of care coordinated around this.

GO FURTHER

Visit the following website to view the House of Care model in more detail and identify three ways in which this model can empower individuals living with long-term conditions. www.yearofcare.co.uk/house

WEBLINK:
CARE MODEL

HOW TO PROVIDE PERSON-CENTRED AND COLLABORATIVE NURSING CARE TO PEOPLE WITH LONG-TERM CONDITIONS

The role of nurses to support people with long-term conditions is well recognised. There is a plethora of evidence demonstrating improved clinical outcomes and enhanced experience of people with long-term conditions when they are supported by nurses with enhanced knowledge and skills.

Advanced practice roles for nurses are becoming increasingly common, such as advanced nurse practitioners within GP surgeries, Hospital at Home services and condition-specific nurse specialists. The common factors within these roles are leadership, the ability to undertake a comprehensive assessment, initiate investigations, diagnose and to be an independent non-medical prescriber. Added to this, are the changing expectations of a population who want to be more involved in the decisions and management of their own care and who recognise the contribution nurses have to make.

SELF-MANAGEMENT

Living with a long-term condition can significantly impact upon the individual's quality of life. As an example, Qin et al. (2015) suggest that living with arthritis can have a major negative impact upon the person's ability to participate in social activities, and to continue in paid employment.

There are a number of valuable skills and techniques health practitioners can utilise to facilitate patients' abilities to self-manage their long-term conditions. Embedding evidence-based skills in practice can support patients to engage in the behaviours necessary to optimise self-management and will create a culture where these skills can be sustained. When the focus of the patient interaction is based upon collaborative care planning and the assets or skills the patient may already have, this can help to build confidence and facilitate the sustainable behaviour change to live well with long-term conditions.

So what can nurses do to support self-management?

SEE ALSO
CHAPTER 7

- Health-promoting behaviours – nurses can help patients understand how their lifestyles such as diet, exercise and smoking can impact upon their health and their long-term condition.
- Signpost to easy-to-understand information and educational materials.
- Facilitate small achievable goals and action planning – when making lifestyle changes necessary to improve health many people sometimes fall at the first hurdle because the change they wish to make may be too great to achieve. Nurses can help people break these activities down into smaller, more achievable goals.
- Peer support – nurses can signpost patients to support organisations where they will meet others with similar conditions and circumstances.
- Provide a coaching role – people manage their own conditions most of the time; they spend very little time with healthcare professionals. Therefore, nurses should provide a coaching role – supporting and encouraging people to self-manage.
- Provide support to unpaid carers and recognise the vital role they have.

(NHS Scotland, 2009)

Recognition of the importance of self-management is essential. As a nurse you have a key role to play in ensuring people have the right knowledge, skills and support when they need it. This will enable people to develop the necessary skills and confidence to live well despite having long-term conditions. The Alliance Scotland, previously known as the Long-term conditions Alliance Scotland, has identified five key stages when people need more support to continue to self-manage. The key stages are:

1. on diagnosis
2. living for today
3. progression
4. transitions
5. end of life.

(LTCAS, 2008)

Why don't you check out the self-management resources from the King's Fund and The Health Foundation? There are also some useful films created by NHS Wales showing how self-management can help in the management of a range of conditions.

— GO FURTHER —

For more information on pocketmedic and the conditions covered in these films visit https://vimeo.com/pocketmedic/review/192491822/7ae7a50f49

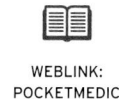

WEBLINK: POCKETMEDIC

When asked, most people will say they self-manage their long-term condition to varying degrees. For some it may be managing complex medication regimens, for others it may involve a technical skill such as administration of insulin or dialysis. They may be confident and capable in some elements of their own care but less confident in other aspects. Self-management support aims to develop the person's knowledge, skills and confidence necessary for successful self-management (Rijken at al., 2008).

HEALTH LITERACY

Health literacy refers to people's knowledge, motivation and competencies to access, understand, appraise and apply health information in order to make judgements and take decisions in everyday life concerning health care, disease prevention and health promotion to maintain or improve quality of life during the life course (WHO, 2013). Poor health literacy is known to be associated with less participation in health-promoting activities and health-screening programmes. People with poor health literacy are also known to take risks associated with their health such as smoking and lack of exercise. For those with long-term conditions this can result in poor management of their conditions which often results in frequent hospital admissions and premature death.

Shared decision-making and self-management interventions are known to be effective in building health literacy skills. Such interventions may include:

SEE ALSO CHAPTER 37

- written information in an easy-to-understand format that supplements clinical consultations
- websites, electronic information sources and virtual support aids
- training for health professionals in communication skills and the use of Teach-back
- coaching and question prompts for patients
- decision aids for patients
- self-management education programmes.

With the right skills, knowledge and confidence, people can often manage their own condition for some time with very little support from healthcare professionals. However, as they age, become frail or their circumstances become more complex, between 15% and 20% of people with a long-term condition will require more input from nurses.

CASE STUDY 18.1: MULTICULTURAL ASPECTS

Your patient has been self-managing their long-term condition for many years. However, now they are becoming frail and require your input.

- It might be easier to first consider these issues in relation to your own beliefs.
- If you have cared for a patient with different religious/cultural beliefs to you, how did their care needs differ?

(Continued)

(Continued)

Jot down your thoughts/considerations in relation to the following circumstances

Table 18.2

	Religion			
Issues	Christian	Islam	Sikh	Judaism
Illness				
Hygiene/contact				
Dietary				
Death and dying				

What have you learned from this exercise?

CONDITION MANAGEMENT AND CARE/CASE MANAGEMENT

Traditionally, services for people with long-term conditions were medically focused and designed to support people to manage the biological aspects of their condition, e.g. HbA1c for those with diabetes. However, there is now recognition of the wider consequences of ill health and the impact this can have on family, employment and mental health. With this in mind and the recognition that a large percentage of people have multiple conditions, the focus is now shifting to a more person-centred approach. For those with complex and frequently changing conditions there is evidence that a coordinated approach to care can improve clinical outcomes for the person and improve their quality of life.

The term Case Management is defined as 'a proactive approach to care focused on identifying high-risk patients and involves assessment, care planning and care co-ordination' (Ross et al., 2011, p.1). Although there has been much debate surrounding this terminology, it is clear that the aim of providing seamless care and support for people with complex health and social care needs is the shared prime objective.

WHAT'S THE EVIDENCE? 18.1

Read the paper by Ross et al. (2011) on the link below and identify three key skills of a care manager. www.kingsfund.org.uk/sites/files/kf/Case-Management-paper-The-Kings-Fund-Paper-November-2011_0.pdf

- What impact does care management have on the patient?
- How would you identify a patient for care/case management?

The core elements of care management include:

- Proactive case finding – using data and other local intelligence to identify patients at risk of hospital admission
- Assessment – a full holistic assessment involving the patient and where appropriate, the family too
- Person-centred care planning – identifying the personal outcomes in relation to care and negotiating/agreeing the actions required to achieve these
- Monitoring and review – especially where the person's condition is continually changing.

As nurses, we are considered well placed to undertake the role of care manager or care coordinator. Of the population with long-term conditions, it is thought that about 5% of people would benefit from care management due to the complex nature of their circumstances.

Care management can be influenced by a number of factors and should be considered in a local context. Services and access to resources may differ as may the health needs of the local population (Smith et al., 2013).

The concept of case/care management is a move away from the task-orientated approach to care to one that involves a change in our way of thinking, our behaviour and culture. It is a move from being reactive, from waiting until there is a crisis before intervening, to an approach which is more proactive, working with the person and their family to identify small changes in the person's condition and to have a clear action plan in place to mitigate and reduce the impact of this and perhaps avoid the need for hospital admission.

Communication with other members of the health and social care team is crucial. Frequent case discussion involving all involved in care (including the person and their family) can help clarify care and treatment strategies and the personal outcomes for the person.

CASE STUDY 18.2

The following scenario is a generic representation of a long-term condition. You will refer to other chapters for specific disorders.

Eddie Thomson, a 58-year-old man, has a long-term condition. He is married to Maggie, 56, and has two daughters ages 32 and 28, both married. His teenage son has just left school and is planning to go to university this year.

Although his condition has steadily worsened over the last number of years, he managed to work in the local factory. However, recently he has been in pain, and mobility and fatigue are becoming more problematic. His wife, a hairdresser, works part-time and increasingly does more around the home.

- Read the following short article and consider how psychosocial issues could affect everyday life in someone with a long-term condition www.nursinginpractice.com/article/managing-psychological-effects-long-term-conditions
- Compare this information with the chapters on respiratory disorder and diabetes
- It would be good to discuss these findings with your colleagues.

Eddie has been admitted to your ward with an unrelated acute illness.

On admission Eddie is anxious and frightened; he is struggling to speak so most of the information will be obtained from his wife.

- Consider six questions that you might want to ask Mrs Thomson to assess Eddie.

(Continued)

SEE ALSO
CHAPTER 24

SEE ALSO
CHAPTER 29

(Continued)

After a couple of days, Eddie's acute condition has resolved; however, he still has pain, mobility and fatigue relating to his chronic disorder.

Thinking about the following activities of living – how might you help care for Eddie in preparation for going home? You should involve other members of the interdisciplinary team.

- Mobility
- Personal hygiene
- Sleeping
- Elimination

Over the following months, Eddie's long-term condition increasingly worsens. Identify potential problems for the following activities of living and outline possible healthcare interventions.

- Work and play
- Maintaining a safe environment
- Expressing sexuality
- Eating and drinking

Eventually, Eddie becomes housebound and restricted in his activities. Consider the involvement of others and potential available resources that could help with the following activities of living.

- Eating and drinking
- Communication
- Breathing
- Dying

Would it have been helpful to anticipate some of Mr Thomson's issues earlier and have plans in place to reduce the impact?

1. Consider how the care for Mr Thomson would change if:
   - He lived on a small island
   - He did not understand English
2. How would your care relate to the NMC Code?

ANTICIPATORY CARE PLANNING

The term 'anticipatory' derives from the Latin term *anticipatus*, or *anticipare*. Anticipatory means taking action ahead of time and, more importantly, 'before it happens'.

The word is often used in the sense of *expecting* a change to occur, through prior knowledge and/or relevant information. An anticipatory plan can help to navigate this journey of preparation for change, through informed understanding and awareness of current and future health (and care) needs.

Anticipatory Care Planning (ACP) demonstrates shared decision-making through a collaborative process that involves relevant conversations between individuals and their care providers

(Department of Health, 2012). This process of meaningful discussion can also help to explore the necessary interventions that may be required for individuals to take a more active role in personal wellbeing, e.g. self-management planning. It can help to support individuals and their carers to plan ahead and be prepared, through a better understanding of health and wellbeing needs, alongside practical and realistic management approaches (Liddy et al., 2013). This unique and emerging concept underpins a shared vision and mutual understanding of the key elements that are pivotal to person-centred care. Furthermore, this demonstrates the value of personalised goals and desired outcomes.

Given the opportunity, the right time and place (whether a hospital setting or within the person's home environment), nurses should encourage people to think ahead and take this proactive lead in their care decisions. This can be achieved through early or opportunistic discussions between professionals, the person and their family. In essence, this conversation should also be about promoting health and wellbeing, preventing ill health and reducing possible crises. Such an approach is the cornerstone of the ACP process.

As nurses and student nurses we have the opportunity and privilege of getting to know our patients and their carers very well over time and we are ideally placed to ensure the right support is provided at times of need. Nurses need to be competent and confident in having ACP conversations at the right time, while supporting individuals to explore their desired outcomes. This requires a change in nursing behaviour, practice and culture. Nurses should facilitate and coach individuals to manage their own health and wellbeing, especially when they are faced with living with long-term and complex conditions.

GO FURTHER

Watch the following video on YouTube and identify three triggers for starting the ACP conversation. www.youtube.com/watch?v=gHzJ_3Z7Iwk

The ACP process has many benefits, such as being holistic, person focused and informative through the very nature of the process. This can be defined as a proactive and mutually collaborative approach. ACP also incorporates a step-by-step style that empowers individuals (and their carers) to identify early changes in their health and wellbeing, and consider what is important to the individual (Steel and Campbell, 2013). More importantly, ACP provides the toolkit for effective communication, through a person-centred dialogue that can help to establish personal choice and practical need. This key information can then be shared and communicated (with agreed consent) to those who provide care.

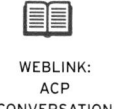

WEBLINK:
ACP
CONVERSATION

UNDERTAKING ACP WITH INDIVIDUALS AND THEIR CARERS

ACP discussions should never be undertaken as a tick box exercise. The process involves sensitive and (at times) emotive discussions, including the exploration of deeply held values and beliefs; these areas take time, and indeed patience, to develop.

Principles of ACP

Knowledge and understanding (through provision of the required information) improve when health professionals actively engage with individuals in their care, leading to better outcomes.

The principles of ACP can be categorised as follows:

- **Collaborative**: Individuals and carers are at the centre of their ACP conversations
- **Ethical**: Respect for the person's values, beliefs and preferences for care, by including what matters to them
- **Comprehensive**: Clear communication of key information (e.g. individuals or care providers involved in care or support requirements)
- **Informative communication**: Establishes a robust pathway of communication sharing (including e-sharing), which can be helpful to other colleagues, care providers or agencies involved in care. Improving individuals' understanding of their health and well being (health literacy) is essential to person-centred care models which incorporate effective communication, self-management and essentially patient safety (The Patient Rights (Scotland) Act 2011, Department of Health, 2012)
- **Self-management approach**:
  o Demonstrates the unique symptoms the person may experience and simple actions they can take to address them
  o Enables early identification of health change or health needs, and relevant interventions required to support recovery or reduce crisis
- **Personal**: Information that is important to the individual or carer
- **Relevant**: Highly important matters, e.g. Do Not Attempt Cardiopulmonary Resuscitation (DNACPR) status or Power of Attorney
- **Realistic**: Recovery goals that reflect the individual's hopes, aspirations and preferences, e.g. 'Things that I must do to keep well' or 'What is important to me and why?' Such measures may help to facilitate *hope* and encourage active participation in the ACP process
- **Carer considerate**: Enabling alternative arrangements or contingency plans in the event of the carer becoming unwell, thereby reducing the need for acute admission to hospital.

The ACP process and conversations are completely voluntary and are undertaken over time, a process that is continually evolving. Some people may not wish to engage with the relevant discussions or may experience anxiety when discussing their future care. Vocalising and anticipating such needs may challenge a person's coping styles or raise issues about their illness and their future; for some, this will address the concept of dying. These are areas that some individuals may not be ready to think about. Such challenges must always be recognised and respected during the ACP process.

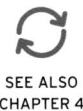

SEE ALSO CHAPTER 4

It is vitally important to consider a person's mental health capacity or ability to make particular decisions about their care and treatment. The Nursing and Midwifery Council (NMC) *Code* standards 4.2 and 4.3 underpin ethical and professional duties to ensure 'properly informed consent is gained' and that this is documented 'before carrying out any action' (NMC, 2015). The *Code* also mandates that nurses must understand 'all relevant laws about mental health capacity' which exist in 'the country of practice', to ensure that the 'rights and best interests of those who lack capacity are still at the centre of the decision-making process' (NMC, 2015).

Anticipatory Care Planning embraces the care of people *with or without capacity* to make preferred decisions relating to their future care. When a person lacks the capacity (or ability) to make such decisions, care must focus on determining their *best interests. This can be achieved through discussion with their carer(s), or those close to them* and key professional care providers.

POWER OF ATTORNEY

Power of Attorney (PoA) safeguards an individual's interests in the event that they lose the capacity to make their own decisions. In Scotland this person is referred to as 'the Granter' (www.publicguardianscotland.gov.uk, 2015). In the rest of the UK, the person giving another individual the power to act on their behalf is known as the 'Donor' (www.gov.uk/power-of-attorney).

PoA is a legal document that appoints another, specific, individual to make care decisions on behalf of the Donor or Granter. This can include paying bills, collecting pensions and other money, or dealing with other financial matters and accounts, subject to any restrictions or conditions that the Granter wishes to include.

Legal institutions in the UK (e.g. banks) recognise two main types of PoA:

- Ordinary Power of Attorney or General Power of Attorney:
    - For temporary use while the Donor/Granter is unavailable
    - Created for a set time period or for a specific purpose
    - Ends at a specified time, or at the request of the person granting PoA, or when the person granting PoA loses mental capacity
    - May be useful if a person is going abroad and requires another individual to look after their affairs in their absence
- Continuing, Lasting Power of Attorney (which replaced Enduring Power of Attorney)
    - For use when the Donor/Granter has lost the capacity to manage their own affairs (www.clickdocs.co.uk/power-of-attorney). Allows another individual to manage a person's legal, financial and health affairs should the Donor/Granter lose capacity in future
    - If the Donor or Granter is diagnosed with, or thinks they may develop, a mental illness (e.g. a degenerative brain disease leading to mental incapacity, such as Alzheimer's disease) and requires another individual to manage their financial affairs and or health and welfare, either now or in the future.
    - A PoA can only be used after it has been registered with the Office of the Public Guardian (OPG).

In Scotland, permanent PoA is referred to as 'Continuing' or 'Welfare Power of Attorney'. Elsewhere in the UK, the equivalent PoA is granted through a 'Lasting Power of Attorney'.

Laws governing PoA in the rest of the UK are different from those in Scotland, and different legal forms are used in the various areas. Broadly, PoA documentation must include a certificate signed by a suitably qualified independent person (such as a GP or a solicitor) confirming that the Donor or Granter fully understands the significance of their PoA. More importantly, there is a requirement to confirm that no undue pressure or fraud has been involved in the making of the Lasting PoA (including Continuing and Welfare).

GUARDIANSHIP AND SAFEGUARDING ORDERS

In Scotland, 'Guardianship' is a court order or appointment that authorises a person to act and make decisions on behalf of an adult with incapacity. Elsewhere in the UK, safeguarding legislation is detailed within the Care and Support Statutory Guidance Policy (www.gov.uk safeguarding policy, 2015).

Guardianship orders apply to anyone over 16 years of age and who is classed as having incapacity, e.g. not able to look after their own affairs (gov.uk safeguarding policy, 2015).

The application for guardianship is granted on the basis that it is *appropriate* and *beneficial* to the adult. Legal obligations or duties include powers that allow the guardian to look after the adult's affairs. Guardianship can be requested to deal with the adult's property and/or financial affairs and to also make decisions about their personal welfare, based on individual circumstances and conditions.

It is usual for orders to be granted for a period of 3 years, although they can be granted for a longer time, in some cases for the lifetime of the adult. Several people can be involved in the application process, including:

- family member
- carer of the adult
- professional person (solicitor, accountant, etc.)
- chief social work officer.

The guardian is also expected to fulfil administrative responsibilities as part of their legal requirements (www.publicguardian-scotland.gov.uk).

In summary, to minimise potential health and welfare dilemmas in the future, the sooner the process of ACP discussions and relevant interventions such as PoA are undertaken, the better. Planning ahead for future care and peace of mind can be important for everyone.

GO FURTHER

WEBLINK:
PATIENT
STORY

Watch the following Patient Story www.youtube.com/watch?v=GXeJKISL4kA

- Who had Power of Attorney for Alice and why?

CHAPTER SUMMARY

- Almost half the population live with a long-term condition.
- With an ageing population, multimorbidity is becoming the norm.
- Living with multiple conditions can lead to the use of many medications; this is called polypharmacy.
- Nurses have an important role in coordinating the care of people with long-term conditions.
- Nurses have a key role in supporting people to self-manage their long-term condition and ensure they have the confidence and skills necessary.
- Planning ahead and having an anticipatory care plan can improve the experience of someone living with a long-term condition and reduce the risk of unnecessary hospital admission.

GO FURTHER

Books

- http://sk.sagepub.com/books/long-term-conditions
- https://us.sagepub.com/en-us/nam/nursing-adults-with-long-term-conditions/book245376#description

FURTHER
READING:
JOURNAL
ARTICLES

Journal Articles

Go to https://study.sagepub.com/essentialadultnursing for free online journal articles related to this chapter. If you are using the interactive ebook, simply click on the book icon in the margin to go straight to the resource.

Weblinks

FURTHER
READING:
WEBLINKS

Go to https://study.sagepub.com/essentialadultnursing for further weblinks related to this chapter. If you are using the interactive ebook, simply click on the book icon in the margin to go straight to the resource.

- www.kingsfund.org.uk/projects/time-think-differently/trends-disease-and-disability-long-term-conditions-multi-morbidity
- www.myacp.scot
- www.health.org.uk/publication/enabling-people-live-well
- www.improvingchroniccare.org/index.php?p=The_Model_Talk&s=27

ACE YOUR ASSESSMENT

ONLINE
QUIZZES

Revise what you have learned by visiting https://study.sagepub.com/essentialadultnursing

- Test yourself with multiple-choice and short-answer questions
- Do the chapter activities in the book and check your answers online

REFERENCES

Allen, K. and Glasby, J. (2013) 'The billion dollar question': Embedding prevention in older people's services – 10 'high impact' changes. *British Journal of Social Work*, 43: 904–24.

Carrier, J. (2009) *Managing Long-term conditions and Chronic Illness in Primary Care. A Guide to Good Practice*. London: Routledge.

Coulter, A., Roberts, S. and Dixon, A. (2013) *Delivering Better Services for People with Long-term Conditions. Building the House of Care*. London: The King's Fund.

Dantic, D.E. (2014) A critical review of the effectiveness of 'teach-back' technique in teaching COPD patients self-management using respiratory inhalers. *Health Education Journal*, 73 (1): 41–50.

Department of Health (2012) T*he Mandate: A Mandate from the Government to the NHS Commissioning Board*: April 2013 to March 2015. [Online]. Available at: www.wp.dh.gov.uk/publications/files/2012/11/mandate.pdf

Henly, S.J., Wyman, J.F. and Findorff, M.J. (2011) Health and illness over time: The trajectory perspective in nursing science. *Nursing Research*, 60 (3) (suppl) S5–S14.

Kaufman, D.W., Kelly, J.P., Rosenberg, L., Anderson, T.E. and Mitchell, AA. (2002) Recent patterns of medication use in the ambulatory adult population of the United States: The Slone survey. *JAMA*, 287 (3): 337–44.

Liddy, C., Johnston, S. and Irving, H. (2013) The community connection model: Implementation of best evidence into practice for self-management of chronic diseases. *Public Health*, 127(6): 538–45. ISSN: 0033-3506 Available at: http://sfx-44nhss.hosted.exlibrisgroup.com/44nhss?issn=0033-3506&isbn=&volume=127&issue=6&pages=538-545&date=2013&doi=&atitle=The community connection model : implementation of best evidence into practice for self-management of chronic diseases.&aulast=Liddy, C.; Johnston, S.; Irving, H.&rft.jtitle=Public Health

Long-term Conditions Alliance Scotland (LTCAS) and Scottish Government (2008) *Gaun Yersel! The Self-management Strategy for People with Long-term Conditions in Scotland. People not Patients*. Edinburgh.

Lynch, J. and Davey Smith, G. (2005) A life course approach to chronic disease epidemiology. *Annual Review Public Health*, 26: 1–35.

Margereson, C. (2010) Trajectory and impact of long-term conditions. In Margereson, C. and Trenoweth, S. (eds) (2010) *Developing Holistic Care for Long-term Conditions*. Abingdon: Routledge.

McCorkle, R. and Pasacreta, J.V. (2001) Enhancing caregiver outcomes in palliative care. *Cancer Control*, 8 (1): 36–45.

National Prescribing Centre (2007) *A Competency Framework for Shared Decision Making with Patients. Achieving Concordance for Taking Medications*. London: Department of Health.

NHS Scotland (2009) *Long-term conditions Collaborative, Improving Self-management Support*. Edinburgh: Scottish Government.

NHS Scotland (2010) *The Healthcare Quality Strategy for NHS Scotland. Edinburgh*: Scottish Government.

NHS Scotland. Anticipatory Care Planning Booklet. Joint Improvement. Improving Lives Across Scotland. Patients, carers and practitioners speak of the impact of Anticipatory Care Planning. www.jitscotland.org.uk (Accessed July 9 2016)

Nursing and Midwifery Council (2015) *The Code: Professional standards of practice and behaviour for nurses and midwives*. Available at: www.nmc.org.uk/standards/code/

Office of Public Guardian (Scotland) www.publicguardian-scotland.gov.uk (Accessed July 8 2016)

Onder, G., Palmer, K., Navickas, R., Jureviciene, E., Mammarella, F., Strandzheva, M., Mannucci, P., Pecorelli, S. and Marengoni, A. (2015) Time to face the challenge of multi-morbidity. A European perspective from the joint action on chronic diseases and promoting healthy ageing across the life cycles (JA-CHRODIS). *European Journal of Internal Medicine*, 26 (3): 157–9.

Qin, J., Theis, K.A., Barbour, K.E., Helmick, C.G., Baker, N.A. and Brady, T.J. (2015) Impact of arthritis and multiple chronic conditions on selected life domains, United States, 2013. *Morbidity and Mortality Weekly Report*, 64 (21): 578–82.

Rijken, M., Jones, M., Heijmans, M. and Dixon, A. (2008) Supporting self-management. In E. Nolte and M. McKee (eds) *Caring for People with Chronic Conditions. A Health System Perspective*, Chapter 6. Maidenhead: McGraw Hill.

Ross S., Curry, N. and Goodwin, N. (2011) *Case management, what it is and how it can best be implemented*. London: The King's Fund.

Salisbury, C.J., Mercer, S.W. and Fortin, M. (2014) *The ABC of Multimorbidity*. Oxford: Wiley-Blackwell.

Smith, A., MacKay, S. and McCulloch, K. (2013) Case management: Developing practice through action research. *British Journal of Community Nursing*, 18 (9): 452–9.

Steel, S. and Campbell, J. (2013) *NHS Lanarkshire. Anticipatory Care Planning. Empowering, Enabling and Enhancing Care. Leading the Way to Better Health Care in Lanarkshire. Project Evaluation Report. May 2013*. Available at: www.nhslanarkshire.org.uk/.../ACP%20Project%20Evaluation%202013.pdf

Tinetti, M.E., Fried, T.R. and Boyd, C.M. (2012) Designing healthcare for the most common chronic condition – multi-morbidity. *The Journal of the American Medical Association*, 307 (23): 2493– 4.

Tseng, H., Lee, C., Chen, Y., Hsu, H., Huang, L. and Huang, J. (2016) Developing a measure of medication related quality of life for people with polypharmacy. *Quality of Life Research*, 25 (5): 1295–302.

Tuzun, H., Aycan, S. and Ilhan, M.N. (2015) Impact of co-morbidity and socioeconomic status on quality of life in patients with chronic diseases who attend primary health care centres. *Central European Journal of Public Health*, 23 (3): 188–94.

Wagner, E. (1998) Chronic disease management: What will it take to improve care for chronic illness? *Effective Clinical Practice*, 1 (1): 2–4.

Williams, A., Manias, E. and Walker, R. (2008) Interventions to improve medication adherence in people with multiple conditions: A systematic review. *Journal of Advanced Nursing*, 63 (2): 132–43.

World Health Organization (WHO) (2011) *Global status report on non communicable diseases 2010*. Geneva: WHO.

World Health Organization (WHO) (2013) Policy brief. *Where are the patients in decision making about their own care*? ISSN 1997-8073 Available at: www.euro.who.int assessed 10.07.2016

Zhang, M., Holman, C.D.A.J., Price, S.D., Sanfilipo, F.M., Preen, D.B. and Balsara, M.K. (2009) Comorbidity and repeat admission to hospital for adverse drug reactions in older adults: retrospective cohort study. *BMJ*, 338: a2752.

CARE OF THE ADULT WITH MENTAL HEALTH ISSUES

19

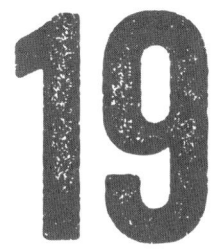

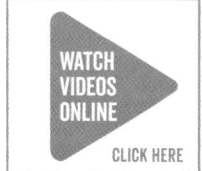

WATCH VIDEOS ONLINE — CLICK HERE

ANGELA QUIGLEY

THIS CHAPTER COVERS

- The concepts of mental health and illness
- The concept of recovery in contemporary mental health care
- An introduction to common mental health disorders
- Alcohol and substance misuse.

> On my public health placement in second year my mentor and I visited a young mother and her child who had moved into the area from another part of the country. The mother explained how she was struggling to care for her child whilst also looking for work and trying to run her house. She had no friends or family in the area and no respite from the stress she was under. She explained that she had been thinking about suicide, as she just couldn't cope with her low mood anymore. My mentor and I offered all the immediate support we could, and amongst other things, with her permission we contacted a local support group. Upon leaving the mother's mood had temporarily improved and she was thankful for our help. This experience increased my awareness of the mental health issues people face out in the community, and made me conscious of the kinds of environments I will be discharging service users back into in the future.
>
> This was particularly relevant on my following placement, where a normally very high-spirited service user developed an uncharacteristically low mood on the day of their discharge. I was aware the service user lived alone and so I asked about their feelings regarding returning home. They informed me that they had really enjoyed socialising in the ward and didn't want to return home. My mentor, the service user and myself spoke to the service user's next of kin about the issue and they agreed that other residential options needed to be explored to improve the service user's mental health. As a result of these experiences I will now make a conscious effort when discharging patients, to thoroughly asses the social environment I am discharging them back into, and consider how this may impact on their holistic health.
>
> **James Matthews, Year 2 Adult Nursing student**

INTRODUCTION

The Nursing and Midwifery Council (2014) set out the standards of competence expected for registered nurses and require that they meet the essential mental and physical needs of all those within their care, across the lifespan, regardless of which field of nursing they practice within. This means as a student nurse it is important that you have an understanding of mental health and illness, and you are able to recognise and respond to the needs of those who come into your care.

Mental and physical health are inextricably linked. Indeed, the diagnosis of an acute illness, living with long-term consequences of illness and long-term conditions, can and do have a significant impact on the mental health of the person as they seek to cope and adjust to their circumstances and manage their conditions. For example, cancer treatment is advancing and with increased survival rates more is known about the impact of the disease on the individual and the potential late and long-term effects of treatment. In terms of mental health, Macmillan (2013) estimate that there are currently around 240,000 survivors living with conditions such as anxiety, depression and post-traumatic stress disorder as well as physical health effects. This means an increased role for primary and secondary care after the initial cancer treatment.

SEE ALSO CHAPTER 22

Furthermore, the links between poor physical health and premature morbidity rates with people living with a serious mental illness are also established (Glasper, 2016). For example, the effects of anti-psychotic medication and lifestyle factors including smoking, diet and inactivity are known to increase the risk of cardiovascular disease, metabolic syndromes and respiratory conditions in people with mental illness. Therefore, in order to assess and care for a person holistically, you must consider the impact that any physical condition might be having on their mental health and vice versa.

THE CONCEPTS OF MENTAL HEALTH AND MENTAL ILLNESS

One view of mental health and illness is that they exist at either end of a continuum. This would suggest that we experience one or other at any given time across the range. However, this could be considered a simplistic and narrow view as it does not take into account the concept of mental well being. Mental wellbeing does not necessitate the absence of illness, but does embrace a more positive perspective to include the person's subjective experience, their personal and community resources, relationships and the attainment of goals. In this view, mental health and illness are seen as two different, but interdependent processes that influence one another (see Figure 19.1). From this standpoint, it is possible that a person with a diagnosis of mental illness can experience positive mental health. Taking this view creates a shift from a deficits perspective to one of resources and capabilities, and opens up possibilities for health promotion, treatment and self-management. It also acknowledges that mental health is universal and not the sole concern of those with a diagnosis of mental illness, thus reducing the 'them and us' stance, which contributes to the issue of stigma.

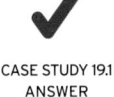

CASE STUDY 19.1 ANSWER

CASE STUDY 19.1: MIKE

My name is Mike and I am 57 years old. I have been living with a diagnosis of bipolar disorder since I was hospitalised with an episode of mania in my early 20s. Initially I found it difficult to accept this diagnosis and the effect it might have on my future. I was reluctant to use medication as it got in the way of my life, particularly when I felt well, and I did not like the side effects. Over the next ten years or so I went through cycles of both mania and depression, often resulting in hospital admissions.

Gradually I began to realise that I would need to make changes to manage my condition and stay out of hospital, which was my main goal. I have been working on my recovery ever since.

Around 10 years ago I was diagnosed with diabetes type II. I knew vaguely that I was at increased risk of physical health problems due to my mental health condition, but it was still a shock. I had been feeling very tired, dizzy and had been experiencing headaches for a while and began to think I was heading for depression. Although I was incredibly thirsty, I did not associate this with the other symptoms and put it down to the medication I was taking for bipolar disorder. I learned that this is common with other people who have mental health problems; we or others attribute any symptoms to that rather than question what else might be going on. When I did speak to my GP about this, he thankfully did investigate further and came back with my diagnosis.

Now I see my psychiatrist and diabetes specialist nurse every six months, and my GP and practice nurse when needed to help monitor and maintain my health. I work on a part-time basis which keeps me occupied and busy, I try to eat healthily and take daily exercise by walking my dog to manage my weight and blood pressure. This also helps my mood. Another important factor for me is to ensure that I get enough sleep. On a day-to-basis I generally feel well but I am aware that my health needs might change.

1. How would you describe Mike's health?
2. What factors did you take into account when doing this?
3. What else might you want to know to help you in assessing his health?

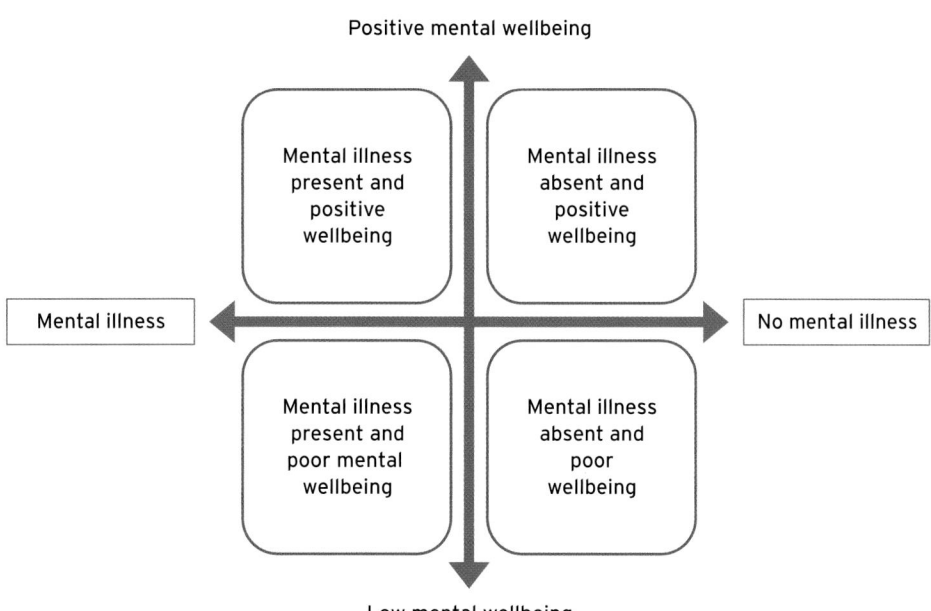

Figure 19.1 Two-continuum model of mental health

Adapted from the Scottish Government's working paper: Towards a Mentally Flourishing Scotland (2007). Reproduced under the terms of the Open Government Licence.

MODELS OF MENTAL ILLNESS

There is a diverse range of models that go some way to increase our understanding of mental illness (Box 19.1); however, no single model provides a definitive explanation. An integrated biopsychosocial approach reflects the interplay of various models and the complex nature of the development of mental health problems. A person's understanding and beliefs about how mental illness develops, for example depression, is important as not only does this influence their choices and expectations of treatment (Khalsa et al., 2011), but knowing this provides a foundation for partnership working towards the person's goals by developing a shared understanding. For example, a person with a diagnosis of irritable bowel syndrome (IBS) with co-existing anxiety may take the view that the anxiety occurred as the result of the IBS or vice versa. This knowledge may be helpful to you as a student nurse to engage the person in treatment, facilitate behaviour change and to improve self-management of the condition.

BOX 19.1: MODELS OF MENTAL ILLNESS

Biological model: Linked to medical model. Mental illness is viewed as a disease process caused primarily by physical and chemical changes that occur in the brain, and also from hereditary factors. Mental illness is identified objectively from diagnostic tests and distinguishable from other disorders by classification of consistent signs and symptoms. Treatment might involve medication or electroconvulsive therapy.

Social model: This suggests that societal influences are the predominant factor in the development of mental health problems. This perspective considers a wide range of factors in which the individual lives, for example their community, family and relationships; and how their socioeconomic status, ethnicity, culture, gender influences their mental health. It recognises how these differences can result in inequalities in health and opportunities for individuals and communities.

Cognitive model: In this model, the person's world view is determined by their thinking. In other words, it is how they interpret events and the beliefs that they hold about themselves and others as a result that influences mental health. It supposes that mental health problems occur as a result of thinking errors and biases that lead to a negative outlook.

Psychodynamic model: Emotional and mental distress is thought to be as a result of early relationships and childhood experiences which in turn affects behaviour, and largely occurs unconsciously.

Behavioural model: In this model, it is understood that a person's symptoms are as a result of maladaptive learning or conditioning. These behaviours are then maintained by a process of rewards or punishments in the environment. For example, a person experiencing anxiety in a supermarket may discover that this reduces on leaving, therefore will adopt this approach to manage future anxiety by either leaving again or avoiding going if possible.

THE CONCEPT OF RECOVERY IN MENTAL HEALTH

> People can and do recover from even the most serious mental health problems. Recovery means being able to live a good life, as defined by the person, with or without symptoms (Scottish Recovery Network, 2016).

In contrast to explanatory models of mental health and illness, recovery emerged from grassroots movements, initially in the USA in the 1950s as a response to dissatisfaction with psychiatry, de-institutionalisation, and the consumer/survivor movements. Service users who had previously been stigmatised and excluded were finding their voice, sharing their narratives and reclaiming their identities and rights as citizens outwith services. Emerging evidence from longitudinal studies revealing that people did recover from schizophrenia strengthened this view. This was counter to the dominant view that many mental illnesses had a chronic and degenerative trajectory. Recovery in this context is not an explanatory model, nor is it about cure. Recovery is a process that is unique to the person, and enables them to live a life in which they are satisfied and are able to contribute to society. People tend to see recovery as a lifelong journey of growing and learning, managing setbacks and celebrating successes, rather than just an end point.

Recovery is now a prominent and influential force in policy making, service delivery and treatment approaches and is coherent with human rights approaches, values-based practice, asset-based approaches and person-centred care rather than the traditional treat and cure model of healthcare. Recovery orientated services and practice are about facilitating and enabling the process of recovery. In working in a recovery-focused way, the nurse's relationship and role here is to travel alongside the person offering support and guidance ensuring control remains with the person and enabling them to take the lead in their care.

ACTIVITY 19.1: REFLECTIVE PRACTICE

Take a few moments to reflect on a recent care experience where you have been involved in caring for a person with a long-term condition.

1. How did you or could you have found out what was important to the person in working together?
2. In what ways did you enable the person or could have enabled the person to take the lead in their own care?
3. How did you or could you have found out about the person's strengths and resources; and how did you or could you have included these in the care plan?

ACTIVITY 19.1
ANSWER

The key elements of recovery include hope, meaning and purpose, control and choice, self-management, risk taking and the importance of relationships. Leamy et al. (2011) offer a conceptual framework of people's experience of recovery resulting in the acronym of CHIME (connectedness, hope, identity, meaning and empowerment) that capture these key components and provides an empirical basis for further research and practice in this area. The following link provides practical guidance in regard to recovery: www.scottishrecovery.net/what-helps/

CASE STUDY 19.2: PETER

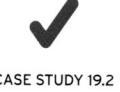

CASE STUDY 19.2
ANSWER

Peter is a 25-year-old man who was admitted to an acute ward with a chest infection. He has a diagnosis of Crohn's disease. His condition has led to frequent admissions to hospital throughout his adult life. He has been unemployed since leaving school and spends most of his time at home. When able to go out he spends his time with friends at the pub. He has no contact with family as he has been an accommodated child brought up in care due to the family's addiction issues. He has not been in touch with his friends since his admission as he is very private and does not want them to know about his health problems.

(Continued)

(Continued)

Peter spends most of his time in the ward reading. Although allowed to leave the ward for short periods to go to the hospital shop or café he rarely does so. The ward staff have given him information on useful websites and contacts he can make. They have also given him information about the activities he could be involved in within the community, but Peter appears disinterested and all he wants is to be allowed to go home and be by himself.

1. What impact does nursing people who have lost hope have on you?
2. How might this impact on the person you are caring for?
3. If you were one of the staff involved in Peter's care, how might you engage with him in a way that would inspire hope?

Summary of key points:

- Mental health and physical health are inextricably linked.
- Mental health includes the concept of mental wellbeing and illness, and they are not mutually exclusive. We all have mental health.
- Explanatory models of mental health may be helpful in assisting a person gain an understanding of how their problems developed.
- Recovery enables the person and others to take a more holistic perspective and focus on living well rather than focusing on illness.

AN INTRODUCTION TO COMMON MENTAL HEALTH DISORDERS

The following is intended to give you a brief overview of the more common mental health disorders that a person may present with while in your care.

Mood disorders

Mood disorder is a general term to describe a state of health where the predominant mood is viewed as distorted or inappropriate. Mood disorders can be understood as occurring across a spectrum, ranging from mild, moderate to severe and can happen across the lifespan. The change to mood is usually accompanied by a change in the overall level of activity, for example in depression it is likely that there will be a reduction in activity levels as opposed to an elated mood which will generally see a significant increase in activity.

Depression

Depression is the leading cause of disability worldwide (WHO, 2017) and is often accompanied by anxiety. There is disruption to the person's functioning and ability to take care of their everyday responsibilities to varying degrees, dependent on the severity of the illness. Depression is treatable but often goes unrecognised and undiagnosed, and can become chronic or recurrent. To receive a diagnosis, the person will present with low mood and a loss of pleasure in activities occurring for at least a two-week period (NICE, 2007). There is a range of accompanying symptoms including:

- disturbed sleep
- decreased or increased appetite and or weight
- fatigue or loss of energy
- agitation or slowing of movements
- poor concentration or indecisiveness
- feelings of worthlessness or excessive or inappropriate guilt
- suicidal thoughts or acts.

WHAT'S THE EVIDENCE 19.1?

Access NICE guidelines [CG90] on www.nice.org.uk/guidance/CG90 related to recognition and management of depression in adults and answer the following questions:

- What might alert you to the possibility of depression in someone you have been caring for and what might the barriers to recognising and identifying depression be? Consider as many factors as possible.
- Find out what two questions you could ask if you suspect a person may be experiencing depression.
- If you gain an affirmative response, what would be your next step or steps?

You will also find guidance here on the stepped care model to treating depression.

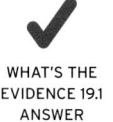

WHAT'S THE
EVIDENCE 19.1
ANSWER

Depression in people with long-term physical health conditions is common due to pain, functional impairment and disability. These co-occurring conditions are likely to exacerbate symptoms of both, which impacts to the detriment of the person's overall quality of life. There can be difficulties in recognising depression in this group as there is sometimes an overlap in the symptoms meaning this is missed, or symptoms appear sub-threshold or mild so go unrecognised and untreated. Recognition is key to ensuring that the person's health is maximised and they are able to access the right treatment.

Anxiety

Anxiety is a functional response to threatening situations. When a person perceives danger the body's flight or fight response is activated: this is an automatic physiological response that is about safety and survival. It is normal to experience some anxiety when, for example, facing an exam, going into a new social situation or interview or when dealing with life stressors. Indeed, anxiety in these situations can be useful as it can heighten awareness and sharpen responses in order to manage these situations. However, when this response is overly sensitive and the person becomes anxious without any obvious threat, then this can be intolerable. It has the effect of interfering with the person's functioning on a day-to-day basis and causes distress. This could be considered as an anxiety disorder. Table 19.1 provides a brief overview of some anxiety-related conditions.

Table 19.1 Brief overview of anxiety-related conditions

Panic Disorder – the person will experience frequent panic attacks, often without an obvious cause. The onset of these panic attacks is sudden, and the person experiences frightening and overwhelming physical and psychological symptoms including palpitations, nausea, sweating and trembling. This is accompanied by feelings of apprehension and dread.

Phobias – the person experiences an extreme or irrational fear of an object, event, place or animal. Common phobias are around flying in an aeroplane, riding in a lift or fear of spiders.

Post Traumatic Stress Disorder (PTSD) – the person will experience severe and distressing physical and psychological symptoms, including anxiety, flashbacks (where the person re-experiences the events), nightmares and intrusive thoughts in relation to a traumatic event or events, and dissociative states (a feeling of being switched off or disconnected from reality). Potential causes may include childhood sexual abuse and witnessing or being subjected to violence. Trauma is complex and what one person may view as traumatic, another may not.

Obsessive Compulsive Disorder (OCD) – the person may experience obsessive thoughts which cause significant distress and intolerable discomfort. The person is then compelled to carry out a behaviour or mental ritual to alleviate this distress and may believe that should they resist there would be catastrophic consequences.

Generalised Anxiety Disorder (GAD) – the person experiences symptoms of anxiety around a wide range of situations rather than related to one specific event. The person experiences worry, restlessness, poor concentration, irritability and difficulties with sleeping. Accompanying physical symptoms include headache, dizziness and muscle tension; as well as the acute symptoms of anxiety such as sweating, palpitations, trembling and shaking.

As well as the physiological response of anxiety, the person also experiences psychological changes; for example, pervasive worry and unhelpful thinking patterns and changes to behaviour. The person may adopt safety or avoidance behaviours intended to reduce feelings of anxiety but this often only adds to the maintenance of anxiety. Please refer to Box 19.2 for a descriptive example. The treatment of anxiety disorders usually focuses on breaking these cycles using a cognitive behavioural approach.

BOX 19.2: DESCRIPTIVE EXAMPLE OF ANXIETY

Peter aged 25 is experiencing anxiety. His increased vulnerability may be due to family and social factors (refer to Activity 19.3) and physical health condition (IBS). Peter worries when out about regarding access to toilets and eating in public. He fears that he may have 'an accident' and soil himself in public, despite this never having happened before. When Peter is out, he is in a state of hyper-vigilance (increased watchfulness), which means he is more sensitive to normal bodily experiences and symptoms of anxiety. He is therefore more likely to misinterpret and attribute these sensations as an urgent need to go to the toilet, thus increasing anxieties.

In an effort to manage these intense and distressing feelings, Peter uses a number of strategies to cope. Although these do temporarily reduce his anxiety, in the long term, they serve to maintain or increase anxiety as he is not given the opportunity to test his fears and prove them unfounded. These strategies include avoidance (not going out at all) and safety behaviours (planning outings around toilets, particular times, and using antidiarroheal medication). Peter then attributes not soiling himself to the strategies he has employed, thus maintaining the fear.

WHAT'S THE EVIDENCE? 19.2

In anxiety a stepped care approach is recommended for GAD according to NICE (2011a). Step one suggests that following identification and assessment, low intensity psychological intervention is recommended. Commonly this includes non-facilitated and guided self-help approaches or psycho-educational groups aimed at overcoming anxiety using an evidence-based approach, typically based on cognitive behavioural principles. Please take some time to find out where you would access evidence-based programmes locally.

Bipolar disorder

Bipolar disorder is characterised by repeated episodes in which the person's mood and activity levels are significantly disturbed, with on some occasions, an elevation of mood and increased energy and activity (mania) and on others a lowering of mood, decreased energy and activity (depression). This can occur with or without psychotic features in either a depressive or manic phase, but thoughts are typically coherent with the presenting mood. For example, when a person is severely depressed, they may experience delusional thoughts featuring guilt or loss and believe themselves responsible for some terrible event. Conversely, when the mood is elevated, the person may believe themselves to have special powers, express grandiose plans or have ideas that they have some special status.

There are two main types of bipolar disorder: types I and II. Bipolar II has hypomania as a feature; this can sometimes go unrecognised with some individuals and the cause for the change in behaviour being attributed to something else, for example if the person is drinking or using drugs, which is common to this condition. Additionally, the person experiencing this state may not view it as a problem as they may enjoy the feeling of energy and elation, and the sense of productivity. However, delays in diagnosis and treatment are likely to have a detrimental effect on the person's relationships, employment and functioning. The person will also experience episodes of depression.

Hypomania symptoms include:

- increased activity and talkativeness
- difficulty in concentration
- decreased need for sleep
- increased sexual activity
- mild overspending or other types of reckless behaviour
- overfamiliarity.

In mania, the symptoms are similar but significantly more prominent and severe causing disruption to functioning relationships, and displaying delusional and expansive thinking. The person may present as aggressive and hostile, particularly if they feel limited by others. Mania almost always requires hospital admission and management as the person is likely to be vulnerable, at risk of harm or exploitation and neglect with loss of self-care including eating, drinking, sleep and hygiene needs. As healthcare professionals we need to consider safeguarding principles, policy and legislation to ensure that the person is safe and has their rights protected.

The following link provides some useful information to increase understanding with regard to bipolar disorder: www.time-to-change.org.uk/category/blog/bipolar

In summary, these are among the most common mood and anxiety disorders that impact on the mental health of the adult population, and it is important as a student nurse that you are able to recognise these in the people you care for. This provides the basis for a conversation around the person's holistic health needs.

Psychosis

Psychosis is a state in which the person experiences a disconnection from reality. The onset, severity and duration of the symptoms experienced by the person, how they perceive, interpret and respond to them, and the impact that it has on functioning determines to an extent whether there is deemed to be a psychotic disorder. Psychotic disorders include schizophrenia, delusional disorders, schizoaffective disorder and brief psychotic disorder. Other presentations of psychosis may be related to mood disorders as previously stated, related to trauma, induced by alcohol or drugs or could be related to a physical cause, for example a brain tumour. Psychosis affects around 3 in 100 people; for some this will be one episode in a lifetime, and for others they may experience a reoccurrence. For approximately 1%, they will go on to have a diagnosis of schizophrenia.

The most common and recognisable symptoms associated with schizophrenia are delusions in which the person may hold a strange belief; and hallucinations, in which they may hear voices, see, feel or smell something that others do not. Within a medical model, these are often classified as positive symptoms (Table 19.2). It is important to note that these experiences are within the realms of normal human experience and not in themselves indicative of psychosis as around quarter of the population have heard voices or held suspicious thoughts. Schizophrenia is also associated with other symptoms including low mood, decreased energy and motivation and disturbances in sleep, which can adversely impact on the functioning of the person. These are commonly referred to as negative symptoms (Table 19.2).

Table 19.2 Positive and negative symptoms associated with schizophrenia

Positive symptoms – distortions of normal functioning
Hallucinations
Delusions
Thought Disorder

Negative symptoms – loss of normal functioning
Loss of **volition**
Poverty of thought and speech

Mental health conditions, particularly schizophrenia and bipolar disorder, carry significant risk of physical health issues, including cardiovascular disease, metabolic syndromes, and sexual health and blood disorders. The reasons for this are complex socio-political factors including: exclusion and stigma which leads to reduced choices and access; treatment factors, for example medication used to treat the disorder can be harmful and have long-term effects; and factors related to the condition that contribute to an unhealthy lifestyle, for example smoking and lack of exercise. Compared with the general population, people with these serious mental health conditions have a reduced life expectancy by approximately 10 years, making this a group who experience significant health inequalities.

CASE STUDY 19.3: JOHN

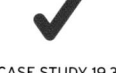

CASE STUDY 19.3
ANSWER

You are currently on placement in an A&E department when you see a man, John, waiting to be seen. He is on his own and looks unkempt in appearance. You notice that he is talking to himself, looks a little distressed and is making odd movements. His arms and legs are jerky. He is tucked in the corner of the waiting area: he appears to be avoiding others and they him. You see on his records that he has a diagnosis of schizophrenia.

1. If you were one of the staff involved in John's care, how might you engage with him in a way that would provide a safe and secure environment for him and others?
2. What impact could John's psychosis have on him, what symptoms could he be experiencing and how can they be managed?
3. What impact could John's psychosis have on the department you are working in?

GO FURTHER

www.ted.com/talks/eleanor_longden_the_voices_in_my_head This link takes you to a TED talk of a personal experience of voice hearing that challenges conventional assumptions about psychosis.

WEBLINK:
TED TALK

PERINATAL MENTAL HEALTH

Largely considered a happy event in society, pregnancy and childbirth entails many changes for a woman; for example, to her body as the pregnancy progresses, during childbirth and adjusting to the new role of being a mother with the increased responsibility and changing relationships with partners and other family members. It is thought around one in five women experience mental health problems during pregnancy and the following year. While for some this may be due to an existing mental condition or previous condition, for others it is this life event that precedes the problem and pregnancy is the single highest risk period for the onset of mental health problems in women generally. Although all women have a potential risk, life stressors, particularly complex and cumulative social factors, for example domestic violence, substance misuse and previous problems in pregnancy increase vulnerability.

Perinatal mental health (PMH) refers to the mental health of women during pregnancy and up to one year postpartum. Specialist PMH services are concerned with prevention, identification and treatment of mental health problems within this population; however, as a student nurse it is essential that you develop awareness of this important aspect of health care.

Three years ago today I knew there was something wrong with me. I didn't know what it was but I felt I was on a very fast downward spiral to a very dark place. Little did I know what a journey I would go through? Scared I wouldn't be my normal self again. I was told I wouldn't be the same person again. I would be stronger. I didn't believe them at the time but these words were true. I've got through an extremely challenging time.

Sally Tyrrell, founder of Lanarkshire postnatal support and awareness,
www.facebook.com/groups/LanarkshirePostNatalDepressionSupportandAwar

The following podcast link provides an insight into postnatal depression: www.rcpsych.ac.uk/default.aspx?page=13589

The consequences of untreated mental health problems can have a devastating impact on the woman and her family, and are linked to family breakdown, depression in partners, developmental issues in children and not least, maternal death. Deaths from mental health disorders are commonly by suicide, and predominately occur between 6 weeks and the first year postpartum, accounting for the largest proportion of deaths in women during this period. Despite a downward trend in overall maternal deaths for physical causes, those related to mental health within the United Kingdom remain unchanged since 2003 making this an area of priority (Knight et al., 2015).

As a student nurse, it is likely that you will be in contact with women, infants and families during the perinatal period while on placement with health visitors. Recognising that this may be a particularly vulnerable time in a woman's life, and being able to identify her emotional and mental health needs and communicating this as early as possible, are key to ensuring the appropriate support, treatment and services are put in place. It may be helpful for you while on placement to discuss this with your mentor and find out about what the local joint working policies and guidelines are for PMH.

The following are red flag signs, which are from some of the lessons learned from the MBRRACE-UK report (Knight et al., 2015), which may be indicative of more urgent intervention. Should you recognise these in the women you see, they must immediately be referred to the specialist PMH team for urgent assessment.

- New thoughts of violent self-harm
- Sudden onset or rapidly worsening mental symptoms
- Persistent feelings of estrangement from their baby.

It is important that these signs are followed up and not dismissed or minimised.

> As a mental health nurse I am aware of the stigma a lot of families feel around mental health during the perinatal period. Fear of their baby being removed from them or being judged as an unfit mother can lead to women not disclosing that they are having difficulty. Spending time with them to explore attitudes to emotional difficulties can assist in identification of potential illness and the value of intervening early to reduce risk of deteriorating mental health whilst improving outcomes of a mother, her child and her family.
>
> Liz, RMN

Attachment describes the quality of the relationship between parent and child, which has a profound effect on an infant's early development. Maternal mental illness can negatively impact the mother–infant attachment as she may be unable to respond to and meet the needs of the infant. A secure attachment, in which the infant feels safe and secure, fosters healthy growth and development in the child; whereas inconsistent and unresponsive patterns of attachment lead to anxiety and ambivalence in the child which impacts on their ability to experience, regulate and express their emotions and form and maintain relationships into adult life. Although the focus of this book is the care of adults, it is important to recognise that all nurses have a responsibility for the welfare and safeguarding of children. Where there is concern about the welfare of the child, and difficulty engaging with the woman, it is important that this information is shared in accordance with local guidelines. Early intervention improves outcomes for both mother and infant during this crucial stage.

Summary of key points:

- Depression is the leading cause of disability worldwide and those with long-term physical and mental conditions are at increased risk.
- Mental health disorders are treatable, and early identification improves outcomes for the person and their families.
- Pregnancy and childbirth carries increased vulnerability for women and their mental health, and the consequences of going unrecognised can be devastating.

SEE ALSO CHAPTER 4

SELF-HARM AND SUICIDE

Self-harm is not a clinical diagnosis but is a description of behaviour that commonly, but not exclusively, includes cutting, burning or poisoning by taking medication. Historically, self-harm has also been linked to attempted suicide although current thinking recognises that the act of self-harm is often not intended to end life. Nevertheless, there is an increased risk that people who self-harm are more likely to die of suicide, highlighting that self-harm is dangerous and should not be minimised regardless of what is perceived to be the intent.

Self-harm can be difficult to understand and some perceptions of self-harm are unhelpful. They convey negative stereotypes, framing the person as an attention seeker, or the behaviour as a 'cry for help', or an attempt to manipulate others which leaves the person feeling stigmatised. This, coupled with the notion that people seeking help for their injuries are time wasting and using valuable resources that could be directed to people who have not caused themselves harm, can sometimes generate poor responses in others, including nurses (Karman et al., 2015). People who have self-harmed and sought treatment report sometimes judgemental attitudes and punitive approaches to their treatment from staff; for example, no offer of anaesthetic prior to stitching which results in further pain, a negative care experience and further distress. It is important to note that a person who self-harms does not enjoy pain and does feel the pain acutely, and that unhelpful responses may contribute to further self-harming.

However, in seeking to understand self-harm from the person's perspective, Tofthagen and Fagerstrøm (2010) propose that it is a mechanism in which mental pain is expressed by infliction of physical pain as a method of alleviating distress. Although self-harm is associated with a range of mental health disorders, it is not always related to mental illness and can be as a result of various psychosocial stressors, including relationship difficulties, bullying and trauma. Where it is related to mental illness, this should be treated. Self-harm can be the person's way of coping, and stopping this without having another way of coping is extremely difficult.

Below, you will find suggestions about how to help someone who presents with self-harm; however, it is important that you work within the scope of your role and ensure that the person has a full psychosocial assessment (Box 19.3)

BOX 19.3: SUGGESTIONS FOR WORKING WITH PEOPLE WHO SELF-HARM

- Listen, learn and understand what has led to the self-harm from the person's perspective without judgement and with compassion. Do not assume that it is for the same reason as before if they are already known to you.
- Acknowledge and validate the distress the person is experiencing, and help them describe the emotions attached (in their words) – demonstrate empathy.

(Continued)

(Continued)

- Ask the person what they would like help with.
- Reduce/minimise harm – adopt a collaborative approach, provide unbiased information to the person regarding risks, assist the person to think about minimising risk of harm, injury and prevent death.
- Provide information/education on how to manage wounds and when to seek help.
- Help them to recognise the triggers to self-harm: what are the first signs that they are feeling distressed, pressured, numb, and/or angry? Be patient – this may take time.
- Help the person identify alternatives to self-harm that are acceptable and useful to them – match to the emotion, get creative! What are their current strengths, supports, and helpful ways of coping, problem-solving strategies? What other resources are out there? Signpost them to services and self-help resources.
- Remember recovery can take time and setbacks are not uncommon.

Suicide is a complex issue, often closely linked with mental illness but also with significant personal factors that lead the person to the final step of taking their own life. For every death by suicide the consequences are far reaching within the family, community and beyond. The Samaritans have collated national figures and report that 6,581 people in the United Kingdom and the Republic of Ireland took their own life in 2014 (Scowcroft, 2016). Despite targeted strategies across the UK (HM Government, 2012; Department of Health, Social Services and Public Safety, 2012; Scottish Government, 2013; and Welsh Government, 2015) aimed at preventative measures, such as training the workforce, supporting people in distress, raising awareness in communities and reducing stigma and taboos; suicide rates are still variable and are not following a consistent downward trend in all sections of society. Further research is required to evaluate what is working and what is not in the drives to reduce suicide at strategic and operational levels, for example, what interventions are effective and for whom in order to reduce suicide rates (Kutcher and Wei, 2016). However, what is known is that the problem cannot be tackled by a single agency, the consequences of suicide are devastating and that anyone seeking help should be taken seriously, and treated with compassion, dignity and respect.

ALCOHOL AND SUBSTANCE MISUSE

As a student nurse, you are very likely to encounter people who experience alcohol and substance misuse issues in every healthcare setting, sometimes unknowingly. In England alone in 2014/15, 1.1 million hospital admissions were related to alcohol disease and just under a fifth of these were for mental and behavioural disorders, second only to cardiovascular disease (Health and Social Care Information Centre, 2016). In Scotland, there were 7,054 drug-related admissions to acute general hospitals and 1,451 in patient mental health admissions (ISDS, 2015).

However, this problem goes beyond health as the wider societal effects of alcohol and substance misuse includes loss of functioning and productivity, for example parenting, caring and work responsibilities; aggression, conduct, criminality and legal problems; and interpersonal and relationship problems. Many people do not seek help from health or social services for a variety of reasons including stigma, exclusion and shame, and concern around consequences of their drug and alcohol misuse and what that might mean. For example, involvement of police, social services or loss of job or home; and for some the nature of their problem means that getting their next drug becomes their priority leaving little time for anything else. The problem is vast and requires coordinated strategic and operational multi-agency and disciplinary approaches to address these issues. As future registered nurses, it is important to make the most of every healthcare encounter and act in a way that is respectful and promotes health and recovery, to take a holistic perspective and to recognise that the person is likely to have multiple needs that also need to be addressed.

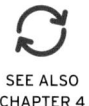

SEE ALSO
CHAPTER 4

Alcohol misuse can be defined as:

- Harmful drinking – a pattern of drinking that directly causes problems to health, including physical and psychological issues and accidents.
- Alcohol dependence – craving, tolerance, a pre-occupation with alcohol and continued drinking regardless of the harmful consequences.

NICE (2011b) clinical guidance states that healthcare professionals working within all areas are able to identify and assess the need for intervention in relation to alcohol misuse.

ACTIVITY 19.2: HEALTH PROMOTION

ACTIVITY 19.2
ANSWER

You are in placement with the practice nurse at a GP surgery, and you see Margaret, a 52-year-old woman who is having her blood pressure monitored and also has back and joint pain. During the appointment she tells you that she has some difficulty sleeping and feels low in mood at times. During the conversation with her she tells you that she will sometimes have a few glasses of wine in the evening to help with her sleep but does not appear to view this as a problem. She is also taking medication for pain.

- What are the opportunities for health promotion here?
- Which area will you focus on and why?

Substance misuse is a broad term that includes the misuse of legal and illegal drugs, including alcohol and prescribed drugs, that is problematic and causes damage to health. According to WHO (2012), of the illegal drugs used in Europe, cannabis is most common followed by cocaine, amfetamine-type stimulants and opioids including heroin. They also report worldwide gender differences in drug misuse with greater numbers of young men having problematic patterns and dependency issues, except in the illicit use of tranquilizers and sedatives where women significantly exceed this. Novel psychoactive substances or so-called 'legal highs' have also gained specific attention due to the increased risks with the name of the product giving no suggestion of what it contains, variable potency and harm, including toxicity, and the typical age of the users being young (Advisory Council on the Misuse of Drugs, 2011).

GO FURTHER

If you are interested in exploring trends, the World drug report by WHO (2012) provides information related to trafficking, production, consumption and consequence of drug misuse from a global perspective. It can be found by following this link: www.unodc.org/documents/data-and-analysis/WDR2012/WDR_2012_web_small.pdf

WEBLINKS

Patterns of use range from recreational to dependency, with some people having a preference for one drug, and others the use of more than one substance, sometimes to counter or enhance the effects of another drug (commonly referred to as polydrug misuse). In terms of health the consequences of the misuse of drugs are significant. The following link provides an accessible overview of these effects: www.drugabuse.gov/related-topics/health-consequences-drug-misuse

ACTIVITY 19.3 ANSWER

ACTIVITY 19.3: REFLECTION

1. Make a list of all of the stereotypes, judgements and labels you can think of related to people who misuse drugs, even if they are not your own views.
2. Consider the impact this might have on the person as broadly as you can.
3. Consider how you can challenge this stigma and discrimination in your everyday life and work – make a list.
4. Finally, consider what difference this might make to you, your colleagues and most importantly the person with a drug misuse problem.

CO-EXISTING SEVERE MENTAL ILLNESS AND SUBSTANCE MISUSE

There is an established inter-relationship between mental health and substance misuse issues, and the co-existence of both (also referred to as dual diagnosis) is thought to occur in a third of people with mental health disorders. This is a complex issue as the person is likely to experience multiple disadvantages, and present with multifactorial needs. Outcomes for this population tend to be poorer in terms of health, relationships and economic costs; treatment is more complex with a lack of specialist or integrated services available and low levels of optimism from healthcare professionals regarding the person's ability and willingness to engage in treatment. This population group often experience poor attitudes and stigma in healthcare settings from staff.

There are various ways of understanding the development of co-existence. For instance, it could be considered that the primary mental health disorder leaves the person more vulnerable to developing an alcohol or substance misuse issue; for example, by attempting to control, alleviate or escape distressing or difficult to manage symptoms. Or, the use of alcohol or drugs triggers the mental health disorder perhaps because of the mode of action of the alcohol or drug. Nevertheless, no matter what our understanding, a person with these co-existing conditions will have complex needs that require to be addressed holistically in order to improve outcomes and reduce risk of relapse in future. This calls for an integrated and coordinated approach that addresses mental and physical health needs, with housing and other social needs, including benefits.

PREPARATION FOR PRACTICE PLACEMENTS 19.1

As already stated, we all have mental health needs and in order to make sure that we can meet the needs of others, it is important that we are self-aware and look after our own mental health. Prior to going to your next practice placement, take some time to think about what you need to maintain and improve your own mental health. For example, walking the dog and seeing my friends. Write this down. Think about what gets in the way of this for you. For example, time factors such as deadlines for assignments. Write it down. What do you first notice when you are not quite feeling on top of things? For example, comfort eating, feeling a bit irritable. Write it down. Think about the ways you might be able to overcome this and who supports you to do this. For example, prioritising exercise or family or buddying-up for activities. Write it down. Finally, there is evidence to suggest that particular things have been shown to improve mental health including connecting with others, being active, learning, giving to others and being mindful www.nhs.uk/Conditions/stress-anxiety-depression/Pages/improve-mental-wellbeing.aspx. Think about how this information might be of use to you in your next placement.

CHAPTER SUMMARY

- Mental health and physical health are inextricably linked and these co-morbidities lead to poorer outcomes for the person.
- Recovery in mental health means living a meaningful life as defined by the person in the presence or absence of illness.
- Knowledge and the ability to identify mental health and substance misuse problems early leads to a more holistic approach to care and improved access to treatment.
- Recovery-focused care and person-centred care principles are complementary and essential in the care of people with mental health and substance misuse issues.
- Integrated and coordinated care with other professionals and agencies is vital in meeting the complex needs of this client group.

GO FURTHER

Go to https://study.sagepub.com/essentialadultnursing for a further case study related to this chapter. If you are using the interactive ebook, simply click on the book icon in the margin to go straight to the resource.

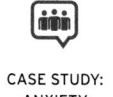

CASE STUDY:
ANXIETY

Books

- Norman, I. and Ryrie, I. (2017) *The Art and Science of Mental Health Nursing: Principles and Practice* (4th ed). London: Open University Press.
  This is a comprehensive text for mental health nurses, students and any healthcare professional interested in working with people with mental health issues.
- Morrisey, J. and Callaghan, P. (2011) *Communication Skills for Mental Health Nursing*. New York: Open University Press.
  This book is aimed at improving communication skills that are useful in nursing practice.

- Nash, M. (2014) *Physical Health and Well-being in Mental Health Nursing.* New York: Open University Press.
  This book looks at the physical health concerns of people with mental health conditions. Although aimed a mental health nurses, it is applicable to adult nurses too.

Journal Articles

FURTHER READING: JOURNAL ARTICLES

Go to https://study.sagepub.com/essentialadultnursing for further free online journal articles related to this chapter. If you are using the interactive ebook, simply click on the book icon in the margin to go straight to the resource.

- Dury, R. (2016) COPD and emotional distress: Not always noticed and therefore untreated. *British Journal Of Community Nursing*, 21(3): 138–41. This article highlights the issue of under-diagnosis of mental health issues in the long-term condition COPD.

The following two journal articles provide practical examples of how nurses within the adult field provide care for people with mental and physical health needs.

- Hardy, S. (2015) Mindfulness: Enhancing physical and mental wellbeing. *Practice Nursing*, 26(9): 450–3.
- Shuttlewood, E., Wignal, A., Wijesundare, S. and Gable, D. (2015) Caring for people with physical and mental health needs: A case example from a diabetes service. *Journal Of Diabetes Nursing*, 19 (8): 309–13.

Weblinks

FURTHER READING: WEBLINKS

Go to https://study.sagepub.com/essentialadultnursing for further weblinks related to this chapter. If you are using the interactive ebook, simply click on the book icon in the margin to go straight to the resource.

- www.brief-encounters.org/introduction/ This website is an excellent resource, with practical advice aimed at assisting nurses to develop relationships with individuals who are emotionally vulnerable.
- www.mentalhealth.org.uk/ This is a good resource that provides a wealth of resources including mental health promotion for you, and to signpost others to research and policy information and contemporary mental health issues.
- www.nationalelfservice.net/mental-health/ This website contains blogs which can help you to keep up to date with important and reliable mental health research and guidance. Evidence based and accessible.

ONLINE QUIZZES

ACE YOUR ASSESSMENT

Revise what you have learned by visiting https://study.sagepub.com/essentialadultnursing

- Test yourself with multiple-choice and short-answer questions
- Do the chapter activities in the book and check your answers online

REFERENCES

Advisory Council on the Misuse of Drugs (2011) *Consideration of the Novel Psychoactive Substances ('Legal Highs').* London: Home Office.

Department of Health, Social Services and Public Safety (2012) *Protect Life: A Shared Vision. The Northern Ireland Suicide Prevention Strategy.* Belfast: Department of Health, Social Services and Public Safety. (www.dhsspsni.gov.uk)

Glasper, A. (2016) Improving the physical health of people with mental health problems. *British Journal of Nursing*, 25 (12): 696–7.

Health & Social Care Information Centre (2016) *Statistics on Alcohol*. Available at: http://content. digital.nhs.uk/catalogue/PUB20999/alc-eng-2016-rep.pdf

HM Government (2012) *Preventing Suicide in England. A cross government strategy to save lives*. London: Department of Health.

Information Services Division Scotland (ISDS) (2015) *Drug-Related Hospital Statistics Scotland 2014/15*. Available at: www.isdscotland.org/Health-Topics/Drugs-and-Alcohol-Misuse/Publications/2015-10-13/2015-10-13-DrugHospitalStatistics-Report.pdf

Karman, P., Kool, N., Poslawsky, I.E. and Meijel, B. (2015) Nurses' attitudes towards self-harm: a literature review. *Journal of Psychiatric and Mental Health Nursing*, 22: 65–75.

Khalsa, S., McCarthy, K.S., Sharpless, B.A., Barrett, M.S. and Barber, J.P. (2011) Beliefs about the causes of depression and treatment preferences. *Journal of Clinical Psychology*, 67: 539–49.

Knight, M., Tuffnell, D., Kenyon, S., Shakespeare, J., Gray, R. and Kurinczuk, J.J. (eds) on behalf of MBRRACE-UK (2015) *Saving Lives, Improving Mothers' Care – Surveillance of maternal deaths in the UK 2011–13 and lessons learned to inform maternity care from the UK and Ireland Confidential Enquiries into Maternal Deaths and Morbidity 2009 -13*. Oxford: National Perinatal Epidemiology Unit, University of Oxford.

Kutcher, S. and Wei, Y. (2016) *The vexing challenge of suicide prevention: research informed perspective on a recent systematic review*. Available at: www.nationalelfservice.net/mental-health/suicide/vexing-challenge-suicide-prevention-research-informed-perspective-recent-systematic-review/

Leamy, M., Bird, V., Le Boutillier, C., Williams, J. and Slade, M. (2011) Conceptual framework for personal recovery in mental health: Systematic review and narrative synthesis. *The British Journal of Psychiatry*, 199: 445–52.

Macmillan (2013) *Throwing a light on the consequences of cancer and its treatment*. Available at: www. ncsi.org.uk/wp-content/uploads/MAC14312_CoT_Throwing-light_report_FINAL.pdf

National Institute for Health and Care Excellence (NICE) (2007) *Depression in adults: Recognition and management*. Clinical Guidance 90. Available at: www.nice.org.uk/guidance/cg90

National Institute for Health and Care Excellence (NICE) (2011a) *Generalised anxiety disorder and panic disorder in adults: management*. Clinical Guidance 113. Available at: www.nice.org.uk/guidance/cg113

National Institute for Health and Care Excellence (NICE) (2011b) *Alcohol-use disorders: Diagnosis, assessment and management of harmful drinking and alcohol dependence*. Clinical Guidance CG115. Available at: www.nice.org.uk/guidance/cg115

Nursing and Midwifery Council (2014) *Standards for Competence for Registered Nurses*. London: NMC.

Scottish Government (2007) *Towards a Mentally Flourishing Scotland*. Available at: www.gov.scot/Resource/Doc/201215/0053753.pdf

Scottish Government (2013) *Suicide Prevention Strategy 2013–2016*. Scottish Government.

Scottish Recovery Network (2016) *Making Mental Health Recovery a Reality for All*. Available at: www.scottishrecovery.net/

Scowcroft, E. (2016) *Suicide Statistic Report 2016*. Samaritans. Available at: www.samaritans.org

Tofthagen, R. and Fagerstrøm, L. (2010) Clarifying self-harm through evolutionary concept analysis. *Scandinavian Journal Of Caring Sciences*, 24 (3): 610–19.

Welsh Government (2015) *Talk to me 2. Suicide and Self Harm Prevention Strategy for Wales 2015–2020*. Available at: http://gov.wales/docs/dhss/publications/150716strategyen.pdf

World Health Organization (WHO) (2012) *World Drug Report*. World Health Organization. Available at: www.unodc.org/documents/data-and-analysis/WDR2012/WDR_2012_web_small.pdf

World Health Organization (WHO) (2017) *Depression*. World Health Organization. Available at: www. who.int/mediacentre/factsheets/fs369/en/

CARE OF THE ADULT WITH DEMENTIA

20

MARGARET BROWN AND HELEN FOX

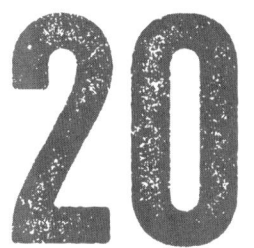

WATCH VIDEOS ONLINE
CLICK HERE

THIS CHAPTER COVERS

- An overview of dementia
- Diagnosis and person-centred assessment in dementia care
- Current models and frameworks in dementia care

- Evidence-informed interventions for the person with dementia
- Living and dying well with dementia.

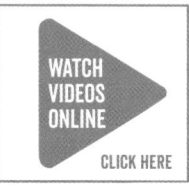

> " I'm still same person – I haven't become somebody different or somebody new – I've just got an extra problem to deal with.
>
> Ian, a person living with dementia
>
> (Sharp, 2017) "

INTRODUCTION

In this chapter you will explore concerns about the person living with dementia throughout their illness. In an exploration of the syndrome of dementia, the impact on the person and family is examined, including the concept of living well. Assessment and care needs of the person are reviewed and the role of the student nurse is highlighted. Dementia is caused by a range of diseases that result in cell death within the brain. As dementia progresses the person requires an increasing range of interventions, especially in relation to healthcare needs. Most people who develop dementia are likely to be older and that means they are also at risk of developing multiple health conditions. As a student nurse you will care for the person with dementia in a range of settings, in hospital, community and care homes. Care is often complex and requires skills and knowledge based on a biopsychosocial, cultural and spiritual framework.

Globally, the number of people who live with dementia is 47.5 million, increasing each year by 7.7 million (World Health Organization (WHO), 2016). In developing countries, these numbers are rising too, as more and more people reach old age. Prevalence in the UK is currently 850,000 and this will increase to over 1 million by 2025 and 2 million by 2051 (Prince et al., 2014).

It is impossible to truly understand what it might be like to experience dementia but it is vital for you to develop awareness of the impact of dementia on the person, the family and the people who support them. One of the most important learning activities is reflection and here I explain how I learned from one experience. When I was a community mental health nurse for older people I was asked to see Patricia who had advanced dementia. She struggled to find her way around her house and she could say few words. During the visit she suddenly saw the keyboard set up in her sitting room, sat down and played beautifully from a range of musical styles. Then she turned and said clearly, 'This is me!' This experience challenged all my previous beliefs; I now think I had at that time a very narrow understanding of how individual the experience of dementia could be. Every time I meet a person with dementia, I remember Patricia.

AN OVERVIEW OF DEMENTIA

By examining some of the beliefs about dementia we will now discuss a few myths about this illness, so prominent in the media and health and social care.

Dementia happens to an individual, whether old or young, rich or poor, educated or not. Therefore, each person needs to be approached in a person-centred way. Of course there are commonalities – no one would suggest otherwise – and some of these are due to similar changes within the brain. However, dementia happens to a unique human being and that means that each person is different. Older age is a risk factor but not all older people have dementia: it is not considered to be part of normal ageing. Dementia can occur at a much younger age and some people are more likely to develop this, including people who have Down's syndrome.

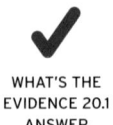

WHAT'S THE
EVIDENCE 20.1
ANSWER

WHAT'S THE EVIDENCE? 20.1

Can a person live well with dementia? This may seem a strange statement to make about an illness that is life limiting, yet this way of perceiving life with dementia has been driven by people who are experiencing dementia. Now what do you think about using the term 'suffering' from dementia? Is this common language used about a person living with dementia?

What is the evidence about the concept of 'living well with dementia' and how it sits alongside the idea that the person is 'suffering'?

CRITICAL THINKING STOP POINT 20.1

Read and reflect on the Deep Guide and the following paper:

The Dementia Engagement and Empowerment Project (2014) Dementia words matter: Guidelines on language about Dementia. Available at: http://dementiavoices.org.uk/wp-content/uploads/2015/03/DEEP-Guide-Language.pdf

Bartlett, R., Windemuth-Wolfson, L., Oliver, K. and Dening, T. (2017) Suffering with dementia: the other side of "living well". International psychogeriatrics, 29(2), pp.177-179. Available at: https://www.kmpt.nhs.uk/downloads/get-involved/the-other-side-of-living-well-article.pdf

Consider this:

1. What impact does language have on the provision of care?
2. What are the consequences of a lack of reflection on key concepts such as 'suffering'?

The concept of living well with dementia began to be used more widely after the publication of dementia strategies in the UK (Department of Health, 2009; Scottish Government, 2010). These documents referred to living the best life possible with dementia. Words such as hope, recovery and optimism were used instead of calling this tragic or devastating (Clarke et al., 2011). Living well is a concept also driven by people with dementia, who do not want to be considered unable to manage their lives. The Scottish Dementia Working Group is comprised of people with dementia who are a political action group and are represented on most of the decision-making forums in Scotland, including the Scottish Government www.sdwg.org.uk.

WHAT IS DEMENTIA?

The term dementia does not refer to a single disease but a syndrome or collection of clinical features that are the result of a variety of illnesses. The World Health Organization (2016) defines dementia as 'a syndrome in which there is deterioration in memory, thinking, behaviour and the ability to perform everyday activities'. While memory impairment is certainly the most prominent feature in most people with dementia, further changes occur in language, comprehension, behaviour and function.

There are a number of causes of dementia and the four most common are Alzheimer's disease (62%), vascular dementia (17%), dementia with Lewy bodies (4%) and frontotemporal dementia (2%). It is also possible to have more than one of these conditions, called mixed dementia (10%) (Prince et al., 2014). These different forms of dementia can affect different parts of the brain, often with a different rate and pattern of progression over time.

Alzheimer's disease is characterised by a steady, progressive decline in memory, language ability and visual spatial abilities. The person will gradually develop more and more difficulty thinking, communicating and carrying out daily living activities. Because progress is normally slow, it can be difficult to identify when the person begins to have symptoms. It is thought that a person can live from about 2.5–12 years with this condition.

Vascular dementia is caused by problems with blood circulation to the brain. The person is more likely to experience slowed thinking and low mood. This form of dementia is often related to high blood pressure, stroke and diabetes. Progression is likely to be more closely linked to physical health problems and the person will have episodes of rapid deterioration, followed by stable periods. It is difficult to predict how long the person will live with this illness, because of the other physical health problems.

Dementia with Lewy bodies is linked to Parkinson's disease. These Lewy bodies are abnormal structures in the brain cells. Difficulty with memory is one of the first signs, together with slowed thinking. Word finding and visuospatial difficulties also occur early in the condition. The person has difficulty problem solving and making decisions. A key sign is fluctuation in consciousness and hallucinations are common. Parkinson-like symptoms occur, mainly related to gait and movements; less often there is tremor. Falls are frequent. Progression can be rapid. The person is likely to be very sensitive to antipsychotic medication, often prescribed for treatment of hallucinations. These can increase the severity of the movement disorder, leading to falls.

Frontotemporal dementia (Pick's disease) occurs more often in a younger age group. This affects specific areas in the frontotemporal area of the brain and while the person may not experience memory problems associated with other presentations, they may have changes in behaviour, emotional responses and communication.

Mixed dementia can also occur and this can involve overlapping of symptoms and responses in the person who has more than one illness. The most common of this mixed presentation is Alzheimer's disease and vascular dementia.

While there is no doubt that the person living with dementia has damage to their brain, how they respond to this will vary and impact on the way they behave and react. Like all of us, the person with dementia who is upset or distressed will respond to that emotion. If another person teases, condescends or ignores them, this will also cause a response. The danger of focusing on the brain damage or biological causes of dementia can lead to diagnostic overshadowing, when an illness is blamed for all the person's responses and behaviours. A holistic approach to dementia is vital to developing an understanding of the experience of dementia and contributes to supporting the person in living well.

WORKING TO PREVENT DEMENTIA

Table 20.1 The causes of dementia are varied and can include:

Demographics	Presence of long-term conditions	Lifestyle factors
Older age	Diabetes	Smoking
Female gender	Cardiovascular disease	Low levels of activity
Lower education	Stroke	Loneliness
Lower socioeconomic level	Hypertension	Poor diet
	Depression	

Recent epidemiological studies report that the numbers of people developing dementia may be stabilising, in Europe at least. This may be the result of lifestyle and health modifications, together with improved management of long-term and cardiovascular conditions (Wu et al., 2016). This change has resulted from a greater understanding of some of the causes of dementia as shown in Table 20.1. Keeping active, eating well and staying connected to others and the community is not only a good recipe for cardiovascular health but also for preventing dementia.

SEE ALSO
CHAPTER 25

ACTIVITY 20.1
ANSWER

ACTIVITY 20.1: HEALTH PROMOTION

Make a list of all health promotion activities that you can think of that could help prevent dementia. Write beside each item on the list your own health behaviours. You may find some that are unavoidable such as gender and ageing but how many could you influence? What might you change to reduce your risk of developing dementia?

DIAGNOSIS AND PERSON-CENTRED ASSESSMENT IN DEMENTIA CARE

A timely diagnosis of dementia can be a way to improve choice and extend the period of independence, by improving support and information for the person, family and friends. This has led to an emphasis on improving diagnostic rates of dementia. Consequently, there is an expectation that there will be provision of post-diagnostic support. The Alzheimer's Society has produced the *Dementia Guide* for all people diagnosed with dementia to provide information and advice to support living well (Alzheimer's Society, 2013).

In Scotland, the Five Pillars Model (Alzheimer Scotland, 2013) guides the process of post-diagnostic support. Scotland is the only country in the UK that provides such a structured approach to support the person after diagnosis. These Five Pillars are:

- planning for future decision-making
- supporting community connections
- peer support
- planning for future care
- understanding the illness and managing the symptoms.

ASSESSMENT OF DEMENTIA

Diagnosis of dementia can only be made if the person has multiple cognitive deficits including memory and functional impairment, but no disturbance of consciousness. This must be a change from the person's previous level of functioning and be of long duration (over six months) (Thomas, 2008).

Assessment of the person with dementia should be an integrated multi-professional process and the role of the nurse is a key component. This team will include medical staff and psychiatrists specialising in older people. Other disciplines are generally involved, such as psychologists, occupational therapists, speech and language therapists and social workers. Other practitioners will be needed for specific issues and these may include pharmacists, physiotherapists, podiatrists, dentists, housing and third sector staff. As a nurse you can be core to supporting the person and their family when they are engaged with the wider team, by coordinating what can be an overwhelming experience. For the nurse who spends a good deal of time with the person, there is an opportunity to answer any questions, clarify what has been discussed and ensure that the dignity and choices of the person and family are maintained.

The focus on person-centred assessment means getting to know what matters to the person, the family and wider network, in addition to the person's past and present health and social history. The person should be asked if they wish to know their diagnosis and with whom this information might be shared. A comprehensive assessment should include:

- Clinical history from the person and family
- Physical health assessment including routine blood tests, blood pressure and other appropriate investigations determined by the clinician. This process will rule out other causes of the person's symptoms, such as folic acid and vitamin B12 deficiency or an underactive thyroid.
- Psychological assessment will include using rating scales including those that provide information on cognition such as ACE III (www.fom.gla.ac.uk/aceiiitrainer/) or the Montreal Cognitive Assessment, MoCA (www.mocatest.org/).
- A review of medication, including over the counter medicines that may have adverse effects that could reduce cognition.

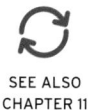

SEE ALSO
CHAPTER 11

Source: National Institute for Health and Care Excellence (NICE) 2006. Reproduced with permission under the NICE UK Open Content Licence.

Dementia can be difficult to diagnose and particularly in older people, who can have a number of other conditions that can cause similar symptoms. These can range from Vitamin B and folate deficiency, hypoactive thyroid, untreated diabetes or cardiac disease to the misuse of medication or alcohol.

Two of the most common conditions confused with dementia are depression and delirium. This is often termed the three Ds – Dementia, Delirium and Depression – these are particularly hard to differentiate, especially in older people. To complicate the situation, the person can be experiencing one, two or all three of these at the same time. Table 20.2 shows some of these differences:

Table 20.2   Dementia, Delirium and Depression: A quick guide

	Dementia	Delirium	Depression
History of the illness	Slow onset over months or years	Sudden, abrupt onset	Slow onset over a period of weeks or months
Awareness	Normally not affected	Person is distracted and this can change rapidly	Can have difficulty concentrating
Sleep	Usually stable over time	Definite change from normal pattern	Problems getting to sleep or early morning awakening
Memory	Recent memory more likely to be affected. Finds difficulty retaining new information	Current and recent memory changes and problems	The person reports that memory is worse but others may not notice
Cognition	Difficulty reasoning, planning and understanding	Disordered thinking. Going from one subject to another	Slowed thinking, feelings of hopelessness

Adapted from Acute Care Dementia Learning Resource, NHS Education for Scotland. © NHS National Services Scotland. Reproduced with permission. You can access the full document utilising this link: www.nes.scot.nhs.uk/media/350872/acute_dementia_interactive_2011.pdf

Below is an example of how an older person may present in a hospital setting. Consider how this person may behave and respond to care.

ACTIVITY 20.2
ANSWER

ACTIVITY 20.2: CRITICAL THINKING

Mr Murphy is being cared for in hospital following an episode where he is found walking around in his street during the night, wearing his nightclothes. He is found to have a urinary tract infection and is experiencing delirium. Using Table 20.2, could you write a short description of how Mr Murphy might behave and respond?

Assessment is not all about identifying deficits. It is just as important to investigate the person's strengths and assets. A timely diagnosis of dementia can be a way to improve choice and enable the person and family to make decisions about now and the future.

GO FURTHER

A robust assessment should always include what matters to the person living with dementia and some useful tools have been developed to capture this important information. These are free to use and family members can be involved in the process if the person consents.

"This is Me" is provided by the Alzheimer's Society: www.alzheimers.org.uk/site/scripts/download_info.php?downloadID=399

"Getting to Know Me" is available from Alzheimer Scotland:
www.alzscot.org/assets/0001/9836/Getting_to_know_me_form_single_pages.pdf

WEBLINKS

CURRENT MODELS AND FRAMEWORKS IN DEMENTIA CARE

In dementia care these frameworks include person-centred and relationship-focused care; these share a core theme of being centred on the person, together with those who provide care and support.

Person-centred care is a concept identified with Tom Kitwood (Kitwood, 1997). He was a key figure in the move away from a medical model of care to a more holistic and individual approach to meet the needs of the person with dementia. He identified in the 1990s that the care of most people with dementia was task oriented. He advocates an approach where the person is valued, their needs addressed and their care individualised. The person's life history and previous personality becomes key to care.

Nolan et al. (2006) developed this person-centred approach further, by focusing on relationships in dementia care. This framework is called the SENSES, using the six senses called security, continuity, belonging, purpose, achievement and significance. These six senses are applied to all care partners and the person with dementia. Recent research in care homes found that using the senses framework improved the quality of life for residents (Brown Wilson et al., 2013).

The current drive towards integrated care may lead to new ways of working and supporting the person. A central aim of integration is to shift the balance of care to the community setting, ensuring that resources can be better employed to meet the needs of the person.

THE JOURNEY OF DEMENTIA

As dementia progresses, the person's need for support and care will increase. This progression is often described in stages. However, it is important to remember that individuals can progress at different rates and depends on age at onset, other health conditions, form of dementia and external conditions such as care, medication, diet and psychological state.

Early stage

The person begins to have difficulty with daily tasks and activities. Planning and organising may become challenging. Memory may be affected, usually for recent events. The person may begin to withdraw from social events and activities.

Middle stage

The person may start to have difficulty finding their way around, losing possessions. Daily personal care may be less fastidious. A sense of time and place may diminish. Eating, drinking and sleeping may be affected. This period may also include changes in behaviour, mood and responses. The person may see and hear things that are not apparent to others.

Late stage

The person needs assistance with all activities of living and may become less mobile. Verbal communication begins to fail and increasingly the person depends on non-verbal communication and touch. Not everyone with dementia reaches this late stage; normally up to a third of people survive (Nilsson et al., 2012).

EVIDENCE-INFORMED INTERVENTIONS FOR THE PERSON WITH DEMENTIA

There are a number of interventions for the person living with dementia and it is important that these are offered in a timely and appropriate way. For the person in the earlier stages of the illness, where language is preserved, there is a range of therapeutic approaches to maintain and support remaining strengths. As the person becomes less able to connect with complex interventions these can be modified. In the later stages, interventions may focus on aspects of daily living and the use of sensory approaches.

Effective communication supports all interventions with the person. Communication skills deteriorate progressively for most people with dementia and it will take the person more time and effort to communicate. Together with word-finding difficulties, the person may also have problems articulating language and it is important to match the person's communication. Use short sentences containing a single idea and give the person time to understand and answer. Position yourself at the same level as the person and ensure they can hear and see you before you speak. Use all the senses to communicate with the person as this increases the chance of getting the messages across. Non-verbal communication is key, particularly as the person moves to a more advanced stage and can lose the ability to communicate verbally.

Throughout the course of the illness it is important to try and understand the person's reality and respond to how they might be feeling. This can help avoid distress and anxiety. No matter how advanced the dementia, it is important to address the person directly and not talk over them to others.

Tips for communicating effectively: see, hear, then touch

- To gain attention, move into the person's visual field and make sure you can be seen.
- Introduce yourself clearly.
- Use short sentences containing one idea at a time.
- Avoid questions that challenge the person's difficulty with memory.
- Try not to use negatives like 'don't go in there' or 'no you can't', redirect or distract the person.
- Touch should be used when you have the person's attention and permission.
- Smile and use other positive non-verbal behaviour: the person will respond to the emotion.

A SUPPORTIVE ENVIRONMENT

The environment can support the person's remaining abilities and strengths. Increasing light, decreasing sound and making the environment understandable can promote independence and improve interaction.

Dementia design guidelines are widely available (Dementia Services Development Centre, 2013; King's Fund, 2015). These outline how to design or adapt living spaces to maintain the independence of people with dementia. Some examples of dementia-friendly design include non-glare surfaces and having good colour contrast, which can compensate for some of the brain changes affecting vision, as well as problems associated with the ageing eye. The older person needs up to three times the light level of a young adult as the older eye deteriorates and lighting should be shadow free as this can lead the person to misperceive the environment.

CASE STUDY 20.1: JIM

CASE STUDY 20.1
ANSWER

Jim, aged 81 years, was admitted to hospital for a few days following a period of sudden memory impairment and confusion. He was found to have a chest infection. Jim had been living at home with his wife and cared for her as she had dementia. He had been a farmer and was generally fit and well for his age, although he had developed cataracts in both eyes. He was asking to go home saying he was worried about his wife. He was in a single room at the end of the ward near the entrance. One evening he was found stroking the air at his feet and talking to himself. When staff tried to get him to bed he became angry and refused finally saying he was staying with his dog.

- Reflect on what might be causing Jim to think there was a dog in the room.
- Identify some interventions that could improve Jim's situation.

Many older people also have a degree of hearing loss. Dementia can make this worse as damage can affect how sound is processed, distorting what is heard. The challenge of processing sounds and understanding what they might mean can be overwhelming. The multiple noises of care environments present too many demands on their limited resources.

INTERVENTIONS AND TREATMENT

There are some medical interventions that may have an effect on the symptoms of dementia, but there are none that provide a cure. Consequently, psychosocial interventions should be considered as part of the care approach. A psychosocial intervention is a non-pharmacological method using purposeful human interaction in a wide range of therapeutic approaches (Hunter et al., 2016). These interventions, for example, may include cognitive stimulation therapy, reminiscence approaches and life story work.

Cognitive stimulation therapy

This approach involves stimulating the person's remaining cognitive abilities by using specific and planned group activities for set times on a weekly basis. These include word and number games, in addition to discussions about a range of themes such as food or family. The outcome is to maintain or improve cognition (Woods et al., 2012).

Reminiscence approaches

This involves working with the person in remembering past experiences. This activity can be carried out with an individual or in groups. Objects, film, music or art are used to provide stimulation and increase pleasure. There are some considerations that need to be identified, such as being aware of aspects of the person's life that could cause distress. Many older people, having lived a long life, may have some memories that are unhappy and a good knowledge of the person's history is very important.

Life story work

Used with reminiscence or alone, this approach may involve life story books or memory boxes. Working with life story can identify needs, help understand behaviours and support meaningful activity. The process of creating a life story may involve family, friends and care staff and is a way of connecting the person with others.

ACTIVITY 20.3
ANSWER

ACTIVITY 20.3: REFLECTION

Consider what you would put in a life story box or book. This may include objects, photographs or letters. You can include anything that would stimulate conversation about your life. Make a short list and explain what these mean to you.

Now consider if you were an older person with dementia, what would you wish to show a student nurse? Is there anything you might not want to share?

This exercise is a useful way to prepare to care for the person with dementia and think about how you can provide support to ensure their choices are respected.

MEDICATION AND DEMENTIA

There is no cure for dementia, and management using medication is available only for Alzheimer's disease. Two groups of medicines are licenced; acetylcholinesterase inhibitors (donepezil, rivastigmine and galantamine) and N-methyl-D-aspartate receptor antagonist (memantine). Donepezil, rivastigmine and galantamine are licensed for the person with mild to moderate Alzheimer's disease and memantine for the person with severe dementia. These medicines are used to support and maintain cognition and treat a range of symptoms including hallucinations, delusions, marked agitation and behavioural distress (NICE, 2011).

GO FURTHER

WEBLINK:
DEMENTIA
MEDICATION

More information on the range of medications used in dementia can be found here: www.alzheimers.org.uk/info/20162/drugs/106/drugs_used_to_relieve_behavioral_and_psychological_symptoms

SEE ALSO
CHAPTER 13

Medication should be used with caution in older people with dementia and polypharmacy, where the person is taking multiple different medications, can increase the risk of adverse effects. There are particular concerns about the use of antipsychotic medication used to treat agitation in people with dementia, where there is limited evidence of any benefit (Corbett et al., 2014).

> Mum reacted badly to any medication, she just didn't tolerate drugs well. I expressed my disappointment at the lack of information before she started this drug. The nurse took this on board and had an information leaflet produced explaining all about the drug for new patients.
>
> **Norma, daughter**

STRESS AND DISTRESS

Dementia creates stress in the person and when this stress is not managed carefully, then this can lead to distress. These distressed behaviours are very like our own when we are overcome with stress and have no control.

ACTIVITY 20.4: REFLECTION

ACTIVITY 20.4
ANSWER

1. Write down a few things that can make you stressed.

These will include a range of physical, psychological and interpersonal situations.

2. Now write down what you do when you become stressed.

These will probably include some form of emotional release and may involve anger or tears.

Reflect for a moment about your reasons and responses to stress. Stress can most often be caused by the way other people behave with us, by personal worries about our health or welfare or by feeling insecure, unhappy or undervalued. This could make us react by being tearful, angry, agitated, withdrawn or aggressive. The causes and reactions of the person with dementia to stress are the same as yours. The main difference is that you have more control over much of your life and can usually find a way to reduce stress. What might happen if you were not able to exert control? Now imagine this:

> You are in a large supermarket outside your usual area and you have your own or a friend's children with you. Suddenly you cannot see the children and you know it is time for them to be home as it is well past dinnertime. You search frantically, abandoning your trolley of food. A couple of store workers come over and when you tell them about your situation offer to take you for a cup of tea. They tell you that you are too old for children or that your children are grown up. How would that feel? Would you be happy to do that? How would you respond?

What is the source of your distress here? Is it the loss of the children, the unfamiliar environment or the response of the staff? Perhaps it is all of these?

Now consider a care setting where a similar experience can be even more distressing.

SAFETY AND SECURITY

The need to manage risk should be considered within an enablement approach to help the person to live well with dementia. Using enablement principles brings the focus to what the person can still do and support the person to function at an optimum level.

The law has provided guidance to safeguard the person with dementia in the Mental Capacity Act 2005 in England and Wales (Department of Health, 2005) and The Adults with Incapacity Act in

Scotland 2000 (Scottish Government, 2000). These Acts set out the concept of capacity and provide a legal framework to safeguard the person's health and social and financial wellbeing. The core principles shared by both of these Acts are:

- First that it is important to assume the person has capacity unless there is evidence to show otherwise.
- The person should be supported to make decisions as far as is possible even if they are considered to lack capacity.
- People have the right to make decisions that are not considered to be the same as others may make.
- Any decisions made by others for the person who cannot make these must be in their best interests.
- The decision made for the person must be the least restrictive possible.

**SEE ALSO
CHAPTER 4**

Positive risk-taking by the person with dementia can conflict with the risk averse or safety first culture that happens in some settings. So these two models of risk may cause conflict between safety and enablement (Clarke et al., 2011).

ACTIVITY 20.5: CRITICAL THINKING

Peter - rights and risks

Peter is an independent man; never married, he has lived alone since his parents died. At 76 he is physically fit but lately he has been avoiding family and friends. He has stopped attending his local church and rarely leaves home. His sister is worried about him.

Consider this situation from the perspective of the two models of risk, between safety first and enablement and independence.

At the heart of issues of safeguarding are safety and autonomy. While safeguarding the person is a key role of the nurse, respect for autonomy and consideration of the legal directives should be included in all considerations to provide a balanced approach to risk in dementia.

LIVING WELL WITH INCREASING NEED FOR SUPPORT BY OTHERS

As dementia progresses the person will need increasing support from others. The person may move to a very sheltered care setting or a care home. The person with dementia may find this extremely stressful and a close consideration of risk must be part of this process. Moves to hospital are particularly stressful.

> Mum broke her hip and had to be admitted to hospital at an advanced stage of the disease. I prepared a help sheet for the nurses with information about mum and the strategies we used when a difficult situation arose. I also spoke to the consultant. The nurses were very grateful for this and the Doctor wrote to me to say they had decided to make it policy, that the memory clinic should ask relatives for an information sheet about the person with dementia which could be kept on file and then used if they had to be admitted to hospital. It is important for nurses to ask about the patient with dementia in order to be able to care for him/her effectively.
>
> **Norma, daughter**

> The lady in our ward had been admitted to hospital due to deteriorating health and to establish her on new medication. She had been diagnosed with Alzheimer's disease a few years previous and lived at home with her husband. During her time in hospital, I was able to get to know this lady. We sang a lot and listened to the music she enjoyed, drinking tea on the couch. The stories she recalled of her childhood, however recent they were to her mind, brought her great joy. As I spent time with her over the weeks we were able to incorporate new ways of helping her to feel safe and at ease. This was a great help to her husband who was eager to learn about some of these activities we engaged with in the ward, for example Reminiscence Therapy and Doll Therapy, which were new to him. It was a privilege for me to be a part of caring for this lady, being allowed into her and her husband's life.
>
> **Megan, student nurse**

Of course, as dementia progresses the person may need increasing support with fundamental activities of living and these include eating and drinking, personal care and moving around. All of these activities can potentially be a source of distress for the person where care is not provided sensitively and in a way that engages with the person.

LIVING AND DYING WELL WITH DEMENTIA

Having dementia includes the need not only to live well, but also to die well. As dementia progresses, care needs and settings will be subject to change and each transition will bring new challenges. Understanding care of the person with dementia includes being able to care for the person who is dying. It is suggested that a palliative care approach may be adopted even at the point of diagnosis (NICE, 2006). Therefore, nurses should have appropriate knowledge and skills in supportive and palliative care. By adopting a palliative care approach for the person with dementia who is dying, the nurse affirms life and accepts death is a normal process, works to reduce distress, integrates the biopsychosocial and spiritual aspects of care and supports families (van Der Steen et al., 2016).

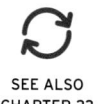

SEE ALSO
CHAPTER 23

The person with dementia has a need for support and care throughout the illness and this should include consideration of the spiritual aspects. These are particularly difficult to support as dementia progresses and the person is no longer able to talk about their spiritual or religious life, and family and friends can support you to help during this time (Ødbehr et al., 2014).

PAIN AND DISTRESS

Pain is a common symptom, often missed in the person who has dementia, particularly when this becomes advanced (Closs et al., 2016). Pain is a subjective experience and only the person can know their experience of pain. However, when a person has advanced dementia they will have a limited ability to express what they are experiencing. If pain is poorly managed then it will impair the person's general health and wellbeing and may cause a range of behaviours that can be misunderstood as shown in the case study about Mary.

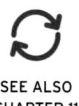

SEE ALSO
CHAPTER 11

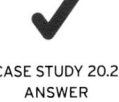

CASE STUDY 20.2
ANSWER

CASE STUDY 20.2: MARY

Mary at 84 has advanced dementia and no longer speaks. She is usually quiet and accepts all help from the staff in her care home with little reaction. However, over the past week she has been making loud growling noises when she is approached, she only takes food reluctantly and is not sleeping. She has now developed a rash on her upper back, which has small blisters.

A few days later the doctor saw Mary and diagnosed herpes zoster (shingles). It is likely she has been experiencing severe pain for some time, due to nerve damage caused by this common condition in older people.

- What might have been done to avoid this situation?

FAMILY AND CARERS

The total number of unpaid care hours in the UK for the person with dementia is £1.34 billion (Prince, 2014). While the family and friends of the person living with dementia are considered throughout this chapter, it is important to take time to think about their needs. Over time, the person may need increasing support and family and friends may find themselves in the role of carers. While an important role it can also be a very stressful one and carers can become ill as a result of caring over time. It is important, therefore, to understand key concerns and maintain good communication with carers.

I do not know how we would have survived the four years mum was in care without the support we received from the unit manager. We developed complete trust in her judgement. Someone like her, who always had time for relatives, had excellent nursing skills and sought solutions to problems, was such a benefit to relatives and she was a role model for her staff.

Norma, daughter

GO FURTHER

WEBLINK:
ALZHEIMER'S
FACTSHEET

The Alzheimer's Society provides a range of factsheets and advice for carers. https://www.alzheimers.org.uk/get-support/publications-factsheets-full-list

So now you are preparing to care for the person with dementia. Your role as a student nurse in dementia care is important: first, because of the regulation, education and training of the nurse and second, for the range of skills nurses possess in both interpersonal and body processes which means they can provide effective and safe care.

> As a nurse working with patients living with dementia it is important to see the person not the illness. By recognising the 'individual' we strive to deliver person-centred care. Involving families and carers as key partners in the person's care is invaluable. We should be able to deliver a high standard of complex care showing empathy and understanding at all stages of their illness, and within any environment. Really we should treat others the way we would expect to be treated.'
>
> Margaret, mentor

Despite this person-centred approach advocated by the mentor, some nursing students may feel unprepared to care for the person with dementia, or may have unrealistic expectations about exactly what they need to know.

> In preparation for practice, I was convinced I needed to possess an in-depth knowledge of the various medication used in the treatment of dementia. I therefore focused on cholinesterase inhibitors, medication used to relieve behavioural and psychological symptoms, antipsychotics and even those used in the treatment of sleep disturbance. In truth – as a first-year student – the knowledge of pharmacological treatments was undoubtedly useful; however, more fundamental elements to care should have taken priority at this early stage in my student journey. A good understanding of how dementia can impact on the person can help the student see – to a degree – the patient's perspective. Good basic communication skills are vital – use short simple sentences. Exercise patience – stay calm and allow time to respond. Ask for advice if you are not sure and try to be as consistent as possible.
>
> Paul, student nurse

The vision for the nurse's role in dementia care (Department of Health, 2016) clearly shows the importance of learning and developing excellence in practice in dementia care. This key role includes health promotion, communication and relationships, dementia education, reduction of stigma and safeguarding.

CHAPTER SUMMARY

- Dementia is a complex syndrome caused by a diverse range of different disease processes.
- An integrated and holistic approach will be more successful in meeting care needs.
- Person-centred and relationship-focused approaches are key to supporting the person living with dementia, family and supporters.
- Safeguarding the person living with dementia should also include risk enablement to allow choice and respect.
- Thorough assessment is vital, not only to identify the person's needs but also remaining assets and strengths.
- Evidence-informed care to support living and dying well with dementia requires a wide and comprehensive range of knowledge and skills for nurses.

CASE STUDY:
ISOLATED
LIFESTYLE

GO FURTHER

Go to https://study.sagepub.com/essentialadultnursing for a further case study related to this chapter. If you are using the interactive ebook, simply click on the book icon in the margin to go straight to the resource.

Books

- Barker, S. and Board, M. (2012) *Dementia Care in Nursing*. London: Learning Matters/SAGE Publications
  This is a very useful text for student nurses and links with your practice learning in a range of settings.
- Downs, M. and Bowers, B. (2014) *Excellence in Dementia Care: Research into Practice*. England: Open University Press/McGraw-Hill Education
  This book contains a range of interventions that are evidence informed for practice.

FURTHER
READING:
JOURNAL
ARTICLES

Journal Articles

Go to https://study.sagepub.com/essentialadultnursing for further free online journal articles related to this chapter. If you are using the interactive ebook, simply click on the book icon in the margin to go straight to the resource.

ONLINE
QUIZZES

ACE YOUR ASSESSMENT

Revise what you have learned by visiting https://study.sagepub.com/essentialadultnursing

- Test yourself with multiple-choice and short-answer questions
- Do the chapter activities in the book and check your answers online

REFERENCES

Alzheimer Scotland (2013) *5 Pillars Model of Post Diagnostic Support*. [Online] Available at: www.alzscot.org/campaigning/ [Accessed 02/03/18]

Alzheimer's Society (2013) *The Dementia Guide*. [Online] Available at: www.alzheimers.org.uk/dementiaguide [Accessed 02/03/18]

Brown Wilson, C. Swarbrick, C., Pilling, M. and Keady, J. (2013) The senses in practice: enhancing the quality of care for residents with dementia in care homes. *Journal of Advanced Nursing*, 69(1): 77–90 https://doi.org/10.1111/j.1365-2648.2012.05992.x

Clarke, C.L., Keady, J., Wilkinson, H. and Gibb, C.E. (2011) *Risk assessment and management for living well with dementia*. Jessica Kingsley Publishers.

Closs, S.J., Dowding, D., Allcock, N., Hulme, C., Keady, J., Sampson, E.L., Briggs, M., Corbett, A., Esterhuizen, P., Holmes, J. and James, K. (2016) Towards improved decision support in the assessment and management of pain for people with dementia in hospital: A systematic meta-review and observational study. *Health Service and Delivery Research*, 4(30).

Corbett, A., Burns, A. and Ballard, C. (2014). Don't use antipsychotics routinely to treat agitation and aggression in people with dementia. *British Medical Journal*, 349(g6420): 25368388.

The Dementia Services Development Centre (2013) *Improving the design of housing to assist people with dementia*. Stirling: University of Stirling. [Online] Available at http://www.cih.org/resources/PDF/Scotland%20general/Improving%20the%20design%20of%20housing%20to%20assist%20people%20with%20dementia%20-%20FINAL.pdf (accessed May 2018)

Department of Health (2005) *Mental Capacity Act*. London: HMSO [Online] Available at: www.legislation.gov.uk/ukpga/2005/9/pdfs/ukpga_20050009_en.pdf [Accessed 02/03/18]

Department of Health (2009) *Living Well with Dementia: A National Dementia Strategy*. [Online] Available at: www.gov.uk/government/uploads/system/uploads/attachment_data/file/168220/dh_094051.pdf [Accessed 02/03/18]

Department of Health (2016) *Dementia Nursing Strategy*. [Online] Available at: www.gov.uk/government/uploads/system/uploads/attachment_data/file/554296/Dementia_nursing_strategy.pdf [Accessed 02/03/18]

Hunter, A., Keady, J., Casey, D., Grealish, A. and Murphy, K. (2016). Psychosocial intervention use in long-stay dementia care: A classic grounded theory. *Qualitative Health Research*, 26(14): 2024–34.

King's Fund (2015) *Enhancing the Healing Environment: Environments of care for people with dementia*. London, King's Fund. [Online] Available at https://www.kingsfund.org.uk/projects/enhancing-healing-environment/ehe-in-dementia-care (accessed May 2018)

Kitwood, T. (1997) *Dementia Reconsidered: The person comes first*. Maidenhead: Open University Press.

National Institute for Care Excellence (NICE) (2006) *Dementia: Supporting people with dementia and their carers in health and social care*. [Online] Available at: www.nice.org.uk/guidance/cg42 [Accessed 02/03/18]

National Institute for Care Excellence (NICE) (2011) *Donepezil, galantimine, rivastigmine and memantine for the treatment of Alzheimer's disease*. [Online] Available at: www.nice.org.uk/guidance/ta217 [Accessed 02/03/18]

Nilsson, K., Gustafson, L. and Hultberg, B. (2012) Survival in a large elderly population of patients with dementia and other forms of psychogeriatric diseases. *Dementia and Geriatric Cognitive Disorders*, 32(5): 342–50.

Nolan, M.R., Brown, J., Davies, J., Nolan, J. and Keady, J. (2006) *The Senses Framework: Improving care for older people through a relationship-centred approach. Getting Research into Practice (GRiP) Report No 2. Project Report*. Sheffield, UK: University of Sheffield.

Nursing and Midwifery Council (2010) *Standards for Pre-registration Nursing Education*. [Online] Available at: www.nmc.org.uk/standards/additional-standards/standards-for-pre-registration-nursing-education/ [Accessed 02/03/18]

Ødbehr, L., Kvigne, K., Hauge, S. and Danbolt, L.J. (2014) Nurses' and care workers' experiences of spiritual needs in residents with dementia in nursing homes: A qualitative study. *BMC Nursing*, 13(1): 12.

Prince, M., Knapp, M., Guerchet, M., McCrone, P., Prina, M., Comas-Herrera, A., Wittenberg, R., Adelaja, B., Hu, B., King, D., Rehill, A. and Salimkumar, D. (2014) *Dementia UK: Update* (2nd ed.). London: Alzheimer's Society.

Scottish Government (2000) *Adults with Incapacity (Scotland) Act*. [Online] Available at: www.legislation.gov.uk/asp/2000/4/contents [Accessed 02/03/18].

Scottish Government (2010) *Scotland's Dementia Strategy*. [Online] Available at: www.gov.scot/Resource/Doc/324377/0104420.pdf [Accessed 02/03/18]

Sharp, B.K. (2017) Stress as experienced by people with dementia: An interpretative phenomenological analysis. *Dementia*, p.1471301217713877.

Thomas, A. (2008) The syndrome of dementia. In: Jacoby, R., Oppenheimer, C., Dening, T. and Thomas, A. (eds) *The Oxford Textbook of Old Age Psychiatry*. Oxford: Oxford University Press, pp. 423–4.

van der Steen, J.T., Radbruch, L., de Boer, M.E., Jünger, S., Hughes, J.C., Larkin, P., Gove, D., Francke, A.L., Koopmans, R.T., Firth, P. and Volicer, L. (2016) Achieving consensus and controversy around applicability of palliative care to dementia. *International Psychogeriatrics*, 28(01): 133–45.

World Health Organization (WHO) (2016) *Dementia*. [Online] Available at: www.who.int/mediacentre/factsheets/fs362/en/ [Accessed 02/03/18]

Wu, Y.T., Fratiglioni, L., Matthews, F.E., Lobo, A., Breteler, M.M., Skoog, I. and Brayne, C. (2016) Dementia in Western Europe: epidemiological evidence and implications for policy making. *The Lancet Neurology*, 15(1):116–24.

CARE OF THE ADULT WITH A LEARNING DISABILITY

21

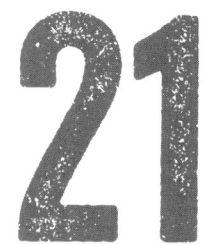

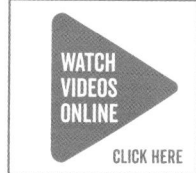

WATCH VIDEOS ONLINE
CLICK HERE

ROBERT STANLEY

THIS CHAPTER COVERS

- What is a learning disability?
- The health needs of people with a learning disability
- Issues of consent and capacity within the acute adult nursing environment

- Consideration for when adults lack capacity
- Strategies and considerations in making reasonable adjustments.

"

The Carer's Voice

Alan MacDonald died suddenly in Lister Hospital, Stevenage, on 20 December 2009, aged 53. Alan had lived independently with his wife, supported by carers. Alan had Down's syndrome and a moderate learning disability, and was considered by his family to have a 'full and active life'. He enjoyed going to the day centre and local cricket club. Three days before admission to hospital, Alan was noted by his family to be 'in fine form'. However, on 15 December 2009, he was admitted to hospital with abdominal pain and diarrhoea. From the time Alan was admitted, his family felt they had to 'beg' staff to treat him, only to be met with 'hostility'. On one occasion, for example, a member of Alan's family who is a doctor asked nurses to give him paracetamol intravenously to treat his dangerously high temperature. She said that this request was 'again met with hostility'. Summing up her feelings about Alan's nursing care at the hospital, she said: 'I felt the nurses on the ward did not respect a gravely ill patient with special needs and a grieving family. Instead of using respect, tact, care and understanding, I and the rest of Alan's family were faced with hostility, disrespect and no consideration for the distressing situation.' The cause of death was multiple organ failure, sepsis and bronchopneumonia. After a protracted complaint against it by Alan's family, the hospital has finally apologised for the attitude of some of its nursing staff. But, for the family, the lack of respect shown for their loved one is something that will never be forgotten.

(Mencap, 2012: 3)

"

This chapter provides information that will help you, as a student, to deliver high-quality healthcare to people with a learning disability. It is estimated that there are 1.4 million people in the UK with a learning disability (Emerson et al., 2011). **All too frequently healthcare for people with a learning disability is characterised by a lack of understanding of the needs, and a lack of reasonable adjustment to respond to those needs**. As this chapter will demonstrate, this is a health inequality that has resulted in poorer health for people with a learning disability. This chapter assists you in preparing for clinical placements and to consider how to deliver a person-centred approach and, therefore, effective nursing care to adults with a learning disability. Everyone deserves good quality healthcare.

WHAT'S THE EVIDENCE? 21.1

There is no definitive record of the number of people with learning disabilities in the UK. No agency or department has the responsibility of collecting information of the prevalence or incidence of learning disability in the population. It can only be estimated (Emerson et al., 2012).

Do you think there should be a definitive register for people with a learning disability? If so, how do you think it should operate? What would be the advantages and disadvantages of it?

WHAT IS A LEARNING DISABILITY?

The World Health Organization (WHO, 1980) has defined impairment as any loss or abnormality of structure or function. A disability is defined as a restriction resulting from an impairment, and a handicap is the disadvantage to an individual resulting from an impairment or disability.

A learning disability is a reduced intellectual ability and difficulty with everyday activities – for example, household tasks, socialising or managing money – which affects someone for their whole life. People with a learning disability tend to take longer to learn and may need support to develop new skills, understand complex information and interact with other people.

A diagnosis of learning disability will give little insight about the individual as there is a huge span of ability and disability across the learning disabled population. The level of support someone needs depends on individual factors, including the severity of their learning disability. For example, someone with a mild learning disability may only need support with things like getting a job. However, someone with a severe or profound learning disability may need full-time care and support with every aspect of their life – they may also have physical disabilities.

People with learning disabilities do not constitute a single homogeneous group. The definition can vary between professions, and countries. Please consider this in What's the Evidence? below.

WHAT'S THE EVIDENCE? 21.2

Three widely used definitions of learning disability are:

1.   Valuing People (Department of Health, 2001: 14):

'Learning disability includes the presence of: A significantly reduced ability to understand new or complex information in learning new skills (impaired intelligence), with:

- a reduced ability to cope independently (impaired social functioning),
- which started before adulthood, with a lasting effect on development.'

2. DSM-V (American Psychiatric Association, 2013)

The DSM-V definition of 'Intellectual Disability' refers to limited functioning in three areas:

- social skills (e.g. communicating with others)
- conceptual skills (e.g. reading and writing ability)
- practical ability (e.g. clothing/bathing oneself).

www.dsm5.org/Documents/Intellectual%20Disability%20Fact%20Sheet.pdf

3. ICD-10 (WHO, 2010)

'... a condition of arrested or incomplete development of the mind, which is especially characterised by

- impairment of skills manifested during the developmental period,
- which contribute to the overall level of intelligence, i.e. cognitive, language, motor and social abilities.'

How would you define a learning disability? Why do you think there is not one definition of learning disability?

Thus, a person with a learning disability has difficulty in learning new skills or applying the skills that they do have to new situations. People with learning disabilities can learn new skills but may take longer to do this and need more help to develop their skills and understand information that they find complex.

Possible impact of learning disability:

- difficulty following instructions
- difficulty in understanding and processing information
- difficulty in understanding abstract concepts such as time or directions
- repetition of phrases in a conversation without expanding the content.

ACTIVITY 21.1: IMPLICATIONS FOR YOUR NURSING PRACTICE

How might you recognise someone has a learning disability?
Take a look at: www.youtube.com/watch?v=HwxjoBQdnOs
How does this challenge your preconceptions about people with a learning disability?

ACTIVITY 21.1
ANSWER

VIDEO:
RECOGNISING
DISABILITY

The causation of a learning disability may be either genetic or environmental across four distinct periods: pre-conceptual, prenatal, perinatal and postnatal. A few of the causes are listed below; however, bear in mind that most individuals do not have a known cause for their disability:

- chromosomal abnormality (**trisomy**, deletion, sex chromosome abnormality)
- metabolic (amino acid, carbohydrate, lipid)
- cerebral degeneration
- cerebral malformations
- intrauterine (nutritional deficiency, congenital infection)
- malnutrition
- toxic agents (drugs, alcohol)
- trauma
- extreme neglect: sensory and social deprivation.

ACTIVITY 21.2: CRITICAL THINKING

TERMINOLOGY

What are the differences or similarities between the following terms?

- Idiot
- Imbecile
- Moron
- Mental subnormality
- Mental handicap
- Learning disability
- Mental retardation

- Mental impairment
- Mental deficiency
- Intellectual disability disorders
- Cognitive disability
- Special Needs
- Developmental disability

Consider why there may be so many different terms, and why do terms change?

What are the implications when different professions and governments use different terms?

What are some other, more unpleasant terms you may have heard?

Which term do you think should be used to describe this group of people and why?

Please read: www.mencap.org.uk/blog/words-i-find-offensive for an insider's view.

Please read: www.campbellmgold.com/archive_esoteric/morons_imbeciles_idiots.pdf for an understanding of some of the history of these terms.

GO FURTHER

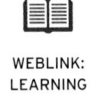

WEBLINK: LEARNING OBSERVATORY

The Improving Health and Lives: Learning Disabilities Observatory document 'A working definition of learning disabilities' is a good starting point to explore the differences and similarities between 'Learning Disability', 'Learning Difficulty' and 'Intellectual Disability' http://webarchive.nationalarchives. gov.uk/20160704162453/http://www.improvinghealthandlives.org.uk/uploads/doc/vid_7446_2010-01WorkingDefinition.pdf (Emerson and Heslop, 2010). Additionally, the terms 'Learning Disability', 'Autism' and Other Disabilities or impairments are also considered.

Since the early part of the twentieth century a classification was made between those who were mildly, moderately or severely disabled based on IQ scores. This classification of severity of learning disability has moved away from tests of intelligence to consider functional abilities including social, conceptual and practical skills. People with a learning disability can be seen as falling on a spectrum of ability. People who are able to be independent in many areas of their lives but need assistance with specific areas such as finances, occupation or social skills may be viewed as having a mild learning disability. Individuals who require support in all domains of their daily life have a severe or profound learning disability. This has been depicted in Table 21.1 below:

Table 21.1 American Psychiatric Association (2013) classification of Learning Disability

	DSM-5 Adaptive functioning score	Indicators	Prevalence (>1 million people)
Mild learning disabilities	55-70	Compared to same age peers, often difficulties in academic skills, abstract thinking, understanding social cues, managing money.	~40%
Moderate	40-55	Simple sentences, poor risk assessment/decision-making skills, needs repeated attempts to learn new skills.	~31%
Severe	25-40	Illiterate, understands and/or uses key words/signs, needs support in activities of daily living skills.	~21%
Profound	<25 across multiple domains	Co-morbid physical disabilities often limit functioning, dependent on others for ADL, limited understanding of symbolic communication.	~8%

Reproduced with permission of the American Psychiatric Association.

The notion of this or other classifications is to note the level of impact the learning disability has upon the individual. Characteristic of the environment of changing terminology, there has been an inconsistent application of this classification within this country and internationally. In the UK two, and occasionally three categories of learning disability are used. In 1999 the Department of Health acknowledged the use of the four categories, although in 2001 (DH) used the subcategories only of severe and mild/moderate.

An individual's quality of life cannot be assumed from judgements made regarding the impact of their level of disability. Many individuals who have a severe or profound disability can live fulfilled and meaningful lives. Quality of life can be assessed by taking the time to talk to the individual, and those that know them well, to ascertain what they enjoy, their goals and aspirations and how their disability affects them, and how we can support them to overcome barriers that prevent them from reaching these goals.

CRITICAL THINKING STOP POINT 21.1 ANSWER

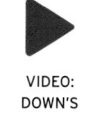

VIDEO: DOWN'S SYNDROME

CRITICAL THINKING STOP POINT 21.1

Please now take a few minutes to watch the video clip about a girl who has Down's syndrome. www.youtube.com/watch?v=pk-5qJ4qJK0

Do you think this girl has a profound, severe, moderate or mild level of learning disability? Why? How important is this distinction?

THE HEALTH NEEDS OF PEOPLE WITH A LEARNING DISABILITY

Healthcare services are designed to meet the needs of the general population, and not specifically the needs of people with a learning disability. It is important for you to have an accurate understanding of the ways that health needs for people with a learning disability are different from the population as a whole as it will enable you to respond to those needs effectively.

It is reasonable to ask if the pattern of ill health is the same as the general population. It isn't. As noted, there is an increased prevalence of some conditions, and associated co-morbidities. There is an increased incidence of:

- gastrointestinal cancer
- leukaemia in children with Down's syndrome
- psychiatric disorders, schizophrenia and challenging behaviours
- dementia (see case study – Max)
- epilepsy
- sensory impairments (e.g. hearing or vision)
- dysphagia (see case study – Abdul).

(Emerson at al., 2012).

CRITICAL THINKING STOP POINT 21.2

WHY THE DIFFERENCE?

List some reasons why you think people with a learning disability have a greater risk of poorer health than the main population. You may want to use Dahlgren and Whitehead's (1991) modelling of health determinants (www.bridgingthegap.scot.nhs.uk/understanding-health-inequalities/introducing-the-wider-determinants-of-health.aspx).

WEBLINK:
HEALTH
MODEL

It is appropriate to ask why is the pattern of health different for people with a learning disability. The Improving Health and Lives Learning Disabilities Public Health Observatory (IHaL) identified five broad determinants of health inequalities for people with learning disabilities (Emerson et al., 2012):

- social determinants
- genetic and biological determinants
- communication difficulties and reduced health literacy
- personal health behaviour and lifestyle risks
- deficiencies in access to and quality of health provision.

(Atkinson et al., 2013).

It is the vulnerability to each of these five determinants that, for people with a learning disability, infers a different pattern of ill health in comparison with the rest of the population. This is seen in Table 21.2 below. The consequences of these different patterns is important as the median age of death for someone with a learning disability is 67 years, with this decreasing as the level of learning disability increases.

Table 21.2 The determinants of health

Social determinants	People with learning disabilities are more likely to be exposed to poverty, poor housing conditions, unemployment, social isolation and hate crime.
Genetic, biological and environmental determinants	People with moderate to profound learning disabilities are more likely than the general population to die from congenital abnormalities. In addition, a number of syndromes associated with learning disabilities are also associated with some specific co-morbidities.
Communication and health literacy determinants	People with learning disabilities can have limited bodily awareness and may have atypical pain responses. In addition, limited communication skills may reduce their ability to convey health needs to relatives, friends, paid support workers.
Personal health risks and behaviours determinants	Over 80% of people with a learning disability do not engage in the recommended amount of physical activity, and those in restrictive environments are at increased risk of inactivity. Additionally, there is a widespread lack of knowledge about healthy eating leading to an increased risk of obesity, which is associated with an increased risk of diabetes.
Access to and the quality of healthcare and other services	There are a number of barriers to accessing quality healthcare • scarcity of appropriate services; • failure to make 'reasonable adjustments'; • lack of expertise and experience among healthcare staff; • 'diagnostic overshadowing'.

ACTIVITY 21.3

Consider each of the determinants in Table 21.2 in turn. How could you positively improve someone's health that was adversely affected by each determinant?

GO FURTHER

Please see: **The A–Z of health issues affecting people with learning disabilities**. Available at: www.2gether. nhs.uk/files/azhealth.pdf. This gives a very brief overview of some of the health needs for adults with a learning disability. Use this as a basis for making further investigations to inform your practice.

WEBLINKS

Please refer again to CRITICAL THINKING STOP POINT 21.2. What are some issues you think Libby might typically face across her lifespan?

Please take a look at:

http://www.learningdisabilities.org.uk/support-us/stories/mitchells-story/

Things to think about:

Within the scope of your work how could you positively improve someone's health that was adversely affected by this determinant?

Please take a look at http://www.gmc-uk.org/learningdisabilities/200.aspx#206

Please look at this video:

http://www.gmc-uk.org/learningdisabilities/50.aspx

Consider why the poor experiences happened in this way.

CASE STUDY 21.1: ABDUL

Abdul Barzani is a 29-year-old gentleman from a Pakistani background. Abdul has a profound learning disability and has epilepsy manifested by tonic-clonic seizures. He lives in supported living where he receives 24/7 support.

Weight   51.69 kg
Height   1.77 cm
BMI   16.5
Respirations 15 rpm

Medication:

- sodium valproate 1.25 b.d.
- lamotrigine 25 g b.d.
- lactulose 20 ml o.d.

Abdul's general health and wellbeing is greatly impaired. In terms of his epilepsy, the frequency of his seizures is increasing and there is no reported triggering factor. He also had three diagnosed episodes of bronchitis, one episode progressing into a double bronchial pneumonia.

He is a wheelchair user due to his condition; he has a progressive scoliosis, arthritis and tendonitis. He has a history of pressure sores on his ankles. Currently his left ankle is showing signs of redness.

Abdul has both urinary and faecal incontinence. His food and dietary intake are impaired due to his dysphagia and motility issues. He often takes 30 minutes to eat two teaspoons of food and 50 ml of water if tolerated. He experiences overflow faecal incontinence as a result of constipation arising from an insufficient dietary fibre and fluid intake.

Abdul shows a dysarthria and has impairment of voluntary movement of the lips, tongue and palate; there is heavy oral dribbling. He appears to have a recognition of familiar voices and his vocalisations are prevocal. His mother always speaks to him in Urdu, his siblings in English. He shows a heightened sensitivity to noise and some forms of touch, particularly around his face.

Abdul's BMI has reduced from 18.5 to 16.5 in a six-month period. His support workers are finding it increasingly difficult to support his nutrition and fluid intake. The consultant has agreed an elective admission.

Plan: For admission today for insertion of a percutaneous endoscopic gastrostomy

1. What steps should you take to support Abdul and his family for this surgery?
2. For ideas take a look at this video: www.gmc-uk.org/learningdisabilities/282.aspx, and the resources section at the end of the chapter.
3. How are the determinants of health noted above impacting upon Abdul?
4. Using a framework such as the Activities of Daily Living, identify Abdul's needs and prioritise them.

SEE ALSO
CHAPTER 9

ISSUES OF CONSENT AND CAPACITY WITHIN THE ACUTE ADULT NURSING ENVIRONMENT

As an adult nurse you will need to consider the capacity and ability of your patient with a learning disability to give informed consent, which may mean undertaking a further assessment to determine capacity. This, of course, applies to all patients but is particularly pertinent to patients with learning disabilities. When assessing capacity you will need to:

- communicate effectively (please refer below to the section on communication in 'Strategies and Considerations in Making Reasonable Adjustments')
- effectively assess and understand what the current health needs are;
- allow time to let the patient make her or his own choice wherever possible;
- remember – the patient has the right to have an advocate present, if necessary.

The core principle of consent to treatment is that treatment and nursing care must not take place without permission. The law recognises that adults have a right to determine whether or not to accept treatment. Dame Elizabeth Butler-Sloss stated in Re MB (Caesarean Section) [1997] 2 FLr 426 (CA):

> The right to determine what shall be done with one's own body is a fundamental right in our society. The concepts inherent in this right are the bedrock upon which the principles of self-determination and individual autonomy are based. Free individual choice in matters affecting this right should, in my opinion, be accorded very high priority.

This core concept applies to all individuals who have the capacity (the ability to understand, retain, weigh up and communicate) to decide the particular decision. For individuals with a learning disability this can mean there may be some decisions they can make, whereas others they cannot. **It does not mean, however, that because someone has a learning disability they are automatically presumed not to have capacity.**

The most important point to remember when considering consent and working with people who have a learning disability is that consent should be viewed as a 'process' and not a one-off event. The importance of this is that capacity can change on a daily basis – or even more frequently. Particularly in a learning disability capacity it is dynamic and fluid. It is important to revisit understanding, to check for understanding, and to consider if further adjustments need to be addressed.

Time and Support are, therefore, key in this process. Each time that consent is required then the person's capacity and understanding should be reviewed and applied to each individual situation. Consider Critical Thinking Stop Point 21.3 below. Within this exercise consider the difference between consenting to having a wash and consenting to a major operation. The nursing action must be how best to support the patient to understand the information and express his or her wishes.

SEE ALSO
CHAPTER 4

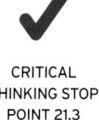

CRITICAL
THINKING STOP
POINT 21.3
ANSWER

CRITICAL THINKING STOP POINT 21.3

A 30-year-old man with moderate learning disabilities is living in a residential home with three other people. He has refused to wash or have a bath for over two months and the staff and residents have begun to complain to his consultant psychiatrist and community nurse. Some members of the team believe that the best thing to do is to section him under the Mental Health Act 1983 and essentially 'force' him to wash.

- What do you think are the key issues here?
- If you were the community nurse, what might you need to consider?

For consent to be valid a person must be:

- capable of taking that particular decision (in other words 'competent')
- acting voluntarily and not under coercion, duress or pressure from others
- provided with enough information to enable them to make a decision.

People with capacity can refuse treatment at any time, even if to do so is detrimental to their health and wellbeing. Legally, it is irrelevant whether a person signs a form to give consent, or does so orally or non-verbally. If a patient with a learning disability has had capacity to consent to a procedure, and is withdrawing it because he/she is finding it unpleasant, that withdrawal of consent must be followed. To do otherwise would be unlawful. The key factor in valid consent is whether the person has capacity. Succinctly, for people to give valid consent for treatment they must be able to:

> Comprehend and retain information relevant to the decision, particularly in relation to the consequences of having or not having the treatment, and use and consider this information in the decision making process. (Department of Health, 2005)

Nurses and others should view consent and ascertaining capacity as a process that involves person-centred ways of explaining treatments. This can be done via augmented communication methods, using easy-to-understand language, pictorial guides, or conveying information through a close carer or family member.

WHEN ADULTS LACK CAPACITY

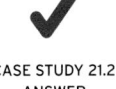

CASE STUDY 21.2
ANSWER

CASE STUDY 21.2: MAX

Max is 53 years old, has Down's syndrome and has been diagnosed with early onset dementia; he takes memantine 5mg o.d. He has been living with Andrew (his brother, who is his main carer) his whole life. Andrew has two grown-up children, and is divorced.

Max's disease has been progressing in the nine years since diagnosis. He is increasingly confused and now needs constant supervision. Mostly he cannot hold a conversation and he will easily forget what is said and repeat the same questions again and again. This can be frustrating for Andrew. He needs help with personal hygiene and with eating and drinking. Currently Max will only eat ice cream.

You are on placement with the district nursing team. When you and the district nurse arrive to see Max, you are shocked by the state of the house: it is filthy, and smells strongly of urine. Andrew says he has rather given up on most things.

Andrew introduces both of you to his brother Max. Max is unable to retain any information, and when you ask him questions, he is unable to answer you, just saying 'is it raining today, is it raining today, is it raining today'. Around half way through the meeting, Max stands up, and shouts at you, 'Andrew's shoes, Andrew's shoes'. He becomes very distressed, shouting at Andrew. He clings to Andrew, crying saying, 'Don't go, I'm good, don't go, I'm good, don't go, I'm good', and eventually urinates on the carpet. Andrew excuses himself and takes Max upstairs. Andrew comes downstairs and starts to cry. He says it is like this every day.

Andrew has asked for this visit. He wants to put Max into a nursing home.

Things to consider:

- Does Max have the capacity to agree or refuse this decision?
- How might Max be best supported in this, and what nursing actions are necessary for this?

THE MENTAL CAPACITY ACT

The Six Lives Progress Report (DH, 2010) received worrying evidence of failure to comply with the Mental Capacity Act including examples of Do Not Resuscitate orders being placed on patients' records without discussion with the individual or family, and family carers being asked to sign consent forms for adults.

Following this report the NHS Operating Framework 2010/11 suggests:

> particular emphasis should be given to ensuring staff are trained to make reasonable adjustments, communicate effectively and follow the Mental Capacity Act (2005) Code of Practice in all their interactions with patients with learning disabilities to ensure full compliance with the law in respect of capacity, consent and best interest decision making (Department of Health & NHS Finance, 2009: 41).

The main aim of the Act is to provide a statutory framework to empower and protect people over the age of 16 who may lack capacity to make some decisions for themselves. Section 1 of the Act sets out five underpinning principles:

- **A presumption of capacity** – every adult has the right to make their own decisions, and they must be assumed to have capacity to do so unless it is proved otherwise.

Nursing considerations: This means that if someone has a diagnosis of early onset dementia, such as the case of Max noted above, or a learning disability, do not presume that person does not have capacity to make that particular decision. There may be many decisions Max cannot make, but there may some smaller ones he can. The skill of nursing is ensuring he retains the ability to have those decisions heard and supported.

- **Individuals being supported to make their own decisions** – an individual must be given all practicable help before anyone treats them as not being able to make their own decisions.

Nursing consideration: People with learning disabilities have a wide range of communication needs. Nurses must take an individualised approach to communicating using communication aids as necessary. In order to do this, nurses will need to understand about alternative communication techniques and tools and know whom they should contact if they cannot communicate effectively.

- **Unwise decision** – just because an individual makes what could be considered to be an unwise decision, such as deciding not to wash as discussed above, they should not be treated as lacking capacity to make that decision.

Nursing considerations: An unwise decision may not be indicative of a learning disability, but simply the patient's preference.

- **Best interests** – an act done or decision taken under the Act for or on behalf of a person who lacks capacity must be done in their best interests.

Nursing considerations: Where there are complex, life-changing decisions that cannot easily be made it is likely a best interests meeting will be called. This provides a venue for the full range of opinions and views as well as ensuring the legal interests of the person are protected. Typically a best interests meeting is called if there is a lack of consensus about what is in the best interests of the person. In the cases of Max given above, or Joan discussed below, it is certain a best interests meeting would be called.

- **Least restrictive option** – anything done for or on behalf of a person who lacks capacity should be the least restrictive of their basic human rights and freedoms.

Nursing considerations: There is an expectation when acting on behalf of another person to respect their known wishes, their preferences, and always to consider how best to support the individual. If someone, such as Max, is wandering in the night, the least restrictive option is not necessarily locking them in their bedroom.

CRITICAL
THINKING STOP
POINT 21.4
ANSWER

CRITICAL THINKING STOP POINT 21.4

A person is unable to make a decision, and considered to be lacking in capacity if they cannot:

- understand
- retain the information
- weigh-up the benefits and consequences of that decision
- and communicate the decision.

What communication techniques might a nurse use to enable a patient to understand, retain, weigh-up and communicate a decision?

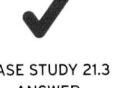

CASE STUDY 21.3
ANSWER

CASE STUDY 21.3: JOAN

Date of birth:	06/06/1985
Weight:	124.7 kg
Height:	182 cm
BMI:	37.6
Waist circumference:	114.3 cm
Pulse:	100 bpm
Respirations:	30 rpm
Medication:	Metformin 200mg once daily

Joan has a mild learning disability. Joan lives independently in her own flat and is supported three hours per day with general household chores. She has **Prader-Willi syndrome** and is obsessional about eating which previously has involved her stealing from stores. Joan has a history of challenging behaviours and can have significant mood swings. Characteristic of her syndrome, Joan will obsessively pick at her arms and face. This is particularly manifest when she is stressed or upset. There has been a frequent history of the sores infecting, and the healing of them is becoming more problematic.

Joan has type 2 diabetes that is very poorly controlled because of her lack of dietary compliance due to her obsessional eating. For the last two months she has had a large open, infected sore on her arm that she regularly/obsessively picks at.

You are on placement with the practice nurse who sees Joan every fortnight to monitor her diabetes. On your placement you feel you have developed a good relationship with Joan, but you are concerned that her health is deteriorating in the time you have known her. At this morning's clinic she told you she had a whole box of cereal, three jam sandwiches and a whole Victoria sponge cake with ice cream for breakfast. Additionally, she had three chocolate bars on the way to the clinic. You have read that the best options for individuals with Prader-Willi syndrome is to control all access to food (www.nhs.uk/Conditions/prader-willi-syndrome/Pages/Management.aspx). You are wondering if this is the best option for Joan's wellbeing.

1. Does Joan have capacity to be making the unwise decisions concerning her dietary management?
2. How does Joan's learning disability make this case different?
3. Should Joan be moved into an environment with restricted access to food?
4. What can you, as the student working with the practice nurse, do to support Joan's wishes?
5. Which members of the multidisciplinary team do you think would be useful contacts in this case?

BEST INTERESTS

Some people with learning disability lack the capacity to give valid consent for a particular decision; however, it is possible for treatment to be lawfully provided if the treatment is deemed to be in the person's best interests. No one can give consent on behalf of an adult who lacks the capacity to give consent, and this includes their parents, unless they have been appointed by the person with the learning disability with Power of Attorney.

Legally it is the health professional responsible for the treatment who decides whether the treatment is in the person's best interests. In practice, most decisions taken by the responsible professional will be after discussion and agreement from a multidisciplinary team, carers and family. A decision on what is in a person's best interest should not be based on medical treatment/intervention alone. Matters such as general wellbeing, relationships, social issues, and spiritual/religious beliefs should also be considered. When a proposed treatment is controversial, e.g. sterilisation, and interested parties strongly oppose it, then the doctor responsible for the treatment can and should seek a court decision on best interest.

STRATEGIES AND CONSIDERATIONS IN MAKING REASONABLE ADJUSTMENTS

What are reasonable adjustments?

Under the Disability Discrimination Act, and more recently under the Equality Act, all public sector services have a legal duty to make '**reasonable adjustments**' to the way they make their services available to people with learning disabilities, to make them as accessible and effective as they would be for people without disabilities. Many of us may be familiar with ramps being installed to facilitate access of wheelchair users to service areas. Reasonable adjustment must also consider making whatever alterations are necessary to policies, procedures, staff training and the way the service is delivered to ensure that they work equally well for people with learning disabilities.

This legal duty for health services is 'anticipatory'. This means that health service organisations are required to consider **in advance** what adjustments people with learning disabilities will require, rather than waiting until people with learning disabilities attempt to use health services to put reasonable adjustments into place.

CRITICAL THINKING STOP POINT 21.5

ANTICIPATORY DUTY

When you are on placement consider how accessible the environment is to someone with a learning disability, and what improvements could be considered.

WHY ARE REASONABLE ADJUSTMENTS IMPORTANT FOR PEOPLE WITH LEARNING DISABILITIES?

Over the past 20 years, the substantial and wide-ranging health inequalities experienced by people with learning disabilities have become increasingly well documented. Common problems noted have been with safeguarding procedures, access to advocates, care planning, staff training, institutional regimes and rigorous scrutiny of service quality. Adults with a learning disability have died while in hospital because of poor care.

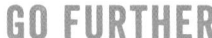

GO FURTHER

WEBLINK: DEVELOPMENTAL DISABILITY HEALTH

Please read http://cddh.monash.org/assets/death-by-indifference.pdf. This and evidence from other inquiries resulted in the Department of Health setting up an independent inquiry into the healthcare experienced by people with learning disabilities, which reported in 2008 (Michael, 2008).

This report reinforced the findings of previous inquiries, stating that 'There is a clear legal framework for the provision of equal treatment for people with disabilities and yet it seems clear that … services are not yet being provided to an adequate standard' (Michael, 2008: 55). People are dying because reasonable adjustments are not being put into place.

There are known barriers to delivering an effective healthcare service for people with a learning disability, however a range of strategies have been devised to overcome these barriers:

1. **Not being included in health screening including**: cervical screening tests; breast screening; dental check-ups; epilepsy checks and sensory impairment assessments. Additionally, there are syndromes associated with learning disability where there are known health risks that are not

regularly and consistently screened. Individuals with Down's syndrome are not always routinely screened for dementia, thyroid function or cardiac function. These are some of the issues facing Libby across her lifespan (Critical Thinking Stop Point 21.1).

Nursing consideration: Regular health screening of people with learning disabilities through co-operation between specialist learning disability teams, GPs and primary health care teams improves health status and access to other mainstream health services (Cassidy et al., 2002; Martin et al., 1997).

2. **Health promotion materials not being accessible** for people with a learning disability.

Nursing consideration: Low levels of literacy among people with learning disabilities means that access to information in text is problematic for many. Strategies for simplifying printed matter have been devised by Mencap (Mencap, 2009). Similar guidelines have also been produced by the European Commission and CHANGE (2009). Strategies include:

*   covering only one idea per sentence;
*   use of active rather than passive verbs;
*   avoidance of abstract concepts.

GO FURTHER

The business of producing easy-to-read documentation is growing steadily. Here are examples from the British Institute of Learning Disabilities: www.bild.org.uk/easy-read/easy-read-information/ and from the Foundation for People with Learning Disabilities: www.learningdisabilities.org.uk/our-work/health-well-being/easy-read-guides-health-conditions/

Take a look at information within your practice area, and consider how it could be made accessible.

Also, be aware easy-read information is only an option. There are a high number of adults with a learning disability who will be unable to read anything. How would you support their needs for information?

WEBLINKS

---

3. **Environmental barriers**, that is the person with a learning disability is unable to access health services independently.

Nursing consideration: Where appropriate, e,g. in primary care, consider offering extended or double appointments where this would assist to support effective communication. Consider offering a choice of appointment time, for example the first or last appointment may suit particularly anxious patients or those who find sitting in busy waiting areas difficult.

4. **Communication impairments** are commonly associated with learning disabilities, whether with regards to expressive communication or comprehension. Difficulties in communication can impact in many ways. Unmet communication needs can lead to challenging behaviour. People with learning disabilities often have difficulty adapting to new situations. This means that for planned or unplanned admissions there is potential for challenging behaviour.

Nursing consideration: Across the last 15 years the UK Government has issued documents stressing importance of inclusion (DH, 2001, 2009), but where does communication come in? Although communication was not identified as one of the core principles of the two white papers, it is acknowledged that it is central to the consideration of rights, social inclusion, choice and independence (Jones, 2000).

- Allow plenty of time for the person to understand and respond. It is important to be prepared to wait much longer.
- Take into account the knowledge, skills and experience of the person with learning disabilities. Obtain insight into the person's past.
- Ideas or information should be presented in the order in which they are to happen or have happened.
- Consider using visual support such as photographs, objects of reference, symbols or signing, e.g. Makaton. Combining several of these approaches is often the most effective.
- When new information or difficult concepts are discussed, keep the number of information-carrying words per sentence or phrase to two.
- Make it clear you have finished discussing a topic before introducing any new ideas.
- Say exactly what is required or needs to be done rather than using figurative language, metaphors or idioms. For example, rather than saying, 'Hop on the scales' say, 'Stand on the scales'.
- Words such as negatives 'can't', 'don't', 'won't', 'never' are more difficult to understand. If you have to use a negative word or phrase support it visually with either a photograph or gesture.
- Pronouns such as 'he', 'she', and 'it' are more difficult than real nouns or names, e.g. say, 'The Nurse will do your blood test. The Nurse will take your blood after breakfast.'
- Vocabulary – communicate using simpler words and concepts where possible, e.g. 'house'/'home' instead of accommodation/residence; 'use' instead of utilise/operate.
- Be aware of the impact the environment has on interactions – background noise and people can distort or make thinking extremely difficult for the person.

ACTIVITY 21.4: REFLECTIVE PRACTICE

van der Gaag (1998) identified a number of core principles considered critical to establishing a positive communication environment:

- The communication needs of the individual are at the heart of all practice.
- The involvement of significant others in the individual's environment is critical.
- The focus is on partnership communication and therefore considers not only communication skills use of service users but also that of significant others.

Reflect on one of your practice placements and consider if it demonstrates a positive communication environment. What was good about the communication environment? How could it be improved?

Other than individuals with a learning disability, who else would benefit from a positive communication environment?

---

5. **Diagnostic overshadowing** where a change of behaviour or change in physiology is attributed to the learning disability rather than an underlying ill health. This can also be informed by atypical manifestations of pain or discomfort. Difficulties in communication can impact in many ways. Unmet communication needs can lead to challenging behaviour. People with learning disabilities often have difficulty adapting to new situations. This means that for planned or unplanned admissions there is potential for challenging behaviour.

Nursing consideration: Nurses should ask: 'What would I do if I was in a strange place, with strange people, who do not talk with me?' As long as nurses lack insight and understanding about people with a learning disability, there is potential for discrimination and stigma. Use the hospital passport to enable an accurate assessment and recording of information.

CHAPTER SUMMARY

The impact of the learning disability upon the adult with a learning disability means:

- communication difficulties, both in understanding and expression
- lack of awareness of what health services exist, and how to access them
- lack of awareness of the various screening programmes available, and the impact this could have on their health
- a potential for a diminished understanding of the ability to understand, retain and weigh-up consequences of health decisions
- a risk of having a range of social needs associated with increased health needs.

Across the UK a range of policies have been put in place to support people with a learning disability and enable their inclusion within the community. Broadly, the policies since 2001 have been endeavouring to create opportunities in citizenship, empowerment, decision-making, equality and social inclusion (Department of Health 2009; Department of Health and Social Security, 2005; Scottish Government, 2013).

In terms of addressing and responding to health needs and health services there has been a consistent response which is instrumental in directing nursing actions in all fields:

- effective communication with patients, carers, family members and clinicians
- collaborative working between general and specialist services
- enabling access to general services with support from specialist services
- developing healthcare staff on understanding the needs of people with a learning disability
- ensuring all people with a learning disability are registered with a GP
- delivering individualised, person-centred care to the person with a learning disability
- ensuring inclusion in health screening and health promotion campaigns.

This is how to care for the adult with a learning disability.

GO FURTHER

Go to https://study.sagepub.com/essentialadultnursing for a further case study related to this chapter. If you are using the interactive ebook, simply click on the book icon in the margin to go straight to the resource.

CASE STUDY: LEARNING DISABILITY

Journal Articles

Go to https://study.sagepub.com/essentialadultnursing for further free online journal articles related to this chapter. If you are using the interactive ebook, simply click on the book icon in the margin to go straight to the resource.

FURTHER READING: JOURNAL ARTICLES

FURTHER
READING:
WEBLINKS

Weblinks

Go to https://study.sagepub.com/essentialadultnursing for further weblinks related to this chapter. If you are using the interactive ebook, simply click on the book icon in the margin to go straight to the resource.

- Atkinson, D., Boulter, P., Hebron, C. et al. (2013) The Health Equalities Framework (HEF): An Outcomes Framework. Available at: www.ndti.org.uk/uploads/files/The_Health_Equality_Framework_final_word.pdf.
  The Health Equalities Framework (HEF) works by monitoring the degree and impact of exposure of people with learning disabilities to acknowledged, evidence-based determinants of health inequalities.
- Heslop, P., Blair, P., Fleming, P., Hoghton, M., Marriott, A. and Russ, L., (2013) CIPOLD Confidential inquiry into premature deaths of people with learning disabilities (CIPOLD) : final report. Bristol: Norah Fry Research Centre, 2013. Available at: https://www.bristol.ac.uk/media-library/sites/cipold/migrated/documents/fullfinalreport.pdf
  CIPOLD was tasked with investigating the avoidable or premature deaths of people with learning disabilities through a series of retrospective reviews of deaths. The aim was to review the patterns of care that people received in the period leading up to their deaths, to identify errors or omissions contributing to these deaths, to illustrate evidence of good practice, and to provide improved evidence on avoiding premature death.
- www.youtube.com/watch?v=IyV1v-nib38
  In this short film, volunteers from the project Getting It Right – From The Start talk about communication. They share some of the things you should keep in mind when communicating with people with a learning disability.

ONLINE
QUIZZES

——— ACE YOUR ASSESSMENT ———

Revise what you have learned by visiting https://study.sagepub.com/essentialadultnursing

- Test yourself with multiple-choice and short-answer questions
- Do the chapter activities in the book and check your answers online

REFERENCES

American Psychiatric Association (2013) *Diagnostic and Statistical Manual of Mental Disorders* (5th ed.). Arlington, VA: American Psychiatric Publishing.

Atkinson, D., Boulter, P., Hebron, C., Moulster, G., Giraud-Saunders, A. and Turner, S. (2013) *The Health Equalities Framework (HEF): An Outcomes Framework*. Available at www.ndti.org.uk/uploads/files/The_Health_Equality_Framework_final_word.pdf (Accessed 02/03/18)

Cassidy, G., Martin, D.M., Martin, G.H.B. and Roy, A. (2002) Health checks for people with learning disabilities: Community learning disability teams working with general practitioners and primary health care teams. *Journal of Learning Disabilities*, 6: 12–136.

Dahlgren, G. and Whitehead, M. (1991) *Policies and Strategies to Promote Social Equity in Health*. Stockholm, Sweden: Institute for Futures Studies.

Department of Health (2001) *Valuing People: A New Strategy for Learning Disability for the 21st Century. Towards Person Centred Approaches: Planning with People*. London: Stationery Office. Available at: www.gov.uk/government/uploads/system/uploads/attachment_data/file/250877/5086.pdf (Accessed 02/03/18)

Department of Health (1999) *Once a day one or more people with learning disabilities are likely to be in contact with your primary healthcare team – how can you help them?* Available at: http://webarchive.nationalarchives.gov.uk/+/www.dh.gov.uk/en/publicationsandstatistics/publications/publicationspolicyandguidance/dh_4006868?PageOperation=email.

Department of Health (2009) *Valuing People: Now.* Available at: www.gov.uk/government/uploads/system/uploads/attachment_data/file/215891/dh_122387.pdf. (Accessed 02/03/18)

Department of Health & NHS Finance (2009) *The Operating Framework. For The NHS In England 2010/11.* Available at: http://systems.hscic.gov.uk/infogov/links/operatingframework2010-2011.pdf. (Accessed 02/03/18)

Department of Health (2010) *Six Lives Progress Report.* Available at: www.gov.uk/government/uploads/system/uploads/attachment_data/file/212292/Six_lives_2nd_Progress_Report_on_Healthcare_for_People_with_Learning_Disabilities_-_full_report.pdf. (Accessed 02/03/18).

Emerson, E. and Heslop, P. (2010) *A Working Definition of Learning Disabilities.* Durham: Improving Health and Lives Learning Disabilities Observatory.

Emerson, E., Baines, S., Allerton, L. and Welch, V. (2011) *Health Inequalities and People with Learning Disabilities in the UK: 2011.* Durham: Improving Health and Lives: Learning Disabilities Observatory.

Emerson, E., Hatton, C., Robertson, J., Baines, S., Christie, A. and Glover, G. (2012) *Health Inequalities and People with Learning Disabilities in the UK: 2012.* Durham: Improving Health and Lives: Learning Disability Observatory.

Great Britain. *Mental Capacity Act 2005: Elizabeth II. Chapter 9* (2005) Available at: www.legislation.gov.uk/ukpga/2005/9/pdfs/ukpga_20050009_en.pdf (Accessed 02/03/18)

Jones, J. (2000) A total communication approach to meeting the communication needs of people with learning disabilities. *Tizard Learning Disability Review,* 5: 2026.

Martin, D.M., Roy, A. and Wells, M.B. (1997) Health gain through health checks: Improving access to primary health care for people with intellectual disability. *Journal of Intellectual Disability Research,* 41: 401–8.

Mencap (2009) *Am I Making Myself Clear? Mencap's guidelines for accessible writing.* Available at: www.mencap.org.uk

Mencap (2012) *Death By Indifference: 74 Deaths And Counting: A Progress Report 5 Years On.* London: Mencap.

Re MB (Caesarean Section) [1997] 2 FLr 426 (CA).

Michael, J. (2008) *Healthcare for All: The independent Inquiry into Access to Healthcare for People with Learning Disabilities.* Emerald Group Publishing Limited. https://doi.org/10.1108/13595474200800036

Scottish Government (2013) *The Keys to Life – Improving Quality of Life for People with Learning Disabilities.* Available at: www.gov.scot/resource/0042/00424389.pdf. (Accessed 02/03/18).

van der Gaag, A. (1998) Keynote review: Communication skills and adults with learning disabilities. *British Journal of Learning Disabilities,* 26 (3): 88–93.

World Health Organization (WHO) (1980) *International Classification of Impairments, Disabilities, and Handicaps. A manual of classification relating to the consequences of disease.* Geneva: World Health Organization.

World Health Organization (WHO) (1992) *International Statistical Classification of Diseases and Related Health Problems, 10th Revision (ICD-10).* Geneva: World Health Organization.

CARE OF THE ADULT WITH CANCER

22

MAURA DOWLING AND ELIZABETH MEADE

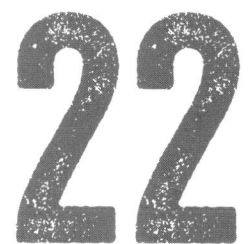

WATCH VIDEOS ONLINE · CLICK HERE

THIS CHAPTER COVERS

- Introduction to cancer
- Cancer staging
- Treatment of cancers and their side effects

- The physical, psychological, emotional and spiritual needs of the patient with cancer and the provision of patient-centred care.

Caring for patients who have cancer made me feel anxious when I first started my nursing training. I found it challenging to find the right thing to say to these patients who are enduring such a vulnerable time in their lives. Most patients love to see a student coming as we tend to have that small but extra time to deliver care, which means there is more time to get to know the patient. Many patients suffer from cancer-related fatigue. I feel this can be one of the hardest things for the patients to deal with as they feel they are well enough to do loads of things but their energy levels just don't allow them to do so. I found on placement that reassuring patients that what they are feeling is normal for their situation and the use of goals are really helpful. For example, one of my patients had more energy after lunch so she preferred to have a shower in the afternoon. Allowing for her shower to occur later in the day she felt she had accomplished something big as she wasn't feeling overwhelmingly fatigued.

Lynn Muldowney, third year undergraduate nurse

Caring for cancer patients can cause anxiety for students, especially around communication. This is evident in Lynn's comment above. Lynn wrote this comment in third year but when we met her again in the fourth year of her programme, her confidence in communicating with cancer patients had increased hugely. Equipping student nurses with good communication skills, especially the art of listening, helps to improve the patient's quality of life.

On my first week's placement on the oncology unit in third year, I was overwhelmed by the volume of cancer jargon and specialised terminology being used by nurses at handover. Initially, this hindered me in my communication with patients. However, over the following weeks, I gradually began to understand what many of the more common terms being used meant, and became more relaxed in my interactions with patients on the unit. What helped was the booklet for students on the unit which had a list of common terms used in cancer care and explanations. This was developed by the clinical placement facilitators assigned to the cancer unit and the link lecturer from my university. The clinical facilitators and link lecturer were very helpful in checking my understanding with me and asking me questions that promoted me to seek clarifications. I kept a list of questions I had in a small notebook and that also helped me stay focused on meeting my learning needs on the placement. My preceptor and the ward manager were also significant to my learning. They made me feel part of their team from the first day and regularly reminded me to keep asking questions and that no question was not relevant to my learning. The welcoming atmosphere on the unit helped my learning a lot and my level of comfort in communicating with patients.

Lynn Muldowney, third year undergraduate nurse

INTRODUCTION

The last three decades have seen remarkable progress in the prevention, detection and treatment of cancer. Diagnosis is now more precise, surgery is less mutilating and radiotherapy is now more targeted. The selection of patients with some cancers (for instance, breast and bowel cancer) for **adjuvant chemotherapy** is based not only on prognostic and predictive factors but on newer molecular profiling which will ensure that chemotherapy is given to the patients who need and respond to chemotherapy. This has led to dramatic increases in cancer survivors worldwide. Traditionally, standard treatments included surgery, radiation, chemotherapy and hormone therapy, but now with a better understanding of cancer biology new **targeted agents** and **immunotherapy** are part of the standard of care for many cancers. These developments all provide a more tailored approach to cancer management.

The management of cancer involves a multidisciplinary team approach in order to provide the highest standard of care for patients throughout their cancer journey from diagnosis through treatment and into follow-up care. The multidisciplinary team include surgeons, medical oncologists, radiotherapists, specialised oncology trained nurses and allied healthcare professionals (such as social workers) who all put the patient at the centre of their care and decision making.

The diagnosis of cancer for any patient is potentially life changing and can come as a huge shock. Patients have worries about their diagnosis, prognosis, treatment and side effects and the impact of cancer, not only on themselves, but also their families. The social, psychological and financial impact of cancer can have longstanding effects depending on the stage of the cancer and the prognosis as well as the duration of treatment(s). It is a very stressful time, and a person-centred approach is central to the care provided to patients and their families.

Many patients and their families are overwhelmed by the diagnosis and treatment, which can affect their ability to actively engage in important discussions regarding diagnosis, treatment and prognosis. Oncology trained nurses have the knowledge and skills to help reduce the patients' stress and help them and their families to navigate their way through their treatment(s).

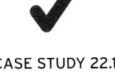

CASE STUDY 22.1
ANSWER

CASE STUDY 22.1: MARY

Mary was diagnosed with high-risk breast cancer. She underwent a mastectomy and axillary lymph dissection, adjuvant chemotherapy for six months and radiotherapy for six weeks. Mary was 'devastated by her diagnosis' and the 'shock of hearing the word cancer' and all that it implies. She is a separated mother of three children. Two of her children have experienced severe mental health issues. Her main concerns were her children and the impact that her illness would have on their lives and her ability to care for them. She was determined that she would continue her normal routine and stated that she 'did not have time to be sick'.

Mary is typical of many women with children living with cancer. Mothers with cancer often experience significant worry and stress over concerns about their children and a need to protect their children from seeing them ill.

It is important for nurses to give women like Mary opportunities to talk about these worries and tease out any strategies that may help, such as seeking out support from a local cancer support group or service.

Cancer care can often be fragmented. This happens because cancer patients are often cared for by different teams and sometimes in different hospitals. The clinical nurse specialist (CNS) plays a very important role in minimising fragmented care and providing person-centred care. The CNS coordinates each patient's care and acts a patient advocate, as they navigate the healthcare system. The CNS also provides information, education and support regarding the patient's treatment options and management of treatment side effects.

It is essential to ascertain the family supports available to each patient as this can have a significant impact on the patient's ability to cope during their treatment. Oncology nurses offer practical advice on coping with cancer and treatments as well as information on supportive services available. Close involvement with the patient's general practitioner (GP) is also essential in order to improve continuity of care and support from community services.

Student nurses receive mentoring and advice from oncology trained nurses while on clinical placement. Mentorship from specialist oncology nurses contributes greatly to students' positive experience and learning on placement.

> The oncology staff are very knowledge. Many have a postgraduate qualification and have great amounts of knowledge. Being allocated to a nurse for each shift allowed me to create a learning relationship with the nurse in order to gain invaluable experience and confidence in providing care to oncology patients whilst on clinical placement.
>
> **Lynn Muldowney, third year undergraduate nurse**

PROVIDING PERSON-CENTRED, HOLISTIC CARE TO A PATIENT WITH CANCER

A diagnosis of cancer is life altering. Issues about life and death predominate in a person's search to find a cause for their cancer. Many people diagnosed with cancer do cope well with their diagnosis and treatment, and do not display abnormal levels of distress. However, others may not be equipped with sufficient emotional reserves or social support and experience psychological distress.

Those people who cope better than others do so for a number of reasons, including: marital satisfaction, religious sources, good problem-solving skills, higher education attainment, and social support (next of kin play a vital role). These people can experience what is called 'post-traumatic growth' and this is a current area of much interest for researchers (McDonough et al., 2014). However, a minority of cancer patients and their families develop post-traumatic stress symptoms (PTSS) and post-traumatic stress disorder (PTSD) (Cordova et al., 2017). This can result in heightened symptom distress and reduced quality of life. Risk factors for PTSD include a prior trauma, a pre-existing psychiatric condition and poor social support (Cordova et al., 2017). It is important for nurses to acknowledge that each person living with a diagnosis of cancer will react in their own unique way and how they cope will be influenced by many factors, including how well they have coped in the past with major life challenges and their support systems.

Cancer and its treatments and side effects can affect patients in a variety of ways including physically, emotionally and mentally. Most patients with cancer will require nursing care at some time in their cancer journey. Many patients require ongoing follow-up care after completion of treatment as over half of patients survive their cancer. Nurses caring for patients with cancer have the potential to improve the quality of care provided and patient outcomes. Patient-centred care is now an integral part of care where a partnership is developed between healthcare providers, patients and their families.

It aims to help patients participate in decision making to improve their health outcomes. Nurses caring for patients with cancer need to be able to recognise the impact of cancer on all aspects of a patient's life and address these concerns.

A diagnosis of cancer also has implications for the patient's family, with potential changes in family roles, financial pressure and the worry, stress and uncertainty associated with caring for a loved one who is unwell. Nurses play a very important role as patient advocate and are ideally placed to ascertain the patient's knowledge and understanding regarding their diagnosis and cancer treatment(s). Information needs vary between patients and different stages in the cancer journey. It is essential, therefore, to assess each patient's information needs and tailor information and support to suit these needs. Patients should receive accurate information provided in a sensitive manner and feel that they are being listened to and heard and are involved and supported in their decision making. Summarising the information provided and checking the patient's understanding will help them to become more active in their care.

It is essential that students appreciate the centrality of person-centred care for cancer patients and their families. Students can play an important role in this care. On placements, students have more time to spend with cancer patients and patients value greatly opportunities to communicate with students. Often the conversations are about sport or TV because cancer patients want to take time away from being a 'patient with cancer' and feeling some way a bit 'normal'. Out of the 'small talk' between nurses and patients emerges the opportunity for patients to seek advice. If patients seek advice, it is important that students seek assistance from their specialised oncology trained colleagues if they have a deficit in knowledge or skills. Through the provision of advice on the management of specific side effects at different stages throughout the patient's cancer journey, patients' quality of life is improved.

CANCER PATHOPHYSIOLOGY AND EPIDEMIOLOGY IN CANCER PREVENTION

Epidemiology is a science that is very important in understanding cancer. Epidemiology is used to track the occurrence of cancer, paint a picture of the natural history of cancer and identify causes of cancer. Therefore, epidemiology is very important in guiding cancer prevention and early detection (through **screening** measures). After diagnosis, most patients want to know why they developed cancer; a knowledge of pathophysiology therefore provides the student nurse with essential information on the various different causes of cancer.

WHAT'S THE EVIDENCE? 22.1

Lee, D.H., Keum, N. and Giovannucci, E.L. (2016) Colorectal cancer epidemiology in the nurses' health study. *American Journal of Public Health*, 106(9): 1599-607.

Colorectal cancer (CRC) is the second most commonly diagnosed cancer in women and the third in men worldwide. In 2012, an estimated 1.36 million new cases of CRC were diagnosed worldwide, which accounted for 9.7% of total cancers, excluding non-melanoma skin cancer. The rates of CRC, however, vary more than 10 times across the world, with high-income countries showing approximately 2.5 times higher rates than low-income countries.

This study was a narrative review of research studies published from the Nurses' Health Study between 1976 and 2016. The Nurses' Health Study is a large, prospective cohort study from the USA.

The review reported that red and processed meat, alcohol, smoking and obesity were associated with an increased risk of CRC. A decreased risk of CRC was associated with folate, calcium, vitamin D, aspirin and physical activity. In addition, modifiable factors, such as physical activity, vitamin D, folate, insulin and insulin-like growth factor binding protein-1, and diet quality, were identified to be associated with survival among CRC patients.

Now read this article and reflect on what health promotion advice you would give to someone asking about colorectal cancer risk.

Epidemiologic studies show patterns of cancer occurrence within countries and comparisons across countries. For instance, epidemiological studies on ovarian cancer in the UK reveal a fall in death rate but the death rate is still higher than in other European countries and the USA (Doufekas and Olaitan, 2014). In addition, five-year survival estimates range from 12% in parts of Africa compared to almost 90% in the USA, Australia and Canada. These differences have been linked to a combination of early detection, access to treatment services and cultural barriers.

Epidemiologic studies have also helped us understand the role of infections in cancer. We now know that infections associated with cancer are more common in developing countries, and as many as one third of cancers worldwide are associated with microbial infections. **Helicobacter pylori** is associated with gastric cancer. Other infections associated with cancer include **clonorchis sinensis** and **opisthorchis viverrini**, which are linked with bile duct cancer, and **enterotoxigenic bacteroides fragilis**, which is associated with colon cancer. Under normal conditions, an acute inflammatory response is self-limiting but with chronic inflammation, **cytokines** can induce **DNA** damage, which can result in the development of cancer.

Alterations in our genes can also result in the formation of cancer. While an inherited predisposition to cancer does not mean that someone will definitely get cancer, it does greatly increase the risk of getting cancer. Examples of mutated genes that can cause cancer include **BRCA1** and **BRCA2** genes, which account for 5–10% of all breast cancers. The BRACI and BRAC2 genes are both associated with an increased risk of breast cancer and ovarian cancer.

Another example of a genetic change that results in cancer is what happens when a translocation occurs at cellular level and a 'fusion gene' develops. The 'Philadelphia translocation', a translocation between chromosomes 9 and 22 (written as follows: t(9:22)), is one such gene and occurs in 90–95% of cases of chronic myeloid leukaemia (CML). Other examples include **KRAS** and **NRAS**, which are **oncogenes** present in colon cells and associated with colorectal cancer.

It is essential that nurses have an awareness of the potential causes of cancer. This is important because not only will every nurse at some stage in their career care for a patient with cancer, but also because of all the opportunities nurses can use for health promotion on preventing cancer. Nurses can impact on all elements of cancer control from prevention, treatment, survivorship and palliative care. Nurses are central to the delivery of high-quality cancer services as they have an important role in encouraging healthy lifestyle in the prevention of cancer, promoting screening and early detection, and maintaining healthy lifestyle in survivorship care.

HEALTH PROMOTION

While we cannot change some risk factors for cancer (age, gender and family history), we can change our lifestyles to reduce our risk of cancer. Lifestyle activities that can reduce our risk of cancer include:

- not smoking
- eating a healthy diet: limiting intake of food high in calories, fat and sugar, red and processed meat and salt. Eating more fruit and vegetables, wholegrain and pulses
- being active and exercising
- maintaining a healthy weight
- keeping within normal recommended alcohol intake
- avoiding ultraviolet sun exposure (be sun smart).

Despite our knowledge on the contributing factors to the development of cancer, some people choose to ignore health promotion advice. These are often people who are fatalistic about cancer. Fatalism is a belief that events are fixed in advance for all time in such a manner that humans are powerless to change them. In the context of cancer, fatalism is a belief that death is inevitable when cancer is present.

SCREENING FOR CANCER

CASE STUDY 22.2: PAULINE

Pauline is 32 years old but never attended for a cervical cancer screen until this year. She has been invited many times since the age of 25 (the age at which women in UK are first invited) but never attended. Pauline is quite fatalistic and is of the belief that if you get cancer it's too late anyway so why bother to attend for screening. Pauline has had asthma since childhood but it has been managed well. However, eight weeks ago she developed a bad wheeze so attended a local GP surgery where her inhalers were reviewed and she was commenced on a course of oral steroids. While Gina, the practice nurse, was questioning Pauline on her general health and educating Pauline on the steroid and inhaler use, she also ascertained that Pauline had never attended for a smear test and arranged for Pauline to return the following week when her period was finished to have a smear and HPV test (human papilloma virus test).

Pauline's smear was abnormal so the laboratory also undertook a test for the human papilloma virus (HPV). The HPV test was positive so she was referred to the colposcopy clinic. At the colposcopy clinic, the trained colposcopy nurse treated the abnormal surface cells on the cervix under local anaesthetic using a very fine heated wire loop. This procedure is known as LETZ (large loop excision of the transformation zone). A sample of the cervical tissue was then sent to the laboratory for further analysis.

HPV is also associated with other cancers besides cervical cancer. Can you identify one of these cancers?

What reasons might be contributing to Pauline's fatalistic attitude to cancer?

DIAGNOSIS AND STAGING

ACTIVITY 22.1: REFLECTIVE PRACTICE

Before reaching a diagnosis of cancer, patients must undergo many tests. These tests are often repeated after a course of treatment to determine if the cancer has responded to the treatment. Waiting for test(s) results is a time of intense anxiety for patients and their families. Nurses play a key role in providing information on what patients need to do in preparation for these tests and what the tests entail.

Reflect for a moment on what tests you think are undertaken to check if someone has cancer or to see if a person has responded to their cancer treatment. To help you answer this question, think about the tests you may have seen patients have when you were on placement.

SEE ALSO
CHAPTER 22

When a person is suspected of having cancer, they must undergo many tests. These tests are not only to accurately diagnose the type of cancer the person has but also to stage the cancer so that the person's response to treatment can be monitored by follow-up tests. Initially, a biopsy is taken in order to get a **histological** diagnosis and to differentiate the type of cancer and the presence or absence of predictive markers. These include oestrogen, progesterone and **HER2/neu** status in breast cancer patients, **RAS (biomarkers)** status in colon cancer patients and **EGFR (epidermal growth factor receptor)** in lung cancer. This analysis will then be utilised in the selection of treatment for patients. It is important to remember that not all cancers are the same and we now have a greater understanding of cancer biology and the molecular differences inherent in many cancers.

STAGING

Once a cancer is diagnosed, the cancer must be 'staged' in order to classify the extent of its spread within the body. This information also often influences the choice of treatment. Moreover, accurate staging is important for records on treatment outcomes for each type of cancer and each stage of cancer. This information is useful in developing cancer guidelines for treatment.

The tumour-node-metastasis (TNM) system of the American Joint Committee on Cancer (AJCC) is the preferred staging system for solid tumours such as breast, lung and colon. However, non-solid tumours (blood cancers) cannot be classified by TNM.

The letters represent the following: **T** = the tumour's size, depth of invasion, and involvement of surrounding structures. **N** = the presence or absence of involved nodes and the size and the number. **M** = the presence or absence of metastases (spread to other organs). A number is also added to each letter to indicate the size or extent of the tumour and the extent of tumour spread. For instance, prostate cancer T2 N0 M0 means that the tumour is located only in the prostate and has not spread to the lymph nodes or any other part of the body.

The results of the TNM results determine the stage of the cancer. Most cancers have four stages: stages I (one) to IV (four). Some cancers also have a stage 0 (zero).

Stage 0. This stage describes cancer in situ, which means 'in place'. Stage 0 cancers are still located in the place they started and have not spread to nearby tissues. This stage of cancer is often highly curable, usually by removing the entire tumour with surgery.

Stage I. This stage is usually a small cancer or tumour that has not grown deeply into nearby tissues. It also has not spread to the lymph nodes or other parts of the body. It is often called early-stage cancer.

Stages II and III. These stages indicate larger cancers or tumours that have grown more deeply into nearby tissue. They may have also spread to lymph nodes but not to other parts of the body.

Stage IV. This stage means that the cancer has spread to other organs or parts of the body. It may also be called advanced or metastatic cancer.

Cancers are also '**graded**' to determine how similar the tumour is to normal tissue. Grading is *not the same* as staging of a cancer. Grading refers to how abnormal the tumour cells look when viewed under a microscope. It gives an indication of how quickly a tumour is likely to grow and spread. If the cells of the tumour and the pattern of the tumour's tissue closely resemble those of normal cells and tissue, the tumour is called 'well-differentiated'. A well-differentiated tumour tends to grow and spread at a slower rate than tumours that are 'undifferentiated' or 'poorly differentiated' which have abnormal-looking cells and may not have normal tissue structures. Most cancers are assigned a numerical 'grade'; however, the factors that determine the tumour's grade can vary between different types of cancer.

Staging investigations tests include **CT (computed tomography) scans**. However, CT is limited in its ability to differentiate between normal and cancer tissue. Therefore, MRI (magnetic resonance imaging) is also used. MRI is especially useful in imaging of the brain, spine, peripheral limbs and joints, neck and pelvis. Another important diagnostic test is the PET scan. PET is the abbreviation for **positron emission tomography**, which is a form of nuclear medicine scan using a specially designed scanner. FDG-PET denotes a specific radioactive material, F-fluorodeoxyglucose, given one to two hours before PET. This is particularly useful in cancer because of its ability to discern malignant disease in multiple organs, at multiple sites. Immunoscintigraphy is another form of nuclear medicine scan which produces images revealing the presence of cancer. With immunoscintigraphy, a radioactive material is injected intravenously along with monoclonal antibodies (these are often referred to as 'magic bullets') specific to a tumour type. **Tumour markers** are also used in the diagnosis of cancer. These markers are searched for in the person's blood sample. For instance, CA-125 (Cancer Antigen 125) is present in greater concentration in ovarian cancer than in other cells; PSA (prostate specific antigen) is specific for prostate cancer.

The diagnosis and staging of cancer may take many weeks. This is a very difficult and anxious time for patients and their families. The staging will determine whether the cancer is potentially curable or incurable which will have serious implications for patients and their families. Good communication is essential at this time. Patients should be provided with written and verbal information regarding proposed investigations. Nurses can provide realistic time frames for when results will be available, explaining why it can take weeks for some results to become available. Patients should be advised to bring a family member to their consultation and to write down any questions they may have in advance. Listening to patients and allowing them time and space to voice their fears and worries helps to support them through this distressing period and can help to improve their cancer experience. The student nurse can at this time build up a rapport with the patient, finding out about their social, domestic and work life and their social supports. Good communication can also help improve self-management and reduce the distress associated with a diagnosis of cancer.

TYPES OF CANCERS

There are many types of cancers that are classified as solid tumours (or non-haematological) or haematological (Table 22.1).

GO FURTHER

The Cancer Research UK website lists all cancers by type and key information on each one. Visit the site as you review Table 22.1.

www.cancerresearchuk.org/about-cancer/type/

WEBLINK: TYPES OF CANCER

Table 22.1   Types of cancer

Non-haematological cancers (solid tumours)	Haematological cancers
Breast	Leukaemia (acute and chronic)
Lung	Lymphoma (Hodgkin's and Non-Hodgkin's)
Skin	Multiple myeloma
Genitourinary (prostate, testicular, bladder)	Myelodysplastic syndromes
Head and neck	
Gynaecologic (ovarian, cervical)	
Gastrointestinal	
Sarcomas	
Brain tumours	
AIDS-related malignancies	

CANCER TREATMENTS

Cancer can be treated in many ways and those with cancer are often treated with more than one form of therapy. The cancer treatment journey takes many months and nurses play a key role in supporting patients on that journey.

Surgery is a treatment option for solid tumours. For early stage cancer, surgical resection remains the mainstay of curative-intent treatment. Sometimes, chemotherapy and/or radiotherapy is given before surgery (this is called neo-adjuvant chemotherapy/radiotherapy) to shrink a tumour's size.

Radiotherapy is another major treatment option in cancer. It can be used to cure cancer, (e.g. Hodgkin's lymphoma), as an adjuvant treatment (i.e. used with another cancer treatment, in for instance, breast cancer) or as palliation (to relieve symptoms, e.g. pain from an enlarged tumour site pressing on surrounding tissue). Radiotherapy is the process of using radiation, which damages deoxyribonucleic acid (DNA) and, as a result, causes cell death. Cancer cells undergo frequent division and growth, so are more vulnerable to radiation damage than cells that do not divide, or do so infrequently. Therefore, most cancers are sensitive to radiation effect, and this sensitivity is known as radiosensitive or radioresponsive. However, some types of cancers are radioresistant. This radioresistance can be overcome by giving chemotherapy at the same time as radiotherapy, higher than usual doses of radiotherapy, or more daily treatments in smaller doses.

There are three main methods of delivery for radiotherapy: external beam radiation, **brachytherapy** and systemic isotope therapy.

Planning for external beam radiotherapy is crucial. Patients must be treated in the same position every day as this minimises the risk of damage to surrounding tissue. Therefore, before starting radiotherapy, an x-ray machine called a simulator is used to plan treatment. Brachytherapy involves the placement of radioactive sources within tissues/tumours or body cavities. This allows very high doses of radiation to be delivered directly to the immediate area where the radiation sources are placed. Brachytherapy is commonly used to treat prostate cancer.

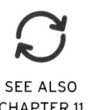

SEE ALSO CHAPTER 11

Systemic isotope therapy is another form of cancer treatment. The best example is the use of iodine-131 in the treatment of thyroid cancer.

The side effects of radiation therapy are mostly related to the area being treated. Two common acute symptoms experienced by patients receiving external radiotherapy are skin reactions and fatigue.

HEALTH PROMOTION

Fatigue following radiotherapy treatment is a major cause of worry and distress for patients and they will ask you what they can do to alleviate their fatigue.

You can tell patients that something simple like taking short walks each day will help their fatigue. Another form of exercise that has been proven to help alleviate fatigue is yoga. Both walking and yoga are safe and effective forms of exercise that most cancer patients can engage in.

WHAT'S THE EVIDENCE? 22.2

In a review of the literature, Glover and Harmer (2014) outline that up to 85% of patients will experience some skin damage from external beam radiotherapy.

They outline measures to manage skin reactions and self-care measures to prevent skin damage for patients who are undergoing external beam radiation.

Read this article and identify what advice you can give to patients to prevent skin damage and nursing interventions when skin damage occurs.

Glover, D. and Harmer, V. (2014) Radiotherapy-induced skin reactions: Assessment and management. *British Journal of Nursing*, 23(4), S28, S30-35.

ANTI-CANCER MEDICINES

The major classes of anti-cancer agents are as follows: cytotoxic drugs, targeted agents and hormonal agents.

Cytotoxic agents are more commonly referred to as '**chemotherapy**'. More than one cytotoxic agent is given to ensure the tumour cells are attacked at all phases of the cell cycle. Cytotoxic agents are classified as cell-cycle-nonspecific or cell-cycle-specific. The most common routes of administration are intravenous and oral.

GO FURTHER

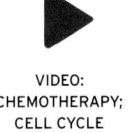

VIDEO:
CHEMOTHERAPY;
CELL CYCLE

This YouTube clip explains the cell cycle and how chemotherapy works on different phases of the cell cycle. You need to understand the cell cycle in order to understand how chemotherapy works. Take some time out to view this useful resource. www.youtube.com/watch?v=VRhz3DhjG5M

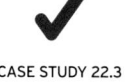

CASE STUDY 22.3: AMANDA

Amanda is a 32-year-old mother of two children (Max, 5 and Ruth, 3). She was diagnosed with Acute Myeloma Leukaemia (AML) when she went for investigations for a history of feeling very tired, flu-like symptoms, bruising, loss of appetite, dizziness and passing out.

Amanda was commenced on induction chemotherapy with high-dose Cytarabine (Ara-C) and following this chemotherapy treatment went into complete remission (CR). Complete remission in AML means that her neutrophil and platelet counts had recovered to near normal levels and she did not need to have red cell transfusions. Also, her bone marrow biopsy showed no clusters of what are known as 'blast cells' (immature blood cells). Amanda then commenced on consolidation therapy (post-remission therapy) to ensure she would stay in remission.

Amanda experienced a range of side effects on chemotherapy. She lost her hair (alopecia), had nausea, lost weight, had a metal-like taste in her mouth, was constantly tired (fatigue), and her brain felt 'foggy' (chemo brain). Amanda loved reading so found the chemo brain a big challenge.

What advice can nurses give to Amanda about managing 'chemo brain'?

CASE STUDY 22.3 ANSWER

ACTIVITY 22.2: REFLECTIVE PRACTICE

Consider the fact that cytotoxic drugs have most effect on the rapidly dividing cells in the body. The rapidly dividing cells are those of the bone marrow, gastrointestinal tract, skin and hair. What side effects will a person experience because of this? And what nursing interventions can help patients manage those side effects?

ACTIVITY 22.2 ANSWER

Did you know that cytotoxic agents fall under the heading of a 'high-alert medication'? The many variations in chemotherapy prescriptions can result in errors (dosing is individualised and there are many routes of administration). It is, therefore, important that guidelines are in place that provide recommendations for the safe prescribing, dispensing and administration of chemotherapy in the treatment of cancer (Meade, 2014). Safety measures to avoid errors in chemotherapy administration include the use of computerised prescriptions, which are reported to be safer than manual order sheets (Kulberg et al., 2013).

Nurses are trained to administer chemotherapy intravenously in specialist cancer centres. Many patients have a cannula inserted by the nurse and are then given their chemotherapy. Some patients have a long lasting catheter inserted for their course of chemotherapy. These include a PICC line (peripherally-inserted central catheter), which is a flexible catheter inserted into a vein in the arm and with the tip sitting in the atrium of the heart. PICC lines can be left in position for a number of months. Central lines are also used for some patients. These are catheters inserted through the skin in the chest into a major vein. These can be left in place for many months. A portacath has a small reservoir implanted under the skin of the upper chest wall and needles can be inserted into this reservoir to administer the chemotherapy. Portacaths can stay in place for as long as is needed.

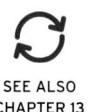

SEE ALSO CHAPTER 13

—————————— **GO FURTHER** ——————————

VIDEOS

Competence in accessing and de-accessing portacaths is essential for all oncology nurses.

Watch this excellent YouTube video showing how to access a portacath step by step. www.youtube.com/watch?v=Sx2dfSUNoCU

This is an excellent YouTube video showing how to de-access a portacath step by step. www.youtube.com/watch?v=Rqkerfex5ql

Nursing care is planned, coordinated and delivered within the multidisciplinary framework to meet patients' needs across diverse settings throughout their cancer journey. Nurses' practice varies and includes nursing assessment, delivery of an intervention, patient education, coordination and evaluation of care. Nurses play a central role preparing patients and their families for treatment, helping them to understand and manage their disease, treatment and possible side effects and counselling patients at all stages of their cancer journey including palliative care for complex symptom management. Regular holistic assessment of the patient's needs throughout the cancer journey is essential in the delivery of high-quality nursing care.

Cancer is now a chronic illness for many people. These patients have to manage their symptoms at home and attend oncology day units for review, usually by a specialist or advanced practice oncology nurse. A major aspect of cancer management is now the use of oral chemotherapy. However, patients often find the side effects difficult and may not adhere to the treatment. Nurses play a central role in educating patients on how to manage the side effects of oral chemotherapy (Komatsu et al., 2014). Nurses also play a central role in following up these patients by telephone in between clinic visits.

CRITICAL THINKING STOP POINT 22.1

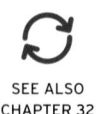

SEE ALSO CHAPTER 32

CRITICAL THINKING STOP POINT 22.1

Imatinib is an oral chemotherapy (see chapter 32, activity 32.6).

Another oral chemotherapy drug is capecitabine (Xeloda), used to treat a range of cancers (breast, colorectal, stomach, pancreatic and oesophageal cancer). Nurses play a key role in educating patients who are taking oral chemotherapy. Many cancer centres now have nurse-led oral chemotherapy clinics where patients are reviewed and educated by experienced oncology nurses.

Go to the Cancer Research UK site below:

www.cancerresearchuk.org/about-cancer/cancers-in-general/treatment/cancer-drugs/capecitabine

Review the common side effects of capecitabine and consider how patient-centred care can be delivered to patients on this oral chemotherapy drug.

TARGETED AGENTS

There are a variety of **targeted agents** available to treat cancer. These include Monoclonal antibodies (MoAbs), which are antibodies that can recognise, and bind to tumours. Many MoAbs halt tumour growth (cytostatic), as opposed to the cells being destroyed by chemotherapy (cytotoxic). However, some MoAbs are not only capable of recognising tumour cells but also of destroying them with assistance from cells of the immune system. A very important example is Herceptin (trastuzumab) which binds to the antigen of the epidermal growth factor receptor 2 **(HER2)** overexpressed on many cancer cells, for instance in breast cancer.

CASE STUDY 22.4: DEIRDRE

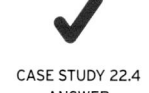

CASE STUDY 22.4
ANSWER

Deirdre is a 44-year-old practice nurse who was diagnosed with left breast cancer. She has two young sons and her husband works away from home. She had a large rapidly growing mass measuring 6cm on mammogram with positive axillary lymph nodes on ultrasound. Biopsy showed ductal carcinoma, grade 3 ER/PR negative and Her2/neu positive. CT scan showed no evidence of metastatic disease. She received neoadjuvant chemotherapy to shrink down the tumour and allow breast-conserving surgery which is the standard of care. Her chemotherapy consisted of 4 cycles of Adriamycin (doxorubicin)/cyclophosphamide every 2 weeks followed by paclitaxel chemotherapy weekly for 12 weeks with Herceptin every 3 weeks. She proceeded to surgery where she had a pathological complete remission. Following surgery she had adjuvant radiotherapy to the breast and continued Herceptin for 1 year.

Deirdre found her chemotherapy the most difficult part of her treatment. She found it very difficult to cope with the fatigue and myalgias associated with chemotherapy as it affected her ability to work and care for her children.

Doxorubicin (Adriamycin) and Herceptin are potentially cardiotoxic. What follow-up advice and health promotion education should Deirdre receive?

Haemopoietic growth factors are a type of **cytokine** (glycoprotein messengers that mobilise white blood cells to defend the body). An example of one is granulocyte-colony stimulating factors (G-CSFs) which is given to some patients to reduce the complications of neutropenia (low white cell count following chemotherapy), minimise neutropenic complications and help in the delivery of chemotherapy at full dose and on schedule.

More recent developments in the field of targeted therapies include developments in **immunotherapy**. Immune therapy is changing the treatment paradigm for many cancers by helping to unleash the patient's own immune systems against their tumour. An important part of the immune system is its ability to tell between normal cells in the body and those it sees as 'foreign'. This lets the immune system attack the foreign cells while leaving the normal cells alone. To do this, it uses 'checkpoints' – molecules on certain immune cells that need to be activated (or inactivated) to start an immune response. Cancer cells can often find ways to use these checkpoints to avoid being attacked by the immune system. Recent developments in the use of 'checkpoint inhibitors', which target these checkpoints, are showing great promise in the treatment of cancer. However, these drugs can allow the immune system to attack some normal organs in the body, which can lead to serious side effects in some people. Common side effects of these drugs can include fatigue, cough, nausea, loss of appetite, skin rash and itching. Less often they can cause more serious problems in the lungs, intestines (colitis), liver (hepatitis), kidneys, hormone-making glands, or other organs.

ANTI-ANGIOGENESIS AGENTS

These agents prevent the development of blood vessels and, therefore, prevent one way for cancer to spread. One example is lenalidomide (Revlimid), a thalidomide-derived drug that is used in treating multiple myeloma (this is taken orally by patients).

Hormonal agents are used extensively in treating cancer. These include glucocorticoids (prednisolone), selective oestrogen receptor modulators (e.g. tamoxifen) (used as an adjuvant treatment to extend survival in women with breast cancer) and aromatase inhibitors (e.g. letrozole) used as an adjuvant treatment to extend survival in postmenopausal women with breast cancer.

CRITICAL THINKING STOP POINT 22.2

Standard international treatment for postmenopausal breast cancer survivors is to take an aromatase inhibitor for 10 years after they finish their cancer treatment. These agents have many side effects and nurses play a central role in advising women on what to expect and what measures they can take to minimise the side effects.

Both Norma and Brona (pseudonyms) are postmenopausal women who were treated for breast cancer and are now taking letrozole. The excerpts below are taken from a conversation they had with the authors (MD and EM) in a focus group interview with a group of women as part of a research study (Meade et al., 2017). Hormonal treatment was debilitating for these women and many felt that they had not been warned enough of the side effects they would experience.

No matter how hard I try now I can't exercise because my knees have completely seized up. And my mobility is nil. Now I know I had arthritis starting off at the beginning but it's really bad now. Definitely that tablet [letrozole]. (Norma)

I found when I was put on my tablet [letrozole] my arthritis went very, very bad and my weight started to go on. I have 4 stone on now at the minute which I don't want because it's bad, my knees are gone, my back, I have problems with my back and I'm trying to lose get this weight off now. I got on alright, I got through the chemo and radium and everything else but it was afterwards that everything started to set in. (Brona)

It is vital that nurses ask patients about their side effects each time the patient attends for review. Patients feel cared for if asked and given the opportunity to talk about their side effects and discuss self-care measures that they can engage in.

GO FURTHER

Prednisolone is commonly used in cancer treatments. Go online and find out what role prednisolone plays in cancer treatment.

HEALTH PROMOTION

The doses of steroids prescribed to cancer patients can be high, resulting in disturbing symptoms for some patients. Nurses should advise patients and their families that while the steroids do cause patients to feel a sense of energy and even euphoria, steroids also adversely affect patients' sleep and some patients can even experience hallucinations. Nurses should also emphasise to patients that they will experience a drop in mood once the prescribed course of steroids has been completed.

Haematopoietic stem cell transplantation (HSCT) is an inclusive term used to describe multiple sources of donor stem cells available for transplantation, i.e. bone marrow, peripheral blood, and cord blood. This treatment is used extensively in the management of blood cancers, for instance, multiple myeloma. The goal of HSCT is to rescue the marrow from the toxic effects of chemotherapy, with or without total body irradiation (TBI). This allows the administration of higher and potentially more curative doses of chemotherapy.

SYMPTOM MANAGEMENT

Cancer patients often experience multiple symptoms, and these are now more commonly grouped into symptom clusters. Symptom clusters are where a patient has two or more concurrent symptoms that are related. Managing symptom clusters requires a holistic approach because these multiple symptoms affect the patient's overall quality of life and their ability to continue on their treatment, which ultimately affects their prognosis. A person-centred approach is essential in the management of patients' symptoms.

The symptom cluster of insomnia, depression and fatigue has been found to be the cluster that caused the most effect on patients' functioning (Oh et al., 2012). Cytokine activity is believed to be involved in the development of symptom clusters, whereby their activity increases in stressful physical and psychosocial events, such as a cancer diagnosis (Illi et al., 2012). Cytokines are factors released by immune cells that exert an effect on other cells. In breast cancer, cytokine activity has been found to be associated with depression (Kim et al., 2013). This emphasises the importance of psychosocial care for cancer patients and the role this care can play in managing symptom clusters. Moreover, nurses should assess and manage symptoms simultaneously as opposed to focusing on single symptoms (Oh et al., 2012). Fatigue is the most common and distressing symptom associated with cancer and its treatments. It is important to establish the cause of fatigue and discuss with the patient how fatigue can be managed. Management approaches include exercise, rest, psychosocial measures, nutrition, sleep and medications. Accurate nursing assessment of symptoms as well as accurate advice, information and support can help to alleviate some of the symptoms cancer patients' experience.

GO FURTHER

The treatment of cancer continues to evolve as we gain a better understanding of the biology of cancer and its heterogeneity. This has led to a more tailored approach to cancer care resulting in higher cure rates and longer survival for patients with advanced disease. Cancer survivor numbers continue to grow and survivorship care is now seen as an integral component of cancer care. The goal of cancer treatments must not only be to maximise cure rates but also to minimise long-term effects of cancer treatments. Health promotion and education on disease-preventing activities and management of long-term side effects should be central to nurses' care of oncology patients in follow up.

PREPARATION FOR PRACTICE PLACEMENTS 22.1

Students can prepare themselves for placements in oncology settings by becoming familiar with the particular terminology used in in cancer, such as 'staging', 'grading' and reviewing how the rapidly dividing cells of the body are affected by cytotoxic drugs and what advice can be given to patients to help them manage the side effects of their treatments.

When embarking on a placement in an oncology care setting I feel the student should research some bits of information, for example, the effects of chemotherapy such as nausea or mucositis before commencing the placement. Having some awareness of these will make you more comfortable when you start the placement as you will know what to be looking out for in these patients. I feel however from my own experience, the best thing you can bring to the patient's bedside is a warm 'hello', a smile and an understanding of the vulnerable position the patients find themselves in.

Lynn Muldowney, third year undergraduate nurse

CHAPTER SUMMARY

Having read this chapter, the student should have gained an understanding of:

- The causes of cancers and lifestyle activities to minimise risk of cancer.
- The diagnosis and staging of cancer and how it impacts the patient and their families.
- The treatments available in the management of cancer and some of the associated side effects.
- The importance of patient-centred care in all stages of the cancer journey.
- The importance of family and social support for patients with a diagnosis of cancer.

GO FURTHER

CASE STUDY: COLON CANCER

Go to https://study.sagepub.com/essentialadultnursing for a further case study related to this chapter. If you are using the interactive ebook, simply click on the book icon in the margin to go straight to the resource.

Books

- Wilke, G.M. and Barton-Burke, M. (2016) *Oncology Nursing Drug Handbook*. Burlington, MA: Jones & Bartlett Publishing.
  Written especially for nurses caring for patients with cancer, the 2016 *Oncology Nursing Drug Handbook* uniquely expresses drug therapy in terms of the nursing process: nursing diagnoses, a etiologies of toxicities, and key points for nursing assessment, intervention, and evaluation.

Journal Articles

FURTHER READING: JOURNAL ARTICLES

Go to https://study.sagepub.com/essentialadultnursing for further free online journal articles related to this chapter. If you are using the interactive ebook, simply click on the book icon in the margin to go straight to the resource.

- Sturgeon, C.M., Lai, L.C. and Duffy, M.J. (2009) Serum tumour markers: How to order and interpret them. *British Medical Journal*, 339(7725): 852-8.
  This article will provide you with a good understanding of blood tumour markers used when diagnosing cancer.

Weblinks

FURTHER READING: WEBLINKS

Go to https://study.sagepub.com/essentialadultnursing for further weblinks related to this chapter. If you are using the interactive ebook, simply click on the book icon in the margin to go straight to the resource.

- www.cancer.org
  American Cancer Society website – very easy to negotiate. Very detailed accounts of all cancers.
- www.macmillan.org.uk/information-and-support
  Macmillan provides an excellent resource for all types and treatments for cancer.

ACE YOUR ASSESSMENT

ONLINE QUIZZES

Revise what you have learned by visiting https://study.sagepub.com/essentialadultnursing

- Test yourself with multiple-choice and short-answer questions
- Do the chapter activities in the book and check your answers online

REFRENCES

Cordova, M.J., Riba, M.B. and Spiegel, D. (2017) Post-traumatic stress disorder and cancer. *The Lancet Psychiatry,* 4(4): 330–8. doi:10.1016/S2215-0366(17)30014-7

Doufekas, K. and Olaitan, A. (2014) Clinical epidemiology of epithelial ovarian cancer in the UK. *International Journal of Women's Health,* 6(1): 537–45. doi:10.2147/IJWH.S40894

Glover, D. and Harmer, V. (2014) Radiotherapy-induced skin reactions: Assessment and management. *British Journal of Nursing,* 23(4): S28, S30–35.

Illi, J., Miaskowski, C., Cooper, B., Levine, J.D., Dunn, L., West, C., Dodd, M., Dhruva, A., Paul, S.M., Baggott, C., Cataldo, J., Langford, D., Schmidt, B. and Aouizerat, B.E. (2012) Association between pro- and anti-inflammatory cytokine genes and a symptom cluster of pain, fatigue, sleep disturbance, and depression. *Cytokine,* 58(3): 437–47.

Kim, J.M., Stewart, R., Kim, S.Y., Kang, H.J., Jang, J.E., Kim, S.W., Shin, I.S., Park, M.H., Yoon, J.H., Park, S.W., Kim, Y.H. and Yoon, J.S. (2013) A one year longitudinal study of cytokine genes and depression in breast cancer. *Journal of Affective Disorders,* 148(1): 57–65.

Komatsu, H., Yagasaki, K. and Yoshimura, K. (2014) Current nursing practice for patients on oral chemotherapy: A multicenter survey in Japan. *BMC Research Notes,* 7(1).

Kullberg, A., Larsen, J. and Sharp, L. (2013) 'Why is there another person's name on my infusion bag?' Patient safety in chemotherapy care – A review of the literature. *European Journal of Oncology Nursing,* 17(2): 228–35.

Lee, D.H., Keum, N. and Giovannucci, E.L. (2016) Colorectal cancer epidemiology in the nurses' health study. *American Journal of Public Health,* 106(9): 1599–607.

McDonough, M.H., Sabiston, C.M. and Wrosch, C. (2014) Predicting changes in posttraumatic growth and subjective well-being among breast cancer survivors: The role of social support and stress. *Psycho-Oncology,* 23(1): 114–120.

Meade, E. (2014) Avoiding accidental exposure to intravenous cytotoxic drugs. *British Journal of Nursing,* 23(16): S34–S39.

Meade, E., McIfatrick, S., Groarke, A.M., Butler, E. and Dowling, M. (2017) Survivorship care for postmenopausal breast cancer patients in Ireland: What do women want? *European Journal of Oncology Nursing* 28: 69–76.

Oh, H., Seo, Y., Jeong, H. and Seo, W. (2012) The identification of multiple symptom clusters and their effects on functional performance in cancer patients. *Journal of Clinical Nursing,* 21(19–20): 2832–42.

CARE OF THE ADULT AT THE END OF LIFE

23

TONY DUFFY

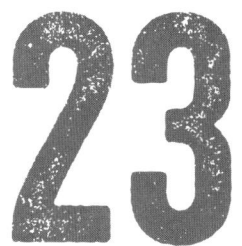

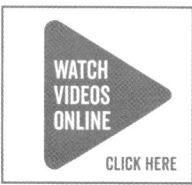

WATCH VIDEOS ONLINE

CLICK HERE

THIS CHAPTER COVERS

- An overview of recent developments in the principles and practice of palliative care in the UK
- An explanation of the recent growth of interest into the meaning and practice of end of life care
- A discussion of the pharmacological knowledge and skills needed by a nurse to manage common symptoms experienced at the end of life
- A discussion of the many practical ways in which a nurse can support a patient who is planning for a good death.

> "
> How people die remains in the memory of those who live on.
>
> Dame Cicely Saunders (1918–2005)
> "

INTRODUCTION

Cicely Saunders is widely regarded as the founder of what has become known as the 'modern hospice movement' (Department of Health England, 2008) and it is an honour to begin this chapter with a fine quotation from her. Dame Saunders was one of many health professionals who, in the final decades of the twentieth century, strove to develop and provide high quality, multi-professional, holistic care to people who were experiencing pain and other distressing symptoms at the end of their lives (du Boulay and Rankin, 2007). We should be very proud of the care provided in the United Kingdom to dying people and their families. International data, allowing for the creation of a Quality of Death Index, has been gathered twice, once in 2010 (Economist Intelligence Unit, 2010) and the other in 2015 (Economist Intelligence Unit, 2015). On both occasions the UK has been recognised as providing the best end of life care in the world.

This chapter will inform you of how this world-leading status has been achieved and what approaches are currently being promoted to further improve end of life care in the UK. This chapter will explore what is commonly understood by the phrase 'palliative care' and how its meaning has been changing in the UK since end of life care strategies started to be published around Britain in 2008. It is important for you as nurses to understand the difference between 'palliative care', 'end of life care' and 'last days of life' care and for you to consider how and when these terms are most appropriately used. Using the correct words and phrases can encourage you to adopt a professional attitude and role when involved with people at the end of their lives and to communicate better with colleagues also involved in achieving the best quality of life and death within British society.

THE CHANGING FACE OF PALLIATIVE CARE

In the UK, palliative care is currently undergoing significant changes with regards to how it is conceived, defined and delivered. In many regards, it is still faithful to the internationally recognised definition and principles of adult-orientated palliative care as provided by the World Health Organization (see Box 23.1). It is holistic in the assessment of people's needs and multi-professional in the delivery of care. It is focused upon promoting quality of life up to the moment of death and then refocuses upon providing support during bereavement.

The WHO definition has been around for nearly 30 years although it has been revised occasionally due to changes in perspective of what palliative care is and who it is for. The original definition grew out of the British hospice movement, which was largely a collection of independent and charity-funded hospices and community care teams established within local communities in the UK. Their aim was to help local people dying of cancer whose needs could not be met by a National Health Service largely structured and funded as a curative organisation (Rivett, 1998). Significant changes to the WHO definition occurred in 1992 where the phrase 'in conjunction with anti-cancer treatment' was removed along with the idea that palliative care was only for those whose disease was not responsive to curative interventions. The term 'palliative care' no longer means just caring for the person dying of cancer, or of anyone in the last few days of life. Indeed, the current definition clearly states that palliative care is applicable to people with life-threatening, rather than life-shortening, illness and is to be delivered much earlier than traditionally believed.

As can be seen by the WHO definition (Box 23.1), *palliative care* and *end of life care* can appear synonymous. In the minds of many nurses, palliative care and end of life care mean the same thing. You may hear some colleagues say 'this patient is now palliative' meaning that the patient is expected to die very soon, maybe in the next few hours. In the UK, especially since 2004, there have been concerted attempts to distinguish between what is meant by *palliative care* and what is meant by *end of life care* (National Council for Palliative Care (NCPC), 2006). Increasingly, the care of people with life-limiting long-term conditions is being considered along the lines of *supportive care* and *palliative care* with palliative care focused upon the high-quality assessment and management of pain and other symptoms caused by a disease process (NCPC, 2015). Although end of life care requires a large amount of palliative care input, it can be regarded as a unique aspect of nursing care with its own aims and objectives. Whereas palliative care is primarily focused upon the promotion of quality of life, end of life care can be regarded as primarily focusing upon those factors that prepare for, and then achieve, quality of death.

BOX 23.1

The World Health Organization definition of palliative care for adults

Palliative care is an approach that improves the quality of life of patients and their families facing the problems associated with life-threatening illness, through the prevention and relief of suffering by means of early identification and impeccable assessment and treatment of pain and other problems, physical, psychosocial and spiritual. Palliative care:

- provides relief from pain and other distressing symptoms;
- affirms life and regards dying as a normal process;
- intends neither to hasten or postpone death;
- integrates the psychological and spiritual aspects of patient care;
- offers a support system to help patients live as actively as possible until death;
- offers a support system to help the family cope during the patient's illness and in their own bereavement;
- uses a team approach to address the needs of patients and their families, including bereavement counselling, if indicated;
- will enhance quality of life, and may also positively influence the course of illness;
- is applicable early in the course of illness, in conjunction with other therapies that are intended to prolong life, such as chemotherapy or radiation therapy, and includes those investigations needed to better understand and manage distressing clinical complications. (WHO, n.d)

Exploring this in more detail, let's look at Figure 23.1. This illustrates the late twentieth-century relationship between the curative approach dominating the NHS and the palliative approach dominating the hospice movement. There are many accounts from this time (for example, see Diamond, 1999) of patients being promised a cure from cancer until all curative interventions had been exhausted. They were then, sometimes quite brusquely, introduced to a hospice or palliative care nurse who was tasked to inform them that they were now 'terminal' The patient suddenly found that they no longer had access to those health professionals they had got to know so well over the previous months (or years) and now needed to form new trusting relationships with a new caring team.

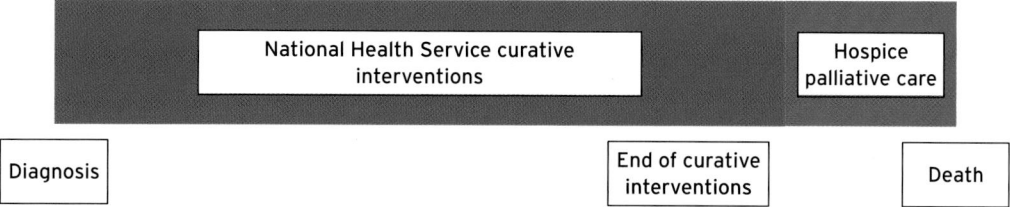

Figure 23.1   The traditional relationship between NHS and palliative care providers

Figure 23.2 illustrates a system of care advocated by the NCPC. Palliative care focuses upon pain and symptom management and is not something to be considered only when the patient is believed to be dying. It is a holistic, supportive and patient-centred philosophy of care which should be applied as soon as any signs or symptoms of disease becomes apparent, even before a clear medical diagnosis has been made. Palliative care can be delivered by all nurses in all care settings supported, when necessary, by small teams of local specialists in pain and/or symptom management. These palliative care specialists would play a larger role the nearer the patient reached the point of death with all its associated complexities of need. Specific end of life care planning should have commenced at least six months before expected death, ideally, 12 months beforehand.

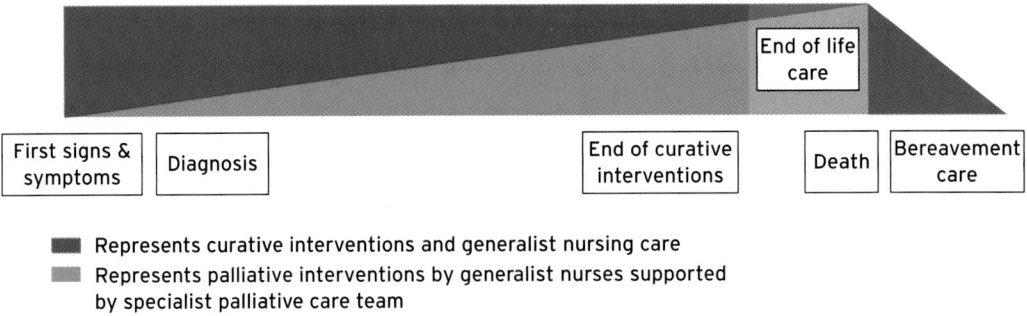

Figure 23.2   The NCPC model of palliative care provision planning

Figure 23.3 attempts to show how palliative care can be incorporated into the care of someone diagnosed with a life-threatening illness but for whom curative interventions prove successful. End of life care would not be needed (although could still be considered and planned for, such as the writing of a Will or identifying attorneys – see later in this chapter) and palliative care interventions would reduce as complex needs reduced. Some specialist interventions, such as anxiety counselling, may continue after the patient has returned home from the hospital although that would depend upon the patient's need and the general practice's access to the service.

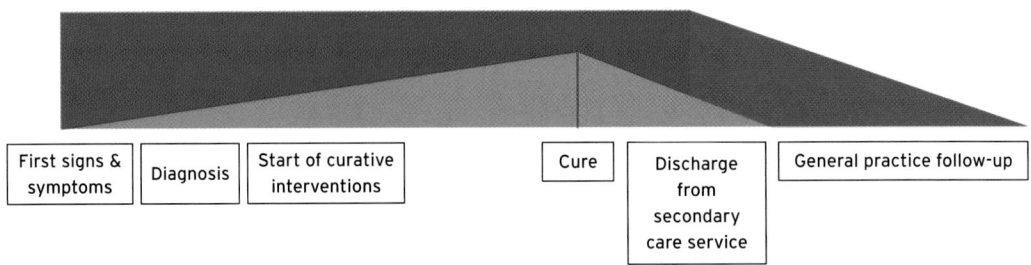

Figure 23.3   The palliative intervention in the cured patient

THE DEVELOPMENT OF END OF LIFE AND LAST DAYS OF LIFE CARE

Although *palliative care* was developed to ease the burden of people dying of incurable diseases, recent national policies and strategy documents are increasingly making a distinction between 'palliative care,' 'end of life care' and 'last days of life care' (see Table 23.1).

Table 23.1 Key components of the principles of care

Palliative care	Focused upon the promotion of **quality of life,** it is centred around impeccable assessment of a patient's holistic needs and aims to alleviate any pain and distressing symptoms caused by a long-term or degenerative disease.
End of life care	Starting 6 to 12 months before expected death (or upon diagnosis if the timespan is shorter), focused upon **planning** for the inevitable to ensure the patient and their family/close friends are holistically **prepared** for when death occurs. Getting ready for *a good death.*
Last days of life care	Commenced when a responsible senior clinician (ideally with the agreement of other doctors and nurses in the team) believes that the patient is entering the terminal phase of life. Focused upon the **alleviation** of pain and other symptoms which may distress the patient and/or attending family members/close friends. This period of time can be anything from an hour to 14 days.

As previously described, the palliation of symptoms related to disease can be delivered to people who are still receiving curative interventions and who may, hopefully, be eventually cured of the disease. Palliative interventions can also be provided by any nurse to any patient with a long-term condition, such as diabetes, which is not expected to shorten their life if well managed.

Since 2008, when specific end of life care delivery strategies started to be published in the nations of the UK, it has become useful to use a new phrase to describe the commissioning and delivery of care required by people whose long-term condition is expected to deteriorate within 12 months to the point that death occurs. This phrase is 'End of Life Care' and, considering that a third of all hospitalised patients are in the last year of their lives (Andrews and Butler, 2014), it is an aspect of adult nursing which should be delivered very frequently.

You may have some concerns about the accuracy of decisions regarding whether someone is expected to die within 12 months. Of course, there is always an element of uncertainty in the decision-making although many decades of research and clinical experience have allowed 'death trajectories' to be created (see Figure 23.4) which allow us to anticipate the level of deterioration someone with a specific illness will experience over the final weeks or months of life. It might be that a patient expected to die within 6 to 12 months lives for another 14 months. It might be the patient dies within three months. The most important part of end of life care is not the accuracy of the 'premonition' (after all, a frail elderly person expected to die due to complications of COPD can still suddenly die of an unexpected infection or heart attack – see Figure 23.5) but the recognition that the patient has entered the final phase of life and that preparations for the achievement of a good death can commence. A good death is one in which the dying person feels as though they remain in control up to the point of death and beyond, that their wishes, beliefs and values are respected, that they die in a place acceptable to them, that any pain and symptoms are well managed in a dignified manner, that they have been given the time and space to say goodbye to important people and that closure has been obtained (Meier et al., 2016; Steinhauser et al., 2000; Ternestedt et al., 2002).

Innovations in end of life care

The nations of the UK are always exploring new approaches and strategies with which to improve the experiences of their people when a natural, expected death is expected soon.

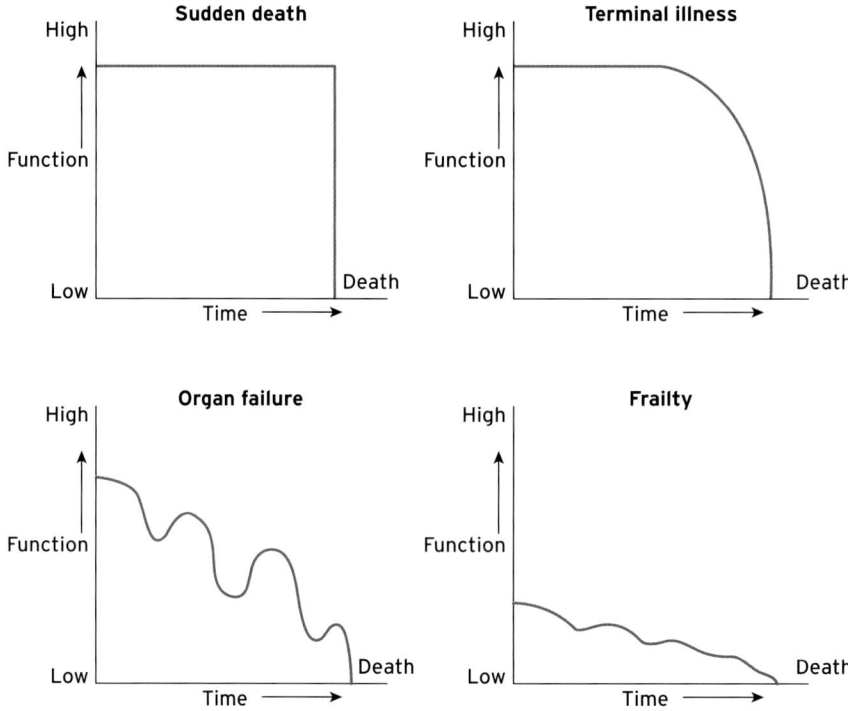

Figure 23.4 Trajectories of dying (RCN, 2015)

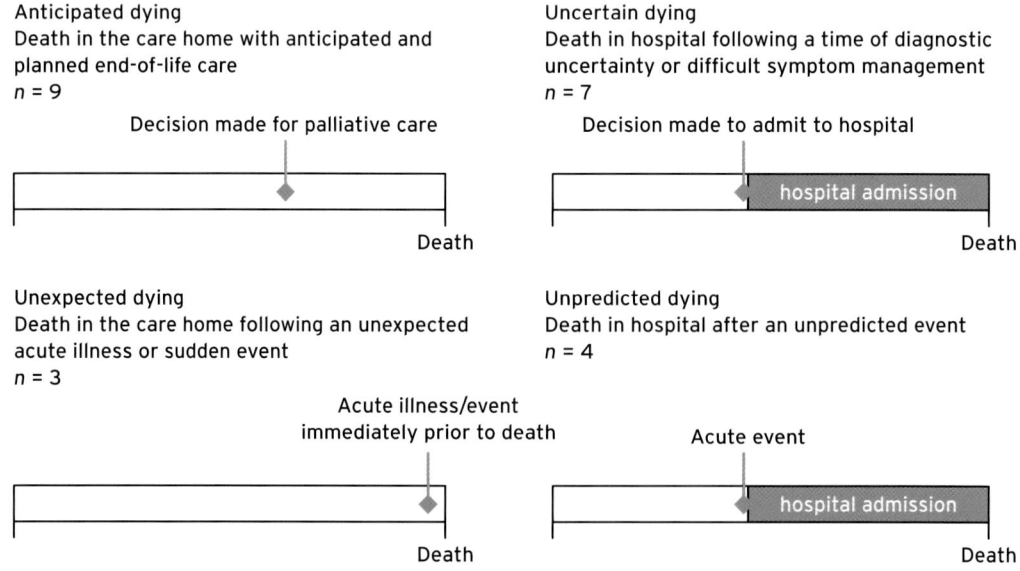

Figure 23.5 Trajectories to death in residential care homes during the last month of life (Barclay et al., 2014)

GO FURTHER

Since the advent of devolution, the four nations which form the UK have been determining for themselves what might be the best way to promote improvement in palliative and end of life care in their population. Enhancing end of life care is a core component of all governments' health policies (Watts, 2012). Below is a list of the current national strategies found in the four nations. Please access and read the one that relates to your area of habitation and work. When reading it, consider how the strategies relate to the traditional idea of palliative care and identify some of the approaches designed to promote a 'paradigm shift' – a change of culture so that people feel more empowered to discuss end of life care issues and engage with processes which encourage planning for a good death. Some of these processes, such as writing Wills, registering Lasting Power of Attorney and considering DNACPR orders are discussed later in the chapter, so you may find it useful to read these sections alongside your nation's document.

England: Leadership Alliance for the Care of Dying People (2014) One chance to get it right. Available at: www.gov.uk/government/uploads/system/uploads/attachment_data/file/323188/One_chance_to_get_it_right.pdf

Wales: Welsh Government (2016) Palliative and End of Life Care Delivery Plan. Available at: http://gov.wales/docs/dhss/publications/170327end-of-lifeen.pdf

Scotland: Scottish Government (2016) Strategic Framework for Action on Palliative and End of Life Care; 2016–2021. Available at: www.gov.scot/Resource/0049/00491388.pdf

Northern Ireland: Health & Social Care Board (n.d.) Transforming Your Palliative and End of Life Care Programme. Available at: www.transformingyourcare.hscni.net/tyc-in-action/palliative-and-end-of-life-care/

WEBLINKS

The **National Institute for Health and Care Excellence** (NICE) is a body charged with the review of the current research literature and to then provide evidence-based recommendations for clinical practice. After the publication of *More Care, Less Pathway* (Independent review of the Liverpool Care Pathway, 2014), it was required to review and update its guidelines on end of life care. I recommend that this new guideline (NICE, 2015), NG31, is read carefully as it highlights the key areas for nursing interventions when caring for a patient and their family in the dying phase of their life. It is available here: www.nice.org.uk/guidance/ng31

One of the better-known innovations was called the Liverpool Care Pathway (LCP) and was developed in the late 1990s and early 2000s in an attempt to expand the excellent aspects of end of life care found in hospices to a variety of English NHS and private care settings where the majority of dying people were receiving too little pain and symptom management (Ellershaw et al., 2001). It is important that you know of this integrated care pathway (ICP) of the dying person because its attempts to improve symptom control in the last 48 hours of life have been recently highly criticised and caused a lot of public concern. The LCP encouraged the development of similar ICPs in other nations (for example, Wales – Fowell et al., 2002) but it is the specific lessons learned from the success and failures of the LCP which will be explored and discussed here, as these lessons currently determine the approaches to end of life care being promoted throughout the UK.

The LCP aimed to stop dying patients from receiving unnecessary investigations and drugs by ensuring the needs of the patient were thoroughly reviewed so that only intervention to reduce distressing symptoms were considered in the final 48 hours of life. It achieved some great things such as encouraging prescribers to ensure commonly used drugs were written on the **PRN** side of drug charts in case the dying patient needed them, instead of waiting until expected pain and symptoms began before considering prescribing the appropriate palliative drug (see Table 23.2 later in this chapter).

In 2014, **NICE** withdrew its support for the LCP following criticism of it within the 'Neuberger Report' (Independent Review of the Liverpool Care Pathway, 2014). Despite its good intentions, the LCP was found to have been implemented poorly in most NHS Hospital Trusts resulting in limited review of care and becoming associated with the terrible phrase 'withdrawal of care'. A 'pathway' approach was also criticised for not encouraging the assessor to identify the *individual* needs of the dying person. It also appeared to encourage some health professionals to regard end of life care beginning only in the final hours of life so that end of life care discussions were not being encouraged over the previous 6 to 12 months.

The LCP was only used in England but the negative publicity was so great that all the other countries of the UK thought it sensible to review their own end of life and last days of life care strategies with England, Wales and Scotland all publishing new strategies since the Neuberger Report (see Go Further above). These new strategies share many key objectives, which aim to ensure that the individual needs of the dying person are assessed, identified and responded to in an appropriate, acceptable and timely manner. They all emphasise that a good death is something which needs to be planned and prepared for, and highlight that nurses and other professionals employed by the NHS need to promote a cultural shift so that British people are more willing to discuss and consider planning for their death, especially if they have a life-threatening or progressively degenerative disease.

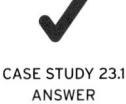

CASE STUDY 23.1
ANSWER

CASE STUDY 23.1

Recollection of an event by a registered nurse of 35 years' experience

"I remember an incident which occurred during my first month as a newly qualified staff nurse on a general medical ward in London, an incident which still makes me feel ashamed. A very sick diabetic man was admitted due to his high blood sugar levels. He had already had a leg amputated due to his diabetes and was in poor cardiovascular health. He had two charming teenage daughters who would visit regularly and they formed a good, open and trusting relationship with the nurses caring for their dad. After being on the ward for a couple of weeks, the patient rapidly deteriorated and died suddenly one afternoon. The daughters were not informed of his death for a couple of hours and by the time they arrived, their dad had been washed, packed and shrouded ready to go to the mortuary. They were very tearful and soon left when the porters came for the body. The next day they returned to the ward to see again the cubicle and bed where their dad had spent his last few days and to talk to those who had cared for him and befriended them. The bed was now occupied by another patient and my colleagues and I stayed away from the daughters, not knowing what to say. Eventually they started crying again. It was at that time that the senior staff nurse in charge that morning gave out a gasp of exasperation and frogmarched them off the ward exclaiming her role was to help the living, not the dead and that they should not return to the ward. I was appalled by that but did and said nothing as I did not really understand the role of the professional nurse at that time. Thirty years of nursing has now given me the knowledge and skills required to understand and meet the needs of people like those two distraught girls but I sometimes wonder why the senior staff nurse did not use her knowledge and skills better at that time. I think it was because she had the wrong attitude to go with it. When nursing dying people, you cannot see them as problematic tasks to be completed and then forgotten as soon as possible. You must see them as people with unique needs and understand how their passing will affect those who love them."

After reading the case study, please write down some answers to the following questions.

1. Why do you think the patient had already been prepared for the mortuary before his family had been given the opportunity to sit quietly with their father?
2. Why do you think the daughters returned to the ward the day after their father died?
3. Where do you think you should primarily look to understand better the role of a nurse and the correct attitudes expected of registered nurses in the UK?
4. If you were the senior staff nurse, what approaches do you think you would have used to address the needs of the two daughters of the deceased patient?

Drug-related palliative interventions in the last days of life

Regardless of diagnosis, age or gender, it is recognised that, in the last days and hours of life, there are common symptoms that can occur which, if not managed well, can cause a lot of distress to the dying person and those around them. Uncontrolled pain may be present which can increase suddenly as the dying person rapidly deteriorates. As levels of consciousness reduce, the person can become very agitated and anxious. Severe feelings of nausea are commonly experienced which may result in vomiting. As death nears and consciousness is lost, secretions can gather at the back of the dying person's throat. It is not believed that this causes the person any pain or discomfort but it is known that the noise, sometimes called a 'death rattle', can cause distress in loved ones waiting nearby for the final moments of life to pass. Individual people may exhibit other signs and symptoms close to death, such as **Cheyne–Stokes respiration** and hallucinations, but pain, nausea, anxiety and respiratory secretions are the most commonly experienced symptoms and they can be effectively managed with pharmacological interventions.

If the person is dying in a community setting, it is increasingly common to find delivered to the home an orange box which many people call the 'just in case' box. Often provided by primary care services, these orange boxes contain drugs which can be administered by the attending nurse when the patient is assessed to be experiencing increased pain, anxiety, nausea or respiratory secretions (see Table 23.2). The route of administration is normally subcutaneous (SC) and doses are recorded on the PRN aspect of the patient's drug chart. A syringe driver may be used to administer SC drugs over a 24-hour period. If the person is dying in hospital, these drugs should be prescribed by the patient's medical team in the PRN aspect of the patient's drug chart as soon as the clinical and nursing teams agree that the person appears to be entering the final days of life. A key role of the nurse is to ensure that the drugs are administered correctly and their efficacy of action is assessed.

Table 23.2 Commonly used PRN drugs and doses during last days of life

Indication	Drug	Dose	Frequency	Route
Pain	Diamorphine	2.5–5 mg or one sixth of the daily dose	2–4 hourly	Subcutaneous (SC)
	Morphine	2.5–5 mg or one sixth of the daily dose	2–4 hourly	SC

(Continued)

Table 23.2   (Continued)

Indication	Drug	Dose	Frequency	Route
Nausea/ vomiting	Cyclizine	50 mg	4 hourly with a maximum dose of 150 mg over 24 hours	SC
	Haloperidol	1.25-1.5 mg	4 hourly	SC
Anxiety/distress	Midazolam	2.5 mg or 5 mg	2 hourly	SC
Respiratory secretions	Hyoscine hydrobromide	400 micrograms	4 hourly with a maximum dose of 2.4 mg over 24 hours	SC
	Glycopyrronium	200 micrograms	4 hourly with a maximum dose of 1.2 mg over 24 hours	SC

It is important for nurses to know how a PRN dose of an opioid is calculated as they are accountable for the safe administration of any drug they administer (Nursing and Midwifery Council, 2015) (see Go Further below). They can also offer advice and guidance to the doctor who may be unfamiliar with prescribing opioid drugs.

GO FURTHER

Table 23.2 lists the name, dose, frequency and route of commonly used drugs with people who are dying. The table does not explain the careful approach required if the patient has never previously received opioids. Such a patient can be regarded as 'opioid-naïve' so an oral (if the oral route is viable) starting dose of 2.5mg to 5mg is advised. This opioid drug is usually morphine in a liquid form (called morphine sulphate elixir) although it may eventually be taken as a tablet (called *morphine sulphate tablet* or MST). If this initial small dose is inadequate it can be repeated after 30 minutes and continue to be repeated until a satisfactory level of pain management is reported by the patient. A simple yet reliable pain assessment tool, such as a numerical or verbal analogue scale (Hjermstad et al., 2011), should be used by the nurse to communicate with the patient and document the results. After 24 hours, the total dose of the opioid drug consumed by the patient should be calculated and then divided by six. This resulting figure is the dose of opioid the patient should be offered every four hours over the next 24 hours and recorded on the 'regular' aspect of the drug chart. If the patient experiences any breakthrough pain then a dose of the drug can be offered from the PRN aspect of the drug chart. The PRN dose should always be one sixth of the daily dose. If several PRN doses are required per day then the total amount of morphine received over 24 hours should be added up and then divided by six to calculate the four-hourly dose the patient is encouraged to take the following day. This process is called **titration**. It is important that opioid-naïve people are given an anti-emetic at the same time as the opioid so to reduce the chance of a common side effect, nausea.

SEE ALSO
CHAPTER 11

Example of a numerical analogue pain assessment tool.

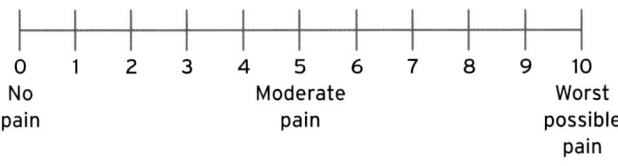

| 0 | 1 | 2 | 3 | 4 | 5 | 6 | 7 | 8 | 9 | 10 |

No pain   Moderate pain   Worst possible pain

WORKING WITH PEOPLE TO PLAN FOR THE INEVITABLE

When people agree to get married, the preparations can often take many months or years to arrange. Many people spend months planning for the birth of a child. However, some marriages do not take place and some babies are not born. Inevitably though, all living people will die but it is well known that in British society, many people do not plan for their death.

Nurses should seek to promote the highest quality of life and death in those people they care for although this can be challenging in a culture in which death is not often discussed within family units. Fortunately, we have been helped recently by the development of approaches which encourage the advanced consideration of factors which, if left unconsidered and undocumented, can result in an unnecessary increase in physical, psychological, social and spiritual distress as the death of a person approaches.

The writing of a Will

The writing of a Will is not a new innovation yet, despite the fact that more than 75% of people in Britain die a natural, expected death at the end of a time of prolonged illness (Office For National Statistics, 2016), 59% of British people have not written a Will and a third of people die **intestate**, leaving no instructions as to what they want to happen to their body and property after death (Unbiased, 2016). As nurses, we should encourage people who are in their last year of life to write a Will, even if they think they have nothing of value to bequeath. We can prepare ourselves to offer appropriate guidance and support at this time by writing a Will of our own so we know the type of discussions and processes required to get it accepted by all and legally recognised. Often, lawyers need to become involved but if your patient is worried about the cost of this, you could help your patient to find out when the latest 'free Will' initiative is available in their local area. A quick 'Google' search normally achieves this. Many health charities recognise the value of having a Will in place upon death and offer to assist in the writing of one. For example, see the Cancer Research UK (CRUK) website page called 'Free Will Service'. It is worth remembering that Wills are only enacted after death and they cannot determine what type of medical and nursing care is received before death.

GO FURTHER

If you live or work in England or Wales, find out more about what is meant by the terms 'Wills', 'probate' and 'inheritance' at GOV.UK (n.d.). This information can help you to prepare to work with your patients and their families in both an educative and supportive role when your patient is believed to be in their final year of life. If you live or work in Scotland, the process is called 'confirmation' and you can find out more at 'Scottish Courts and Tribunals' (n.d.) at: www.scotcourts.gov.uk/taking-action/dealing-with-a-deceased%27s-estate-in-scotland. If you live in Northern Ireland, the process is called 'grant of probate' and you can find out more at NIDirect (n.d.) at: www.nidirect.gov.uk/articles/applying-probate.

WEBLINKS

Lasting Power of Attorney (LPA)

It is very important for all nurses to understand what is meant by an LPA, who can have LPA on behalf of someone else and how it is legally established. With this knowledge, the nurse can educate patients about LPA and assist them to discuss the need for one with other members of the family.

This discussion becomes especially important if it is known the patient may lose the mental capacity to make decisions for a significant amount of time before death occurs as can happen in many neuro-degenerative diseases such as Parkinson's disease or vascular dementia. Basically, someone authorised by the patient and registered as an attorney with the Office of the Public Guardian (OPG) can, when the patient loses mental capacity, make all the necessary decisions regarding the care the patient receives, just as if the attorney *was* the patient.

If the patient and their family believe that the registering of an attorney would help ensure that the patient receives the type of care which respects their values and beliefs, you should direct the patient to the GOV.UK website (see Go Further below). You may find that a patient might like you to look at the information with them so they can ask questions that they may not be yet ready to ask other members of their family.

You must remember to enquire with all patients admitted to hospital whether or not they have registered an LPA. If they do, you must speak to the attorney otherwise you may make inappropriate and illegal decisions on behalf of the patient. You should know that whereas a Will starts upon the death of a patient, an LPA ends at the same point of time.

GO FURTHER

WEBLINK: POWER OF ATTORNEY

All the information necessary to record and register a LPA with the OPG can be found on the GOV.UK website at www.gov.uk/power-of-attorney. I advise you to access this site and read about this increasingly popular initiative so you can facilitate high-quality and informed discussions with the patient. Please note that there are two types of LPA, one for health and wellbeing and the other for property and finance. Both can be set up at the same time or just one (with the other maybe set up later, if the patient wishes it).

Currently it costs £82 to register an LPA (although discounts are available). I suggest you carefully consider protecting your more vulnerable patients and families by advising them that they do not need to access the aid of a lawyer, solicitor or commercial firm to write and register an LPA as they can charge an additional fee on top of the £82, which can be anything between £200 and £1000.

Advance Care Planning

Since the Mental Capacity Act of 2005, nurses are encouraged not so much to act as advocates for patients but to find ways to enable and empower patients to obtain louder, stronger voices in decision-making processes. We should encourage all patients at the end of their lives to consider writing an advance care plan (ACP). Basically, these are documents in which patients write down the type and level of healthcare intervention they would like to receive if they lose mental capacity or consciousness. Many charities provide information and templates for ACPs and you should access and read this information on their websites to prepare yourself for ACP-related discussions with your patients and their families. An ACP is not legally binding as it may contain instructions which are illegal or impossible but, if one has been written which is reasonable, measured, and completed before mental capacity has been lost, it would take a very brave doctor to dismiss it. The existence of an ACP should be documented in the patient's clinical record and the patient should be encouraged to keep it where it can be easily found. A good place to keep it is in a container in the fridge as paramedics are increasingly looking there for health-related information and drugs (Lions Club International, 2018). If you know that an ACP exists for a person but that clinical and nursing decisions are not respecting it, you should raise you concerns according to local policies and procedures.

GO FURTHER

A good place to find out more about what is meant by an ACP and what it tries to achieve is the Gold Standards Framework website. Another excellent site is provided by the Alzheimer's Society (see References for weblinks for both sites). As a nurse, you can conduct your own Google search and see whether there is a particular site which provides valuable and simple-to-read information for patients considering writing an ACP.

Funeral Plans

It is estimated that a basic funeral in the UK costs approximately £6000 (Fairer Finance, 2017). When someone dies, the sudden shock of this cost and the difficulty in finding the money to pay for a 'decent send-off' is not what is needed. Considering that a large percentage of people who die in the UK do so after a long illness, you can use this time to encourage the patient and their family to consider the financial burden of funerals and to plan for it. Some diagnoses allow for more time to make an effective funeral plan. For example, if nursing someone newly diagnosed with Parkinson's disease, that person can have up to 15 years to save and organise a funeral plan. Nurses must be part of a cultural shift within society to encourage a population to be aware of the costs many years in advance of a time when illness or disease may threaten life.

There has been a significant increase in the number of funeral plans taken out in the UK recently with 1.2 million people now holding such a plan (Fairer Finance, 2017). Nurses should make patients aware of the high costs of dying but also that, as in any growing industry, some unscrupulous activities can occur and that the small print should always be read (NAFD, 2017). Nurses should have the knowledge and skill to assist people to understand the issues and make sense of the documentation involved.

Someone newly diagnosed with advanced, aggressive lung cancer may have only weeks to live and may not have the savings to pay for a basic, traditional £6000 funeral. You should know that there is a growing trend for what is being known as 'direct funeral', which was what David Bowie decided on for himself (Millard, 2016). These meet national legislation requirements and because they cut out all the trappings of a traditional funeral with hearses and church services, they can cost as little as £900. You should advise poorer families to explore this option, as it might be the preferred option over taking out a substantial loan from a lender.

Cultural, religious and spiritual needs

Traditionally, nurses ask a patient a question about their religion so it can be recorded in their nursing notes. The reply may be the name of a religion or 'none'. I suggest you should not just record this reply and move on but probe deeper, especially if working in a multi-ethnic, multi-cultural area. People who do not identify with any particular religion still have spiritual needs which need to be assessed to determine whether any nursing intervention is required. It is well known that many nurses are confused as to the difference between religion and spirituality and that this lack of understanding can result in inadequate assessment and care (Rogers and Wattis, 2015). I advise all nurses to understand the difference so to better fulfil their role of being holistic practitioners (NMC, 2015).

A problem which can occur in the last days of life, and which nurses should be aware about much earlier than the final few hours of a person's life, is related to nursing in a fluid and experimental multicultural society (see Case Study 23.2).

CASE STUDY 23.2

Multi-faith, multicultural lives

Barbara was born in Cardiff in 1951, the second of three daughters. Her parents were Christians and she was baptised into the Roman Catholic church when two weeks old. Along with her sisters she attended the local Catholic school until she was 16 after which she left home to work in Birmingham as a theatre seamstress. During this time she stopped attending church. When Barbara was 19 she fell in love with Sohail, a Muslim man for whom she converted to Islam to get married and start a family. They had two sons but when their children were teenagers, the marriage began to fall apart and they divorced when the youngest son reached his 16th birthday.

Barbara moved from Birmingham to Manchester where she began to explore and embrace Buddhism. At this time she fell in love with a Buddhist, Issan, eventually marrying him and giving birth to a son and daughter. They spent many happy years together until the children left home. Barbara kept in contact with her sons from her previous marriage and occasionally travelled to Birmingham to see them but her old and new families never met. When she was 63, Issan suddenly died and was cremated according to his Buddhist and cultural traditions.

Barbara began to feel very lonely as a widow and re-established contact with her younger sister, eventually moving back to Cardiff to be nearer her sibling. The sister had always attended the local Catholic church and Barbara started to attend with her. She liked the mass as this reminded her of a happy childhood and much-missed parents. After a diagnosis of advanced ovarian cancer, Barbara started to accept communion again. One afternoon Barbara was admitted to a hospital ward via A&E after a fall at home. Two days later she experienced a major stroke and lost consciousness for the final time.

The nurse in charge called the numbers she had been given by Barbara when asked for next of kin. The next morning the two sons from her first marriage arrived, soon followed by the children from her second marriage. All were told that Barbara was not expected to live more than a few more hours. All the children were upset by this news and tried to do what they thought was best for their mother. Unfortunately, this caused great arguments and conflict. The two Muslim sons wanted certain words and phrases to be repeatedly said into Barbara's ear until death occurred. The other two children wanted to start Buddhist rituals based upon establishing a peaceful environment. Just when the nurse in charge was trying to prevent a loud argument from descending into physical violence, Barbara's sister arrived telling everyone that Barbara had recently started to attend Church again and that she had called for a priest to administer the sacrament of the last rites. As they argued, Barbara died.

Situations like Barbara's are not unknown in modern Britain and many nurses can provide anecdotal accounts of similar incidences. No one wants this to happen. It is important that we encourage people in the last year of life who have had families with more than one partner, especially if those families have been brought up in very different cultures, to clearly state whatever bells, smells, oils, rites, rituals and words will be acceptable to them when death occurs. Ideally, these wishes should be clearly discussed with relevant family members and reinforced by inclusion in an advance care plan and Will.

CHAPTER SUMMARY

- Providing end of life care is a common aspect of adult nursing in all settings.
- Palliative care improves the quality of life of patients facing life-threatening illness.
- End of life care focuses upon preparing for and achieving quality of death.
- Pain, nausea, anxiety and respiratory secretions are the most common end of life symptoms and can be effectively managed with pharmacological interventions.
- Patients should also be encouraged to think about legal, financial and spiritual planning for their death.

GO FURTHER

Go to https://study.sagepub.com/essentialadultnursing for a further case study related to this chapter. If you are using the interactive ebook, simply click on the book icon in the margin to go straight to the resource.

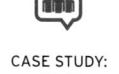

CASE STUDY:
COPD

Books

- Bardy, S. (2016) *Choosing End of Life Nursing*. Australia: ATF Press.
  An interesting exploration into why nurses choose to work in palliative care.
- Nicol, J. and Nyatanga, B. (2017) *Palliative and End of Life Care in Nursing* (2nd ed.). London: SAGE.
  This book discusses some of the key aspects of palliative and end of life care and is aimed at pre-registration nursing students.
- Pettifer, A. (2012) *End-of-Life Nursing Care*. London: SAGE.
  An accessible book which will help you to prepare for the challenges faced when caring for dying patients and supporting their families.

Journal Articles

Go to https://study.sagepub.com/essentialadultnursing for further free online journal articles related to this chapter. If you are using the interactive ebook, simply click on the book icon in the margin to go straight to the resource.

FURTHER
READING:
JOURNAL
ARTICLES

- Bussooa, K. and North, E. (2016) Personalised care plans in the last days of life. *Nursing Times*, online issue 9: 7-9.
  Findings from the piloting of a tool to help ensure nurses consider the priorities of care for the dying person when caring for patients who are in the last days of life.
- Kononovas, K. and McGee, A. (2017) The benefits and barriers of ensuring patients have advance care planning. *Nursing Times*, 113 (1): 41-4.
  This article explores the pros and cons of advanced care planning.
- Thomas, C. (2017) Improving hospital discharge for patients at the end of life. *Nursing Times*, 113 (10): 53-6.
  An evaluation of palliative care nurses coordinating fast-track discharges at the end of life to help ensure patients can be cared for, and die, in their preferred place.

FURTHER
READING:
WEBLINKS

Weblinks

Go to https://study.sagepub.com/essentialadultnursing for further weblinks related to this chapter. If you are using the interactive ebook, simply click on the book icon in the margin to go straight to the resource.

- www.rcn.org.uk/clinical-topics/end-of-life-care
  A great online toolkit full of end of life care resources for all nurses.
- www.dyingmatters.org/
  This is a public-facing website which aims to help people talk more openly about dying, death and bereavement, and to make plans for the end of life.
- www.resus.org.uk/dnacpr/decisions-relating-to-cpr/
  Resuscitation Council, British Medical Association and Royal College of Nursing guidance for decisions relating to cardiopulmonary resuscitation.

ACE YOUR ASSESSMENT

ONLINE
QUIZZES

Revise what you have learned by visiting https://study.sagepub.com/essentialadultnursing

- Test yourself with multiple-choice and short-answer questions.
- Do the chapter activities in the book and check your answers online.

REFERENCES

Alzheimer's Society (2018) *Decision-making, Advance Care Planning and the Mental Capacity Act 2005.* Available at: www.alzheimers.org.uk/info/20091/what_we_think/767/decision-making_advance_care_planning_and_the_mental_capacity_act_2005/4

Andrews, J. and Butler, M. (2014) *Trusted to Care.* Available at: http://gov.wales/docs/dhss/publications/140512trustedtocareen.pdf

Barclay, S., Froggatt, K., Crang, C., Mathie, E., Handley, M., Iliffe, S., Manthorpe, J., Gage, H. and Goodman, C. (2014) Living in uncertain times: Trajectories to death in residential care homes. *British Journal of General Practice,* 64 (626): e576–e583.

Cancer Research UK [Online] *Free Will Service.* Available at: www.cancerresearchuk.org/support-us/donate/leave-a-legacy-gift-in-your-will/free-will-service

Department of Health England (2008) *End of Life Care Strategy: Promoting high quality care for all adults at the end of life.* Available at: www.gov.uk/government/uploads/system/uploads/attachment_data/file/136431/End_of_life_strategy.pdf

Diamond, J. (1999) *Because Cowards Get Cancer Too.* London: Vermilion.

du Boulay, S. and Rankin, M. (2007) *Cicely Saunders: The Founder of the Modern Hospice Movement.* London: SPCK.

Economist Intelligence Unit (2010) *The Quality of Death: Ranking end-of-life care across the world.* Available at: https://graphics.eiu.com/upload/eb/qualityofdeath.pdf

Economist Intelligence Unit (2015) *The 2015 Quality of Death Index: Ranking palliative care across the world.* Available at: www.eiuperspectives.economist.com/sites/default/files/2015%20EIU%20Quality%20of%20Death%20Index%20Oct%2029%20FINAL.pdf

Ellershaw, J., Smith, C., Overill, S., Walker, S.E. and Aldridge, J. (2001) Care of the dying: Setting standards for symptom control in the last 48 hours of life. *Journal of Pain and Symptom Management,* 21(1): 12–17.

Fairer Finance (2017) https://www.fairerfinance.com/campaigns/funeral-plans

Fowell, A., Finlay, I., Johnstone, R. and Minto, L. (2002) An integrated care pathway for the last two days of life: Wales-wide benchmarking in palliative care. *International Journal of Palliative Care*, 8 (12): 566–73.

Gold Standards Framework [Online] *Advanced Care Planning*. Available at: www.goldstandardsframework. org.uk/advance-care-planning

GOV.UK [Online] *Wills, probate and inheritance*. Available at: www.gov.uk/wills-probate-inheritance

Health & Social Care Board [Online] *Transforming Your Palliative and End of Life Care Programme*. Available at: www.transformingyourcare.hscni.net/tyc-in-action/palliative-and-end-of-life-care/

Hjermstad, M.J., Fayers, P.M., Haugen, D.F., Caraceni, A., Hanks, G.W., Loge, J.H., Fainsinger, R., Aass, N., Kaasa, S. and the European Palliative Care Research Collaborative (EPCRC) (2011) Studies comparing numerical rating scales, verbal rating scales, and visual analogue scales for assessment of pain intensity in adults: A systematic literature review. *Journal of Pain and Symptom Management*, 41 (6): 1073–93.

Independent Review of the Liverpool Care Pathway (2014) *More Care, Less Pathway: A review of the Liverpool Care Pathway*. Available at: www.gov.uk/government/uploads/system/uploads/attachment_data/file/212450/Liverpool_Care_Pathway.pdf

Leadership Alliance for the Care of Dying People (2014) *One chance to get it right*. Available at: www.gov.uk/government/uploads/system/uploads/attachment_data/file/323188/One_chance_to_get_it_right.pdf

Lions Club International (2018) [Online] *Message in a bottle*. Available at: www.lions105d.org.uk/projects/miab.html

Meier, E.A., Gallegos, J.V., Montross-Thomas, L.P., Depp, C.A., Irwin, S.A. and Jeste, D.V. (2016) Defining a good death (successful dying): Literature review and a call for research and public dialogue. *The American Journal of Geriatric Psychiatry*, [Online] 24 (4): 261–71. Available at www.ncbi.nlm.nih.gov/pmc/articles/PMC4828197/

Mental Capacity Act (2005) [Online]. Available at: www.legislation.gov.uk/ukpga/2005/9/pdfs/ukpga_20050009_en.pdf

Millard, R. (2016) I'm glad people – including David Bowie – are starting to opt out of their own funerals. It's about time. *Independent* newspaper article. Available at: www.independent.co.uk/voices/im-glad-people-including-david-bowie-are-starting-to-opt-for-direct-cremation-funerals-are-outdated-a6939516.html

National Council for Palliative Care (2006) *End of Life Care Strategy*. Available at: www.ncpc.org.uk/sites/default/files/NCPC_EoLC_Submission.pdf

National Council for Palliative Care (2015) *Palliative Care Explained*. Available at: www.ncpc.org.uk/palliative-care-explained

National Institute for Health and Care Excellence (NICE) (2015) *Care of dying adults in the last days of life*. Available at: www.nice.org.uk/guidance/ng31

NIDirect [Online] *Applying for Probate*. Available at: www.nidirect.gov.uk/articles/applying-probate

Nursing and Midwifery Council (2015) *The Code: Professional standards of practice and behaviour for nurses and midwives*. London: NMC.

Office for National Statistics (2016) *Deaths*. Available at: www.ons.gov.uk/peoplepopulationandcommunity/birthsdeathsandmarriages/deaths

Rivett, G. (1998) *From Cradle to Grave: 50 Years of the NHS*. London: King's Fund.

Rogers, M. and Wattis, J. (2015) Spirituality in nursing practice. *Nursing Standard*, 29 (39): 51–7.

Royal College of Nursing (2015) *Typical Death Trajectory*. Available at: http://rcnendoflife.org.uk/the-patient-journey/typical-timeline-of-conversation/

Scottish Courts and Tribunals [Online] *Dealing With a Deceased's Estate in Scotland*. Available at: www. scotcourts.gov.uk/taking-action/dealing-with-a-deceased%27s-estate-in-scotland

Scottish Government (2016) *Strategic Framework for Action on Palliative and End of Life Care; 2016–2021*. Available at: www.gov.scot/Resource/0049/00491388.pdf

Steinhauser, K.E., Christakis, N.A., Clipp, E.C., McNeilly, M., McIntyre, L. and Tulsky, J.A. (2000) Factors considered important at the end of life by patients, family, physicians, and other care providers. *Journal of the American Medical Association*, 284 (19): 2476–82.

Ternestedt, B-M., Andershed, B., Eriksson, M. and Johansson, I. (2002) A good death. Development of a nursing model of care. *Journal of Hospice and Palliative Nursing*, 3: 153–60.

Unbiased (2016) *Fewer people in the UK have Wills in place than last year, with nearly four in ten over 55s having no Will at all*. Available at: https://business.unbiased.co.uk/press-releases/fewer-people-in-the-uk-have-wills-in-place-than-last-year-with-nearly-four-in-ten-over-55s-having-no-will-at-all-26-9-2016

Unbiased [Online] *Making a Will*. Available at: www.unbiased.co.uk/life/family-matters/write-your-will/

Watts, T. (2012) Promoting health and wellbeing at the end of life: The contribution of care pathways. *International Journal of Palliative Nursing*, 18 (7): 348–54.

Welsh Government (2016) *Palliative and End of Life Care Delivery Plan*. Available at: http://gov.wales/docs/dhss/publications/170327end-of-lifeen.pdf

World Health Organization (WHO) (Online) Definition of Palliative Care. Available at: www.who.int/cancer/palliative/definition/en/

MANAGING NURSING CARE OF ADULTS WITH SPECIFIC CONDITIONS

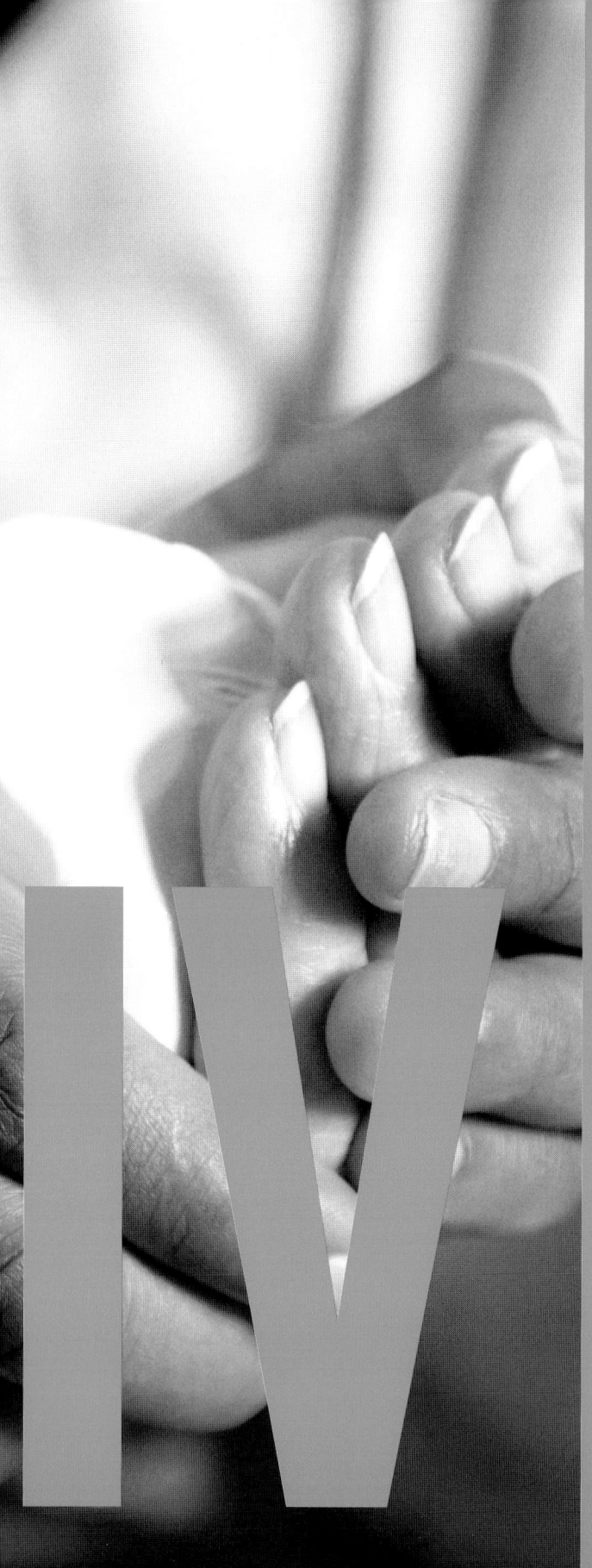

IV

CARE OF THE ADULT WITH A RESPIRATORY CONDITION

24

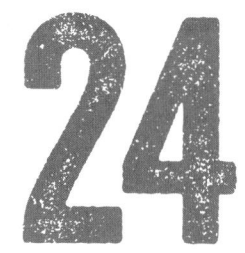

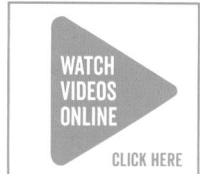

WATCH VIDEOS ONLINE · CLICK HERE

RACHEL BOWATER AND SARAH LEYLAND

THIS CHAPTER COVERS

- An overview of the anatomy and physiology of the respiratory system
- Respiratory assessment
- Clinical characteristics and underlying pathophysiology of two common respiratory conditions (asthma and chronic obstructive pulmonary disease)

- Common diagnostic procedures and clinical investigations
- Nursing assessment, care and management of the adult presenting with common respiratory conditions.

" Hi! I have recently been diagnosed with asthma, which has surprised me as my symptoms were that of a persistent cough and tight chest rather than a wheeze. My symptoms have been somewhat difficult to manage, but are now improving, and I have been reviewed by my GP and attended the asthma clinic on a regular basis.

(Patient voice)

"

" Respiratory assessment may on the surface appear as simple observation that nurses can follow guidelines on. However, on greater analysis many of the components of a respiratory assessment can appear in both health and illness depending on the context, so presence or absence is not necessarily something that can just be simply observed for. Therefore, when student nurses are learning this skill it is useful to reflect on episodes of care with more experienced colleagues.

(Practitioner voice)

"

INTRODUCTION

> When we are healthy, we take our breathing for granted, never fully appreciating that our lungs are essential organs for life. But when our lung health is impaired, nothing else but our breathing really matters. (Forum of International Respiratory Societies, 2013: 4)

Worldwide, the mortality and morbidity associated with lung disease is quite simply staggering, and asthma and COPD are two of five respiratory conditions which contribute to this global burden. It is estimated that 235 million people suffer from asthma and more than 200 million people have COPD (Forum of International Respiratory Societies, 2013: 4). According to the British Lung Foundation (2015), 700,000 hospital admissions are associated with lung disease each year and this accounts for 8% of all hospital admissions. COPD is seen to be one of the leading causes of death within the UK (30,000 deaths/year) and although asthma mortality is considerably lower (1,200 deaths/year) it is the highest in Europe and significant for a controllable disease. The two diseases may cause similar symptoms; however, the table (24.1) below may assist in differentiating between asthma and COPD.

Table 24.1   Clinical features of asthma and COPD (NICE, 2010)

	COPD	Asthma
Smoker or ex-smoker	Nearly all	Possibly
Symptoms under age 35	Rare	Often
Chronic productive cough	Common	Uncommon
Breathlessness	Persistent and progressive	Variable
Night-time waking with breathlessness and/or wheeze	Uncommon	Common
Significant diurnal or day-to-day variability of symptoms	Uncommon	Common

Reproduced with permission under the NICE UK Open Content Licence.

   This chapter covers how to care for an adult with a respiratory condition and its aim is to provide you with a knowledge and understanding of what you should consider when assessing a patient, how to undertake an accurate respiratory assessment and your role as a nurse in the provision of timely and appropriate interventions both in the acute and community setting. Respiratory assessment is fundamental in the provision of effective nursing care and it is essential that you are able to recognise and differentiate between the norm, and the signs and symptoms associated with respiratory deterioration.

   Specific focus will be placed on two of the most common respiratory conditions that you may encounter in practice: asthma and COPD. The underlying pathophysiology, clinical characteristics and assessment of these conditions will be discussed in more detail and clinical investigations will be considered. Case studies and scenarios will be used to further support learning and additional resources accompanying this chapter can be found on the companion website.

ACTIVITY 24.1: CRITICAL THINKING

Have you had the opportunity within clinical practice to undertake a respiratory assessment? What things do you need to consider before doing so? Reflect on your experience and knowledge gained so far and discuss this with your mentor.

ANATOMY AND PHYSIOLOGY

Anatomically, the respiratory system is made up of the upper and lower respiratory tract. The upper consists of the nose, mouth, pharynx and larynx whereas the lower consists of the trachea, bronchi, respiratory bronchioles, alveolar ducts and alveoli (Tu et al., 2013).

Air entry occurs via the nose through the external nares or nostrils as they are known. When air enters the nasal cavities it is warmed, filtered and humidified by a system of nasal turbinate bones and a dense capillary network, which ensures further mixing of inspired air as it passes onto the pharynx. The mucous membrane lining the nasal cavity traps debris, and hair-like projections known as cilia propel dust particles towards the pharynx where this is swallowed or expectorated. The pharynx, or throat as it is more commonly known, sits behind the nasal cavity and mouth and extends to a point where the larynx and oesophagus divide. The larynx can be found between the pharynx and trachea and sits anteriorly to the oesophagus. A flap of cartilage known as the epiglottis is attached to the entrance of the larynx and on swallowing, the entrance to the larynx is blocked and food is directed into the oesophagus.

The lungs sit within the thoracic cavity and the heart, major vessels and anatomical structures of the mediastinum can be found between them. A protective membrane lines the wall of the thoracic cavity (parietal pleural membrane) and another surrounds the lungs (visceral pleural membrane). The narrow cavity that exists between the two layers is known as the pleural space and it contains a small amount of fluid which lubricates the two surfaces allowing them to move freely against one another during breathing. The diaphragm separates the thorax and the abdominal cavity and its action is essential to the inflation and deflation of the lungs. On inspiration, the diaphragm contracts and flattens and the ribs are pulled upwards and forward by the contraction of the external intercostal muscles. As the chest dimensions increase, **intrathoracic pressure** changes and air is drawn into the lungs. On expiration, the diaphragm relaxes and air flows out of the lungs and intrathoracic pressure returns to normal.

The lower respiratory tract is commonly known as the tracheobronchial tree, which subdivides into a series of branches: primary, secondary and tertiary bronchi, which increasingly narrow and shorten. In its simplest sense, this network allows air to be conducted or transported to the alveoli via the trachea, bronchi and bronchioles. As their primary function is that of conduction they are not involved in gas exchange, and this is often referred to as the anatomical dead space (Creed and Spiers, 2010).

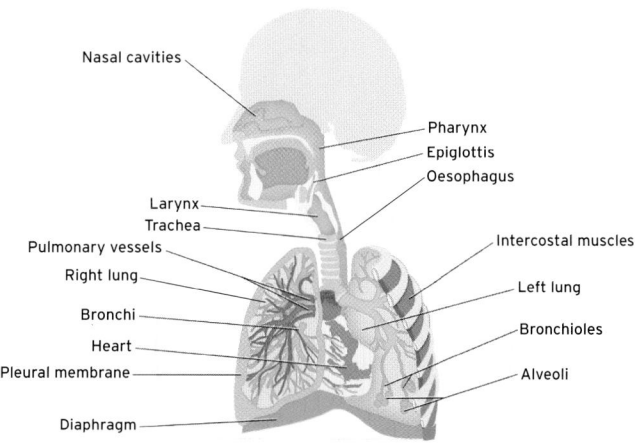

Figure 24.1 Organs of the respiratory system

Source: Boore et al. (2016). Illustrated by Shaun Mercier, © SAGE Publications.

CONTROL OF BREATHING

The respiratory centres are found within the medulla oblongata and pons, which form part of the brainstem. They control the rate and depth of breathing and the rate at which this occurs will change according to oxygen demand and the body's needs.

Gas exchange

Respiration is the process by which oxygen (O_2) is delivered to the tissues (cells) from the atmosphere and carbon dioxide (CO_2) is then removed. There are four distinct phases involved in this process, although only two relate to the respiratory system:

- pulmonary ventilation
- external respiration
- oxygen transport
- internal respiration

Pulmonary ventilation

Pulmonary ventilation is a mechanical process that relates to the movement of oxygen into and carbon dioxide out of the lungs, and in order for this to occur there needs to be a change in intra-pleural pressure (Figure 24.2).

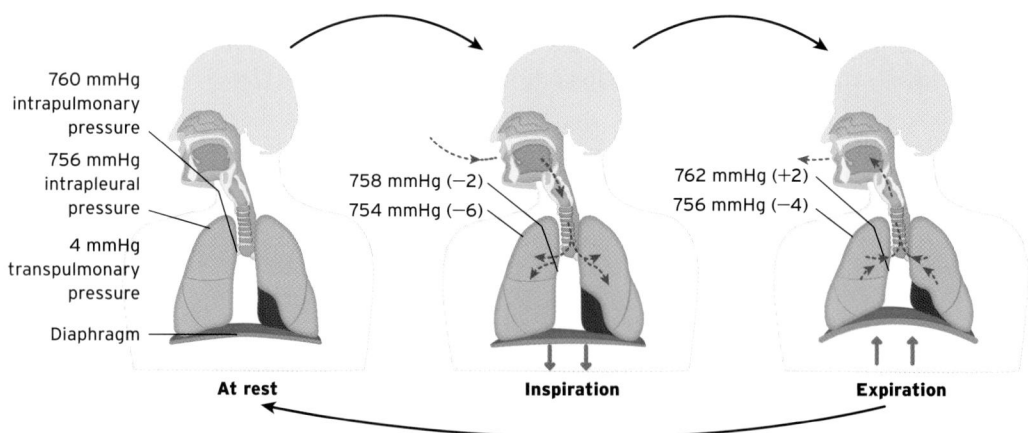

Figure 24.2 Inspiration and expiration

Source: Boore et al. (2016). Illustrated by Shaun Mercier, © SAGE Publications.

At rest, atmospheric and intrathoracic pressures are equal but during inspiration the pressure falls (sub-atmospheric) as the thorax expands and the diaphragm contracts, and air flows from an area of high to low pressure until an equilibrium is reached and inspiration ceases. Expiration is a passive process and is due to the elastic recoil of the lungs which forces air out of the lungs and back into the atmosphere (Peate and Nair, 2011).

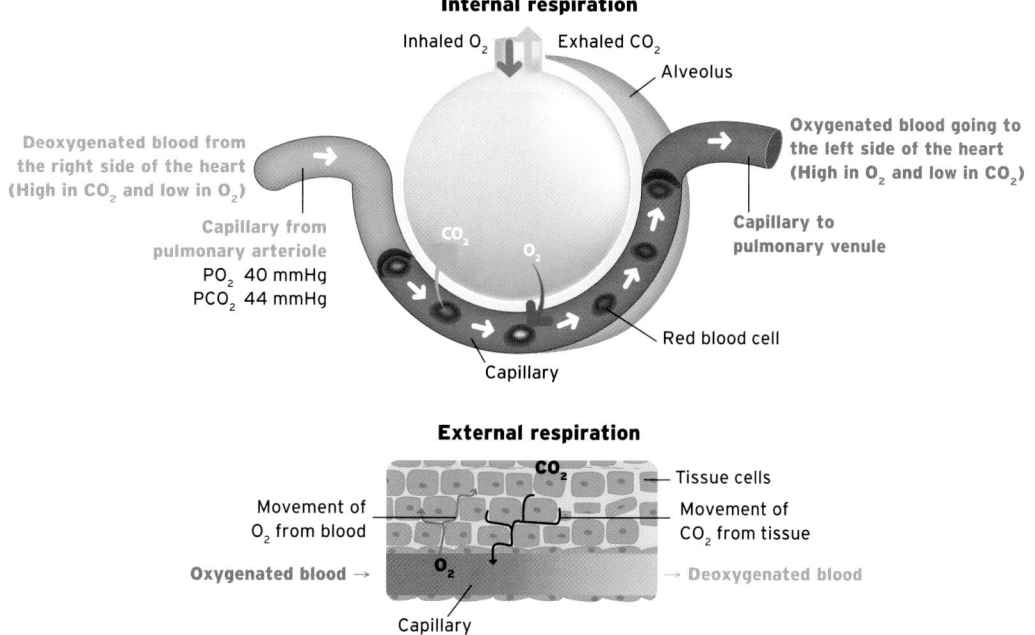

Figure 24.3   Internal and external respiration

Source: Boore et al. (2016). Illustrated by Shaun Mercier, © SAGE Publications.

External respiration

An adult lung contains approximately 300 million alveoli (Peate and Nair, 2011; Creed and Spiers, 2010) each of which is 0.2 mm in diameter and which are surrounded by a network of capillaries (Figure 24.4).

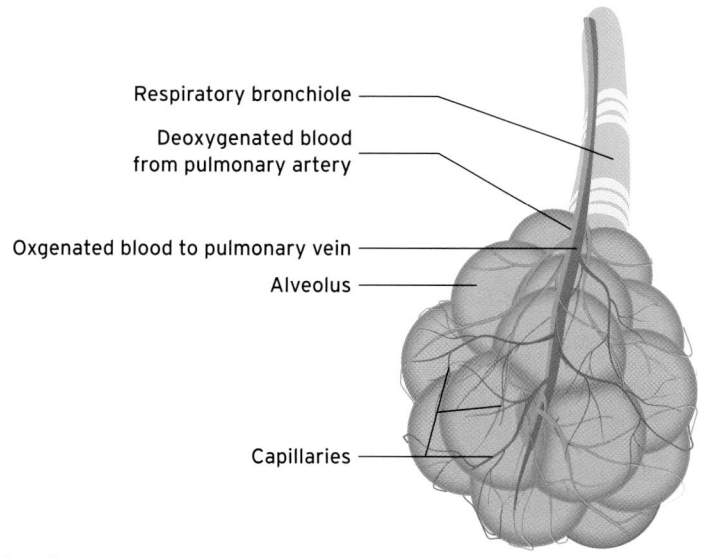

Figure 24.4   Alveoli

Source: Boore et al. (2016). Illustrated by Shaun Mercier, © SAGE Publications.

External respiration (Figure 24.3) is the process by which oxygen diffuses across the alveolar capillary membrane and into the pulmonary circulation. Gaseous exchange and **diffusion** occur because of the concentration gradient that exists between the alveoli and the pulmonary capillary. Deoxygenated blood returning to the lungs, from the right side of the heart, has a higher content of carbon dioxide and lower content of oxygen than that of alveolar air and oxygen moves accordingly into the blood and carbon dioxide moves into the alveoli. The effectiveness of external respiration is dependent on an adequate supply of both oxygen and blood being delivered to the alveoli capillary membrane (Peate and Nair, 2011; Creed and Spiers, 2010).

Breathlessness and the load capacity drive relationship

In health, the complex mechanisms described above maintain respiration and ventilation over a wide range of activities. However, during illness different factors affect the ability of the lung to function and maintain adequate gas exchange. Imbalances may lead to respiratory failure. According to Hess and Kacmarek (2014) respiratory failure can either be hypoxaemic (failure to oxygenate i.e. low PaO_2) or hypercapnic (inadequate ventilation i.e. high $PaCO_2$).

The ventilatory system can be described as a 'pump' consisting of the diaphragm and chest wall muscles, and the neural control of these muscles. If any of the above components (pump) deteriorate, hypercapnic respiratory failure may result.

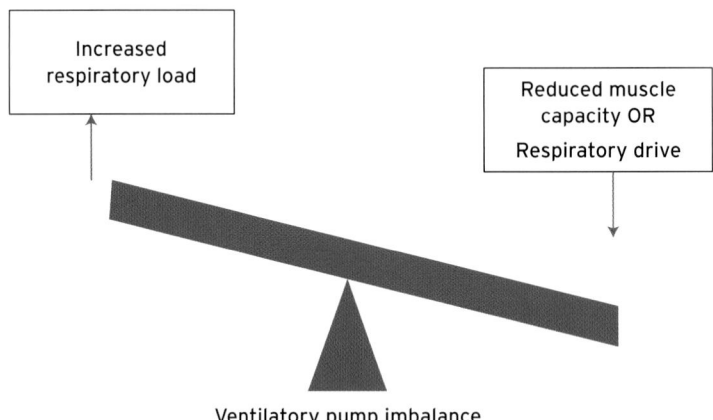

Figure 24.5   Load, capacity and drive

Source: Boore et al. (2016). Illustrated by Shaun Mercier, © SAGE Publications.

According to Moxham and Jolley (2009) the respiratory load is the pressures that need to be generated for the lungs to expand and achieve **ventilation**. If the patient has an underlying condition such as lungs that are inelastic (fibrosed, pulmonary oedema), or the lungs are hyperinflated, or airways are obstructed by conditions such as asthma or cystic fibrosis, the respiratory muscles have a greater load to overcome. Chest wall deformities, including obesity and ascites, will also increase respiratory load.

If the load (Figure 24.5) on the respiratory muscles is increased, respiratory muscles require additional effort to breathe adequately. Hess and Kacmarek (2014) also describe secretions, mucosal oedema and **bronchospasm** among factors that cause excessive ventilatory muscle load. Some factors described above are reversible, such as management of secretions and bronchospasm by appropriate therapies, physiotherapy or patient positioning to reduce load on respiratory muscles.

Respiratory capacity is the ability of the respiratory muscle 'pump' to function (Moxham and Jolley, 2009). Respiratory muscle function is reduced if the patient's lungs are hyperinflated, due to respiratory muscle fatigue, which also impairs gas transfer. Hess and Kacmarek (2014) describe several factors that may result in inadequate muscle function. These include electrolyte imbalances, malnutrition, pharmacologic agents, muscle atrophy and fatigue.

Drive can be abnormally high or low. Neural drive can be abnormally high, for example, in patients with COPD, as they have a flattened diaphragm and reduced muscle capacity, which results in dyspnoea. Conversely, neural transmission can be impaired and also cause respiratory failure, for example, in patients with a spinal cord injury. Central neural drive may be impeded by pharmacologic agents (sedatives or narcotics), hypothyroidism or brainstem injury (Hess and Kacmarek, 2014).

ACTIVITY 24.2: CRITICAL THINKING

Consider a patient that you have been involved in providing care for in relation to their respiratory history and symptoms. Are there any elements that you can optimise with regard to the load/capacity/drive relationship? What strategies would you use?

RESPIRATORY ASSESSMENT

Higginson and Jones (2009) suggest: inspection, palpation, percussion and auscultation. The 'Inspection' stage should include a 'Look, Listen and Feel' approach. Palpation, percussion and auscultation are all advanced skills that require specific training.

Look: The practitioner can gain a lot of assessment data as they approach the patient and observe them.

Colour – What do you notice about the patient's skin and mucus membrane colour? Is **cyanosis** present? – this *may* provide an indication of haemoglobin saturation. However, presence of cyanosis is a late sign that a patient has low oxygen saturations; conversely, cyanosis may be present chronically in those with long-term lung or heart conditions (Jevon and Ewens, 2007). Cyanosis should be assessed centrally – such as lips and buccal mucosa – as peripheral cyanosis may also be due to poor perfusion, not necessarily a respiratory cause.

Ability to speak – Can the patient talk to you in full sentences without appearing breathless? Increased effort/inability to speak, use of short sentences or monosyllables may indicate difficulty in breathing.

Use of accessory muscles – Do you notice use of abdominal muscles, sternomastoid and scalene muscles? This is normally only seen in someone with respiratory distress or increased exertion. In health or with normal activity levels, the diaphragm and intercostal muscles facilitate the patient achieving adequate volumes without the use of additional muscles.

Rate, rhythm and depth of breathing – What do you observe about how the patient is breathing? What is the respiratory rate? Above or below the normal range of 12–18 bpm can indicate respiratory difficulty and would normally trigger an Early Warning System (EWS). The rhythm of breathing can be observed: is the patient's breathing shallow, normal or deep? Shallow or deep breathing needs to be taken in the context of other parameters; for example, deep breathing may be normal during exercise and shallow breathing normal during sleep – but both can also be signs of respiratory distress.

In health, people breath in (Inspiration) and out (Expiration) at a ratio of 1:2 (Higginson and Jones, 2009). Breathing in for longer (with a short expiration) or breathing out for longer (a longer expiration) may indicate respiratory distress or illness.

Chest movement – What do you observe about the how chest is moving? In health, the chest moves symmetrically, therefore asymmetry may be a sign of pathology. Do you see any paradoxical movements such as chest moving opposite the abdomen or sternum moving inwards? These are not seen in health.

According to Welch and Black (2017), not being able to talk in sentences, sweating or cold clammy skin, altered level of consciousness (including restlessness and confusion) may be due to a greatly increased effort in breathing or inadequate respiratory support.

Does the patient have physical signs of a chronic lung condition? These include a 'barrel shaped chest', this may be noted as the nurse observes chest movement, the anterior–posterior diameter is enlarged and **clubbing** of the fingers (Moore and Woodrow, 2009).

Do you notice additional factors that may be observed during respiratory assessment, e.g. productive cough, pursed lip breathing and nasal flaring? Does the patient need to sit upright and lean forward to assist their breathing? Again, these are not present in health.

Listen: Can you hear added sounds as you assess the patient's breathing? Turbulent airflow causes added sounds. Jevon and Ewens (2007: 37) provide a summary of those sounds that are audible without the aid of auscultation:

- *Stridor:* 'croaking' respirations which are louder during inspiration; caused by laryngeal or tracheal obstruction, e.g. foreign body, laryngeal oedema or laryngeal tumour.
- *Wheeze*: noisy musical sound caused by turbulent flow of air through narrowed bronchi or bronichioles, more pronounced on expiration; causes include asthma and chronic obstructive pulmonary disease (COPD).
- *'Rattly'* chest: e.g. chest infection, pulmonary oedema and sputum retention.
- *Gurgling*: caused by fluid in the upper airway.
- *Snoring*: snoring sounds may be associated with the tongue blocking the airway in an unconscious patient.

It is of note that not all respiratory difficulties are accompanied by a sound. A completely silent chest/breathing may indicate an obstructed airway or absent movement of air and this is a medical emergency.

Feel: With permission, by placing both hands gently on either side of the patient's chest the nurse may ascertain additional information, such as sputum retention, **surgical emphysema** and rise, fall and depth of breathing (Higginson and Jones, 2009). Again, this is an element of respiratory assessment with which senior nurses, physiotherapists or doctors can assist you in interpreting findings.

In addition, the following parameters might be useful to add for completeness:

The British Thoracic Society (BTS) (O'Driscoll et al., 2017) recommends utilising SpO_2 as the 5th vital sign. However, it is important that those monitoring SpO_2 are aware of the limitations and factors that can affect accuracy: SpO_2 monitoring does not provide data on the patient's pH, PCO_2, or haemoglobin levels. Therefore, a normal saturation level does not mean a patient will not require further tests such as arterial blood gases (ABG).

According to BTS (O'Driscoll et al., 2017), poor peripheral perfusion, skin pigmentation, **motion artefact** and the site of the probe can all affect accuracy of readings. Probe placement on the ear or finger is therefore preferable to toes. Before placing the saturation probe, always remove nail varnish or false nails if present. If the patient has been exposed to carbon monoxide (from smoke inhalation) or has methaemoglobinaemia (after smoking), the SpO_2 reading may appear higher than it really is, and therefore is falsely reassuring. This is because COHb and methaemoglobin are not distinguishable from oxyhaemoglobin by the oximeter.

Higginson and Jones (2009) indicate respiratory assessment should form part of comprehensive assessment and, therefore, also include temperature, pulse and blood pressure. Other sources of data such as drug charts, fluid balance and medical notes may also add to the overall assessment. Moore and Woodrow (2009) suggest assessing the patient's cough and any sputum produced. Sputum that is coloured, frothy, copious or thick may indicate pulmonary oedema or lung pathology.

Once a basic respiratory assessment has been undertaken the nurse must escalate concerns to senior staff/ medical staff and document findings. Depending on the severity of assessment findings this may mean a call for a medical emergency team, or **SBAR** call for a raised EWS. It may be necessary for additional investigations to be carried out, e.g. ABG, chest x-ray.

SEE ALSO
CHAPTER 9

ASTHMA

The prevalence of asthma continues to increase worldwide and despite advances in treatment, there has been a concomitant increase in mortality. In the UK, 5.4 million people are currently receiving treatment and of these, 80% are adults. The cause of this increase in prevalence is not well understood, but one hypothesis (hygiene) suggests that the western lifestyle has reduced our exposure to pathogens and **helminths** in early childhood and that our relationship with cleanliness predisposes us to allergies later in life. Factors that may trigger symptoms and individual response vary, and these may include genetic predisposition, allergens (pollen, dust mites, fungal spores, and dander), environmental factors, diet, stress and exercise (Forum of International Respiratory Societies, 2013).

In 2014, the National Review of Asthma Deaths (NRAD) published a report 'Why asthma still kills'. Despite advances in modern medicine and the development of evidence-based guidelines, the review found that 'major preventable factors were identified in two thirds of all asthma deaths'. There is no gold standard definition of asthma; however, the Global Initiative for Asthma (GINA) (2017: 14) suggests that:

> Asthma is a heterogeneous disease usually characterised by chronic airway inflammation, it is defined by a history of respiratory symptoms such as wheeze, shortness of breath, chest tightness and cough that vary over time and intensity and variable airflow limitation.

Defined as a chronic inflammatory disorder, asthma is characterised by mucosal inflammation, hyperresponsiveness and narrowing of the airways. Episodic and variable in presentation, asthma is a serious condition and can be difficult to treat due to psychosocial issues: patient compliance with treatment, denial, and failure to monitor own symptoms, which can lead to a failure in management (Creed and Spiers, 2010). Causes of asthma and individual response may vary and it can either be atopic or non-atopic in presentation. **Atopic** asthma usually starts in childhood and can be associated with certain identifiable triggers (e.g. dust, pollen, dander) and family history (Kaufman, 2011) whereas non-atopic asthma tends to have a later onset and may develop in adults as a consequence of infection.

Pathophysiology

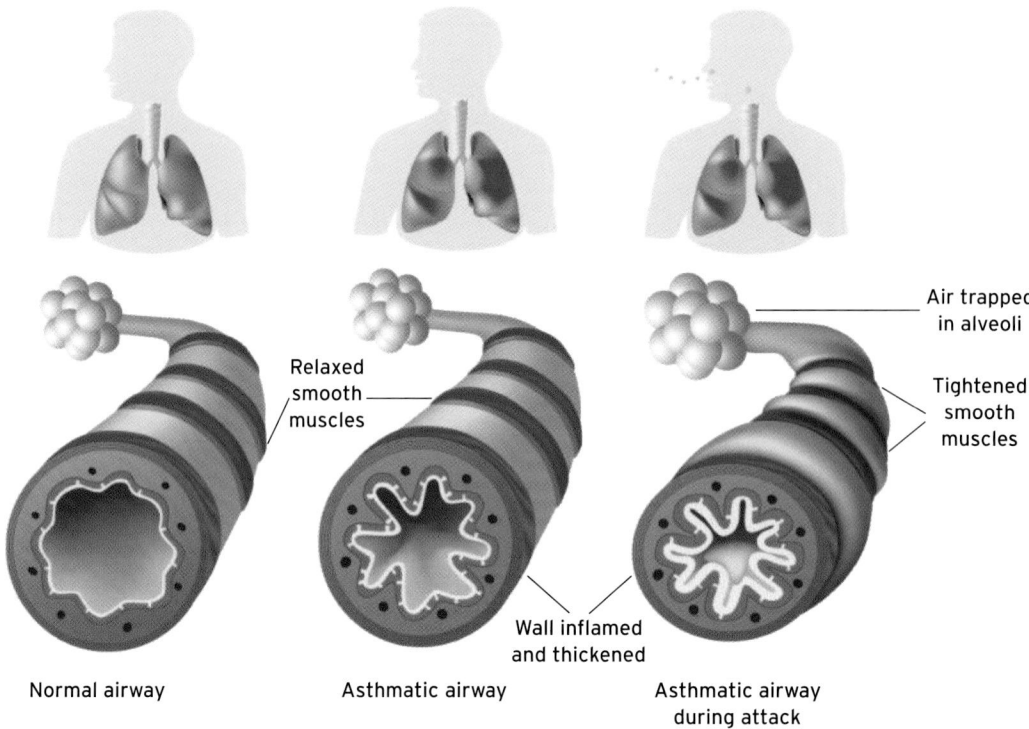

Figure 24.6 Pathology of asthma

Source: Science Photo Library

Asthma can affect the trachea, bronchi and bronchioles and symptoms are caused by reversible changes in the airways. Narrowing of the bronchial lumen as a result of epithelial damage, overproduction of mucous and oedema cause an increase in airflow resistance (difficulty breathing out of the lungs) within the airways and the patient will often present with signs of dyspnoea and wheezing (Cohen and Hull, 2015). The epithelial layer that lines the trachea, bronchi and bronchioles can become damaged and peel away (Kaufman, 2011) and 'shedding' of this protective layer can lead to hyperresponsiveness of the airway. Bronchospasm, which is defined as a sharp contraction of the bronchial smooth muscle, causes the airways to narrow, capillaries to leak and oedema, which impairs mucus clearance and increases mucous production, which can cause 'plugs' that may lead to occlusion of the airway (Figure 24.6). Without proper treatment, airway remodelling (structural changes) can occur within the lower respiratory tract and this can be associated with a progressive loss of lung function and fibrosis.

WHAT'S THE EVIDENCE? 24.1

The recently published NICE (2017) guidelines – Asthma: diagnosis, monitoring and chronic asthma management aims to improve patient diagnosis and control of symptoms.

- Reflect upon the care you have provided to a patient living with asthma.
- Look at the guidelines relating to diagnosis and consider how you can apply your findings to practice.

Structured clinical assessment

The British Thoracic Society and Scottish Intercollegiate Guidelines Network (SIGN) (2016) and National Institute for Health and Care Excellence (NICE) (2017) have devised a series of guidelines relating to the aetiology of asthma and its management. This stepwise approach provides clinicians with an evidence-based guide on the best assessment strategies and available treatment. According to BTS (O'Driscoll et al., 2017), there is no single diagnostic test and diagnosis should be based on clinical assessment and objective tests that assess variable airflow limitation and the presence of airway inflammation (spirometry, peak flow, fractional exhaled nitric oxide (FeNO), **bronchodilator reversibility test,** testing of atopic status and sputum eosinophils). Undertaking a structured clinical assessment to assess the initial probability of asthma should be based on Figure 24.7 on the next page.

Lung function tests

Spirometry is a relatively simple test which assesses lung function and can be used to differentiate between obstructive and restrictive lung disease by measuring forced vital capacity (FVC) and forced expiratory volume (FEV) over a second (Kaufman, 2011). Tests are performed by measuring the volume of air expelled from the lungs following maximum inspiration of air during a single breath: this is done on three consecutive occasions and the highest reading is then recorded (reproducibility of data). The ratio normally declines with age and so actual and predicted measures are used in assessment in spirometry. Poor technique and misinterpretation of results can lead to a wrong diagnosis and inappropriate treatment. It is, therefore, essential that healthcare practitioners have received appropriate training and are competent in the technique.

SEE ALSO CHAPTER 12

Peak expiratory flow (PEF) monitoring is another method used to assess lung function and uses a small hand-held device which measures airflow through the airways on expiration. Although dependent on technique and patient effort, PEF assesses the rapidity of the flow rate during a forced expiration (best of three) and can be used to assess the effectiveness of bronchodilators both pre- and post-treatment. Multiple measurements can be taken over several weeks to assess the variability of airflow using electronic meters and patient diaries; however, reliability is based on individual compliance (BTS and SIGN, 2016).

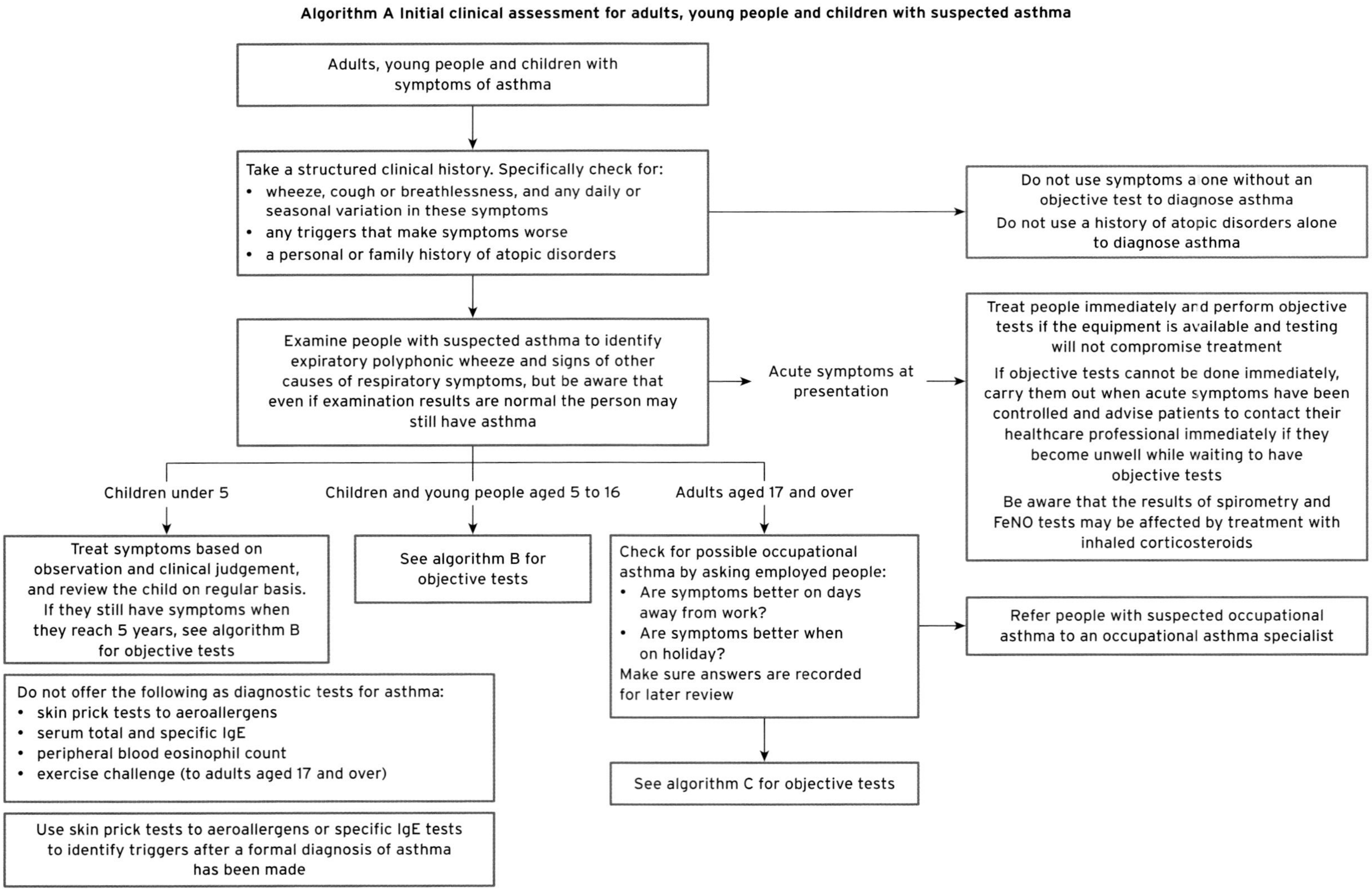

Algorithm A Initial clinical assessment for adults, young people and children with suspected asthma

Figure 24.7 Asthma management (BTS and Sign, 2016).

Reproduced from BTS/SIGN British Guideline on the management of asthma, with kind permission of the British Thoracic Society.

ACTIVITY 24.3: CRITICAL THINKING

We have considered spirometry and peak flow but what other objective tests are available in the diagnosis of asthma? What are the benefits of these tests? How will the results of these tests influence patient care?

Consider utilising the NICE 2017 guidelines when formulating your answers to these questions.

Pharmacological management

The ultimate goal of asthma management is disease control so that patients can remain symptom free and be able to lead a normal life (refer to Figure 24.8).

Complete control of asthma is defined as:

- no daytime symptoms
- no night-time awakening due to asthma
- no need for rescue medication
- no asthma attacks
- no limitations on activity including exercise
- normal lung function (in practical terms FEV1 and/or PEF>80% predicted or best)
- minimal side effects from medication.

Asthma management (BTS and Sign, 2016) Reproduced from BTS/SIGN British Guideline on the management of asthma, with kind permission of the British Thoracic Society.

Pharmacologically a step-wise, age-based approach is currently used to guide asthma management (Figure 24.8). Depending on the severity of the disease, treatment should be commenced at the most appropriate level with the aim to achieve early control. Maintaining control can then be achieved by increasing or decreasing the treatment as necessary according to patient response (BTS and SIGN, 2016). Asthma medication can be divided into two groups: 'preventers' (reduces inflammation and swelling) and 'relievers' (relax airways). Patients may be prescribed one or more of the following:

- Inhaled corticosteroids (ICS): Steroids work by reducing inflammation and swelling in the airways and helping to control symptoms and prevent attacks, e.g. budesonide, beclomethasone
- Leukotriene receptor antagonists (LTRAs): Reduce the body's response to allergens and help relax the airways, e.g. montelukast
- Short acting beta agonists: Known as rescue medicines as they act within minutes providing quick relief. They help to relieve bronchospasm but do not reduce swelling or inflammation within the airways, e.g. Ventolin, Albuterol
- Long acting beta agonists (LABA): These are used to provide long-term control of asthma symptoms rather than quick relief and they are in combination within inhaled steroids, e.g. Symbicort, Serevent.

ACTIVITY 24.4: REFLECTION

Environmental exposure, pregnancy and obesity can all lead to the exacerbation of asthma. What non-pharmacological strategies are available? Make a list and discuss this further with your mentor.

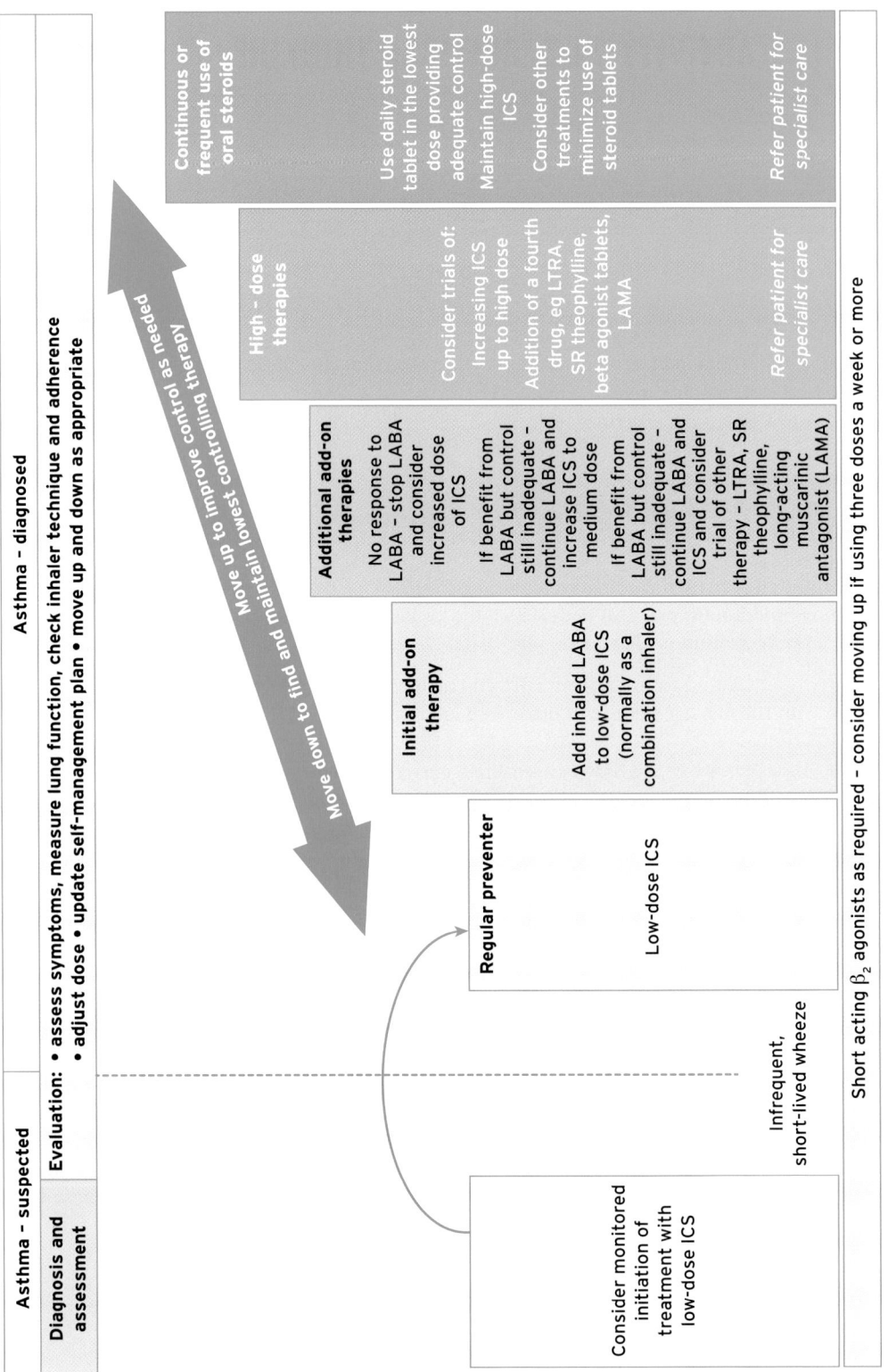

Figure 24.8 Asthma management for adults (BTS and Sign, 2016)

Reproduced from BTS/SIGN British Guideline on the management of asthma, with kind permission of the British Thoracic Society.

Health promotion

Health promotion and patient education play a key role in asthma management by empowering patients to take control and responsibility for their condition. As nurses, we can play a pivotal role in promoting patient self-management by using different approaches and resources that best support patients:

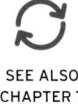

SEE ALSO
CHAPTER 7

- personalised asthma action plans
- self-management education
- monitoring inhaler technique and adherence with asthma treatment
- lifestyle changes: exercise, advice on diet and weight loss interventions, cessation of smoking
- non-pharmacological management: breathing exercise programmes, employing methods for reducing dust mites within the home
- online resources/helplines
- support groups.

ACTIVITY 24.5: REFLECTION

Consider some of the current guidelines with regards to health promotion using the following weblinks:

- British Lung Foundation: www.blf.org.uk
- Asthma UK: www.asthma.org.uk

CASE STUDY 24.1: KATHLEEN

CASE STUDY 24.1
ANSWER

Kathleen is a 44-year-old lady who visits her GP with the following symptoms:

- Persistent, non-productive cough
- Tight chest
- Worsening symptoms at night
- Peak flow 300

    o   What are your initial thoughts?
    o   How would you assess this lady?
    o   Is the peak flow normal?

She is initially started on salbutamol and is reviewed weekly; however, her symptoms do not improve. Her GP prescribes Clenil Modulite.

- What is this and why do you think it was prescribed?

Her symptoms continue to worsen and she requires her 'reliever' on a regular basis.

- What is the difference between a 'reliever' and a 'preventer'? Provide some examples.

(Continued)

(Continued)

A five-day course of oral prednisolone 30 mg once daily is prescribed and she is sent for a chest x-ray which shows mild hyperinflation.

- Why do you think this is?
- What are the benefits and side effects of this medication?
- What does hyperinflation mean? Relate this to the patient.

Kathleen responds to prednisolone and on review her medication is changed to Symbicort (2 puffs, twice a day). This is a combination inhaler, which can be used as both a 'reliever' and 'preventer'. Kathleen attends the asthma clinic for review every two weeks; however, her symptoms remain poorly controlled. The GP decides to start her on montelukast and refer her to a specialist centre for further review.

- What is montelukast?
- Why do you think this was prescribed?
- What advice would you give to Kathleen?
- What other assessments could be undertaken?
- How would you promote patient self-management?

To support you in formulating your answer, refer to the resources available on the companion website and the national guidelines that have been mentioned within this chapter.

CHRONIC OBSTRUCTIVE PULMONARY DISEASE

The Global Initiative for Chronic Obstructive Lung Disease (GOLD) (2017) and NICE (2010) define COPD as a chronic airflow obstruction resulting from long-term exposure to noxious particles. The exposure results in a chronic inflammatory response which causes damage to the parenchyma of the lung (previously referred to as emphysema) and small airways fibrosis (previously referred to as chronic bronchitis) (GOLD, 2017). Often, the particles arise from cigarette smoke, but may be from occupational exposure, burning fuel such as wood (indoors and outdoors) and air pollution.

Steiner et al. (2015: 805) refers to COPD as a 'spectrum of lung pathologies associated with systemic co-morbities and exacerbations'. The heterogeneous nature of COPD can make diagnosis challenging as there is no one specific test (NICE, 2010). A key characteristic of COPD is that the airflow obstruction is not fully reversible; it is a long-term condition that is likely to be progressive.

The physiological changes described above result in deteriorating lung function that often manifests as exercise intolerance. However, MacIntyre (2008) asserts loss of function in patients with chronic lung diseases is multifactorial and the cardiovascular system, skeletal muscle factors, orthopaedic and psychological issues all play a part, which may affect individuals to a greater or lesser degree.

Ventilatory limiting factors

According to MacIntyre (2008), the limiting factor during exercise in health is the cardiovascular system, not the respiratory system. People with COPD develop respiratory limitation due to a load/capacity imbalance, i.e. the mechanical load on the lungs to breathe exceeds the capacity (strength and endurance) of the respiratory muscles to respond (MacIntyre, 2008). The increased airway resistance for inspiration and expiration and possible reduction in compliance significantly increase the work of breathing. Gas trapping in COPD causes hyperinflation of the lungs (air is trapped in the lungs due to airway narrowing or collapse and poor elastic recoil) with greater effort required by the respiratory muscles (MacIntyre, 2008).

As the lungs are chronically hyperinflated the diaphragm is pushed down and flattened which lessens the efficiency, and inflammatory mediators reduce respiratory muscle strength and endurance (MacIntyre, 2008). According to Hess and Kacmarek (2014), if changes to the diaphragm are profound a paradoxical breathing pattern may occur when the diaphragm contracts. The lateral rib cage moves inward rather than outwards during paradoxical breathing (Hess and Kacmarek, 2014). The primary muscle groups are the accessory muscles (intercostal, scalenes, sternomastoid, pectoralis, parasternal). The capacity to breath and the efficiency with which people are able to breath are compromised by physiological changes within the respiratory system.

Cardiovascular factors

MacIntyre (2008) describes the cascade of events that may follow chronic respiratory diseases, but impact on the cardiovascular system. In some patients, pulmonary vascular abnormalities may worsen pulmonary hypertension and right ventricular dysfunction, particularly if hypoxaemia is present (MacIntyre, 2008). The loss of function of the right ventricle reduces cardiac output and, therefore, oxygen delivery to the tissues. Deconditioning of cardiac muscle and dyspnoea lead to a spiral of events – inactivity due to dyspnoea lead to further deconditioning of the heart muscle, which causes reduced exercise ability, which causes further deconditioning.

Skeletal muscle factors

Inflammatory mediators alter protein turnover and the result for COPD patients is a loss of muscle mass significantly adding to loss of function. Another common finding in patients acutely unwell with an exacerbation of COPD is malnutrition. Inadequate nutrition further impairs respiratory muscle function (limiting respiratory muscle capacity). Care must be taken to replace nutrients but not over feed patients as they may lack protein and calories and also have an electrolyte imbalance (Hess and Kacmarek, 2014).

Corticosteroids taken by patients with COPD during exacerbations or long term have a deleterious effect on skeletal muscle protein (MacIntyre, 2008). Acidosis (as might be experienced during an acute episode) also impairs muscle function, therefore the effects are many and varied and all contribute to the spiralling loss of function that is described above.

Co-morbidities that are commonly found in COPD patients

In addition to the physiological changes to body systems that may result from COPD, there are many patients who experience co-existing diseases that significantly impact on COPD prognosis.

The Global Initiative for Chronic Obstructive Lung Disease (GOLD, 2017) has identified several co-morbidities that are commonly found in patients with COPD: generally the management of these disorders is not altered in those with COPD. According to GOLD (2017), these co-morbidities can occur during any stage of COPD and often have similar symptoms, confounding diagnosis.

Diagnosis

According to Vestbo et al. (2013: 350):

> a clinical diagnosis should be considered in any patient who has dyspnoea, chronic cough and/or sputum production, and a history of exposure to risk factors for the disease.

NICE (2010:11) suggests those over 35 with a risk factor and one or more of the following:

- exertional breathlessness
- chronic cough
- regular sputum production
- frequent winter bronchitis
- wheeze.

Due to the common co-morbidities and exhaustive differential diagnosis of COPD symptoms, NICE (2010: 11) also recommend asking about the following factors:

- weight loss
- effort intolerance
- waking at night
- ankle swelling
- fatigue
- occupational hazards
- chest pain*
- **haemoptysis*.**

* These symptoms are not common in COPD and may suggest an alternative diagnosis.

Diagnosis is complex due to the heterogeneous nature of the illness, which affects people differently. However, the primary symptom is breathlessness; therefore, NICE recommend the use of the Medical Research Council (1959) dyspnoea scale to quantify the amount of exertion required to experience breathlessness.

During the initial assessment patients should have a chest x-ray, full blood count (to assess for anaemia or polycythaemia) and calculation of body mass index (BMI) (NICE, 2010). Other investigations might include (Table 24.2):

Table 24.2

Serial domicillary peak flow measurements	To exclude asthma if diagnostic doubt remains
Alpha-1 antitrypsin	If early onset and minimal smoking history or family history
Transfer factor for carbon monoxide ($T_L CO$)	To investigate symptoms that seem disproportionate to the spirometric impairment
CT scan of the thorax	To investigate symptoms that seem disproportionate to the spirometric impairment
	To investigate abnormalities seen on chest radiograph
	To assess suitability for surgery
ECG	To assess cardiac status if features of cor pulmonale
Echocardiogram	To assess cardiac status if features of cor pulmonale

Pulse oximetry	To assess the need for oxygen therapy
	If cyanosis or cor pulmonale present, or if FEV1 <50% predicted
Sputum culture	To identify organisms if sputum is persistently present and purulent

(NICE, 2010)

Reproduced with permission under the NICE UK Open Content Licence.

Reproduced from BTS/SIGN British Guideline on the management of asthma, with kind permission of the British Thoracic Society.

Once a diagnosis is confirmed the next task is to establish the severity of the disease and the impact on the patient's life. The disease has many underlying causes and sequelae (as previously described); therefore, a careful medical and social history are required to assess the impact of the disease and options for reducing ongoing exposure risks such as smoking cessation.

Assessment of severity

Once the diagnosis of COPD has been made it is vital that assessment of severity of illness and the impact on the individual is appraised. Due to the variable nature of both cause and effect this may require assessment of the following:

- Symptoms – this may include a questionnaire to establish breathlessness, wellbeing and impact of disease on daily life.
- Severity of airflow limitation – spirometry can enable a grading system such as NICE (2010) or GOLD (2017) to be utilised to classify severity of illness.
- Exacerbation risk – exacerbation of COPD is when symptoms have worsened to require a change in medication, and management may be community based or require hospitalisation. Exacerbations are classified as mild – a change to inhaled medication, moderate – where an oral antibiotic and/ or oral steroid is required, or severe – support for respiratory symptoms requires hospital admission (GOLD, 2017).

Treatment/Therapeutic options

The goals of therapy are to reduce symptoms and frequency at which exacerbations occur and to improve lifestyle and exercise tolerance (GOLD, 2017). However, it is of note that none of the currently available therapies avert the long-term deterioration in lung function.

GOLD (2017) recommend that patients with COPD are offered vaccination for influenza and pneumococcus. Rehabilitation should also be offered as it may significantly improve people's ability to engage with activities of daily living (GOLD, 2017).

A key goal suggested by both NICE (2010) and GOLD (2017) is smoking cessation; this should be offered to all patients with COPD or, if relevant, reduction of exposure to other pollutants.

Therapeutic options are also broadly categorised as management of stable disease and management of exacerbations. However, therapy is individualised and will vary depending on severity of disease.

Management of stable disease

Inhaled therapy – This is likely to include a short acting bronchodilator to relieve breathlessness (NICE, 2010), short acting or long acting muscarinic antagonists may be required if bronchodilators are not sufficient (NICE, 2010), and inhaled corticosteroids may also be an option for some patients.

These medications may be used in combination. However, it is important the correct delivery device is chosen. Patients need to master inhaler technique in order to deliver the drug effectively; alternative devices such as spacers or nebulisers may be more appropriate.

WHAT'S THE EVIDENCE? 24.2

Reflect upon the care you have provided to a patient living with COPD.

- Look at the guidelines relating to medication and consider how you can apply your findings to practice.

You may wish to utilise the GOLD (2017) guidelines when formulating your answer.

Oral therapy – NICE (2010) provide a summary of oral medication use in COPD patients as part of the overall management guideline. Oral therapy may include oral corticosteroids (this is only for exceptional circumstances and the dose should be kept to a minimum). Oral theophylline is a possible therapeutic agent; however, drug interactions may occur and the plasma level requires to be monitored. Oral mucolytic may be considered for patients with a chronic production of sputum, but are not routinely used.

The use of inhaled and oral medication in combination may be required depending on patient response to therapy.

WHAT'S THE EVIDENCE? 24.3

It may be appropriate for people to receive long-term oxygen therapy; however, there is a risk of respiratory depression. Refer to the BTS (Hardinge et al., 2015) guidelines for home oxygen use in adults and discuss your findings with your mentor.

Non-invasive ventilation (NIV) – If persistent abnormalities exist in arterial blood gas analysis, patients may be referred to specialist centres for assessment for long-term NIV that they manage at home.

This disease is extremely variable between individuals and patient-specific therapy or referral to a specialist is likely. Another consideration is management of co-morbidities. Specialist teams should be established for COPD due to the multifactorial nature and complex management required.

GOLD (2017) suggest patients benefit from pulmonary rehabilitation programmes with improved exercise tolerance and a reduction in breathlessness and fatigue.

Management of exacerbations

Periodically, people may experience an acute worsening of their symptoms and this is described as an exacerbation of COPD (or infective exacerbation of COPD). The deterioration is over and above normal fluctuations of symptoms and often requires a change in medication or support, and is commonly precipitated by respiratory tract infection (GOLD, 2017). An important part of the management of COPD is to prevent occurrence of exacerbations. Exacerbations are significant as they are associated with an acceleration of lung function decline, significant mortality, and long recovery periods that may involve admission to hospital (GOLD, 2017). Patients may be managed in the community or hospital following an assessment of the severity of symptoms and likely need for more advanced respiratory support than they are receiving at home. According to NICE (2010), diagnosis of an exacerbation is made clinically and does not rely on investigation findings. Each individual has a different baseline therefore it is a change from *their* norm.

Exacerbations of COPD are likely to require pharmacological management. Short acting bronchodilators are commonly used to relieve symptoms of breathlessness. Oxygen should be provided and adjusted to achieve a pulse oximetry target range. Arterial blood gases should be measured on admission and repeated to monitor response to treatment. Antibiotics may be prescribed but only if there is a clinical indication such as purulent sputum or chest x-ray changes. If patients do not respond to optimal medical therapy, non-invasive and possibly invasive ventilation may be required in appropriate settings.

Prior to hospital discharge a full assessment of care requirements should take place, including the possible need for long-term oxygen therapy. Follow-up in the community should be provided.

SEE ALSO
CHAPTER 18

Oxygen therapy

Oxygen is an important element of care of patients with a wide range of respiratory conditions. As provision of healthcare develops and initiatives such as Hospital at Home increase, oxygen therapy is increasingly being delivered in community settings.

A subset of patients with COPD may be suitable for management using long term oxygen therapy (LTOT) at home. BTS (Hardinge et al., 2015) define LTOT as 'oxygen used for at least 15 hours a day in chronically hypoxaemic patients'. They require monitoring of this therapy using pulse oximetry. Kelly (2013) states that some community teams also have portable blood gas analysers, sampling ear lobe capillaries to obtain readings. The pH and PCO_2 readings are comparable with arterial samples; however, PO_2 readings will not reflect arterial measurements. Therefore, SpO_2 readings are taken in conjunction to ensure patients are well oxygenated.

Ambulatory oxygen therapy (AOT) may also benefit people who already have LTOT and desaturate during exercise; they would need an assessment to determine suitability.

However, despite the benefits of oxygen therapy there are some important considerations for patients with COPD. NICE (2010) advise patients who have LTOT need to be warned of the dangers of fire and explosion. Oxygen prescription and administration needs to meet the standards required for any medication. Oxygen must be prescribed to meet a target oxygen saturation range recorded on a prescription chart. The current target saturations for patients with hypercapnic respiratory failure are likely to be 88–92%, whereas the target for most acutely ill patients requiring oxygen therapy is 94–98% (O'Driscoll et al., 2017).

Delivery devices are often nasal cannuale or face masks incorporating a venturi system. Nasal cannuale deliver a variable amount of oxygen depending on how much air the patient is also breathing. For example, if the flow is set at 2 l/min and the patient is not entraining much additional air as they breathe they will receive a higher amount of oxygen, or conversely less oxygen if they increase the amount of air they entrain as they breathe. However, nasal cannuale are more easily tolerated. There is less variability in concentration of oxygen received by the patient with a venturi system as the air is blended as it is entrained through the device to give a more reliable amount.

Kelly (2013) described the emerging evidence base for the dangers associated with the use of oxygen therapy as even short episodes of high flow oxygen during ambulance transfers and during emergency treatment may be detrimental (Kelly, 2013). Careful titration of oxygen using a saturation target is required: using criteria such as apparent breathlessness is not appropriate. It may be appropriate to provide patients at risk of hypercapnic respiratory failure with an alert card they can give healthcare professionals.

CONCLUSION

Worldwide, the burden of respiratory disease is ever increasing, as is the need for safe and effective care. As nurses, we must attain the necessary knowledge and skills to care for this patient population and in doing so we will be able to provide appropriate individualised care across a variety of practice settings.

CHAPTER SUMMARY

- Respiratory disease remains a major cause of premature death worldwide, and asthma and COPD are two of five respiratory conditions that contribute to this global burden.
- By having an understanding of the respiratory system, you will be able to relate your assessment findings to your patient and their underlying pathophysiology.
- Respiratory assessment is an invaluable skill that can be used to assess and care for patients whatever the practice setting.
- By learning to undertake an accurate respiratory assessment you will be able to guide patient management and the provision of timely and effective respiratory care.
- Nurses have a vital role to play in health promotion and lifestyle changes, which can help to improve a patient's quality of life.

GO FURTHER

CASE STUDY: RESPIRATORY PROBLEMS

Go to https://study.sagepub.com/essentialadultnursing for a further case study related to this chapter. If you are using the interactive ebook, simply click on the book icon in the margin to go straight to the resource.

Books

- Beachy, W. (2013) *Respiratory Care Anatomy and Physiology: Foundations for clinical practice* (3rd ed.). Missouri: Elsevier.
  Details applied respiratory and cardiovascular physiology and how anatomy relates to physiological functions.
- Bourke, S.J. and Burns, G.P. (2015) *Respiratory Medicine: Lecture notes* (9th ed.). Oxford: Wiley-Blackwell.
  Covers everything from the basics of anatomy and physiology through to information on a full range of respiratory diseases.
- Ward, J.P.T., Ward, J. and Leach, R.M. (2015) *The Respiratory System At A Glance* (4th ed.). Oxford: Wiley-Blackwell.
  An accessible illustrated textbook covering common respiratory conditions.

Journal Articles

FURTHER READING: JOURNAL ARTICLES

Go to https://study.sagepub.com/essentialadultnursing for further free online journal articles related to this chapter. If you are using the interactive ebook, simply click on the book icon in the margin to go straight to the resource.

- Ellis, G. (2018) Factors affecting outcomes in patients receiving acute non-invasive ventilation. *Nursing Times*, 114 (3): 34-7.
  Discussion of a study to ascertain aspects of care that could be improved for patients receiving non-invasive ventilation.
- Holmes, L.J. (2017) Nurses' role in improving outcomes for patients with severe asthma. *Nursing Times*, 113 (4): 22-5.
  Exploration of the adequate assessment, support and treatment required for severe asthma both in primary care and specialist centres.
- Steiner, M.C., Evans, R.A., Greening, N.J., Free, R.C., Woltmann, G., Toms, N. and Margan, M.D. (2015) Comprehensive respiratory assessment in advanced COPD: a 'campus to clinic' transitional framework. *Thorax*, 70 (8): 805-8.
  Discussion of a framework for a structured, systematic and detailed assessment in COPD.

Weblinks

FURTHER READING: WEBLINKS

Go to https://study.sagepub.com/essentialadultnursing for further weblinks related to this chapter. If you are using the interactive ebook, simply click on the book icon in the margin to go straight to the resource.

- www.brit-thoracic.org.uk/
  The website of the British Thoracic Society (BTS) which develops standards to improve care for people who have respiratory diseases: Better Lung Health for All.
- http://goldcopd.org/
  Website of the Global Initiative for Chronic Obstructive Lung Disease (GOLD) which works with health-care professionals to improve prevention and treatment of COPD internationally.
- www.blf.org.uk/
  Public-facing website of the British Lung Foundation which is the only UK charity dedicated to lung health.

——— ACE YOUR ASSESSMENT ———

ONLINE QUIZZES

Revise what you have learned by visiting https://study.sagepub.com/essentialadultnursing

- Test yourself with multiple-choice and short-answer questions
- Do the chapter activities in the book and check your answers online

REFERENCES

BTS and SIGN (2016) British Thoracic Society and Scottish Intercollegiate Guidelines Network British Guideline on the Management of Asthma: A national clinical guideline.

Cohen, B.J. and Hull, K.L. (2015) *Memmler's the Human Body in Health and Disease* (13th edn). Philadelphia: Lippincott Williams and Wilkins.

Creed, F. and Spiers, C. (2010) *Care of the Acutely Ill Adult: An essential guide for nurses*. Oxford: Oxford University Press.

FIRS (2013) *Respiratory Diseases in the World: Realities of Today – Opportunities for Tomorrow*. Sheffield: European Respiratory Society Publications Office.

GINA (2017) Global Strategy for Asthma Management and Prevention.

GOLD (2017) Available at: http://goldcopd.org/

Hardinge, M., Annandale, J., Bourne, S., Cooper, B., Evans, A., Freeman, D., Green, A., Hippolyte, S., Knowles, V., MacNee, W., McDonnell, L., Pye, K., Suntharalingam, J., Vora, V. and Wilkinson, T. (2015) BTS guidelines for home oxygen use in adults. *Thorax*, 70; Supplement 1: i1–i43.

Hess, D.R. and Kacmarek, R.M. (2014) *Essentials of Mechanical Ventilation* (3rd ed.). New York: McGraw Hill Education.

Higginson, R. and Jones, B. (2009) Respiratory assessment in critically ill patients. *British Journal of Nursing*, 18 (8): 456–61.

Jevon, P. and Ewens, B. (2007) *Monitoring the Critically Ill Patient* (2nd ed.). Oxford: Blackwell Publishing.

Kaufman, G. (2011) Asthma: Pathophysiology, diagnosis and management. *Nursing Standard*, 26 (5): 48–56.

Kelly, L.D. (2013) Acute oxygen therapy for patients in the community. *Nursing Standard*, 27 (21): 63–8.

MacIntyre, N.R. (2008) Mechanisms of functional loss in patients with Chronic Lung Disease. *Respiratory Care*, 53 (9): 1177–83.

Moore, T. and Woodrow, P. (2009) *High Dependency Nursing Care: Observation, intervention and support for level 2 patients* (2nd ed.). Abingdon: Routledge.

Moxham, J. and Jolley, C. (2009) Breathlessness, fatigue and the respiratory muscles. *Clinical Medicine*, 9 (5): 448–52.

NICE (National Institute for Health and Care Excellence) (2010) *Chronic obstructive pulmonary disease in over 16s: Diagnosis and management*. Available at: https://www.nice.org.uk/guidance/cg101

NICE (National Institute for Health and Care Excellence) (2017) *Asthma: Diagnosis, monitoring and chronic asthma management*. Available at: https://www.nice.org.uk/guidance/ng80

O'Driscoll, B.R., Howard, L.S., Earis, J. and Mak, V. (2017) BTS guideline for oxygen use in adults in healthcare and emergency settings. *Thorax, 72*, Supplement 1: i1–i90.

Peate, I. and Nair, M. (2011) *Fundamentals of Anatomy and Physiology for Student Nurses*. Oxford: Wiley-Blackwell.

Steiner, M.C., Evans, R.A., Greening, N.J., Free, R.C., Woltmann, G., Toms, N. and Margan, M.D. (2015) Comprehensive respiratory assessment in advanced COPD: a 'campus to clinic' transitional framework. *Thorax*, 70: 805–8.

Tu, J., Inthavong, K. and Ahmadi, G. (2013) *Computational Fluid and Particle Dynamics in the Human Respiratory System*. London: Springer.

Vestbo, J., Hurd, S., Agusti, A.G., Jones, P.W., Vogelmeier, C., Anzueto, A., Barnes, P.J., Fabbri, L.M., Martinez, F.J., Mishimura, M., Stockley, R.A., Sin, D.D. and Rodriguez-Roisin, R. (2013) Global strategy for the diagnosis, management, and prevention of Chronic Obstructive Pulmonary Disease. *American Journal of Critical Care Medicine*, 187 (4): 347–65.

CARE OF THE ADULT WITH A CARDIAC CONDITION

25

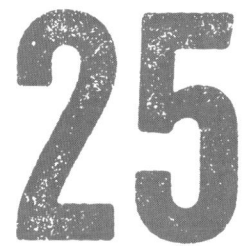

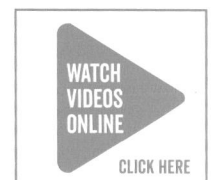

WATCH VIDEOS ONLINE — CLICK HERE

FIONA EVERETT, WENDY WRIGHT AND MEGHAN BATESON

THIS CHAPTER COVERS

- An overview of the anatomy and physiology of the heart
- An explanation of the clinical characteristics and pathophysiology relevant to the most common presenting cardiac conditions
- Nursing assessment of the adult with the most common presenting cardiac conditions
- Health promotion and discharge planning considerations for adults with a cardiac condition.

"

My name is Darshan, I am 83 years old and I have heart failure. I have been admitted to hospital several times over the last few years with breathlessness and loss of appetite. I live with my daughter Amisha, her husband Dinesh and their three children.

I am very happy with the care that I receive both at home and in hospital. I am also grateful to the many people who have looked after me: doctors, nurses, physiotherapists, occupational therapists, radiographers, district nurses and my family.

I feel that I have a team of 'helpers' who support me to remain at home by helping me to manage my symptoms and providing me with information that makes sense and helps me to understand my condition better.

My grandchildren have also introduced me to the Internet and wi-fi, which has given me another means of access to the information advised by the hospital consultant and my GP.

Darshan, cardiac patient

"

"

I am now in my second year and have had one cardiology placement so far in my nursing programme. This placement provided me with a unique learning opportunity as it highlighted the importance of spirituality. I cared for a patient who had experienced a myocardial infarction, who shared their experience with me of having a 'heart attack' and the feeling of 'impending doom'. This made them acutely aware of their mortality and the importance of their religious beliefs and how these beliefs enabled them to look forward to the future. It made me more aware of the importance of listening, of completing nursing documentation and utilising assessment tools which record and capture patients' perspectives, which help to tailor care to meet the individual and holistic needs of each patient.

Sue Carpenter, 2nd year nursing student

"

INTRODUCTION

Nursing adults with a cardiac condition takes place in a variety of care settings ranging from the acute hospital to community setting. It is likely that you either know someone with a cardiac condition or have contributed to his or her care.

Cardiovascular disease (CVD) is a general term, which describes disease of the heart and blood vessels. There are four main types of CVD:

- coronary heart disease
- stroke
- peripheral arterial disease
- aortic disease.

Each person has their own individual set of risk factors, which may be modified or not.

Non-modifiable risk factors:

- age
- gender
- ethnicity
- genetic predisposition
- low birth weight
- diabetes mellitus
- hormonal and biochemical factors.

Modifiable risk factors:

- blood cholesterol
- tobacco smoking
- high blood pressure
- overweight and obesity
- diet
- social class.

Many deaths attributable to CVD are premature but could be prevented by making lifestyle changes, such as exercising regularly, eating healthily and stopping smoking. Many of these habits are established during childhood and can continue into adulthood, which can then result in health issues.

CVD causes over one hundred thousand deaths in the UK each year and is, therefore, considered a public health issue. Nurses have a vital role to play in the prevention and management of this condition across the age continuum. This also includes facilitating public recognition and response to myocardial infarction. Defibrillators are now commonplace within many public areas and enable members of the public to respond should cardiac arrest occur (Resuscitation Council, 2015).

This chapter will focus on three of the most common cardiac conditions that you are likely to encounter within the practice learning environment:

- myocardial infarction
- heart failure
- atrial fibrillation.

GO FURTHER

The British Heart Foundation (BHF) provides a comprehensive range of resources in relation to heart disease and how to prevent it. See the BHF website for more information: https://www.bhf.org.uk/informationsupport/conditions/cardiovascular-disease

WEBLINK:
BHF HEART
DISEASE

Nursing roles may vary depending on the health board, department and geographical area that you work in; for example, venepuncture may be performed by a nurse, doctor, phlebotomist or you if supervised by your mentor. You may already have noticed that there is a cross-over of knowledge, skills and roles between nurses, doctors and other healthcare professionals, which ultimately should result in the provision of high-quality person-centred care. While this chapter mainly explores acute care, reference is also made to ongoing care, which often takes place in the community setting but still may involve follow-up care within the hospital setting.

The following section will focus on the anatomy and physiology of the heart and will provide you with a useful opportunity to revise (Bromfield, 2016).

ANATOMY AND PHYSIOLOGY

Overview

The heart is a muscular organ containing four chambers. Its main function is to pump blood around the circulatory system of the lungs and the systemic circulation of the rest of the body. It must continue its cycle of contraction and relaxation in order to provide a continuous blood supply to the tissues and ensure the delivery of nutrients and oxygen and the removal of waste products.

Location

The heart is located in the chest cavity, between the lungs and is about the size of your fist. Its shape is like a cone, with the apex of the cone pointing forwards and to the left.

Structures of the heart

- heart wall
- chambers of the heart
- valves
- vessels (see Table 25.1).

Blood flow through the heart

Figure 25.1 provides a description of the blood flow through the heart.

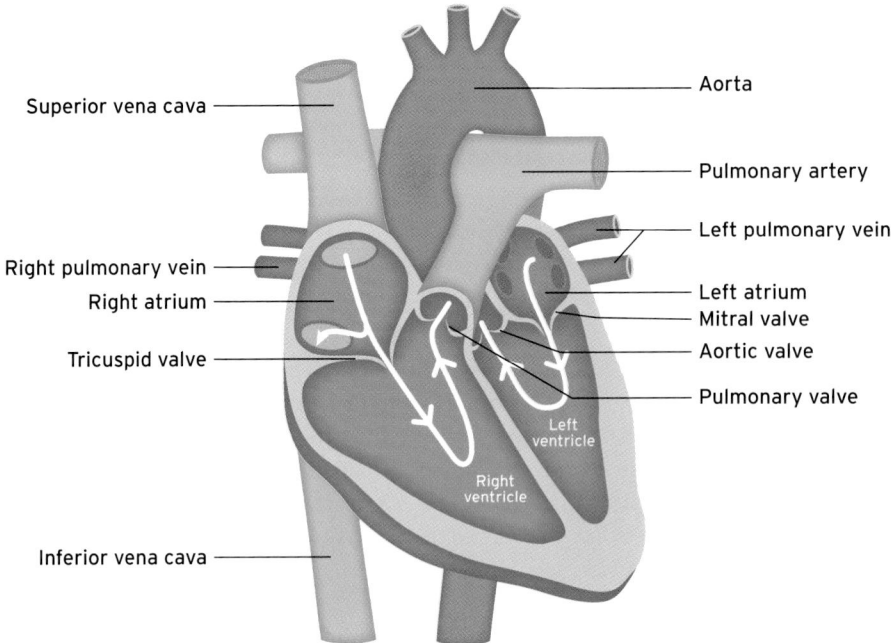

Figure 25.1   Blood flow through the heart

Source: Boore et al. (2016). Illustrated by Shaun Mercier, © SAGE Publications.

Table 25.1   Function of the vessels

Vessel	Function
Superior vena cava	Returns oxygen-depleted blood to the right atrium from the thoracic organs, head, neck and both arms
Inferior vena cava	Returns oxygen-depleted blood to the right atrium from the rest of the body
Pulmonary artery (divides into right and left pulmonary artery)	Takes oxygen-depleted blood from the right ventricles to the lungs
Pulmonary veins (two from the right lung and two from the left lung)	Returns oxygen-rich blood from the lungs to the left atrium
Aorta	Takes oxygen-rich blood from the left ventricle to the whole body
Coronary arteries	Takes oxygen-rich blood to the heart tissues
Coronary veins	Returns oxygen-depleted blood from the heart tissues to the right atrium via the coronary sinus

Conducting system of the heart

The heart has a built-in regulatory mechanism, which produces a coordinated myocardial contraction of the four chambers. This is achieved by the cardiac conducting system, which is composed of:

- the sinoatrial (SA) node
- the atrioventricular (AV) node

- the bundle of His
- the right and left bundle branches
- the Purkinje fibres.

The SA node

The SA node is situated in the right atrium just below the opening of the superior vena cava. It is also known as the pacemaker, so-called because every heart beat is initiated from here. Impulses from the SA node cause the atria to contract.

The AV node

The AV node is a mass of tissue situated at the base of the right atrium. This is the last region of the atria to be stimulated, thus allowing time for the atria to empty the blood into the ventricles before the ventricles start to contract again. This ensures that the blood will flow in one direction only.

Bundle of His

This is a set of fibres that originate from the AV node.

Right and left bundle branches

From the bundle of His the nerves split into the right and the left bundle branches, which carry the electrical signal across the ventricles.

The Purkinje fibres

These tiny nerve fibres surround the ventricles from the endocardium to the myocardium carrying the electrical impulse to the apex of each ventricle.

ACTIVITY 25.1: CRITICAL THINKING

Have you had the opportunity to explore the roles of other healthcare professionals?

In the patient voice at the start of this chapter, Darshan refers to several other healthcare professionals as a team of 'helpers' who have contributed to his care.

Take a few moments to reflect on your experiences so far and discuss with your mentor any gaps in your knowledge with regard to the roles of other professionals and the contribution that they make to patient care.

You may wish to negotiate spending time with other healthcare professionals to fully understand teamworking, as part of your learning plan.

The following section will focus on the clinical characteristics, pathophysiology, nursing assessment, clinical investigations, nursing care implementation and management and evaluation of myocardial infarction.

MYOCARDIAL INFARCTION: CLINICAL CHARACTERISTICS AND PATHOPHYSIOLOGY

Myocardial infarction (MI) is the death of myocardial tissue due to ischaemia (inadequate blood supply) and hypoxia (deficiency in the amount of oxygen reaching the tissues). This is usually caused by a blockage in one of the coronary arteries or their branches. The blockage is often a result of a thrombus (blood clot), which forms following the rupture of an atherosclerotic plaque in the coronary artery. There are other mechanisms that cause disruption of the balance between myocardial oxygen supply and demand resulting in an MI. Table 25.2 provides an outline of the clinical characteristics and pathophysiology of an MI.

Table 25.2 Myocardial infarction: clinical characteristics and pathophysiology

Clinical Characteristic	Pathophysiology
Chest pain	When the coronary arteries become blocked due to occlusion by a plaque or its thrombus oxygen cannot reach the myocardium (heart muscle). This means that the myocardial cells have to switch to anaerobic metabolism (where the cells work without oxygen), which leads to the production of lactic acid (organic compound).
	The lactic acid triggers the pain receptors of the heart, which results in the chest pain.
Nausea and vomiting	This is a common presenting symptom. May be due to stimulation of the sympathetic nervous system (the part of the autonomic nervous system which triggers the fight or flight response).
Tachycardia	Stimulation of the sympathetic nervous system results in a higher heart rate.
Bradycardia	Stimulation of the vagus nerve (tenth cranial nerve, which interfaces with the parasympathetic control of the heart) can reduce heart rate.

It is important that you recognise that not all people experiencing an MI exhibit the signs and symptoms that are usually associated with the event. This is known as atypical presentation. Women and older people are particularly likely to present with atypical symptoms. For example, fewer women than men report chest pain during an MI. This is important as it may contribute to delays in recognition and treatment.

Nursing assessment

Patients presenting acutely unwell with chest pain are more likely to be treated within a hospital setting and should be rapidly assessed using an ABCDE (Airway, Breathing, Circulation, Disability, Exposure/Examination) approach to confirm a diagnosis of MI (Resuscitation Council, 2016). You may already have had the opportunity to undertake this type of assessment through direct patient care or practised this skill in a clinical skills laboratory supported by your mentor or nurse lecturer respectively.

A health history will be obtained as soon as is practical. This should include:

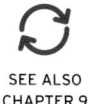

SEE ALSO
CHAPTER 9

- events leading up to admission
- relevant past medical history and family history
- cardiovascular risk factors, such as diet, exercise, recreational drug use and smoking.

The detail of the history will be dependent on the condition of the patient. If the patient is acutely unwell this will be limited to items that are important to the immediate care of the patient.

Physical assessment of the patient will include:

- Assessment of Chest Pain

A specific tool to assess cardiac chest pain should be used. Tools such as the PQRST (Provocation/Palliation, Quality/Quantity, Region/Radiation, Severity, Timing) approach usually include assessment of the location, severity, quality, and radiation as well as what provoked the pain and when the pain started. Again, you may already have had the opportunity to undertake this type of assessment through direct patient care or practised this skill in a clinical skills laboratory supported by your mentor or nurse lecturer respectively.

- Frequent measurement of vital signs

This is important to identify signs of deterioration. Remember to calculate the early warning score if used in your clinical area.

- Continuous ECG (electrocardiogram) monitoring using 3- or 5-lead ECG system

Clinical Investigations

- 12-lead ECG

This should be undertaken as soon as the patient arrives at hospital or, if already in hospital, immediately on complaining of chest pain. This provides information on heart activity from 12 different angles, which enables identification of the exact region of the heart that has been affected. The ECG will be read by a doctor to establish whether the patient is experiencing an MI and where in the heart it is occurring. MIs are classified as STEMI (ST elevation MI) and NSTEMI (non-ST elevation MI).

- Troponin

Troponin (I or T) is released by myocytes (cardiac muscle cells) when they are damaged. A troponin rise plus signs of ischaemia confirms a diagnosis of MI. Because troponin levels peak at 12 to 24 hours after an MI and stay elevated for 10 to 15 days after, troponin can detect an MI which occurred days before the patient presents to hospital.

Troponin (I or T) should be measured on admission/onset of chest pain and 6–9 hours later. If there continues to be suspicion of MI, a third sample may be sent between 12 and 24 hours.

- Physical examination and additional investigations

Monitoring the patient for the development of MI-related complications is important and will include a physical examination, A to E assessment and additional investigations. For example, blood tests will be sent to check:

- urea and electrolytes – allows evaluation of kidney function which may be impacted by the MI or have implications for treatment plans. Also includes measurement of potassium (K^+) levels which, if abnormal, can cause life-threatening cardiac arrhythmias
- random glucose and cholesterol
- full blood count.

SEE ALSO
CHAPTER 9

Nursing care implementation and management

Patients experiencing an MI are likely to be nursed in a Coronary Care Unit (CCU) initially. They will be stepped down to a cardiology ward as soon as they are assessed as fit to move on.

The aim of treatment for MI is to minimise the size of the infarct and return perfusion (oxygenated blood supply) to the myocardium. It is currently recommended for STEMI patients that this is achieved through a primary percutaneous coronary intervention (PPCI). A PPCI is a procedure that is undertaken in the catheterisation laboratories in specialist hospitals to view and unblock the coronary arteries as required. To do this a catheter is threaded up through the femoral or radial arteries into the heart under radiological guidance. Once in place at the blocked vessel the cardiologist will try to unblock the vessel using a stent or other device as appropriate.

Thrombolysis, which requires the administration of medications to dissolve the clot blocking the coronary arteries, may be used if PPCI is unavailable and criteria for inclusion are met. Thrombolysis carries significant risks and, therefore, each patient is individually risk assessed for suitability.

GO FURTHER

WEBLINK:
HEART
CONDITION
TREATMENTS

Information about undergoing a PPCI and receiving thrombolysis is available on the BHF website: https://www.bhf.org.uk/heart-health/treatments

---

Patients experiencing a NSTEMI will be assessed for their need for coronary angiography (x-ray of the heart) and revascularisation (restoration of perfusion). The findings of this assessment will determine optimal treatment and patients may go on to receive coronary angioplasty (widens blocked or narrowed coronary arteries) or coronary artery bypass grafting (a surgical procedure, which diverts blood around narrowed or blocked arteries to improve blood flow and oxygen supply to the heart).

As soon as a diagnosis of MI has been established, a number of medications which reduce the oxygen demand and maximise the oxygen supply to the myocardial tissue (heart muscle) will be prescribed and should be administered immediately. The prescription may include the following medication set known as MONA:

- **M**orphine
  - o   Intravenous morphine relieves chest pain

- **O**xygen
  - o   To treat hypoxaemia and maintain oxygen saturations of 94–98%

- **N**itrates
  - o To dilate coronary arteries
- **A**spirin
  - o Interferes with platelet aggregation
  - o N.B. additional anti-platelet therapy, such as clopidogrel, may be commenced.

Additional supportive measures:

- Immediate bed rest to reduce myocardial oxygen demand until MI treatment is complete. Following this, early mobilisation is encouraged.
- Insertion of a wide bore intravenous (IV) cannula to facilitate administration of intravenous medications such as morphine.
- Frequent observation of vital signs and continuous ECG monitoring. This allows observation for signs of deterioration. Complications such as arrhythmias (irregular heartbeat), left ventricular failure (due to left ventricular systolic dysfunction) and cardiogenic shock (when the heart is unable to pump enough blood to meet the body's needs) can arise after an MI.

Communication and reassurance for patients and families is essential during and after an MI. Shared decision-making is key for cardiac patients to ensure a person-centred approach.

- Depression is common in patients who have experienced an MI and has implications for morbidity and mortality. Patients may be screened for anxiety and depression using a tool such as the Hospital Anxiety and Depression Scale (HADS). There is evidence that patients participating in cardiac rehabilitation experience a reduction in anxiety and depression (Yohannes et al., 2010).

Evaluation

The patient's response to the treatment provided will be monitored closely. They will also be assessed for complications of the treatment or the MI itself.

Some patients will require additional treatment options to optimise their recovery post MI. For example, a person who has undergone a PPCI may go on to require more invasive surgery such as a coronary artery bypass graft.

Development of your nursing assessment skills are key to ensuring that the patient progresses through their recovery period smoothly and provide early recognition of any arising complications. Development of your skills is also key to secondary prevention, the prevention of the patient experiencing further MIs. This is facilitated partly through health education on the ward prior to discharge but, importantly, in the follow-up at cardiac rehabilitation classes which should be available to all appropriate patients post MI.

CASE STUDY 25.1: EUAN

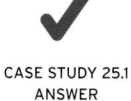

CASE STUDY 25.1
ANSWER

Euan is 50 years old and lives with his wife, Mhairi, in a small village located in the Scottish Borders. They have two children, Gregor and Erin, who both studied at university and have secured jobs in London working in banking and sales and marketing respectively.

Euan holds a senior management position as a Customer Services Manager for an international engineering firm. This is a role that he finds stressful at times but gets tremendous satisfaction from

(Continued)

(Continued)

when he is able to resolve customer queries. Mhairi works part-time as a librarian in the local library, situated in the local town, which is seven miles away from their home.

Euan was admitted to the local district general hospital as an emergency when he developed sudden chest pain, which woke him from his sleep. The pain also radiated down his left arm and made him feel nauseated. His wife Mhairi phoned for an ambulance, as he had not experienced these symptoms before.

Euan spent several days in the Coronary Care Unit. Prior to discharge he and his wife met with the clinical nurse specialist and discussed his lifestyle including: diet, cholesterol, exercise, smoking, alcohol intake and weight.

Euan has realised that there are several changes he can make, which will improve his overall health and wellbeing.

1. What information would you offer Euan and Mhairi in order to support him with lifestyle changes?
2. How could you assist Euan and Mhairi to maintain these changes?

The following section will focus on the clinical characteristics, pathophysiology, nursing assessment, clinical investigations, nursing care implementation and management and evaluation of heart failure.

HEART FAILURE: CLINICAL CHARACTERISTICS AND PATHOPHYSIOLOGY

Heart failure is a complex condition in which the heart can no longer pump blood efficiently to the tissues and organs of the body, thereby reducing oxygen and nutrient provision. Heart failure can develop because of a number of factors. Three common contributing factors are:

1. failure of the pumping mechanism of the heart
2. high resistance in the circulatory system
3. fluid overload.

The most common type of heart failure is left ventricular failure. There are many causes of heart failure but one of the most common contributing conditions is coronary artery disease, which causes myocardial infarction. As medicine has improved, more people are surviving myocardial infarction. This means that more people are now living with heart failure but the death of cardiac tissue during an MI means that the heart cannot pump as well as it once did.

There are many clinical characteristics of heart failure. The difficulty is that many of them are not specific to heart failure and so require a full clinical assessment in order to make a diagnosis. The following clinical characteristics are common but not specific to heart failure, which means that they also occur in other conditions. Table 25.3 provides an outline of the clinical characteristics and pathophysiology of heart failure.

Table 25.3   Heart failure: clinical characteristics and pathophysiology

Clinical Characteristic	Pathophysiology
Dyspnoea (shortness of breath)	There is a range of types of dyspnoea which may be experienced by a person with heart failure. The type of dyspnoea will determine the underlying cause but this may include cardiac insufficiency (inadequate pumping of blood by the heart to the tissues).
Orthopnoea (shortness of breath when lying flat)	One type of dyspnoea. In heart failure the heart cannot cope with the increased volume of blood returning to the heart when the legs are at the same level of the heart. This means that fluid accumulates in the lungs causing orthopnoea.
Ankle oedema	In heart failure the heart cannot pump as much blood out of the heart. This causes a traffic jam for the blood returning to the heart. This traffic jam leads to fluid accumulation in the lower limbs and abdomen. Worsening ankle oedema can be a sign of worsening heart failure.
Fatigue, increased recovery time after exercise	Because the heart cannot pump blood as well as needed, less blood is delivered to muscles and other tissues leading to tiredness. Fatigue is also caused by a reduction in the efficiency of waste removal due to the poorer pumping of the heart.

Nursing assessment

A thorough patient history will be taken and should include information about functional activity to help assess the severity of an individual's heart failure.

Information of particular interest includes:

- How many pillows the patient sleeps with at night or if they sleep upright in a chair. This gives you information about orthopnoea (shortness of breath when lying flat).
- Family past medical history because there can be a genetic component to some types of cardiac failure.
- Assessment of oedema to track improvements or deterioration.

All vital signs will be collected and interpreted according to local policy. All assessment findings will be documented accurately in the patient record.

Clinical investigations

- Chest x-ray

Patients with suspected, acute or new heart failure often have a chest x-ray obtained. This can show if the heart is enlarged, if there is fluid in the pleural space and if there is pulmonary oedema. A chest x-ray will also help with excluding other potential pulmonary causes of the clinical characteristics experienced by the patient.

- Echocardiogram

An echocardiogram (sonogram of the heart) will be undertaken to assess the structure and function of the heart. This can be undertaken either transthoracic (through the thorax) which is non-invasive and performed in a similar way to a pregnancy ultrasound, or transoesophageal (through the oesophagus) which is invasive and performed in a similar way to an endoscopy.

Several measurements will be taken during the echocardiogram but one of the most important is the ejection fraction, which tells us how well the heart is pumping. The ejection fraction is the percentage of the total blood in the heart at the end of diastole, which is ejected from the heart in each beat. A normal heart's ejection fraction is between 50% and 70%. An ejection fraction less than 40% may indicate heart failure.

It is possible to have heart failure with a normal ejection fraction but this is less common.

- 12-lead ECG

This will show any abnormalities in the electrical conduction system through the heart as well as the heart rhythm. If a patient has a completely normal ECG it is unlikely that they have heart failure.

- Blood tests including:
  - urea and electrolytes
  - full blood count
  - liver function tests
  - thyroid stimulating hormone (TSH) (Thyroid disease can mimic heart failure or make it worse)
  - lipid profile
  - glucose
  - B type natriuretic peptide (BNP) or N-terminal pro-B-type natriuretic peptide (NT-proBNP) (natriuretic peptides are a useful aid to clinical decision-making, diagnosis and assessment of severity in heart failure)
- Classification of severity of heart failure.

There are several classification systems available to assess the severity of heart failure. The two most common are the New York Heart Association (NYHA) (2016) Functional Classification and the American College of Cardiology Foundation (ACCF)/American Heart Association (AHA) Stages of heart failure.

Nursing care implementation and management

The key aims of heart failure management are to minimise signs and symptoms, prevent hospital admission, and improve life expectancy.

Patients in heart failure are susceptible to fluid overload and are often on diuretics. Many patients, therefore, require to be weighed daily in order to assess their fluid status and ensure that they are not accumulating too much fluid.

Specialist heart failure nurses help patients manage their condition in the community setting. These nurses regularly follow up patients and can adjust treatment to optimise the patient's condition within the scope of their practice. They can provide expert assessment to recognise and act on signs of deterioration. Heart failure specialist nurses also have a very important education and support role for patients and their families. They can provide support in the context of advanced care planning and palliative care for patients with heart failure although there are also some additional nurses who specifically specialise in palliation for heart failure.

Patients with heart failure will be commenced on a range of medications, such as diuretics, **angiotensin converting enzyme (ACE) inhibitors** and **aldosterone receptor blockers.**

SEE ALSO
CHAPTER 23

Education on their medications is essential to help promote concordance which is important because evidence demonstrates that adherence to treatment guidelines improves outcomes.

Evaluation

Patients with heart failure will be evaluated on an ongoing basis dependent on their clinical condition. This may include regular reviews by a cardiologist. Patients in more advanced stages of heart failure may receive input from a heart failure specialist nurse.

The following section will focus on the clinical characteristics, pathophysiology, nursing assessment, clinical investigations, nursing care implementation and management and evaluation of atrial fibrillation.

ATRIAL FIBRILLATION: CLINICAL CHARACTERISTICS AND PATHOPHYSIOLOGY

People with atrial fibrillation (AF) have an irregular heart rhythm. This can be felt as an irregular pulse. Table 25.4 provides an outline of the clinical characteristics and pathophysiology of atrial fibrillation.

Table 25.4 Atrial fibrillation: clinical characteristics and pathophysiology

Clinical Characteristic	Pathophysiology
Irregular pulse	The atria are in fibrillation, which means they are quivering and not contracting properly.
	This is because there has been a disruption in the electrical pathway through the heart. The nerve impulses are not being reliably conducted through the atrioventricular node into the ventricles. This means that the ventricles are contracting intermittently based on when they receive an impulse from the atria through the atrioventricular node. This results in an irregular heart rhythm, which can be felt as an irregular pulse. The heart rate is often above 100 beats per minute (bpm) but may be lower.
Pulse varies in strength from beat to beat	This is because the length of time the ventricle has to fill will vary due to the irregular ventricular rate. The result of this is that the volume of the blood in the ventricle will vary at each beat because the volume ejected will not be consistent, and the strength of the pulse will vary.
Palpitations	The process by which palpitations are felt is unknown. Some patients will feel every abnormal beat and others do not experience any palpitations.
Dyspnoea (shortness of breath)	Reduction in cardiac output due to the irregular heartbeat occurs. The development of heart failure usually occurs only on exertion.
Syncope (fainting)	When AF is fast (more than 100 bpm), the duration of diastole (when the heart is resting and refilling) is reduced. This means that there is not time for the heart to refill completely and results in a poorer cardiac output leading to reduced cerebral blood flow. This reduction in cerebral blood flow leads to syncope (fainting) as the brain is not receiving enough oxygenated blood to perfuse properly.
Chest pain	The coronary arteries, which deliver oxygenated blood to the heart muscle, fill during diastole (when the heart is resting and refilling). If the AF has a very fast rate the length of diastole is reduced. This reduces the time available for the coronary arteries to fill and therefore reduces oxygen supply to the cardiac muscle resulting in chest pain.

Nursing assessment

A full A to E assessment should be undertaken for any patient who presents acutely unwell. As part of this, the nursing assessment for patients at risk of, or experiencing, AF should include measurement of the heart rate manually for one minute instead of using a pulse oximeter. NICE (2014) recommends that a manual pulse be obtained to check for the possibility of AF in patients presenting with: breathlessness, palpitations, syncope/dizziness, chest pain or a stroke/**transient ischaemic attack (TIA).**

The pulse of a patient with AF will feel irregular. If an irregular rhythm is palpated during the pulse check and this is new or faster than normal, medical staff should be informed and a 12-lead ECG should be undertaken. The ECG will determine if the patient is experiencing AF. If a patient is suspected of experiencing paroxysmal AF, which occurs intermittently, a 24-hour ambulatory ECG monitor or an event recorder ECG can be used to confirm diagnosis.

If the patient is stable enough to answer questions it is important to get a thorough history. Questions will include:

- What are the symptoms they are experiencing? e.g. dizziness, breathlessness, palpitations, etc.
- When did the symptoms start?
- If the symptoms are not ongoing, how long did they last and how often do they occur?
- Did anything trigger the symptoms?
- Family and personal past medical history.
- Lifestyle considerations, e.g. smoking, alcohol, drug use.

Clinical investigations

- Electrocardiogram (ECG)

ECG is utilised in the diagnosis of AF. Figure 25.2 illustrates what a normal sinus rhythm looks like on ECG. If the patient was in AF there would be no distinguishable P waves on the ECG, which would be replaced by lots of chaotic little waves. This is because the normal sinoatrial node to atrioventricular node pathway, which constitutes the P wave, does not exist in AF. You would also notice that the distance between the R waves changes. This is because the ventricles are only receiving impulses intermittently through the AV node.

- Echocardiogram

This enables assessment of the structure and function of the heart muscles and valves. One of the primary concerns in AF is the potential for clotting in the atria.

- Blood tests to check potassium levels, thyroid levels and anaemia

Abnormal levels can lead to arrhythmias and should be checked in order to remedy if required.

Nursing care implementation and management

The key priorities of care of the patient with atrial fibrillation are:

- Rhythm control: restore to normal sinus rhythm

This is usually used for patients with new AF, in younger people and where the person is unresponsive to or unable to tolerate rate control medications. It can be achieved either through electrical or pharmacological approaches known as cardioversion.

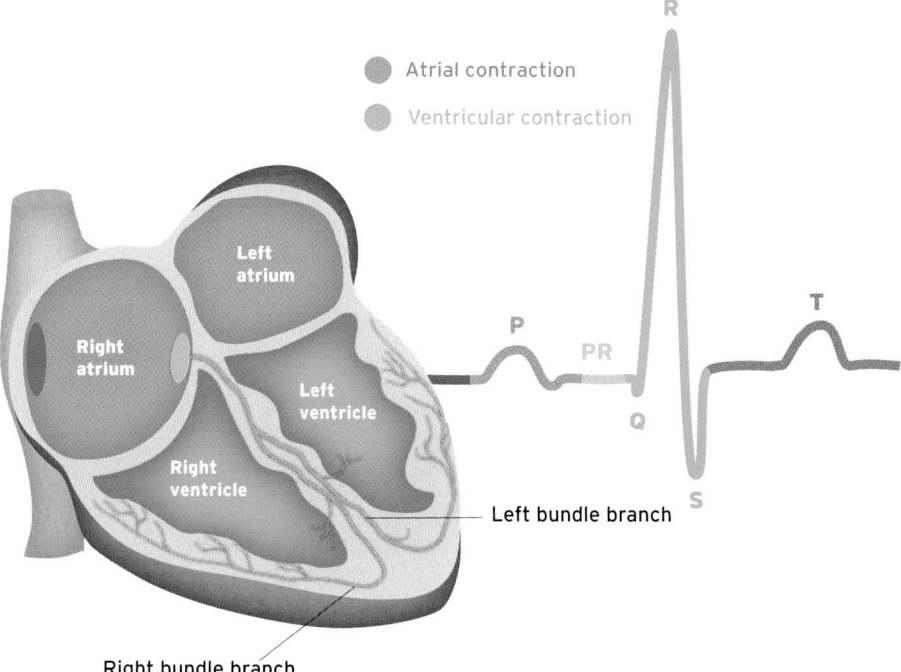

Figure 25.2   ECG: normal sinus rhythm

Source: Boore et al. (2016). Illustrated by Shaun Mercier, © SAGE Publications.

Pharmacological cardioversion uses antiarrythmic agents such as amiodarone to restore sinus rhythm. Such medications are not suitable for all patients and will be risk assessed by medical staff.

Electrical cardioversion uses a defibrillator synchronised to the patient's own ECG to shock their heart back into a normal sinus rhythm. This is the first step in managing AF for a haemodynamically compromised patient. Electrical cardioversion is undertaken in a highly supervised environment such as an intensive care unit with staff who have advanced cardiac life support (ACLS) training. The patient is sedated throughout the procedure. Prior to electrical cardioversion there will be an assessment of whether the patient already has thrombi in the atria and whether anticoagulants should be commenced prior to the cardioversion. Where AF started less than 48 hours ago this may not be required. If there are thrombi in the atria, cardioversion will be delayed since cardioversion could cause them to move resulting in complications such as stroke or pulmonary embolus. Anticoagulation treatment will continue for several weeks after cardioversion.

- Rate control: control the heart rate if sinus rhythm cannot be restored

This can be achieved using medications to control rate such as: beta-blockers, calcium channel blockers, digoxin and amiodarone. For patients who are asymptomatic (i.e. no signs of heart failure) it is recommended that the heart rate be maintained less than 110 bpm. For symptomatic patients the heart rate should be maintained at less than 80 bpm.

- To prevent thromboembolism (blood clots)

People with AF are at high risk of thromboembolism which can lead to stroke (cerebrovascular accident) because the atria are not contracting well, leading to stasis of blood in the atria, increasing the chances of clot formation. Anticoagulants, such as warfarin, are used to prevent thromboembolism.

These have their own risks and require careful and continuous monitoring to ensure the effect is therapeutic and does not lead to additional complications such as bleeding. Both stroke and anticoagulant associated bleeding can be devastating. There are tools available to help medical staff make decisions about what is best for each individual patient. However, the use of factor xa inhibitors known as novel anticoagulants (NOACs) such as dabigatran, rivaroxaban, apixaban and edoxaban are increasingly being used, which do not require the same level of monitoring as warfarin.

GO FURTHER

WEBLINKS

Take a look at some examples of tools utilized in decision-making:

The Scottish Intercollegiate Guidelines Network (SIGN) (2014) *Prevention of stroke in patients with atrial fibrillation*: www.sign.ac.uk/assets/af_publication.pdf

The European Society of Cardiology (2016) *ESC Guidelines for the management of atrial fibrillation developed in collaboration with EACTS:* https://academic.oup.com/eurheartj/article/37/38/2893/2334964

Patients may require radiofrequency catheter ablation to manage AF if they remain symptomatic despite treatment. This is performed in the cardiac catheterisation laboratory by an interventional cardiologist. The ablation effectively rubs out the pathway that is triggering the AF by scarring the tissue at the area of the atria which is causing the AF.

Modifiable risk factors are important in the management of AF. These include smoking cessation, treatment for alcohol or drug misuse, exercise and weight management. Nurse-led services to enable patients to manage their AF have been found to be successful in ensuring that care adheres to guidelines and outcomes (Qvist et al., 2015).

Patients with AF have elevated levels of anxiety and depression when compared with the general population. Services should be made available to them in order to manage this given the impact this can have on quality of life.

Comprehensive patient education is essential in AF, particularly including information about when to seek help.

GO FURTHER

WEBLINKS

Take a look at the following links, which are a useful source of information for patients and carers:

- www.heartrhythmalliance.org/afa/uk/
- www.nhs.uk/conditions/atrial-fibrillation/
- www.stroke.org.uk/what-is-stroke/are-you-at-risk-of-stroke/atrial-fibrillation

---

Evaluation

Patients will be evaluated both acutely and on an ongoing basis following a diagnosis or episode of AF. This evaluation will monitor their heart rate, symptoms and, where appropriate, their

International Normalised Ratio (INR). If it is not possible to return a patient to normal sinus rhythm they will be evaluated on the basis of minimising symptoms to reduce impact on everyday life.

CASE STUDY 25.2: ANNIE

CASE STUDY 25.2
ANSWER

Annie is a 75-year-old widow who lives in the town that she was born and brought up in. She is a retired primary school teacher and Girl Guide leader. She has three daughters and six grandchildren and four great grandchildren. All of her family live within a ten-mile radius of her home. She enjoys reading, voluntary work, playing bowls and spending time with her family and friends.

Over the past several months Annie has experienced several episodes of her heart pounding for a few minutes, which has made her feel dizzy. She usually sits down and this resolves the dizziness fairly quickly. She takes medication for high blood pressure and is due to have her blood pressure checked by the practice nurse at her local GP surgery in a week's time. She has not discussed her symptoms with any of her family or friends, as she does not want to cause them any distress.

1. What information would you provide Annie with in relation to her symptoms?
2. What treatment options may be available to Annie in order to alleviate her symptoms?

DISCHARGE PLANNING

The principles of discharging patients from hospital or other care settings have not changed over many years; however, the process and pace of discharge planning has changed to reflect the complexity of contemporary healthcare, particularly in the context of new services offered outside hospital, for example, intermediate care, and having a population with more older people, who often have complex care needs. Discharge planning must, therefore, be informed by relevant national and local policy and guidance and underpinned by robust principles, which reflect contemporary healthcare service provision and settings.

Effective discharge planning is, therefore, crucial in cardiology to ensure timely discharge and continuity of care. It also helps healthcare providers use limited resources most effectively and unnecessary readmissions to be avoided. Smooth and effective care transfer ensures that health and social care systems are proactive in supporting individuals, their families and carers.

Although nursing roles are distinct in different services and geographical service provision may vary, the role of the nurse in liaising with patients, families and colleagues is central in achieving smooth care transitions.

ACTIVITY 25.2: DISCHARGE PLANNING REFLECTION

ACTIVITY 25.2
ANSWER

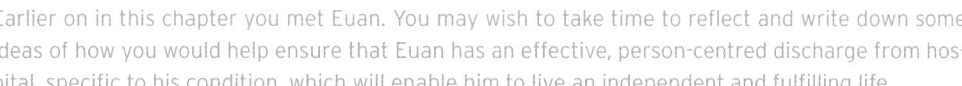

Earlier on in this chapter you met Euan. You may wish to take time to reflect and write down some ideas of how you would help ensure that Euan has an effective, person-centred discharge from hospital, specific to his condition, which will enable him to live an independent and fulfilling life.

(Continued)

(Continued)

Here are some suggestions/hints to get you started:

- Does he require a discharge letter/summary sheet?
- Does he have a specific discharge time?
- Does he require an outpatient appointment?
- Does he require to visit his GP practice or hospital/community clinic?
- Does he require to attend cardiac rehabilitation services?
- Does he require screening/follow up in regard to depression?
- Does he require specific advice in regard to resuming driving?
- Does he require specific advice in regard to resuming sexual intercourse?

HEALTH PROMOTION

All nurses, whatever their practice setting, have a vital role to play in promoting the health of patients, their families/carers.

Promoting health also provides you with a valuable opportunity to develop your understanding of the social and political processes, which not only aim to strengthen the skills and capabilities of individuals living with a cardiac condition, but also bring about change in social, environmental and economic conditions.

Promoting the health of an adult with a cardiac condition encompasses the following:

- cardiac rehabilitation (referral and provision of robust evidence-based information and support)
- diet (promoting healthy eating and referral to the dietician)
- smoking (referral to smoking cessation clinic and provision of nicotine replacement therapy)
- recreational drug use (provision of robust evidence-based information and support)
- alcohol consumption (provision of robust evidence-based information and support)
- exercise (promoting regular healthy levels of exercise)
- medication (provision of robust evidence-based information and support)
- helpline (telephone, web-based, email support options)
- support group (local and national)
- employment (return to work, change of employment).

It is also important that you tailor the advice given to suit the needs of the individual, their family/carers.

SEE ALSO
CHAPTER 7

ACTIVITY 25.3: HEALTH PROMOTION

Take some time out in order to look at the latest guidance in regard to health promotion utilising the following weblinks:

- British Heart Foundation: www.bhf.org.uk
- NHS Choices: www.nhs.uk

Identifying people at risk and providing health promotion advice are integral to your role as a nurse.

WEBLINKS

ACTIVITY 25.4: HEALTH PROMOTION

Keep and complete a diary of your own food intake, physical activity, and smoking and alcohol intake over a seven-day period.

- Can you identify any obstacles which may have prevented you meeting the recommendations, such as time management, for example?
- How would you overcome this obstacle?
- How could you apply this activity to your practice to support a patient or their family/carer to succeed in making a lifestyle change?

PREPARATION FOR PRACTICE PLACEMENTS 25.1

Preparing for your cardiology practice learning experience can help you to alleviate any anxieties that you may have. Your university may already have provided you with some useful information: contact your placement in advance and speak with or arrange to meet with your mentor; revise the learning materials provided, which will allow you to link theory to practice and relate it to what you see and do; speak to other students who have already undertaken a similar placement; and discuss your learning intentions with your lecturer. It is always useful to check transport links, travel times and your duty rota in advance.

You may also find it beneficial if you can track a patient's journey from admission, which will allow you to develop your understanding of observations, specific cardiac investigations, delivering person-centred care, health promotion and discharge planning.

WHAT'S THE EVIDENCE? 25.1

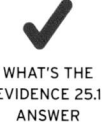

WHAT'S THE
EVIDENCE 25.1
ANSWER

Jaarsma, T. et al. (2014) Research in cardiovascular care: A position statement of the Council on Cardiovascular Nursing and Allied Professionals of the European Society of Cardiology. *European Journal of Cardiovascular Nursing*, 13 (1): 9–21.

Jaarsma et al. examine the complexity of cardiac care and identify knowledge gaps in current research in regard to this provision.

- What are the upcoming challenges and developments in relation to cardiovascular care?
- What recommendations are put forward for future research?

Now read this article and consider whether you would draw the same conclusions as the authors.

─────── **CHAPTER SUMMARY** ───────

- Cardiovascular disease remains a major cause of premature death in the UK.
- Lifestyle changes can make a positive contribution to quality of life and improving cardiovascular conditions.
- Nurses have an important role to play in the prevention, identification and management of cardiovascular conditions.
- Health promotion and cardiac rehabilitation have proven benefits for adults living with cardiovascular conditions.

─────── **GO FURTHER** ───────

**CASE STUDY:
HEART
FAILURE**

Go to https://study.sagepub.com/essentialadultnursing for a further case study related to this chapter. If you are using the interactive ebook, simply click on the book icon in the margin to go straight to the resource.

Books

- Boore, J., Cook, N. and Shepherd, A. (2016) *Essentials of Anatomy and Physiology for Nursing Practice*. London: Sage.
  Introduces the student nurse to the essentials of anatomy and physiology.
- Delves-Yates, C. (ed.) (2018) *Essentials of Nursing Practice* (2nd edn.). London: SAGE.
  A useful resource, which enables nurses to test their knowledge in relation to pathophysiology.
- Rodgers, K.M.A. and Scott, W.N. (2014) *Nurses! Test Yourself in Pathophysiology*. Maidenhead: McGraw Hill.
  An interesting article, which focuses on depressive symptoms

Journal Articles

**FURTHER
READING:
JOURNAL
ARTICLES**

Go to https://study.sagepub.com/essentialadultnursing for further free online journal articles related to this chapter. If you are using the interactive ebook, simply click on the book icon in the margin to go straight to the resource.

- Chung, M.L., Lennie, T.A., Mudd-Martin, G., Dunbar, S.B., Pressler, S.J. and Moser, D.K. (2016) Depressive symptoms in patients with heart failure negatively affect family caregiver outcomes and quality of life. *European Journal of Cardiovascular Nursing,* 15(1): 30-8.
- Frosling, E., Lundqvist, R., Eliasson, M. and Isaksson, R-M. (2015) Health care contact is higher in the week preceding a first myocardial infarction: A review of medical records in Northern Sweden in 2007. *European Journal of Cardiovascular Nursing,* 14(5): 450-6.
- Svavarsdóttir, M.H., Sigurðardóttir, A.K.and Steinsbekk, A. (2016) Knowledge and skills needed for patient education for individuals with coronary heart disease: The perspective of health professionals. *European Journal of Cardiovascular Nursing,* 15(1): 55-63.

Weblinks

**FURTHER
READING:
WEBLINKS**

Go to https://study.sagepub.com/essentialadultnursing for further weblinks related to this chapter. If you are using the interactive ebook, simply click on the book icon in the margin to go straight to the resource.

- National Institute for Health and Care Excellence (NICE)
  www.nice.org.uk/guidance/conditions-and-diseases/cardiovascular-conditions

- NICE guidance accessed via this weblink is an important evidence-based source of information regarding the promotion of cardiac health.
- Scottish Intercollegiate Guidelines Network (SIGN)
  www.sign.ac.uk
  SIGN guidance accessed via this weblink is an important evidence-based source of information regarding the promotion of cardiac health.
- World Health Organization (WHO)
  www.who.int
  WHO guidance accessed via this link is an important evidence-based source of information regarding global recommendations on physical activity for health and the impact of interventions on diet and physical activity.

ACE YOUR ASSESSMENT

Revise what you have learned by visiting https://study.sagepub.com/essentialadultnursing

ONLINE
QUIZZES

- Test yourself with multiple-choice and short-answer questions
- Do the chapter activities in the book and check your answers online

REFERENCES

Bromfield, L.J. (2016) *Anatomy and Physiology Study Guide*. Available at: http://anatomy physiologystudyguide.com/ (accessed 23/02/18).

New York Heart Association (2016) *Classification of Stages of Heart Failure*. Available at: www.heart.org/ HEARTORG/Conditions/HeartFailure/AboutHeartFailure/Classes-of-Heart-Failure_UCM_306328_ Article.jsp (accessed 23/02/18).

NICE (2014) *Atrial Fibrillation: Management*. Available at: www.nice.org.uk/guidnce/cg180 (accessed 23/02/18).

Qvist, I., Hendriks, J.M.L, Moller, D.S, Albertsen, A.E., Mogensen, H.M., Oddershede, G.D., Odgaaard, A., Mortensen, L.S., Johnsen, S.P. and Frost, L. (2015) Effectiveness of structured, hospital-based, nurse-led atrial fibrillation clinics: A comparison between a real-world population and a clinical trial population. Available at: http://openheart.bmj.com/content/openhrt/3/1/ e000335.full.pdf (accessed 23/02/18).

Resuscitation Council (UK) (2015) *Resuscitation Guidelines*. Available at: www.resus.org.uk/ resuscitation-guidelines/ (accessed 23/02/18).

Resuscitation Council (2016) *ABCDE Approach*. Available at: www.resus.org.uk/pages/alsABCDE.htm (accessed 23/02/18).

Yohannes, A.M., Doherty, P., Bundy, C. and Yalfrani, A. (2010) The long-term benefits of cardiac rehabilitation on depression, anxiety, physical activity and quality of life. *Journal of Clinical Nursing*, 19 (19–20): 2806–13.

CARE OF THE ADULT WITH A VASCULAR CONDITION

26

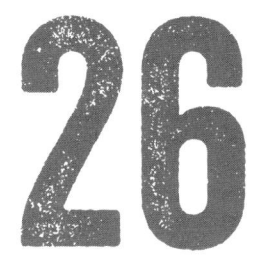

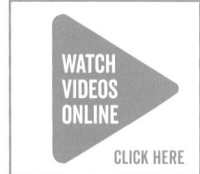

WATCH VIDEOS ONLINE — CLICK HERE

EMMA BOND AND CHRIS JONES

THIS CHAPTER COVERS

- An outline of how you would assess and intervene in the care of patients with the most common vascular problems including: abdominal aortic aneurysm (AAA), peripheral vascular disease (PVD), peripheral arterial disease (PAD) and deep venous thrombosis (DVT)

- Providing advice in regard to lifestyle changes and sustaining them
- Helping the patient come to terms with amputation.

> "
>
> There are more and more people showing up with vascular problems at our clinics and I cannot see this trend reversing anytime soon. The population is growing older and are living with more long-term conditions which affect the blood vessels badly. Sometimes I think that the services are being overwhelmed. As nurses we are doing jobs which were previously being done by doctors because the numbers are so great. And at the same time as we are struggling to manage the problems we have got at the moment, it has to be said that the population at large are not exactly helping. Our patients are getting bigger and bigger by the year and when we do home visits it seems as though nobody ever turns their TV off!
>
> **Francine, vascular nurse specialist**
>
> "

INTRODUCTION

This chapter will cover some but not all of the problems patients face as the result of vascular disease, which is considered a subgroup of cardiovascular disease. The same modifiable and non-modifiable risk factors apply to vascular disease of the heart as to vascular disease elsewhere. Vascular disease is caused by atherosclerosis. This is the progressive narrowing of arteries due to the accumulation of damaging deposits on the walls of blood vessels. These deposits are called atheroma and they will both impede the flow of blood in the vessel and damage the vessel itself and incline to clot formation along their roughened surfaces. Figure 26.1 provides a useful diagram that explains the relationship between atherosclerosis and cardiovascular disease, neurological disease and peripheral vascular disease.

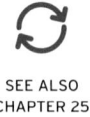

SEE ALSO
CHAPTER 25

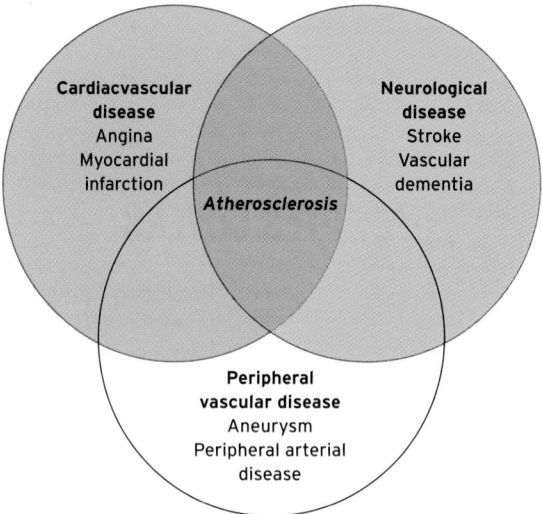

Figure 26.1 The relationship between atherosclerosis and cardiovascular disease, neurological disease and peripheral vascular disease

Nursing in this specialist field can be a very rewarding, frustrating, depressing and deeply gratifying experience all at once. It demands well-developed empathy and an ability to get on with patients and their families who you may see over many years. But it will also require you to be frank with patients to inform them about how much of the management of their condition is in the alteration of their own lifestyle. This might not always be a welcome message. By the time you meet patients they might be heartily sick of a 'stop smoking' message. That does not make its repetition any less worthwhile!

ACTIVITY 26.1: CRITICAL THINKING

- To what extent do you think that individuals are responsible for their own vascular disease?
- Is it their own life choices that have created their disease, or are they the victims of it?
- Is the role of a publicly funded health service to direct people to a healthy lifestyle or simply to help them when their life choices make them ill?

CRITICAL THINKING STOP POINT 26.1

Structure of blood vessels

It is likely that you will have covered the structure of blood vessels in your programme of study so far. However, take a look at Figure 26.2 and the accompanying explanation, which will refresh your learning before proceeding to the section on aneurysm formation.

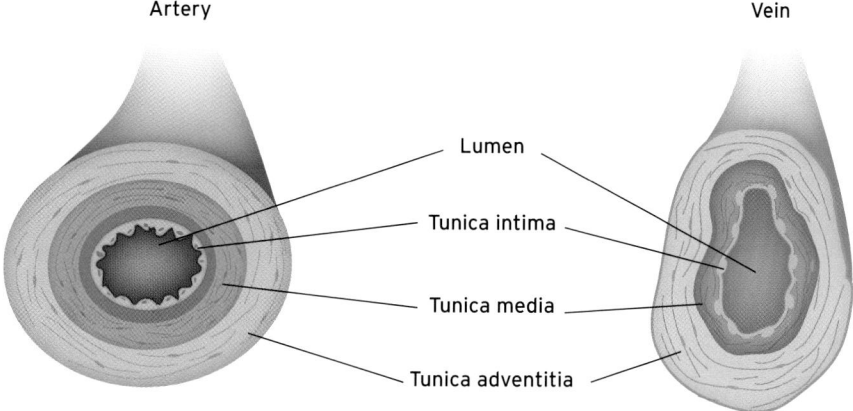

Figure 26.2   Structure of blood vessels

Source: Boore et al. (2016). Illustrated by Shaun Mercier, © SAGE Publications

Arteries and veins have a three-layered structure There is an outer, fibrous layer which gives the blood vessel structure and form. There is a middle muscular layer which allows the blood vessel to dilate and constrict. There is an inner smooth layer which permits the easy flow of blood and which inhibits inappropriate clotting in the vessel.

ANEURYSM FORMATION

Arteries have strong elastic walls, which enable them to withstand the high pressure generated by blood flow within them. Unfortunately, sometimes the walls of the artery develop a weakness. The weakened section begins to bulge. The walls of the weakened section become thinner and can become progressively more fragile and more inclined to bulge further. This process subsequently results in aneurysm formation.

An aneurysm is described as an enlargement of an artery of 50% or more. The process of enlargement can happen because the aorta has become diseased due to systemic illnesses such as:

- atherosclerosis
- hypertension.

Unhealthy lifestyle decisions can also incline a person to aneurysm formation. Smoking is one example of a lifestyle choice associated with aneurysmal disease. Family history can also predict disease (Ye et al, 2016).

More rarely, trauma can cause an aneurysm to form. This type of aneurysm is not caused by the same disease process as those described above. Following a traumatic event an otherwise healthy artery may be damaged and allow blood to leak between its anatomical layers. The artery then swells under the pressure exerted by blood. This type of injury is called a 'pseudo aneurysm'.

Abdominal aortic aneurysms

As a student nurse, this is the likeliest aneurysm you are likely to see especially in an operating theatre or critical care unit. Abdominal aneurysms are often symptom free. Many aneurysms are discovered by accident while the patient is being investigated for another condition. This is especially the case where the investigation involves an ultrasound examination of the abdomen. In this instance a referral will be made to a vascular team for further evaluation.

Since 2013 the National Health Service has offered men over the age of 65 a screening service for abdominal aneurysm. Where no abdominal aortic aneurysm is detected, the man need not be screened again. Where a small aneurysm exists the progress of the disease will be carefully monitored. In the case of a large aneurysm an urgent referral to a vascular surgeon will be arranged.

It was my GP who first spotted it. I was having some pain in my tummy and she thought it might be to do with my ovaries. But when I was being examined she said, 'have you ever noticed this?' and pointed to the middle of my stomach by my belly button. I couldn't see anything but she sent me for some more tests. It turned out that I had a weakness in my main artery and they told me that if it was not treated it might start to leak. I had to go in for an operation which knocked the stuffing out of me to be honest. But since then I seem to be OK, apart from the scar on my stomach.

Cheryl, 59

Aneurysms can be felt as a 'pulsatile mass' in the abdomen and can sometimes be seen to pulsate in the umbilical area. They are more common in men and may be hard to feel if the man carries excess weight around his abdomen. Before the introduction of routine screening for this disease a person might become aware of an aneurysm for the first time when the vessel ruptured. Blood loss following rupture is so severe and rapid that 80% of people who rupture will not survive.

But for the majority of patients with a small (less than 5.5 cm) aneurysm the policy will be 'watchful waiting' (Greenhalgh et al, 1998). This will include regular examinations and ultrasound monitoring. It will also include strict control of blood pressure with **beta blockers** or other antihypertensives. Central to the care of patients will be changes in lifestyle; in particular, emphasis should be placed on the importance of stopping smoking (see Table 26.1).

If the aneurysm grows in size then the next options will be surgical or endovascular procedures. Surgical treatment of aneurysm is not without its own risks. The surgical repair of unruptured

NURSING ADVICE FOR PATIENTS DIAGNOSED WITH ABDOMINAL ANEURYSM

Table 26.1

Problem	Advice
Fear of condition	This is an important consideration in your care of the patient.
	They may have gone from feeling healthy before investigation to now feeling that their abdomen is a 'ticking time bomb'. You should try to reassure them that provided the aneurysm does not grow in size, they need not worry unduly. You should encourage them to self-monitor as it will give them a sense of control.
Lifestyle change	Encourage the patient to STOP SMOKING. You should ensure that they understand why the control of blood pressure is important and how prescribed medication will help in this. Advise the patient to avoid heavy lifting.

aneurysms requires a complex operation. In an older person who may suffer from other medical problems this might prove to be of greater risk. How to balance the risks of surgery against the risks of rupture has been the subject of much research effort. In 1998, the UK Small Aneurysm Trial (UKSAT) indicated that while it was safe to keep aneurysms up to 5.5 cm under regular review, those above this size justified the risk of surgical repair.

SEE ALSO CHAPTER 10

AAAs can be repaired in two ways. The more traditional way is open abdominal surgery, where the aorta is manually repaired by the vascular surgeon using a tube graft. This is stitched into the aneurysmal segment of the aorta. The other option is for a tube (a 'stent') to be mounted on an inflatable catheter. This is then placed into the aneurysmal cavity through a puncture made into the femoral artery. When the catheter is inflated the intra-aortic stent will occupy the lumen of the aorta permitting blood flow. The stent will then relieve the pressure on the aneurysm wall. This will prevent any further growth of the aneurysm and will eliminate or greatly reduce the chance of rupture. The open repair is a much more traumatic operation for the patient and they normally need to spend their first post-operative night in the intensive care unit and have a longer stay in hospital. However, there is little chance of migration or kinking in a fabric graft, which is attached by a sutured **anastomosis.** This fact means that an open procedure requires less post-operative supervision over the months and years. Significantly, this means that the patient will receive less x-ray exposure.

WHAT'S THE EVIDENCE? 26.1

The long-term results of endovascular procedures compared with open procedures have been evaluated: Wilt, T.J., Lederele, F.A., MacDonald, R., Jonk, Y.C., Rector, T.S. and Kane, R.L. (2006) Comparison of endovascular and open surgical repairs for abdominal aortic aneurysm. *Evidence Report/Technology Assessment*, August (144): 1.

Both types of repair have a small risk of damage to the kidneys, blood loss, nerve damage, infection and death and this must be discussed at depth with the patient.

POST-OPERATIVE NURSING OBSERVATIONS OF PATIENTS WITH AN ABDOMINAL AORTIC ANEURYSM REPAIR

- Pain: This operation usually takes some time and requires that the patient has a deep abdominal incision. It is therefore likely that the patient will experience pain. It is important that the patient's level of pain is assessed frequently and appropriately in order that it can be managed effectively. Appropriate prescribed medication should enable the patient to be as pain free as possible. Positioning of the patient carefully can help to minimise pain. If the patient is in pain, they may feel apprehensive about coughing, which may then put them at risk of a chest infection.

- Anxiety: The patient is likely to feel anxious and afraid. They may become clammy and sweaty. It is important to remain with the patient and to avoid leaving them on their own. Consider: is fear and anxiety making their mouth dry? Remember the importance of oral hygiene. Be aware of where the family are and what information they have been given. They will need very careful psychological support in their own right.

- Vital signs: You should be meticulous and repeat these frequently.

  - **A**: Anxiety, pain and morphine may all predispose the patient to vomit. If this is the case prompt action to clear the airway is imperative. Also, if hypotension makes the patient drowsy their ability to defend their own airway might be compromised. Talking to the patient is a useful way of judging the patency of their airway.

  - **B**: Count the patient's respirations. Is the patient capable of speaking in full sentences? Look at the chest. Is it moving equally on both sides? Is the rate normal? What is the patient's oxygen saturation? Do they require oxygen? Have arterial blood gases been analysed? Have the results been reviewed?

  - **C**: What does the trend in pulse rate suggest? Hypovolaemia may result in a 'rapid thready' pulse as the heart compensates to circulate a falling amount of circulating blood volume. Is the blood pressure stable or dropping? If the patient has a central venous line in situ, it is important to understand and interpret what this measurement means. Taking care of the line as per local policy will help to minimise the risk of infection. What is the temperature of the patient's feet? Loss of circulating volume will make them very cold, however, one foot warmer than the other might suggest that a clot may have drifted down one leg from the aneurysm.

  - **D**: Is the patient conscious? Do they know what is happening? Try to remember that the patient has entered a world where strangers are doing incomprehensible things to them in a whirl of activity. As a student nurse your contribution will be invaluable if you try to reassure the patient and be a source of comfort in all the apparent confusion.

  - **E**: If there is a post-operative leak from the graft, blood will pool in the abdomen. Observing the girth of the abdomen will give an early indication of this process. Girth observation should be considered one of the vital observations. The abdomen should be measured with a tape measure and at the same point on the expanding girth.

- Fluid management: Strict assessment and recording of how much fluid has been administered to the patient is essential. Corresponding output is equally essential. How much crystalloid fluid (saline, dextrose) has been infused? How much blood? How much plasma-expanding substances?

- Tissue perfusion: The importance of feeling the temperature of the feet has been discussed in relation to 'C' (Circulation), but other tissues are also at risk. In particular, the kidneys will be very vulnerable to injury because of hypoperfusion. The first sign of injury will be falling urinary output. When did the patient last pass urine? How much was passed? Was it concentrated or clear? Where and how was a record of this kept?
- Spiritual assessment: For the patient, the progress from apparently well to their current state may be a profoundly disturbing experience. What religion are they? Would the family like to speak to a chaplain?

EVALUATION

It will be in the days following the patient's procedure that your observational skills will be most critical. The following are some major signposts you might also look out for, but your observations are integral to the wellbeing and recovery of the patient.

- **Pain.** This should recede over the first few days. If it does not you should look for a reason why it is not. Is the wound healing properly? Is the patient's abdomen distended? If so, why is it?
- **Mobility.** If all is well, the patient should be able to mobilise quickly. It is essential that they are encouraged to do so. Immobility brings innumerable problems in its wake. Constipation is one example and getting to the toilet for the first time will be a welcome milestone for the patient even if it requires support from you.
- **Circulation.** You should feel the patient's feet and assess the pulses in them frequently over the next few days. This will give the clearest indication of the continued patency of the graft.
- **Emotional recovery.** You should be careful to evaluate the patient's emotional state as they recover. They may feel traumatised by the events which have overtaken them. Observe how they relate to their family and friends at visiting time and take the time to speak with the patient's family to gain their opinion.

CRITICAL THINKING STOP POINT 26.2

If this is the first time you have been involved in the delivery of post-operative care in relation to vascular surgery, ask yourself how well you feel you have grasped its essentials? Was there any theory you felt you lacked? Do you consider that this practice experience has filled those gaps?

Reflection

If you have looked after a patient undergoing this level and type of surgery already, what did you find more challenging - the technical aspects of care or the emotional support the patient required? Do you find it easy to engage with patients who are so alarmed? Or are you tempted to focus on the technical elements of care and hope that the emotional aspect will take care of itself?

Ask your mentor how she/he manages these issues. Ask other students how they have managed them.

PERIPHERAL ARTERIAL DISEASE (PAD)

> I started smoking when I was 14 and I thought that I was one of the lucky ones who managed to avoid the health problems. I thought all I had to worry about was lung cancer. But when I became diabetic at the age of 63 I realised that the damage from smoking was already done to my legs. Since that day the state of my legs has got worse and worse. I can't walk more than a couple of hundred yards any more, and at that very slowly. And do you know what the strangest thing is? I still can't stop smoking.
>
> Frank, 69

One of the most common manifestations of arterial disease that you will meet in practice is peripheral arterial disease. This is a painful and unforgiving condition, which most commonly affects the lower limbs. It results from atheromatous arterial plaques, which were described earlier in the chapter. The presence of arterial disease in the legs should indicate to you that the patient is at high risk of problems in the arteries of the heart and brain. They may already be present.

Peripheral arterial disease is a common condition. It is estimated that 20% of over 60s will have this condition to one extent or another. Of this group, 20% will go on to show symptoms up to and including **critical limb ischaemia**.

CLINICAL FEATURES AND PATHOPHYSIOLOGY

The signature symptom of PAD is pain in the legs when the patient exercises which resolves when they rest. Although it has been described as 'angina of the legs' it is more correctly called intermittent claudication (IC). 'Claudication' is a term only used in the context of peripheral arterial disease. It refers to the reputed limp which afflicted the Roman Emperor Claudius and is suggestive of the quality of the pain which the sufferer undergoes. The pain derives from the accumulation of lactic acid in the muscles. This is due to the abnormal, **anaerobic metabolism**, which the muscles of the leg must adopt in the absence of an adequate supply of oxygenated arterial blood.

Claudication is mostly felt in the calves, but it can also be felt in the thighs and buttocks. The site of the pain will be determined by how far up the arterial supply the blockage is situated. A blocked popliteal artery may give rise to pain in the calf. A lesion in the common femoral artery might cause pain in the thigh and calf. Problems in the aorta might produce pain in the buttocks and the full length of the leg.

The symptoms of PAD are used in classification systems that grade the degree of disease severity. One of the most commonly quoted of these scales is the Fontaine classification. Quantifying the disease in this way helps teams summarise findings to each other quickly and efficiently. You may read in the patient's case notes a reference to one of these scales.

Fontaine classification	
Stage	Symptoms
I	No symptoms
II	Intermittent claudication
III	Pain at rest
IV	Ulceration and/or gangrene

NICE (2012) suggests that patients with mild symptoms of intermittent claudication can be treated in the community with lifestyle advice and supervised exercise. Referral to the vascular team is required if their symptoms do not improve or worsen. An interventional treatment may then be considered.

CASE STUDY 26.1: WILLIAM

William is 58 years old and lives with his wife, Sally. They have two grown-up children who are in their twenties but still live at home with their parents. William works as a lorry driver and Sally is a dinner lady at the local primary school. William has smoked since he was 15 and Sally and their two children also smoke.

Recently, William has started to complain of pain in both calves when he has returned home after walking the dog. This is his only form of exercise. He has made an appointment to see his GP as he is worried about the pain but also realises that he needs to cut back on the number of cigarettes that he smokes.

- What information would you offer William in order to support him with lifestyle changes?
- How could you assist William to maintain these changes?

CLINICAL SIGNS OF PAD

Your observations of the site, quality and behaviour of claudication pain will usually suggest to you that there is a problem with blood supply to the leg (see Table 26.2). However, you should bear in mind that arthritis, sciatic pain and spinal compression can also produce pain which could be confused with arterial disease. Other signs might suggest the presence of arterial disease, which might include poorly healing leg wounds and unexplained leg discomfort. If the patient is diabetic it is always worthwhile to do an assessment of the blood supply to the lower limbs and feet.

A quick and easy nursing assessment of blood supply to the limbs can be performed by feeling for the pulses in the feet. If the pulses of the dorsalis pedis and posterior tibial areas cannot be felt, it may be worth initiating a more careful inspection. In addition to feeling the pulses, you should examine the feet for colour, warmth, comparison to the opposite foot and general appearance of the feet and toes. In diabetic patients any abnormality such as blisters or ulcers should be reported immediately.

Diabetic Foot

Diabetes is associated with a high risk of developing PAD and foot problems. To help reduce the risk, the patient could access the annual foot screening service for diabetics across the UK. Diabetics, especially those with poor glycemic control, can develop altered sensation or numbness (neuropathy). This may result in them not perceiving an injury to the foot. Reduced sensation, or numbness, could lead to the person not being alerted to a stone or a rose thorn in their shoe, and this could lead to ulcer formation. Patients with diabetes must be advised to always wear suitable footwear. Walking barefoot is discouraged as it increases the risk of trauma.

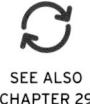

SEE ALSO
CHAPTER 29

Diabetics can also undergo changes to the shape of the foot, and this can lead to areas of high pressure on the sole, which increases the risk of tissue damage and ulceration. It is important to regularly assess the feet of all patients with diabetes while they are in hospital as they are at a greater risk of developing pressure sores than non-diabetics. Many hospitals have a diabetic foot service, where this group of patients will receive specialist treatment.

Table 26.2 Nursing assessment of a person with peripheral arterial disease

Overall appearance	How are they walking? Is there a hint of a limp? How do their hands look? Is there nicotine staining? Is there any odour of tobacco on them? Are they overweight? What does their leg look like? Swollen? Discoloured? Ulcerated? Record your observations accurately utilising appropriate documentation.
Exercise	Ask the patient how far they can walk. Has there been any limitation in their normal activities? If their exercise is limited, what limits it? Is it pain or another problem (such as breathlessness)?
Pain	Where do they get pain? What is the pain like? Do they get it at night? What relieves the pain? What exacerbates it?
Other medical problems	Are they diabetic? For how long? Is it well controlled or chaotic? Do they get chest pain? Are they on any medications?
Smoking	If they smoke, how much do they smoke? For how many years? Have they tried to give up? What happened? Check that they understand the specific problems which smoking causes in their conition.
Foot pulses	Can you find any pulses on their feet? Palpate the posterior tibial and the dorsalis pedis pulses.
Observations	Careful measurement and charting of blood pressure, pulse (rate and regularity) and respiration (pattern and rate) are obligatory parts of this patient's management.

SPECIALIST INVESTIGATIONS FOR PAD

ACTIVITY 26.2

If you have a placement in a vascular service ask your mentor to show you how ankle brachial pressure index (ABPI) is calculated. Under the supervision of your mentor, ask a patient if you can practise your skills on them. It is a pain-free investigation but it yields vital information.

ABPI measures the quality of the flow of blood in the lower limb. It is often performed by district nurses during the assessment of patients with leg ulcers.

ABPI is a cheap and easy to perform measurement which quantifies the degree to which blood flow has been compromised. For this investigation you should ask the patient to adopt a supine position. When relaxed, the patient will have a blood pressure measurement taken from the brachial artery using a sphygmomanometer and a Doppler probe. Following this a blood pressure reading will be taken at the patient's ankle. The ankle systolic pressure is then divided by the brachial systolic pressure.

An interpretation of the results of the ABPI is listed in Table 26.3.

Table 26.3

What you might infer from an ABPI measurement.

Index result
- Interpretation.

Greater than 1.3
- Result hard to interpret due to arteries being in a poorly compressible state because of calcification. This is often the result of damage caused by diabetes.

1.0-1.2
- Normal result.

0.8-0.9
- Indicates evidence of mild PAD.

0.5-0.8
- Evidence of moderate PAD. Referral required.

Less than 0.5
- Evidence of severe PAD. Urgent referral required.

Table 26.4 Provides examples of specialist investigations in relation to a vascular ward placement.

Table 26.4   **Examples of specialist investigations**

Specialist investigations you might see on a vascular ward placement.

Investigation
- Technique
  - Disadvantages

Computed tomography angiogram (CTA)
- In a CT scanner, radio opaque dye outlines arteries, giving very clear images
  - Depends on ionising radiation
  - Dyes can be **nephrotoxic**

Magnetic resonance angiogram (MRA)
- In an MRI scanner, contrast dye outlines large sections of arterial supply. Dyes are much less nephrotoxic. X-rays are not used
  - MRA takes a longer time than CTA. This might be hard to tolerate for patients who are in pain or claustrophobic

Duplex
- Ultrasound scan that measures blood flow in vessels. Identifies stenoses, occlusions and aneurysms. Used on arteries and veins
  - Requires specialist technical support to perform

Angiogram
- Injection of contrast dye into artery. X-ray images are taken to outline arterial map
  - Patients have to lie flat afterwards to prevent bleeding
  - Dye can be nephrotoxic
  - NOT a first line investigation

Drug treatment for PAD is summarised in Table 26.5

Table 26.5 Drug treatment for PAD

Statins:

- Lipid lowering drug intended to prevent build-up of atheromatous plaques in the legs.
  - o Atorvastatin
  - o Simvastatin
    - – Aching legs and cramps
    - – Gastrointestinal disturbances

Anti-platelet drugs:

- These inhibit the first stage of the blood-clotting process: platelet aggregation.
  - o Low dose aspirin
  - o Clopidogrel
    - – Possible abnormal bleeding, especially from the gastrointestinal tract
    - – Indigestion-type discomfort
    - – Dizziness

Anti-hypertensives:

- Control the damage that high blood pressure causes to blood vessel walls. They will only be prescribed if the blood pressure is high.
  - o Angiotensin converting enzyme (ACE) inhibitors
    - – ACE inhibitors have common side effects. The patient should be advised to inform their GP if they develop a dry and debilitating cough and to report any dizziness or fainting when they stand up. The GP may offer alternative anti-hypertensives.

Vasodilators:

- These open up the affected arteries to permit increased blood flow to the limb. This will hopefully reduce pain in the limb.
  - o **Naftidrofuryl oxalate**
    - – Inform the patient that they might experience nausea, some other gastrointestinal disturbances and they may also develop minor rashes

LIFESTYLE ADJUSTMENTS IN PAD

Many of the lifestyle adjustments that the patient will need to make will come as no surprise as they may already have received this advice.

- Smoking cessation. This is especially important and especially difficult among patients with PAD. All specialist vascular nurses will acknowledge that patients often smoke even after an amputation due to vascular disease. That said, referral to smoking cessation services may well produce positive results.
- Weight loss. The fear of inducing pain by walking can mean that a person leads an ever more sedentary lifestyle. This can result in serious weight gain, which will complicate treatment. Fear of leaving the home may also cause the person to become socially isolated.
- Diabetes control. If the patient is diabetic then the close control of their condition is key to managing their limb ischaemia.
- Patients should be advised to contact DVLA about their condition.
- Supervised exercise. The importance of supervised exercise cannot be overemphasised. Exercise produces benefits which affect all aspects of the patient's care, including psychological care.

WHAT'S THE EVIDENCE? 26.2

What's the evidence that exercise programmes improve life in PAD? Al-Jundi, W., Madbak, K., Beard, J.D., Nawaz, S. and Tew, G.A. (2013) Systematic review of home-based exercise programmes for individuals with intermittent claudication. *European Journal of Vascular and Endovascular Surgery*, 46(6): 690-706.

CASE STUDY 26.2: DAVID

David is 72 years old and lives at home alone. His wife died several years ago but his daughter checks on him daily. She helps him with his housework and does his shopping for him. He is a non-insulin dependent diabetic, is overweight, is becoming less mobile and does not monitor his blood glucose levels as regularly as he should. He has an appointment with the practice nurse in order to monitor his diabetic control. His daughter has offered to take him along to the appointment.

- What advice do you think the practice nurse will offer David?
- What advice would you give to David's daughter, as she is aware that her dad does not check his blood glucose levels as regularly as he should?

CRITICAL LIMB ISCHAEMIA (CLI)

When the blood vessels of the legs have blocked to such an extent that there is an inability to supply blood in sufficient quantities to meet the metabolic demands of the limb, the patient is said to have critical limb ischaemia. The patient may suffer constant, intense pain. They may suffer pain when they go to bed, often when they fall asleep and their blood pressure drops. This pain may be reduced if they throw their legs out of the bed and use gravity to assist in perfusion. When the patient has reached this point they will often say that they would prefer to sleep upright in a chair.

At this point, the ABPI will be very low (0.5–0.4) although these figures should be approached with caution as hardened, calcified arteries might produce artificially high results, particularly in diabetics. Unthinking acceptance of a high reading might cause a treatable patient to be missed.

NURSING ASSESSMENT OF CLI, BASED ON 'THE SIX Ps'

Pain

- The patient will have constant gnawing pain in the affected limb. Is the pain exacerbated or relieved by anything at all? Position of limbs for instance? Does sitting upright mean less pain for the patient than lying flat? Does it wake them from sleep? How well, if at all, does their medication help?

(Continued)

(Continued)

Pallor

- What is the colour of the limb? Does the skin blanch if you press it? If you press the nail beds and release the pressure is there any indication of capillary refill, or do the nail beds stay pale?

Pulseless

- Is there any evidence of a pulse anywhere on the affected limb? How do the pulses (or lack of them) on the painful limb compare to those on the other leg?

Perishing cold

- The painful limb has lost its blood supply. It may already have started to look and feel deathly cold. Again, you should compare the temperature of both limbs.

Pins and needles

- This can be a very disturbing symptom that suggests that blood supply to the limb is critically compromised. This is a difficult problem to address utilising conventional analgesia. Referral to a pain specialist/clinic may also be necessary.

Paralysis of sudden onset

- The nerve supply to the limb will be very sensitive to the loss of its blood supply. Pain may be the first indication of nerve damage, but loss of function may also be present.

Invasive treatments for PAD: endovascular procedures

Invasive treatments for ischaemic limbs are comprised of open or closed procedures. Closed procedures involve the use of intra-arterial catheters which are passed down the length of the artery to the lesion. A balloon is then inflated which opens up the artery and permits increased flow of blood to the limb. The technical name for this approach is endovascular because therapy is delivered from inside (endo) the blood vessel. However, balloon angioplasty is often not a definitive treatment for ischaemia. Arteries that have been opened can close again. In this instance the radiologist might use a stent, which is a lightweight metal mesh tube. This will be left in situ to hold the artery open. Stents may be covered in drugs to inhibit the infiltration of tissues through the mesh of the device. Stents of this nature are called 'drug eluting stents'.

Invasive treatments for PAD: surgical procedures

Angioplasty (with or without stenting) is the first treatment for consideration as it is less invasive and carries less cardiovascular risk than surgery. If this is unsuitable or unsuccessful then bypass surgery remains an option. The bypass graft would preferably be fashioned from one of the patient's own veins. Bypass grafts are monitored on a regular basis by duplex scan. This investigation can identify potential problems, such as stenosis of the graft. This can then be treated before the graft can fully occlude (Vartanian and Conte, 2015).

Some patients will not be fit enough to tolerate major surgery or, despite best efforts, the blood supply to their affected leg cannot be improved. In cases such as this, palliative treatment will be required.

Palliative treatment includes ensuring good pain control and excellent wound care where required to reduce the risk of infection. Meticulous foot care will reduce the risk to the foot posed by trauma or from damage caused by careless toe nail cutting or hard skin removal. This approach can sometimes be effective and the patient will not require further surgical intervention. Unfortunately, around 1% of those who develop IC will require an amputation.

Amputation

Amputation is a life-changing and life-limiting experience for patients. It can involve loss of a toe(s), loss of the forefoot, the lower leg, upper leg and in some cases may go as high as the buttock. All patients will require emotional support and it will be your job to provide the support that will carry the patient through this difficult period (Alleway et al., 2014).

For patients who suffer from severe PAD, an amputation of toe(s) or forefoot can have a positive outcome. It can reduce not only pain, but also reduce the risk of infection in the limb and can promote wound healing. However, you must understand that this is seen by many patients as a catastrophic turn of events. Nursing support and empathy at this time are of the utmost importance. The difficulty of this situation is reflected by the fact that, according to the National Confidential Enquiry into Perioperative Deaths, the most common reason for this type of surgery being delayed is because the patient initially refuses to have an amputation.

From a nursing perspective the care of patients following an amputation can present many challenges. From a psychological point of view the sudden change in body image can be very disturbing for a person, and they might struggle to come to terms with it. They might also find it difficult to accept the increase in dependency that an amputation can bring. In the immediate post-operative period, nursing staff will need to be aware that this is a patient at high risk of a fall as they struggle to regain a new sense of balance. All post-operative patients should be re-assessed for risk of falls after their amputation.

Many patients complain of phantom pain after an amputation. Phantom pain describes the sensation of pain in the limb that has been amputated. Patients can describe many unusual sensations from itchiness, to severe pain. There are a number of medications that can treat phantom pain but the psychological impact of feeling pain from a non-existent limb cannot be overemphasised.

Amputation can in many instances lift the psychological burden of a diseased limb from a patient. A limb that has caused intense pain over a long period may suddenly no longer cause the patient any pain. In practice, it is not difficult to find patients for whom the loss of the limb is seen as a liberation from suffering and inconvenience, despite the subsequent difficulties.

Mobilisation after a major amputation can be very difficult. Often the patient is an older person with co-morbidities such as angina, chronic obstructive pulmonary disease (COPD) and arthritis. In some areas of the UK, patients are transferred to a rehabilitation centre that specialises in early mobilisation and has an onsite limb-fitting centre. In other areas, patients will been seen by the limb-fitting team as an outpatient.

Discharge planning at an early stage is key with this patient group as their home environment may no longer be suitable and they frequently need extra support on discharge. Sometimes, the patient's need for intensive support will make a return home impossible and they may require care provision in a nursing home.

Not all patients are suitable for a prosthetic limb. They may be too frail to walk again. The physiotherapists and occupational therapists will assess and advise about what might be possible for these patients. The majority of patients who have had a major amputation will require a wheelchair.

If the patient is not fit for surgery or requests not to undergo an amputation, palliation would be considered. This is discussed at length with the patient and their family to ensure that everybody understands the implication of this decision and that there is shared decision-making.

Evaluation of nursing interventions in PAD

SEE ALSO
CHAPTER 23

- Education. Has the information regarding this condition been understood by the patient? Do they understand the relationship between their lifestyle choices and their condition?
- Prognosis. Does the patient understand the likely options that their condition will present them with? These will be different depending on the level and the stage of their disease.
- Emotional support. Are they coping well with the outlook for the future?

CRITICAL THINKING STOP POINT 26.3

Many nurses find that working in a service for people with PAD is frustrating because patients often find it hard or impossible to comply with lifestyle changes. Also, they may find that attempts to salvage limbs fail despite the commitment and enthusiasm of the service.

Did you feel any of these frustrations? How did you deal with them?

DEEP VEIN THROMBOSIS (DVT)

> I once helped to look after a young woman who had suffered from a pulmonary embolus. She had just got back from America. She responded well to treatment but I was surprised how much pain it gave her and how generally unwell she was. The trained staff told me that hers was not too bad a case too! They said that many people did not make it to hospital at all. The thing that amazed me was the way the whole system fitted together. Her condition was caused by a clot, which formed in her leg and was fired through her venous system into her lungs via her heart. On a theoretical level I knew about the circulation of blood through these systems and everything. But that a problem in one area could cause such serious trouble in another area so quickly still came as a bit of a surprise.
>
> Anna, second year student nurse, A&E placement

Deep vein thrombosis describes the formation of a blood clot (thrombus) in a deep vein of the leg. The thrombus completely or partially obstructs blood flow through the affected vein. Around 1 in 1000 people will sustain a DVT each year. A thrombus can break away and travel to the arteries of the lungs causing a pulmonary embolism. This is a very serious condition that can be fatal due to pulmonary infarction. Refer to Table 26.6, which provides a summary of the nursing assessment of chest pain.

The following are a number of risk factors that increase the likelihood of DVT. But it is worth noting that the unavoidable immobility associated with being a hospital inpatient may itself greatly increase the risk:

- cancer
- previous history of a DVT or other thromboembolism
- surgery

- being a male
- older age (greater than 40 years)
- thrombophilia
- immobility
- hormone treatment
- heart failure
- pregnancy/post-partum
- trauma to the vein
- dehydration.

Refer to Table 26.7, which provides a summary of nursing assessment in relation to DVT.

Table 26.6   Nursing assessment of chest pain: Cardiac or pulmonary embolus (PE)

Reason to suspect PE:
- Sharp, pleuritic pain
- Haemoptysis
- History:
    - Recent travel?
    - Oral contraception?
    - Recent orthopaedic surgery or immobility?
    - Sore leg or DVT?

Reason to suspect cardiac event:
- Central crushing chest pain
- Radiation of pain to arms and/or neck and jaw
- Nausea and vomiting
- Age
- History:
    - Angina?
    - Previous MI?
    - PAD

Table 26.7   Nursing assessment for DVT

- Affected leg: Is the sore leg swollen compared to the other?
- Pain: Is there pain from the leg? Is it sore to touch?
- Colour: Is the limb hot? Is it red?
- Veins: Are there any distended veins in the leg?

The signs and symptoms highlighted in Table 26.7 should increase your suspicion of a DVT, but you should also bear in mind that these signs and symptoms are not unique to a DVT and may be caused by infection, trauma or other pathologies.

Many hospitals have a thrombosis team that assess for the likelihood of a DVT in patients referred by GPs. They will use a pathway such as the Well's Score to assess the probability of a thrombosis and the treatment required (Wells et al., 2001). Refer to Table 26.8, which provides a summary of nursing observations in relation to a DVT.

Table 26.8 Nursing observations for DVT

Pain	Primarily in the leg but observe for AND REPORT
	Chest pain - this will require an ECG
Respirations	Rate
	Pattern
	What is the patient coughing up, if anything?
Pulse oximetry	Is this in the normal range?

NICE (2013) has clear guidance regarding the diagnosis and treatment of a suspected DVT. This includes an ultrasound scan of the leg veins within 4 hours. If this is not achievable then a blood test called a **D-dimer test** should be taken and the patient started on a treatment dose of an anticoagulant. The ultrasound scan can then be performed the next day.

Those assessed as being at low risk of DVT will have a D-dimer test and the thrombosis team will await the result before organising further investigations/treatment.

Those patients diagnosed with a DVT will require at least 3 months of anticoagulation treatment and compression stockings unless contraindicated. Compression is used to reduce the risk of post-thrombotic syndrome (PTS) and patients are advised to use compression stockings for 2 years. In PTS, the damage to the deep veins causes an increase in pressure within the vessel. This can lead to swelling, pain, discolouration, heaviness of the leg, varicose veins, eczema, leg ulcers and 'champagne bottle' legs. This happens in approximately 1 in 3 people who are diagnosed with a DVT. Compression reduces the likelihood of the development of this complication.

Patients are also encouraged to elevate their legs on rest, and take regular walks to stimulate the calf muscle pump. These all reduce the risk of developing PTS after a DVT.

There have been recent developments in the treatment of DVTs, especially where the thrombus is more extensive. One technique involves inserting a catheter into the vein and injecting a thrombolytic agent, which dissolves the clot. Another aims to physically remove the thrombus and restore blood flow. However, thrombolysis has associated risks, which include haemorrhage and stroke, and the treatment is not widely available.

From 2010, the Department of Health has insisted that patients who are admitted to hospital electively or as an emergency should be assessed for DVT risk within 24 hours of admission and re-assessed whenever the clinical situation changes. The assessment tool informs decision-making regarding the use of anti-embolic stockings and/or anticoagulation medication such as low molecular weight heparin (LMWH). Some patients such as those who undergo surgery for cancer or major orthopaedic surgery may be prescribed DVT prophylactic treatment for a number of weeks after treatment to reduce the risk of a post-operative DVT.

Evaluation

The patient with a DVT will be anticoagulated for a long time. Anticoagulation can bring its own problems. It is, therefore, essential to ensure that the patient understands the importance of observing for signs of inappropriate bleeding. This may include bleeding in the gastrointestinal tract. Frank blood or tarry stools may alarm the patient and they should be advised to report this to their GP. Additionally, nosebleeds, extended bleeding from cuts and bleeding gums may all suggest that the anticoagulation regime may need to be reviewed.

CHAPTER SUMMARY

- Vascular disease can be improved by adopting positive lifestyle changes.
- Nurses have an important role to play in the prevention, identification and management of vascular conditions.
- Health promotion can improve quality of life for adults living with vascular conditions.

GO FURTHER

CASE STUDY: HOLISTIC ASSESSMENT

Go to https://study.sagepub.com/essentialadultnursing for a further case study related to this chapter. If you are using the interactive ebook, simply click on the book icon in the margin to go straight to the resource.

Books

- Boore, J., Cook, N. and Shepherd, A. (2016) *Essentials of Anatomy and Physiology for Nursing Practice.* London: SAGE.
- Delves-Yates, C. (ed.) (2015) *Essentials of Nursing Practice*. London: Sage.
- Rodgers, K.M.A. and Scott, W.N. (2014) *Nurses! Test Yourself in Pathophysiology*. Maidenhead: McGraw Hill.

Journal Articles

- Ahmad, N., Thomas, G.N., Gill, P. and Torella, F. (2016) The prevalence of major lower limb amputation in the diabetic and non-diabetic population of England 2003–2013. *Diabetes & Vascular Disease Research*, 13(5): 348–53.
- Anjum, A., Von Allmen, R., Greenhalgh, R. and Powell, J.T. (2012) Explaining the decrease in mortality from abdominal aortic aneurysm rupture. *British Journal of Surgery*, 99(5): 637–45.
- Rose, M.D. (2015) A review of peripheral arterial disease (PAD). *British Journal of Cardiac Nursing*, 10(6): 277–83.

Weblinks

FURTHER READING: WEBLINKS

Go to https://study.sagepub.com/essentialadultnursing for further weblinks related to this chapter. If you are using the interactive ebook, simply click on the book icon in the margin to go straight to the resource.

- Department of Health (2010) *Risk assessment for venous thromboembolism*. [Online] Available at: http://webarchive.nationalarchives.gov.uk/20130107105354/http://www.dh.gov.uk/prod_consum_dh/groups/dh_digitalassets/@dh/@en/@ps/documents/digitalasset/dh_113355.pdf.
- The Royal College of Nursing (2013) *The nursing management of patients with venous leg ulcers*. [Online] Available at: www.rcn.org.uk/professional-development/publications/pub-001269.
- NICE (2013) *Deep vein thrombosis* – NICE CKS. [ONLINE] Available at: https://cks.nice.org.uk/deep-vein-thrombosis#!topicsummary.

ACE YOUR ASSESSMENT

ONLINE QUIZZES

Revise what you have learned by visiting https://study.sagepub.com/essentialadultnursing

- Test yourself with multiple-choice and short-answer questions
- Do the chapter activities in the book and check your answers online

REFERENCES

Alleway, R., Ellis, D., Jarman, D., Kelly, K., Nwosu, E., Protopapa, K., Shotton, H., Smith, N., and Warsame, A., (2014) *Lower limb amputation: Working together* [online]. Available at: www.ncepod.org.uk/2014report2/downloads/WorkingTogetherFullReport.pdf [Accessed 10 Jan 2018].

Department of Health (2010) *Risk assessment for venous thromboembolism.* [Online] Available at: http://webarchive.nationalarchives.gov.uk/20130107105354/http:/www.dh.gov.uk/prod_consum_dh/ groups/dh_digitalassets/@dh/@en/@ps/documents/digitalasset/dh_113355.pdf.

Greenhalgh, R.M., Forbes, J.F., Fowkes, F.G.R., Powell, J.T., Ruckley, C.V., Brady, A.R., Brown, L.C., and Thompson, S.G., (1998) Early elective open surgical repair of small abdominal aortic aneurysms is not recommended: Results of the UK small aneurysm trial. *European Journal of Vascular and Endovascular Surgery.* 16 (6): 462–4

NICE (2012) *Peripheral Arterial Disease: Diagnosis and management.* Available at: www.nice.org.uk/guidance/cg147/chapter/Introduction [Accessed 13 March 2018].

NICE (2013) *Deep Vein Thrombosis* – NICE CKS. [online]. Available at: https://cks.nice.org.uk/deep-vein-thrombosis#!topicsummary [Accessed 23 March 2017].

Vartanian, S.M. and Conte, M.S., 2015. Surgical Intervention for Peripheral Arterial Disease. *Circulation research,* 116(9): 1614–28

Wells, P.S., Anderson D.R., Rodger M., Stiell I., Dreyer J.F., Barnes D.,Forgie M., Kovacs G., Ward J. and Kovacs M.J., (2001) Excluding pulmonary embolism at the bedside without diagnostic imaging: Management of patients with suspected pulmonary embolism presenting to the emergency department by using a simple clinical model and d-dimer. *Annals of Internal Medicine,* 135(2): 98.

Ye, Z., Bailey, K.R., Austin, E. and Kullo, I.J., (2016) Family history of atherosclerotic vascular disease is associated with the presence of abdominal aortic aneurysm. *Vascular Medicine,* 21(1): 41–6.

CARE OF THE ADULT WITH A NEUROLOGICAL CONDITION

27

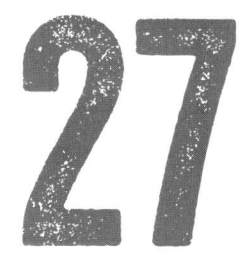

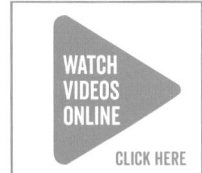
WATCH VIDEOS ONLINE
CLICK HERE

SUE SZCZEPANSKA

THIS CHAPTER COVERS

- Anatomy and physiology of the brain and nervous system
- Clinical characteristics and pathophysiology relevant to Parkinson's disease, multiple sclerosis and stroke
- Nursing assessment and management of the adult with Parkinson's disease, multiple sclerosis and following a stroke
- Discharge planning in relation to the adult with a neurological condition
- Health promotion in relation to the adult with a neurological condition
- Preparation for practice in relation to caring for an adult with a neurological condition.

"

I have come to the end of my second year and I have just completed a placement in a medical ward. This placement provided me with a broad learning opportunity to meet patients presenting with many different conditions. I met a 72-year-old gentleman who had recently been admitted following a fall. He had recently been diagnosed with Parkinson's disease and had fallen in the garden as he had lost his balance when walking down some steps. He told me of the fear he had of the future as he was normally very active playing bowls twice a week, which he has had difficulty doing due to the tremors in his hands. He was also scared that he would not be able to retain his independence if his Parkinson's disease got too bad. This made me more aware of the importance of documenting the patient's activities of daily living and using assessment tools which will allow the patient to retain as much independence as possible.

James Cole, 2nd year nursing student

"

INTRODUCTION

Caring for a patient with a neurological condition takes place in many different clinical settings from neurological intensive care to outpatients. You may have even cared for a patient following a stroke or who has Parkinson's disease or multiple sclerosis.

Neurological disorders can be complex diseases of the central and peripheral nervous system and can include epilepsy, Alzheimer's disease and other dementias, cerebrovascular diseases including stroke, migraine, multiple sclerosis, Parkinson's disease, brain tumours, head trauma, and neurological disorders as a result of malnutrition or alcohol intoxication.

Many bacterial (i.e. meningitis), viral (i.e. Human Immunodeficiency Virus (HIV)), fungal (i.e. *Cryptococcus, Aspergillus*), and parasitic (i.e. malaria) infections can affect the nervous system. Neurological symptoms may occur due to the infection itself, or due to an immune response. As there is such a wide range of neurological conditions it is very important that you have a basic understanding of the brain and nervous system to allow you to confidently care for these patients. Within this chapter the focus will be on the common neurological conditions of stroke, multiple sclerosis and Parkinson's disease, which are some of the conditions you are likely to encounter whilst on placement.

ACTIVITY 27.1
ANSWER

ACTIVITY 27.1: CRITICAL THINKING

Have you had the opportunity to care for a person living with any of the diseases mentioned above? The student voice at the beginning of the chapter discusses the importance of the patient's activities of daily living following the diagnosis of Parkinson's disease.

Take a few moments to reflect on how the activities of daily living would vary in relation to common neurological conditions. When on placement discuss with your mentor what you as a nurse can do to ensure the patient with a neurological condition meets their activities of daily living and what interventions may need to be put in place.

ANATOMY AND PHYSIOLOGY OF THE BRAIN AND NERVOUS SYSTEM

Introduction

The human brain lies in the cranial cavity and weighs approximately 3 lbs. It receives 15% of the cardiac output and has an intricate system of autoregulation ensuring the blood supply is constant despite postural changes.

The central and peripheral nervous system comes under the umbrella of neurology and involves the brain and spinal cord. All the nerves and nerve cells outside the central nervous system make up the peripheral nervous system. Its task is to relay information from the brain and spinal cord to the rest of the body.

The peripheral nervous system (PNS) consists of cranial nerves, which serve the head and neck. It also contains spinal nerves, which branch off from the spinal cord and supply the rest of the body.

The central nervous system (CNS) is made up of the brain and spinal cord. Any response to a stimulus is coordinated by the CNS. It gathers information about, and responds to, changes in the environment.

THE CENTRAL NERVOUS SYSTEM

The CNS is the processing centre for the nervous system. It receives information from, and sends information to, the peripheral nervous system. The brain processes and interprets sensory information sent from the spinal cord.

Central nervous system - brain

The brain is the control centre of the body. It consists of three main components: the forebrain, the brainstem, and the hindbrain. The forebrain is responsible for a variety of functions including receiving and processing sensory information, thinking, perceiving, producing and understanding language, and controlling motor function.

The brainstem controls the flow of messages between the brain and the rest of the body, and it also controls basic body functions such as breathing, swallowing, heart rate, blood pressure, consciousness.

The hindbrain assists in maintaining balance and equilibrium, movement coordination and the conduction of sensory information.

Central nervous system - neurons

All cells of the nervous system are comprised of neurons. Information is passed from neuron to neuron. A typical brain contains something like 100 billion neurons. The axon within the neuron carries electrical impulses and is protected by a fatty sheath called the myelin sheath. The myelin sheath increases the speed at which the nerve impulses are transmitted. Where the axon terminals meet there is a gap called a synapse. The nerve signal will cross this gap to continue onto another neuron to, or from, the central nervous system.

Neurotransmitters

A neurotransmitter is a chemical that is released from a nerve cell, which thereby transmits an impulse from a nerve cell to another nerve, muscle, organ, or other tissue. A neurotransmitter is a messenger of neurologic information from one cell to another.

Central nervous system - spinal cord

The spinal cord is a cylindrical-shaped bundle of nerve fibres that is connected to the brain. The spinal cord nerves transmit information from body organs and external stimuli to the brain and send information from the brain to other areas of the body.

Peripheral Nervous System

The PNS is a division of the nervous system. The primary role of the PNS is to connect the CNS to the organs, limbs and skin. These nerves extend from the CNS to the outermost areas of the body.

The peripheral nervous system is divided into two parts:

* somatic nervous system
* autonomic nervous system.

The somatic nervous system

The somatic system is the part of the PNS responsible for carrying sensory and motor information to and from the CNS.

The autonomic nervous system

The autonomic system is the part of the PNS responsible for regulating involuntary body functions, such as blood flow, heartbeat, digestion and breathing. This system is further divided into two branches:

* the sympathetic system regulates the flight-or-fight responses
* the parasympathetic system helps maintain normal body functions and conserves physical resources.

ANATOMY OF THE BRAIN

Meninges – The meninges cover the delicate nervous tissue offering protection. They also protect the blood vessels that serve the nervous tissue. They contain cerebrospinal fluid and they consist of three tissue layers: dura, arachnoid and pia maters.

Cerebrospinal fluid (CSF) – CSF is produced within the ventricles of the brain and cushions the brain from damage. There is approximately 150 mls of CSF circulating around the brain, in the ventricles and around the spinal cord. The CSF is replaced every 8 hours and has several functions:

1. **Protection**: the CSF protects the brain from damage by 'buffering' the brain.
2. **Buoyancy**: because the brain is immersed in fluid, the net weight of the brain is reduced from about 1400 gm to about 50 gm.
3. **Excretion of waste products**: the one-way flow from the CSF to the blood takes potentially harmful metabolites, drugs and other substances away from the brain.
4. **Endocrine medium for the brain**: the CSF serves to transport hormones to other areas of the brain. (Peate and Nair, 2015)

STRUCTURES OF THE BRAIN

The brain is divided into four anatomical areas, each containing one or more structures:

* cerebrum
* diencephalon
* brain stem
* cerebellum

Cerebrum

The cerebrum is the largest and most highly developed part of the human brain. It is divided into right and left hemispheres that are connected by the **corpus callosum**. The functions of the cerebrum include determining intelligence and personality, thinking, reasoning, producing and understanding language, interpretation of sensory impulses, motor function, planning and organisation and processing sensory information.

Diencephalon

The diencephalon is involved in several functions of the body including directing sense impulses throughout the body, autonomic function control, endocrine function control, motor function control, homeostasis and hearing, vision, smell and taste.

Brain stem

The brainstem is one of the most basic regions of the human brain, yet it is one of the most vital regions for our body's survival. It forms the connection between the brain and the spinal cord, maintains vital control of the heart and lungs, and coordinates many important reflexes.

Three major regions make up the brainstem: medulla oblongata, pons, and midbrain.

The medulla oblongata is the inferior-most region of the brainstem that connects the brain to the spinal cord. The medulla contains autonomic centres such as the cardiac centre, the respiratory centre, the vasomotor centre and the coughing, sneezing and vomiting centre.

Superior to the medulla is the pons, which is larger and structurally more complex than the medulla. The pons works with the medulla oblongata to control the depth and rate of respiration.

Finally, the midbrain forms the most superior and complex region of the brainstem. It contains the nuclei that process auditory and visual information and reflexes. It also maintains consciousness.

Cerebellum

The cerebellum is a structure that is located at the back of the brain. Although the cerebellum accounts for approximately 10% of the brain's volume, it contains over 50% of the total number of neurons in the brain. The cerebellum is involved in the following functions: maintenance of posture and balance, coordination of voluntary movements, motor learning and cognitive functions.

Limbic system

The limbic system is a complex system of nerves and networks in the brain. It controls the basic emotions (fear, pleasure, anger) and drives (hunger, sex, dominance, care of offspring).

Blood supply - Circle of Willis

The circle of Willis is a series of arteries that sit at the base of the brain. It provides multiple pathways for oxygenated blood to supply the brain if any of the principal suppliers such as the vertebral and internal carotid arteries are constricted by physical pressure, occluded by disease, or interrupted by injury.

Blood-brain barrier (BBB)

The blood–brain barrier is a tightly packed layer of cells (endothelial cells) that line the blood vessels in the brain and spinal cord. This barrier prevents large molecules, immune cells and disease-causing organisms (e.g. viruses) from passing from the blood stream into the central nervous system (brain and spinal cord).

Following on from the anatomy and physiology of the brain and nervous system, we will now focus in more detail on Parkinson's disease, multiple sclerosis and stroke.

PARKINSON'S DISEASE: CLINICAL CHARACTERISTICS AND PATHOPHYSIOLOGY

Parkinson's disease is a progressive disease that affects the nervous system (see Table 27.1). It manifests itself by tremors, muscular rigidity and slow, imprecise movement. Parkinson's disease normally affects middle-aged and elderly people but can affect those younger as well. It is associated with degeneration of the basal ganglia of the brain and a deficiency of the neurotransmitter dopamine due to the death of nerve cells in the brain.

Risk factors associated with Parkinson's disease are:

- age – generally manifests in middle to late years of life
- sex – males are more likely to suffer from Parkinson's disease than females
- family history – having one or more close relatives with the disease increases the likelihood that you will get it
- head trauma – research points to a link between damage to the head, neck, or upper cervical spine and Parkinson's.

Table 27.1   Parkinson's disease: clinical characteristics and pathophysiology

Main symptoms of Parkinson's disease	Physical and other symptoms of Parkinson's disease	Mental health and Parkinson's disease
Tremors - normally at rest	Bladder and bowel problems	Anxiety
Slowness of movement (bradykinesia)	Eye problems	Dementia
Rigidity	Falls and dizziness	Depression
Postural instability - leading to the patient falling	Fatigue	Hallucinations and delusions
	Pain	Memory problems
	Restless leg syndrome	
	skin and sweating problems	
	speech and communication problems	
	swallowing problems	

Parkinson's disease is caused by a loss of nerve cells in the part of the brain called the **substantia nigra**. Nerve cells in this part of the brain are responsible for producing the chemical dopamine. Dopamine is a transmitter which acts as a messenger between the parts of the brain and nervous system that help control and coordinate body movements.

If these nerve cells die or become damaged, the amount of dopamine in the brain is reduced. This means the part of the brain controlling movement can't work as well as normal, causing movements to become slow and abnormal.

The loss of nerve cells is a slow process. The symptoms of Parkinson's disease usually only start to develop when around 80% of the nerve cells in the substantia nigra have been lost.

Parkinson's disease diagnosis

The condition is diagnosed clinically, taking into account the medical history. This is often investigated after the appearance of early symptoms such as tremor, slowness of movement, difficulties with handwriting, loss of sense of smell or difficulties in making facial expressions.

MULTIPLE SCLEROSIS

Multiple sclerosis (MS) is an auto-immune disease which attacks the layer that surrounds and protects the nerves, called the myelin sheath. This damages and scars the sheath, and potentially the underlying nerves; due to this, the messages travelling along the nerves become slowed or disrupted.

Risk factors associated with MS are:

- genes – MS isn't directly inherited, but people who are related to someone with the condition are more likely to develop it
- smoking – you are twice as likely to develop MS if you smoke
- viral infections – some viral infections are thought to trigger the immune system leading to MS.

Multiple sclerosis: clinical characteristics and pathophysiology

Table 27.2 Multiple sclerosis: clinical characteristics and pathophysiology

Location	Frequency	Nature of Symptoms
Spinal cord	50%	Motor - weakness, clumsiness, tonic spasm.
		Sensory - numbness, tingling, burning, band-like sensation, altered temperature sensation.
		Sphincter - urinary urgency/hesitancy/retention/incontinence, constipation, faecal incontinence, erectile dysfunction.
Optic nerve	25%	Visual loss, blurred vision, reduced colour vision, pain on eye movement.
Brainstem/cerebellum	20%	**Dysarthria**, dysphagia, **diplopia**, vertigo, facial numbness/weakness, trigeminal neuralgia, deafness, ataxia (trunk and limbs), **nystagmus**, patchy sensory loss, tonic spasms.
Cerebral hemispheres	5%	**Hemiparesis**, hemisensory loss, visual field deficit, dysphasia, seizures, cognitive impairment.

In MS, the immune system, which normally helps to fight off infections, mistakes **myelin** for a foreign body and attacks it. This damages the myelin and strips it off the nerve fibres, either partially or completely, leaving scars known as lesions or plaques.

This damage disrupts messages travelling along nerve fibres – they can slow down, become distorted, or not get through at all.

As well as myelin loss, there can also sometimes be damage to the actual nerve fibres. It is this nerve damage that causes the increase in disability that can occur over time.

SEE ALSO
CHAPTER 12

Investigations for multiple sclerosis

Neurological examination – A physical examination checks for changes or weaknesses in eye movements, leg or hand coordination, balance, sensation, speech or reflexes. While a neurologist may strongly suspect MS at this stage, a diagnosis won't be given until other test results confirm MS.

MRI scan – This is very accurate and can pinpoint the exact location and size of any damage or scarring (lesions). MRI scans confirm a diagnosis in over 90% of people with MS.

Evoked potential – This involves testing the time it takes for the brain to receive messages by placing small electrodes on the head to monitor the brain waves responding to what the patient sees or hears. If myelin damage has occurred, messages to and from the brain will be slower.

Lumbar puncture – A small sample of CSF is taken and checked for abnormalities: patients with MS will be positive for antibodies in their CSF.

Multiple sclerosis disease diagnosis

MS starts in one of two general ways: with individual relapses (attacks or exacerbations) or with gradual progression. Once a diagnosis of MS has been made, the neurologist may be able to identify which type of MS the patient has.

This will largely be based on:

- the pattern of the symptoms – such as whether the patient experience periods when their symptoms get worse (relapses) then improve (remissions), or whether they get steadily worse (progress)
- the results of an MRI scan – such as whether there's evidence that lesions in the nervous system have developed at different times and at different places in the body.

However, the type of MS diagnosis often only becomes clear over time because the symptoms of MS are so varied and unpredictable. It can take a few years to make an accurate diagnosis of progressive MS, as the condition usually worsens slowly.

STROKE - HAEMORRHAGIC AND ISCHAEMIC

There are two main types of stroke – haemorrhagic strokes and ischaemic strokes – which affect the brain in different ways and can have different causes.

Haemorrhagic strokes can also be known as cerebral haemorrhages or intracranial haemorrhages. These are less common than ischaemic strokes. They occur when a blood vessel within the skull bursts and bleeds into and around the brain. The main cause of haemorrhagic stroke is high blood pressure, which can weaken the arteries in the brain and make them prone to splitting or rupture. A mini stroke or transient ischemic attack (TIA) is caused by a temporary disruption in the blood supply to part of the brain. The disruption in blood supply results in a lack of oxygen to the brain. This can cause sudden symptoms similar to a stroke, which resolve themselves within 24 hours.

The causes of developing high blood pressure include:

- being overweight or obese
- drinking excessive amounts of alcohol
- smoking
- a lack of exercise
- stress, which may cause a temporary rise in blood pressure.

Haemorrhagic strokes can also occur when the blood vessels within the brain are badly formed and can balloon and then rupture causing a brain **aneurysm.**

An ischaemic stroke is the most common type of stroke, which occurs when a blood clot blocks the flow of blood and oxygen to the brain. These blood clots typically form in areas where the arteries have been narrowed or blocked over time by fatty deposits known as plaques. This process is known as atherosclerosis.

As we age, there is a certain degree of narrowing within the arteries, but certain things can dangerously accelerate the process.

These include:

- smoking
- hypertension
- obesity
- high cholesterol
- diabetes
- high alcohol intake.

Table 27.3   Stroke: clinical characteristics and pathophysiology

Haemorrhagic stroke	A sudden, very severe headache
	Loss of consciousness
	Nausea and vomiting
	Stiff neck
	Numbness, feeling weak or the inability to move your face, arm or leg on one side of your body
	Dizziness or vertigo
	Blurred vision or sensitivity to light
Ischaemic stroke	Weakness in arm or leg
	Change in sensation in arm or leg
	Facial weakness
	Change in speech or understanding of speech
	Lack of awareness of part of the body
	A loss of coordination
	Visual loss

An ischaemic stroke can be caused by several kinds of disease. The most common problem is the narrowing of the arteries in the head or neck. If the arteries become too narrow, blood cells may collect and form blood clots. These blood clots can block the artery where they are formed (thrombosis) or can dislodge and become trapped in arteries closer to the brain (embolism).

Another cause of a stroke is blood clots coming from the heart, which can occur as a result of an irregular heartbeat, heart attack or abnormalities of the heart valves. While these are the most common causes of ischaemic stroke, there are many possible causes.

When looking at other risk factors, another main one is the heart rhythm atrial fibrillation (AF). This occurs because the atria are fibrillating and not beating in a coordinated way. The lack of sufficient contraction means that the blood in the atria becomes stagnant and can form clots. These clots can break off and travel anywhere in the body, including the brain, and cause a stroke.

SEE ALSO
CHAPTER 25

A haemorrhagic stroke occurs when a blood vessel ruptures and blood accumulates in the tissue around a rupture. This produces pressure on the brain and a loss of blood to certain areas.

SEE ALSO
CHAPTER 12

Investigations for stroke

Blood tests – Routine blood tests are taken from everyone with a possible stroke/TIA, to look at general health. Additional blood tests are also done to look at thyroid gland function, cholesterol levels and glucose levels.

Carotid duplex – This is an ultrasound scan of the major arteries in the neck, which supply blood to the brain. A major cause of stroke is hardening/narrowing of the arteries, caused by atherosclerosis. If narrowing is found on the side that is causing symptoms of stroke, an operation may be offered to clear any plaques that are reducing the blood supply.

CT scan – A CT head scan is usually carried out after a suspected stroke to rule out a possible bleed in the brain. The purpose of carrying out the scan as early as possible is to allow blood-thinning medication to be given more safely (e.g. aspirin).

ECG (Electrocardiogram) – An ECG is a routine investigation that shows the electrical activity of the heart. It provides information on the rate and regularity of the heartbeat. It can also identify old and new heart problems, which may need further investigation (e.g. ECHO).

ECHO (Echocardiogram) – An ECHO is an ultrasound scan which assesses the mechanics of the heart. This can show any heart enlargement (usually caused by high blood pressure) and the degree of any heart failure. Blood clots (which can be a cause of strokes) may also show up on an ECHO.

MRI scan – An MRI head scan may be requested where there is change picked up by CT, but the cause is not clear. It may also be required if the symptoms of the stroke do not 'fit' the changes picked up by the CT. An MRI scan may be used to look at the blood vessels in the neck to rule out any blockage.

Nursing assessment and management of the adult patient with Parkinson's disease, multiple sclerosis or following a stroke

It is important when caring for patients with these complex and debilitating conditions that individualised nursing care is tailored to the patient's needs to give optimal symptom control and improve quality of life.

Key points to remember when caring for patients with Parkinson's disease:

- Around one in 20 people with Parkinson's are under the age of 40.
- The combination of motor and non-motor symptoms can make it difficult to carry out many activities of daily living.

- It is paramount that patients receive their medication on time to give optimal symptom control.
- Parkinson's nurses help patients to manage medications, offer advice and information and provide emotional support.
- The way in which the condition affects patients can vary from hour to hour and day to day.

Key points to remember when caring for a patient with multiple sclerosis:

- Problems with balance, walking and feeling dizzy are very common.
- Bladder problems are very common.
- Constipation and bowel incontinence will be suffered by over 50% of patients at some time through their illness.
- Many patients with MS will experience problems with their vision and it is often an early sign of the disease.
- Overwhelming tiredness is one of the most common signs of MS.
- The emotional effects of MS often go unnoticed.
- About a third of patients with MS will suffer from pain.
- Muscle stiffness and spasticity affects the activities of daily living.
- Between 30 and 40% of patients will experience difficulty with swallowing.

Key points to remember when caring for a patient following a stroke:

- The injury to the brain caused by a stroke can lead to widespread and long-lasting problems.
- Although some people may recover quite quickly, many people who have a stroke will need long-term support to help them manage any difficulties they have and regain as much independence as possible.
- One of the most common psychological problems that can affect people after a stroke are:
  - Depression – many people experience intense bouts of crying and feel hopeless and withdrawn from social activities.
  - Anxiety – where people experience general feelings of fear and anxiety. Sometimes punctuated by intense, uncontrolled feelings of anxiety (anxiety attacks).
- Strokes can cause weakness and paralysis down one side of the body, leading to problems with coordination and balance.
- Stroke can affect swallowing in some patients, increasing the risk of aspiration and lung infections.
- Stroke can damage the part of the brain that receives, processes and interprets information sent by the eyes. This can result in losing half the field of vision.
- Stroke can damage the part of the brain associated with urine and bowel continence.

ACTIVITY 27.2: CRITICAL THINKING

ACTIVITY 27.2 ANSWER

Parkinson's disease is one of the neurological conditions discussed within this chapter. Think about how you would care for that patient and their relatives addressing the physical, psychological and social needs.

- What could you as a nurse do to reassure the patient with a new diagnosis?
- How do you think they may be feeling?

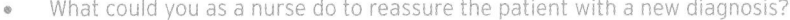

ACTIVITIES OF DAILY LIVING

A patient with a tremor due to Parkinson's disease can find everyday activities such as eating or drinking difficult, and it often becomes more noticeable if the patient you are caring for is anxious or excited. As a nurse you would need to ensure that the patient could eat and drink with assistance as necessary. The patient could be referred to occupational therapy to see what aids could be used to help. The patient who has had a stroke will have to have their swallowing reflex assessed by the speech and language team before they are safe to eat and drink. As a nurse you have to ensure the patient receives adequate nutrition and hydration, which means that they may require nasogastric feeding and an intravenous line for fluids.

Rigidity and **bradykinesia** mean people with Parkinson's can experience problems with turning around, getting out of chairs, turning over in bed or making fine-finger movements, such as writing or fastening a button. Some find posture becomes stooped or that their faces are affected, making facial expressions more difficult. This patient could be at risk of falling and causing themselves harm. The patient would, therefore, need to be assessed to see whether they are safe to get up out of bed or a chair safely themselves. Physiotherapists would be involved in assessing the patient in collaboration with the nurse.

For patients with MS, once the healthcare professional finds the reason for their dizziness and problems with balance they can be addressed and hopefully rectified. Patients with a stroke may not be able to mobilise for a period of time or can suffer from dizziness or lack of balance, which puts them at risk of sustaining a fall. Following a stroke, if the patient is unable to move then the nurse would have to ensure the patient is turned every 2 hours to prevent injury to their skin.

Initiating movement (gait hesitation or freezing) can become more difficult. People with Parkinson's can find it takes longer to do things and get tired more easily. Lack of coordination can also be a problem. This can be the same with some patients with MS and stroke. Patience and reassurance is needed and the facilitation of adequate periods of rest should be enabled.

As well as difficulties with movement, patients can experience symptoms such as tiredness, pain, depression and constipation. These are referred to as non-motor symptoms and can have a negative impact on daily living. It is often these symptoms that people find the most debilitating. As a nurse you need to observe the patient for verbal and non-verbal signs of pain. Allow for regular undisturbed breaks. Assessments such as bowel charts, turning charts, pain assessment charts, etc. all need to be completed accurately and regularly to ensure the patient is pain free and safe from harm.

The combination of these motor and non-motor symptoms can, over time, impair the ability to carry out many activities of daily living, which is why it is necessary to identify the most suitable treatments to manage them. Therefore, nursing and treatment plans need to be unique to each individual.

If patients do not receive their medication on time, the consequences can be serious. Their ability to manage symptoms may be lost; for example, they may suddenly be unable to eat or drink, get out of bed or go to the toilet independently. It is, therefore, very important that medication is administered punctually.

SEE ALSO CHAPTER 11

SEE ALSO CHAPTER 13

ACTIVITY 27.3 ANSWER

WEBLINK: DAILY LIVING CARE

ACTIVITY 27.3: CRITICAL THINKING

Using the Roper-Logan-Tierney Model of Twelve Activities of Daily Living, think about caring for a patient who has had a stroke. Using the model, complete each of the sections and decide how you would plan your care for the patient.

Refer to the following link: www.kindlycare.com/activities-of-daily-living/

Nursing care plan and management of a patient with Parkinson's disease, multiple sclerosis or following a stroke

The nursing goals for patients with Parkinson's disease, MS or following a stroke include improving functional mobility, maintaining independence in performing activities of daily living, achieving optimal bowel elimination, attaining and maintaining acceptable nutritional status, achieving effective communication, and developing positive coping mechanisms.

Nursing interventions for each of the symptoms of Parkinson's disease – muscle rigidity, bradykinesia, tremors at rest and postural reflex abnormalities – are designed to increase the patient's quality of life by minimising symptoms. Nurses are responsible for planning patient medication schedules to maximise drug effectiveness. Constipation is addressed by increasing the patient's fibre and fluid intake and by increasing the patient's mobility. Patient mobility is increased when the patient is taught purposeful activities and to concentrate on the way he/she walks.

In relation to MS, the nurse, as part of the multidisciplinary team, can play a major role in the ongoing support of the patient, as well as in the prevention and management of symptoms. The role of the MS specialist nurse is to provide information, support and advice about the condition from the time of diagnosis and throughout the disease process. Many people will have difficulty coming to terms with the diagnosis, and will be uncertain of the future, and worried about the prospect of disability. All members of the multidisciplinary team can be involved in suggesting relaxation and coping strategies, but sometimes referral to a **neuropsychologist** or counsellor is beneficial. Often symptoms of MS can be treated with drugs, some of which are used in other disorders such as some drugs for epilepsy, which can be used to treat neurological pain in MS patients, and certain antidepressants have been used to treat sensory disturbances that some patients experience.

Fatigue is the most commonly reported symptom in MS and many patients feel this is the most debilitating symptom. MS specialist nurses, physiotherapists and occupational therapists are on hand to advise of fatigue management strategies to try to reduce its effects. There are other symptoms that are silent, such as pain, altered sensation, bladder, bowel and sexual dysfunction, and cognitive problems. One of the most important things is that the nurse discusses them in the initial assessment and that appropriate intervention is carried out in a sympathetic and understanding manner. Many professionals find it difficult to discuss sexual dysfunction, which is a very real problem for many patients with MS, although treatment options are available.

In relation to stroke there is an acute phase and a post-acute phase where the nursing management differs.

During the acute phase, the following needs to be observed and documented in relation to the patient's clinical status:

- observation for a change in the level of consciousness or responsiveness
- presence or absence of voluntary or involuntary movement of extremities
- stiffness or flaccidity of the neck
- eye opening, size of pupils and pupillary reaction to light
- colour of the patient including extremities, temperature and whether the skin is clammy
- ability to speak
- presence of bleeding
- being able to maintain blood pressure (Holbery and Newcombe, 2016).

During the post-acute phase, the following functions need to be assessed:

- the mental status of the patient including memory (short term), attention span, perception, orientation and speech and language
- sensation and perception (usually the patient has decreased awareness of pain and temperature)

- motor control (upper and lower extremity movement)
- ability to swallow safely, nutritional and hydration status, skin integrity, activity tolerance, bowel and bladder function
- continuous monitoring of the patient in relation to the activities of daily living.

CASE STUDY 27.1
ANSWER

CASE STUDY 27.1: JIM

Jim, aged 54, was part of a building crew and was getting out of his work van when he suddenly felt his left leg turn to jelly. 'I fell down, and my workmates got me a chair,' he says. 'They brought me a cup of tea, but I couldn't work out where the handle was to grasp it. Somehow I knew I'd had a stroke and asked them to take me to hospital. I had seen the advert on the telly and I remembered the symptoms.'

'By the time I got there, I didn't have any feeling in the left side of me. I felt like a lump of meat. I could hardly get out of the car.'

Doctors confirmed that Jim was right; he'd had a stroke. He spent the next 27 weeks in hospital undergoing rehabilitation and physiotherapy. 'Luckily, my speech was still all right, though I'm sure my kids and grandchildren sometimes wish I'd be quiet!' he says. 'During my time in hospital I regained around 85% use of my hand and arm. I'm actually very lucky.'

Jim had high blood pressure and was diabetic, which are both risk factors for stroke. However, he had never smoked and, due to his diabetes, was already following the healthy diet recommended for stroke survivors.

'My wife was a chef and she made sure we ate properly,' he says. He was put on antihypertensive medication for high blood pressure and now has regular checks. 'When I had the stroke, I had no idea I had high blood pressure,' he says. Now consider the following:

1. What would have been the priorities for Jim on admission to hospital in relation to diagnosis and treatment?
2. What would have been the priorities in your care plan?

Discharge planning in relation to a patient with Parkinson's disease, multiple sclerosis or following a stroke

- A person should not stay on an acute hospital ward any longer than absolutely necessary.
- Discharge from hospital can only happen when the patient is deemed medically fit for discharge. However, this does not mean that the patient is now 'well' or now has no medical conditions.
- In addition, Health and Social Care Services may also be involved and must be satisfied that the discharge would be safe – which means that there is an appropriate care and support plan in place.
- Hospital staff should be able to estimate the expected date of discharge (EDD). In practice, this often has to be changed/reviewed and any reviews that have an effect on a patient's EDD should be shared with them and their relative/representative.
- Discharge from hospital should be timely and informative. Information should be given to explain how the discharge will be managed. It is the discharge coordinator's job to organise assessments of needs and 'coordinate' the process, i.e. bring the relevant health and social care professionals together, give timescales, etc.

- An assessment of needs will help to identify the patient's ability to manage on leaving hospital and options should be explored and agreed with the individual concerned or their representative.
- A care plan should then be drawn up. This should detail the help and support that is needed and confirm how the care will be delivered.
- All options must be explored with the objective being to maximise a person's independence.

CASE STUDY 27.2: DISCHARGE PLANNING REFLECTION

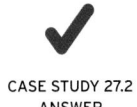

CASE STUDY 27.2
ANSWER

Narianne has an aggressive form of relapsing remitting multiple sclerosis. She experiences debilitating fatigue on a daily basis and has regular relapses.

On her last hospital admission a discussion took place in relation to her starting a monthly infusion of the **disease-modifying drug** (DMD) Tysabri.

'When I was first offered Tysabri, I didn't want it. I'd heard about people who had died on the trial and didn't want to put my life at risk. When my doctor explained how isolated those cases were, and that the treatment had finished trials and had been approved for treating aggressive forms of MS, I decided I would give it a go.'

Narianne had previously taken Copaxone and Avonex - DMDs that are self-injected.

'I had lots of side effects with Avonex and I hated the daily injections with Copaxone. I felt like I was stabbing myself and sometimes had to ask my husband to do it for me. I had been told the monthly infusions for Tysabri were painless and straightforward, and I therefore would no longer have the stress of bad injection site bruises.'

Narianne's MS symptoms include fatigue, mobility and vision problems. 'I'm unable to work because of my fatigue,' she explains. 'I tend to get errands and exercise done in the morning, and then come midday my body starts to shut down, fatigue sets in and I can't do anything other than rest; it's like flicking a switch.'

Tysabri has been known to cause the life-threatening virus **progressive multifocal leukoencephalopathy** (PML), but risk of developing this is small. Potential side effects of the treatment can include infections, headaches, dizziness, vomiting, nausea, liver damage and infusion reactions. Narianne received the first infusions of Tysabri prior to discharge.

- Reflect and write down how you would ensure that Narianne had an effective patient-centred discharge from hospital, specific to her condition.

Consider the following:

- Would Narianne need a discharge letter and who would it be sent to?
- Would she require an outpatient appointment and why?
- Does she require any further input from community services?
- Does Narianne need to have details of who to contact if she wishes to discuss the side effects of the drugs?
- Any other issues you think may come to light at discharge or following discharge?

HEALTH PROMOTION IN RELATION TO A PATIENT WITH PARKINSON'S DISEASE, MULTIPLE SCLEROSIS OR FOLLOWING A STROKE

Student nurses, whether working in hospital or the community setting, have a very important role to play in promoting the health of patients and their families/carers. Traditionally, the focus of health promotion provided by the nurse has been on disease prevention and changing the behaviour of individuals with respect to their health. However, your role as promoters of health may be more complex, since you may have multidisciplinary knowledge and experience of health promotion in practice.

Promoting the health of an adult with a long-term neurological disorder encompasses the following:

Primary care management

- Coordinate care with other primary care health professionals to enable chronic disease management and rehabilitation.
- Be aware of the indications for referral to a neurologist for chronic conditions that require ongoing specialist management and conditions that require early treatment to avoid permanent deficit.

Person-centred care

- Discuss truthfully and sensitively the implications of living with disabling neurological conditions such as Parkinson's disease and multiple sclerosis (Delves-Yates, 2015).
- Demonstrate empathy and compassion towards patients living with disabling neurological conditions.
- Understand the importance of continuity of care for patients with chronic neurological conditions.
- Have an understanding of the anatomy of the nervous system relevant to the diagnosis of the patient.
- Offer health education and promotion to the patient and their family/carer.

Holistic approach

- Recognise that neurological conditions often affect patients during their working lives and consequently have a large impact on the family's social and economic wellbeing.
- Recognise the stigma associated with neurological disease and disability, and how this may differ in different communities and cultures.
- Be cognisant of the key national guidelines and groups (e.g. NICE guidelines; Royal College of Nursing; Department of Health; Parkinson's Disease Society; Multiple Sclerosis Society and Stroke Association) that influence healthcare provision for neurological problems.
- Understand how to access up-to-date information on the management of neurological conditions.

It is important that you tailor the advice to suit the needs of the individual and their diagnosis.

SEE ALSO CHAPTER 7

ACTIVITY 27.4: HEALTH PROMOTION ALERT

Take some time out to look at the latest guidelines in relation to health promotion advice utilising the following weblinks:

- NHS Choices: www.nhs.uk
- Stroke Network: www.strokenetwork.org
- Parkinson's UK: www.parkinsons.org.uk
- MS Trust: www.mstrust.org.uk

WEBLINKS

PREPARATION FOR PRACTICE PLACEMENTS 27.1

Preparing to care for a patient with a neurological condition can help remove any worries you may have. It is advisable to contact your placement in advance and try to arrange to meet with your mentor. Linking theory to practice is really important so it is advisable to gain some knowledge on the patients you will be caring for prior to attending placement.

You may also find it useful to track a patient with a neurological condition from admission, which will allow you to develop your understanding of neurological observations, specific neurological investigations, delivering person-centred care, health promotion and discharge planning.

ACTIVITY 27.5: CRITICAL THINKING

If you were caring for a patient living with multiple sclerosis:

- Consider what phase of their long-term condition they may be experiencing.
- Consider what the priorities of care may be at their stage of the illness.
- How will you prioritise the care for that patient?
- How can you link the information you have gained from this chapter into caring for a patient with a neurological condition, and where are the gaps in your knowledge?

ACTIVITY 27.5
ANSWER

CHAPTER SUMMARY

- Neurological conditions are wide ranging.
- Lifestyle changes can make a positive contribution to quality of life and improve neurological conditions.
- Nurses have an important role to play in the prevention, identification and management of neurological conditions.
- Health promotion has proven benefits for adults living with neurological conditions.

GO FURTHER

Go to https://study.sagepub.com/essentialadultnursing for a further case study related to this chapter. If you are using the interactive ebook, simply click on the book icon in the margin to go straight to the resource.

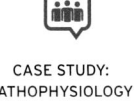

CASE STUDY:
PATHOPHYSIOLOGY
OF STROKE

Books

- Barker, R.A. and Cicchetti, F. (2012) *Neuroanatomy and Neuroscience at a Glance*. Oxford: Wiley-Blackwell. An accessible illustrated neuroscience textbook.
- Hickey, J.V. (2013) *Clinical Practice of Neurological & Neurosurgical Nursing*. Philadelphia: Lippincott Williams and Wilkins. An American core text on neuroscience nursing.
- Woodward, S. and Mestecky, A. (2011) *Neuroscience Nursing: Evidence-Based Theory and Practice*. Oxford: Wiley-Blackwell. An expert overview of UK evidence-based neuroscience nursing.

FURTHER
READING:
JOURNAL
ARTICLES

Journal Articles

Go to https://study.sagepub.com/essentialadultnursing for further free online journal articles related to this chapter. If you are using the interactive ebook, simply click on the book icon in the margin to go straight to the resource.

- Barnes, L. (2017) Parkinson's disease in primary care: an acute deterioration pathway. *Nursing Times*, 113 (5): 55-7.
  Discussion of a pathway to help people with Parkinson's disease manage acute deteriorations in their symptoms while avoiding hospital admissions
- Corcoran, N. and McCullagh, L. (2018) Stroke 5: Health promotion for primary stroke prevention. *Nursing Times*, 115 (3): 53-6.
  An article looking at how nurses can support people to change their lifestyles in order to reduce their risk of stroke. Last in five-part series.
- Roberts, M. (2017) An overview of multiple sclerosis and its holistic management. *Nursing Times*, 113 (1): 19-23.
  A useful overview of MS and its management.

FURTHER
READING:
WEBLINKS

Weblinks

Go to https://study.sagepub.com/essentialadultnursing for further weblinks related to this chapter. If you are using the interactive ebook, simply click on the book icon in the margin to go straight to the resource.

- www.mssociety.org.uk/
  The website of the Multiple Sclerosis Society - a patient-facing organisation
- www.parkinsons.org.uk/
  The website of Parkinson's UK which is a charity that campaigns for better care, treatments and quality of life
- www.stroke.org.uk/
  The website of the Stroke Association which delivers stroke services across the UK, undertakes research and campaigns for better stroke care
- www.who.int/features/qa/55/en/
  Some international resources from the World Health Organization (WHO)

ONLINE
QUIZZES

ACE YOUR ASSESSMENT

Revise what you have learned by visiting https://study.sagepub.com/essentialadultnursing

- Test yourself with multiple-choice and short-answer questions
- Do the chapter activities in the book and check your answers online

REFERENCES

Delves-Yates, C. (ed.) (2015) *Essentials of Nursing Practice*. London: SAGE.

Holbery, N. and Newcombe, P. (2016) *Emergency Nursing at a Glance*. West Sussex: Wiley & Sons.

Peate, I. and Nair, M. (2015) *Anatomy and Physiology for Nurses at a Glance*. West Sussex: Wiley & Sons.

CARE OF THE ADULT WITH A URINARY/ RENAL CONDITION

28

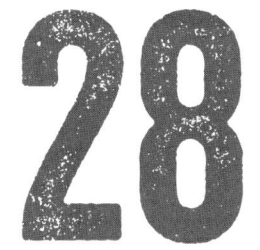

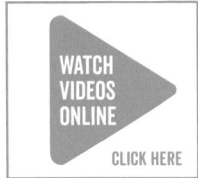

WATCH VIDEOS ONLINE

CLICK HERE

CATHY POOLE AND SUE WOODCOCK

THIS CHAPTER COVERS

- An overview of the anatomy and physiology of the urinary tract
- An explanation of the clinical characteristics and pathophysiology relevant to common presenting urinary/renal conditions

- Nursing assessment and management of the adult with common presenting urinary/ renal conditions.

> "
> There is a perception amongst nursing students that non-acute placements have the potential to be dull and is not 'real' nursing in the way that you imagine when you're watching *24 hours in A&E*. Having a placement in a dialysis unit for 7 weeks completely changed my thoughts of community based nursing and renal nursing, potentially changing the direction of my future career with it.
>
> **Sophie Marshall, 2nd year student nurse, Kingston University**
> "

INTRODUCTION

Nursing adults with a urinary/renal system condition can at first seem confusing. However, if you have a good knowledge and understanding of the normal anatomy and physiology of this system then you will more easily be able to appreciate the consequences of, and symptoms of, urinary/renal disease and understand the nursing care required to meet the individual needs of these patients.

When referring to urinary/renal disorders you will need to take into consideration the whole urinary tract, kidneys, ureters, bladder, and of course the urethra. Conditions that affect the urinary system are often referred to as either upper or lower urinary tract disorders. The management of urinary tract disorders can either be surgical or medical in nature, and in some cases patients need both surgical and medical management.

This chapter will, therefore, begin with an overview of the normal anatomy and physiology of the urinary tract and will then consider some common medical and surgical disorders. It will also provide you with a good insight into the holistic nursing assessment and management of adults with chronic and acute kidney failure, both of which have significant health impacts and are sadly on the increase.

CRITICAL THINKING STOP POINT 28.1

Take a few moments to reflect on what you already know about normal urinary/renal anatomy and physiology. Can you think of any signs and symptoms that may indicate that renal function is deteriorating?

ANATOMY AND PHYSIOLOGY OF THE URINARY/RENAL SYSTEM

The urinary system has a key role in the maintenance of **homeostasis**. The kidney's primary role is to filter waste products from the bloodstream, which are either then reabsorbed back into the bloodstream or excreted in urine. This continuous **filtration, reabsorption** and **excretion** process ensures regulation of water, sodium balance and acid base balance and in essence is an extremely well-designed recycling system. Thankfully, the majority of humans have two kidneys; between them they provide 100% of our kidney function. If one kidney has to be removed (**nephrectomy**) due to injury or disease then the remaining kidney will increase in size and function and will take over 100% of the function. As long as the remaining kidney is not diseased, a solitary kidney can last a lifetime.

The urinary system (see Figure 28.1) consists of the following:

- lower urinary tract
- adrenal gland
- bladder
- right kidney
- left kidney
- ureters
- urethra
- upper urinary tract.

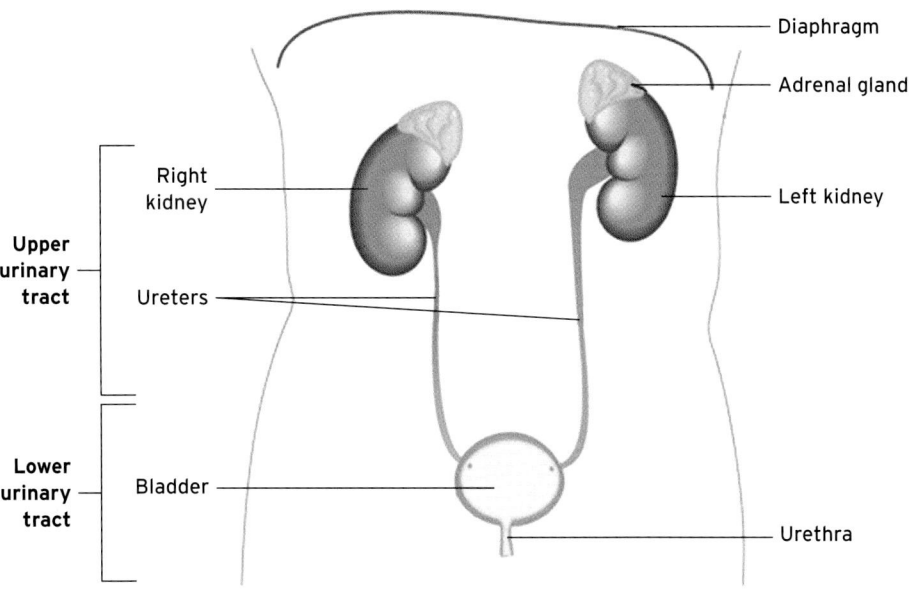

Figure 28.1   The urinary system

Gross structure and location

The kidneys are amazing organs; they are no bigger than fist size and in a day can filter approximately 1800 litres of blood, which results in the production of approximately 1.5 litres of urine which contains water and waste. Kidney development (nephrogenesis) starts during the first week of gestation and continues right up until the 36th week. At birth, babies' kidneys have the full complement of 1 million nephrons in each kidney but they are not fully developed and over the next 4–5 years they mature and reach adult kidney function.

Kidneys are characteristically bean-shaped organs which lie behind the **peritoneum (retroperitoneal)** in the back of the upper abdomen, one on either side of the spinal column at the level of the twelfth thoracic to the third lumbar vertebrae. The right kidney sits slightly lower than the left due to the location of the liver. Each kidney contains between 8–18 **pyramids,** which are conical in shape and contain the **nephrons**; these nephrons are the functional units of the kidney. Each nephron consists of a glomerulus that filters the blood and a tubular structure, which is where **selective reabsorption** and **secretion** takes place during the formation of urine (Mattson Porth and Matfin, 2008).

If you cut a kidney in half lengthways you can clearly visualise the gross structure (Figure 28.2). There are three distinctive areas:

1. the renal cortex = the outermost layer which is a reddish brown colour
2. the renal medulla = the innermost layer which contains the pyramids
3. the renal pelvis = which is a funnel-shaped structure where all the urine drains into before entering the ureter.

Each nephron drains into a collecting duct, and all collecting ducts drain into minor **calyces,** which then converge into major calyces. All the major calyces converge to form the renal pelvis and it is at this point where all the urine flows into the ureter.

The kidney is encased in a tough fibrous layer (renal capsule) and each kidney is surrounded by fatty **adipose connective tissue,** which protects the kidney from mechanical injury and helps, together with the renal blood vessels and **facia,** in keeping the kidney in its anatomical position.

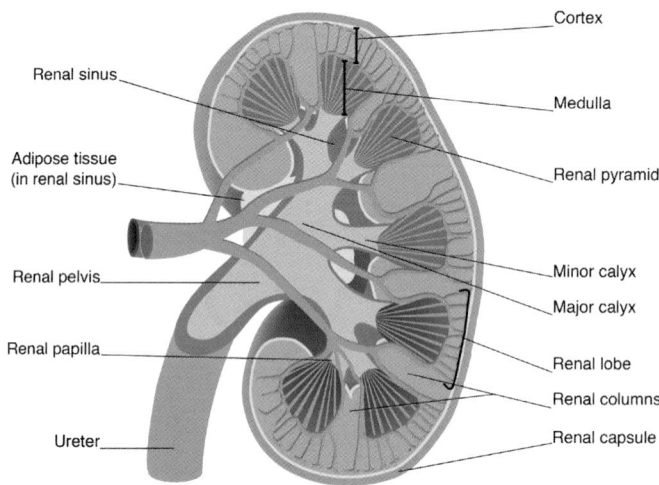

Figure 28.2 Internal structure of the kidney

Source: Boore et al. (2016). Illustrated by Shaun Mercier, © SAGE Publications.

Renal blood supply

In order for the kidneys to continuously filter the blood they need a good blood supply. This blood supply comes from a single renal artery, which arises on either side of the aorta. The renal artery divides several times: each time the diameter of the arteries gets smaller which increases the blood pressure within them, and these arteries culminate in the **afferent arteriole** which is a network of capillaries called the **glomerulus** that sits in the **Bowman's capsule**. At this point the blood supply leaves the glomerulus via the **efferent arteriole** and forms the **peritubular capillaries,** which eventually re-join to form the venous channels through which blood ultimately leaves the kidneys and drains into the inferior vena cava (Figure 28.3).

MICROSCOPIC STRUCTURE

As previously stated each kidney consists of 1 million nephrons, which form the functional part of the kidney.

The nephron

The primary role of the nephron is to form urine. The nephron consists of four parts:

1. Bowman's capsule
2. Proximal convoluted tubule (PCT)
3. Loop of Henle
4. Distal convoluted tubule (DCT)

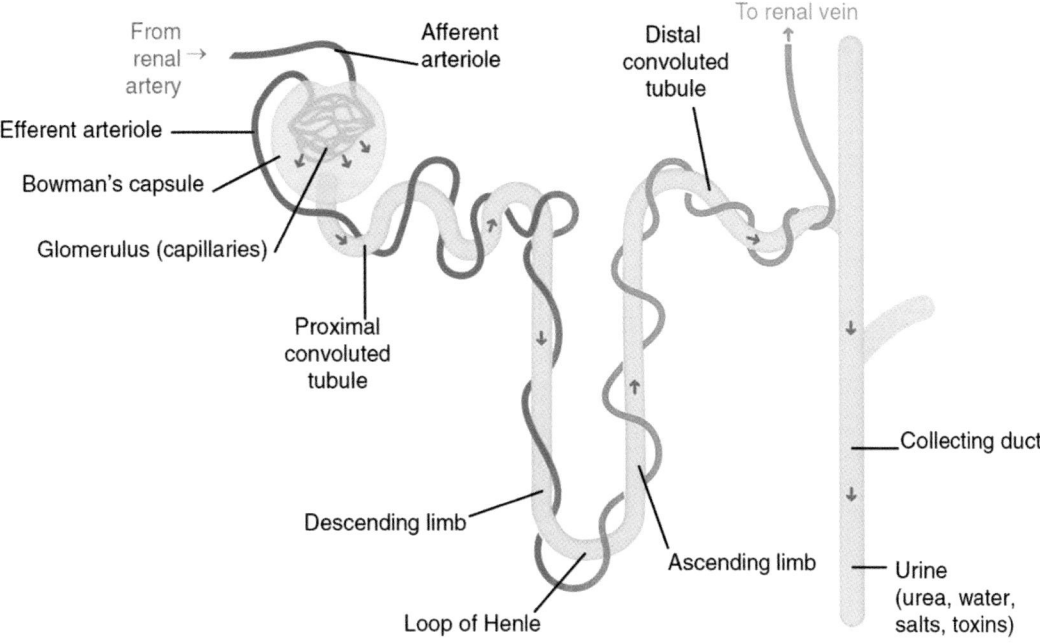

Figure 28.3   Renal blood supply to and from the kidneys

Source: Boore et al. (2016). Illustrated by Shaun Mercier © SAGE Publications.

The mechanism of urine function takes place through three key stages:

1.   glomerular filtration
2.   tubular reabsorption
3.   tubular secretion.

─────────────────── GO FURTHER ───────────────────

In order to understand how the nephron works, watch this YouTube video which provides a handwritten explanation of urine formation and the function of the nephron: www.youtube.com/watch?v=vNvZaGcLzEo

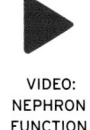

VIDEO: NEPHRON FUNCTION

CRITICAL THINKING STOP POINT 28.2

The following hormones play a major role in fluid homeostasis:

- Angiotensin II
- Aldosterone

(Continued)

(Continued)

- Antidiuretic hormone (ADH)
- Atrial natriuretic peptide (ANP)

Can you explain how these hormones work? Think about what would happen to your hydration status if your kidneys stop working properly.

You may find this weblink a useful resource in helping you to understand the role of these hormones: https://opentextbc.ca/anatomyandphysiology/chapter/26-2-water-balance/

Kidneys play a major role in homoeostasis but they do, however, have two other key functions:

1. Production of **erythropoietin** (EPO) – a hormone needed in the bone marrow to stimulate production of **erythrocytes**.
2. Conversion of **vitamin D** into its active form.

CRITICAL THINKING STOP POINT 28.3

Take a few minutes to reflect on the clinical symptoms associated with a reduction of EPO production and the impact on bone density if vitamin D is not converted to its active form.

Hopefully, you now have a much better understanding of upper urinary tract anatomy and function. Now take some time to consider lower urinary tract anatomy and function by utilising the weblink to an interactive 'innerbody' site, which will help you to understand the lower urinary tract: www.innerbody.com/image_urinov/repo15-new2.html

SEE ALSO
CHAPTER 12

INVESTIGATIONS OF THE URINARY/RENAL SYSTEM

Urinalysis

You may be surprised to know that urinalysis was the first laboratory test done in medicine and has been used for several thousand years. It remains one of the simplest and most cost-effective ways of determining health and illness (Echeverry et al., 2010). In nursing practice, undertaking urinalysis is one of the first clinical skills learned by student nurses and continues to be one of the most common clinical skills still performed in practice across all areas of nursing.

Urine samples are easy to obtain but are known to be unstable, and changes to its composition start to take place straight after micturition. Therefore, the collection, storage, and handling of urine samples are important matters in keeping the integrity of this specimen and thus the reliability of the results.

When obtaining a urine sample you may be asked to obtain one of the following:

- early morning urine (EMU) – first urine passed of the day
- midstream specimen of urine (MSU) – sample of urine from the middle of the voided sample

- 24 hour urine collection – collection of all urine over a 24-hour period
- catheter specimen of urine (CSU) – urine sample obtained directly from a urethral catheter.

Urine is characterised using the following criteria:

- **physical appearance** – normal, fresh urine is pale to dark yellow or amber in colour and clear.
- **chemical composition** – chemical examination of urine using urinalysis strips (Dipstick) includes the identification of protein, blood cells, glucose, pH, bilirubin, urobilinogen, ketone bodies, nitrites and leukocyte esterase.
- **microscopic examination** – this entails the identification of crystals, cells, casts, and micro-organisms.

Renal imaging

Many types of radiological tests are performed to assist the doctors in diagnosing and monitoring patients' kidney diseases; for example (Table 28.1):

Table 28.1 Renal imaging

Type of imaging study	Indication for use
Plain films of the abdomen	Rarely used now, indicated for the evaluation of radiopaque kidney stones (calcium-containing stones, struvite, cystine).
Renal ultrasonography	Excellent as a screening test for urinary tract dilatation (hydronephrosis), a sign of urinary tract obstruction; evaluation of polycystic kidney disease, renal tumours and measurement of kidney size.
Intravenous pyelography (IVP)	Used to detect kidney stones and define the level of obstruction in patients with urinary tract obstruction.
Computed tomography (CT)	Good for diagnosing kidney stones, nephrolithiasis, evaluation of kidney masses/tumours, polycystic kidney disease.
Magnetic resonance imaging (MRI)	Used to provide detailed assessment of the kidney anatomy, for non-invasive assessment of kidney function, estimation of GFR and assessment of congenital anomalies of the kidney, bladder and urinary tract.
Radionuclide scanning	Used to evaluate renal perfusion including renal artery stenosis and thrombosis.
Renal angiography	Used for the direct visualisation of renal blood vessels for the diagnosis and prognosis of renal artery stenosis and renal vein thrombosis.
Retrograde pyelography	Used to localise the site of urinary tract obstruction.
Diuretic renography	Used to identify if a dilated urinary tract is secondary to obstructive lesions (e.g. tumours) or non-obstructive causes (e.g. persistent dilation after relief of a previous obstruction).

Source: Schmitz and Maddukuri (2015)

The choice and frequency of renal imaging studies will be dependent upon the known or suspected urinary/renal disease.

Renal biopsy

When nephrologists (kidney specialists) want to look at kidney tissue to help them determine a renal diagnosis or help them to check and monitor if treatments are improving certain kidney diseases, the only way they can do that is by taking a small sample of kidney tissue, a procedure known as a kidney or renal biopsy. This procedure is usually carried out in the radiology department using ultrasound scanning to carefully locate the position of the kidney. The samples of kidney tissue are examined by a **histopathologist** using very high-powered microscopes in order to diagnose kidney disease or monitor changes. Renal biopsies are usually done under a local anaesthetic as a day case.

Haematology and clinical chemistry

Blood tests are commonly requested for all kinds of diseases; however, for renal patients there is a specific selection of tests, which are undertaken usually on a monthly, three-monthly or six-monthly basis. This is often referred to as a 'Renal Profile' and commonly includes the following (Table 28.2):

Table 28.2   Renal Association Clinical Practice Guidelines 6.1–6.8. Available at: www.renal.org/guidelines/modules/haemodialysis#s6

Blood test	Expected range for renal patients	
Haemoglobin	Maintained within the range 10.0–12.0g/dL	
Calcium	2.1–2.5 mmol/L	
Phosphate	1.1–1.7mmol/L	
Potassium	4.0–6.0 mmol/L for patients receiving haemodialysis therapy	
Sodium	135–145 mmol/L	
Bicarbonate	18–24 mmol/L	
Albumin	< 30.0 g/L	
Ferritin	200–500 ug/L	
iPTH (parathyroid hormone)	14–63 pmol/L	
Urea	2.5–7.0 mmol/L	
Creatinine	Range – Female	50–110 mmol/L
	Range – Male	60–120 mmol/L

It is important to note that laboratories may use different assays and therefore have different normal reference ranges for blood test results.

Due to the nature of dialysis and the potential exposure of blood, patients undergoing dialysis, awaiting renal transplantation or those who are known to require dialysis at some point are also tested for blood-borne viruses (BBV) Hepatitis B, Hepatitis C and Human Immunodeficiency Virus (HIV). Surveillance of the patients' BBV status is carried out in accordance with the Renal Association (2011) clinical practice guidelines.

In the renal environment, the nephrologists pay particular attention to patients' glomerular filtration rate (GFR) as an indicator of renal function. There are several ways GFR can be measured and to assist the diagnosis and management of chronic kidney disease, the Renal Association (2009) has developed an electronic tool to assist in the rapid assessment of an estimated GFR (eGFR).

GO FURTHER

Ask your mentor to show you where to find a creatinine result from relevant patient documentation and try using this eGFR tool which you will find by following this link: https://ukidney.com/nephrology-resources/egfr-calculator

WEBLINK: EGFR TOOL

You will also need to know the patient's age in years. When you have calculated their eGFR consider whether or not they have normal renal function.

COMMON URINARY/RENAL CONDITIONS

Urinary tract obstruction (obstructive uropathy)

Urine should drain freely from the kidneys to the bladder, and there should be no obstruction of urine from the bladder via the urethra. However, for some patients the flow of urine is obstructed. This obstruction causes back flow of urine into the kidneys, which can cause damage to the urinary system (obstructive nephropathy) and causes **hydronephrosis**. According to Preminger (2016), these blockages:

- can be complete or partial
- can lead to kidney damage, kidney stones and infection
- can include pain in the side, decreased or increased urine flow, and urinating at night
- are more common if the blockage is sudden and complete.

The most common causes differ by age; for example, in children obstructive uropathy is usually associated with anatomical abnormalities (e.g. posterior urethral valves, or stenosis at the junction where the ureter enters the bladder (ureterovesical) or at the junction where the pelvis of the kidney and the ureter merge (ureteropelvic). In young adults, calculi (stones) are more common whereas in older adults benign prostatic hypertrophy (BPH), prostate cancer, retroperitoneal or pelvic tumours (including metastatic cancer), and calculi are more common. The prevalence of urinary tract obstruction ranges from 5 in 10,000 to 5 in 1000 depending on the cause (Preminger, 2016).

Treatment is aimed at relief of the obstruction by surgery, either through instrumentation (e.g. endoscopy, **lithotripsy**), or drug therapy (e.g. hormonal therapy for prostate cancer). Swift drainage of **hydronephrosis** is required to preserve renal function, especially if it associated with a urinary tract infection or persistent pain.

Urinary tract infection (UTI)

According to NICE (2015), the incidence of UTI is highest in young women. Around 10–20% of women will experience a symptomatic UTI at some time. Most infections in adult men are complicated and related to abnormalities of the urinary tract. UTI incidence increases with age for both sexes. It is estimated that 10% of men and 20% of women over the age of 65 years have asymptomatic bacteriuria (NICE, 2015). Collection of a clean uncontaminated urine sample is pivotal to the diagnosis of UTI. Most UTIs are caused by bacteria, the commonest organism being *Escherichia Coli*.

Causes of UTI include:

- obstruction of the urinary tract
- not fully emptying the bladder during micturition

- using a condom or contraceptive diaphragm coated in spermicide
- diabetes
- patients who are immunosuppressed are at increased risk (e.g. receiving chemotherapy, post-renal transplantation)
- patients with a urinary catheter are at increased risk
- BPH.

Treatment of UTIs is usually a short course of antibiotics. If the infection involves the upper urinary tract (pyelonephritis) then the course of antibiotics may be prescribed for longer periods of time. It is always worth asking patients about their bowel habits, as often patients who are constipated are more prone to UTIs. A distended bowel full of hard faecal matter pressing on the bladder results in incomplete micturition.

Health promotion – preventing UTIs

There are several actions that patients can be advised to put into place which can help prevent UTI. These include the following:

- Avoid using perfumed bubble bath, soap or talcum powder around your genitals
- Take a shower rather than a bath
- Do not delay going to the toilet to empty your bladder
- Take your time when passing urine to ensure you empty your bladder fully
- Stay well hydrated
- Wipe your bottom from front to back when you go to the toilet
- Avoid using a contraceptive diaphragm or condoms with spermicidal lubricant on them
- Wear underwear made from cotton, rather than synthetic material such as nylon
- Avoid wearing tight jeans/trousers.

Some patients who are at increased risk of UTI may be prescribed low dose prophylactic (preventative) antibiotics. These are usually taken once a day before bed where their action is concentrated in the bladder overnight.

Renal reflux (vesicoureteric reflux)

Vesicoureteric reflux (VUR) is quite a common condition and is commonly diagnosed in babies and young children following UTIs. When people with VUR **micturate** some urine refluxes (squirts) back up the ureters towards the kidneys, and it can be **unilateral** or **bilateral**. Repeated UTIs cause scarring to the kidneys referred to as reflux nephropathy. VUR is graded as follows:

- Grades 1 and 2 are mild – requiring monitoring and the use of prophylactic antibiotics.
- Grades 3, 4 and 5 are more serious – urine refluxes all the way to one or both kidneys, causing **hydronephrosis** and sometimes **megaureter**. In addition to this the bladder may not empty completely. These higher grades are more likely to cause kidney damage and for some patients culminates in chronic kidney disease requiring dialysis and transplantation. Prophylactic antibiotics and/or surgery to correct the VUR may be required for these patients. Surgery is aimed at correcting the reflux and is either done using endoscopic surgery as a day case under general anaesthetic via cystoscopy or by open surgery. During endoscopic surgery, the surgeon can visualise the ureteric orifice and inject a substance, called Deflux®, into the area where the ureter enters the bladder; this helps to prevent urine from refluxing back into the ureter. Alternatively, open surgery is required in the form of ureterteric reimplantation. This involves the surgical removal of the ureter from the bladder, which is then reduced in size and reconnected (reimplanted) into the bladder.

Renal stones (urolithiasis)

Urolithiasis are formed when the urine is heavily saturated with salt and minerals. 60–80% of stones contain calcium, and they can vary considerably in size from small gravel-like stones to large ones which look like staghorns. Large stones can obstruct urinary flow causing **obstructive uropathy** and smaller ones can move within the urinary tract causing severe renal pain (**renal colic**).

The management of renal stones depends on the size of the stone and degree of pain experienced by the patient. Open surgery may be required, or lithotripsy. Lithotripsy involves the use of **extracorporeal** high energy shock waves. These shock waves are passed through the body and break the kidney stones into pieces which are small enough to be excreted during **micturition**.

GO FURTHER

For a more detailed account of the management of renal stones, take a look at the national Kidney Foundation website. www.kidney.org/atoz/content/lithotripsy

WEBLINK: LITHOTRIPSY GUIDE

Kidney cancer

According to NHS Choices (2016), kidney cancer, also referred to as renal cancer, is one of the most common types of cancer in the UK. It is reported to affect adults in their 60s or 70s and is rare in people under 50. These types of tumours can often be cured if diagnosed early. However, cure is less likely if it is not diagnosed until after it has spread beyond the kidney.

GO FURTHER

There are several types of kidney cancer. The most common type is renal cell carcinoma. The Cancer Research UK website has more information about other types of kidney cancer and can be found following this weblink: http://about-cancer.cancerresearchuk.org/about-cancer/kidney-cancer/stages-types-grades/types-grades#other

WEBLINK: KIDNEY CANCER GUIDE

Often, symptoms of kidney cancer are not obvious, and are sometimes identified when patients are being tested for other reasons. Symptoms, if they do occur, can include the following:

- haematuria
- persistent lower back pain or pain in the side just below the ribs
- evidence of a swelling on the patient's side; however, renal tumours are often too small to feel.

As with some other cancers, the precise cause of renal cancer is unknown. There are, however, some risks that can increase the likelihood of renal tumours developing. These risks include (NHS Choices (2016):

- obesity – BMI of 30 or more
- smoking
- hypertension

- family history
- genetic conditions – for example, **Von Hippel–Lindau syndrome**
- long-term dialysis.

Treatment will depend on the size of the cancer and whether it has spread to other parts of the body or not. Treatment may involve the following:

- nephrectomy or a partial nephrectomy
- cryotherapy or radiofrequency ablation – which involves the destruction of cancerous cells by either cold or heat
- chemotherapy
- embolisation – which involves a procedure to cut off the blood supply to the cancer
- radiotherapy.

As with most other cancers, survival is very much related to the type, location and spread of the kidney cancer. NHS Choices (2016) indicate that about 7 in every 10 people survive at least a year after diagnosis and around 5 in 10 live at least 10 years.

Hereditary/congenital urinary/renal disorders

There are a variety of urinary/renal disorders that are hereditary. The advent of antenatal ultrasound screening has greatly improved the early identification of congenital malformations of the renal system. Prior to this, many congenital abnormalities of this nature were not diagnosed until they caused symptoms in infancy, childhood or in some instances in adult life. Improved genetic test techniques have also resulted in improved early diagnosis and management of many genetically inherited renal diseases. Table 28.3 provides an insight into some of these inherited/congenital renal disorders.

Table 28.3   ABC of some inherited/congenital renal disorders

Inherited/congenital renal disorder	Brief description
Alport syndrome	Rare, predominantly X-linked, presents with haematuria, an associated sensorineural deafness and eye defects. Results in chronic kidney disease (CKD).
ANCA-associated vasculitis	A systemic autoimmune small vessel vasculitis syndrome, is associated with antineutrophil cytoplasmic autoantibodies (ANCAs).
Autosomal dominant polycystic disease	Most common inherited cause of CKD. Multiple cysts develop in the kidney, get progressively larger and fill with fluid causing compression of the kidney tissue.
Autosomal recessive polycystic disease	Most common genetic cystic renal disease occurring in infancy and childhood, associated pulmonary hyperplasia due to the size of the kidney cysts. Prognosis is poor often leading to CKD at around 4 years of age.
Bartter's syndrome	Usually diagnosed in childhood or early adolescence, inherited as an autosomal recessive pattern, affecting sodium, potassium and chloride balance.
Congenital (atypical) haemolytic uraemic syndrome	Extremely rare, life-threatening, progressive disease that frequently has a genetic component leading to CKD.

Inherited/congenital renal disorder	Brief description
Congenital nephrotic syndrome	Finnish type which appears during the first year of life: it is however very rare. Heavy proteinuria and generalised oedema that does not respond to steroid treatment.
Genetic amyloidosis	Caused by a gene mutation that produces an amyloid protein that forms into an abnormal shape. These abnormal proteins get deposited in the body's nerves and other organs, i.e. kidneys, and once they build up may affect the function of the kidney.
IgA nephropathy	Most common form of idiopathic glomerulonephritis, which is an autoimmune renal disease, presents with heavy haematuria and also proteinuria leading to CKD.
Reflux nephropathy	Scarring of the kidney due to urine refluxing back up to the kidneys from the bladder, associated with recurrent pyelonephritis, which can culminate in CKD.
Renal dysplasia	A condition where the kidney does not develop normally during embryonic development. Can be detected at antenatal scan.
Obstructive uropathy	For example neuropathic bladder, posterior urethral valves.

Source: Patient: http://patient.info/doctor/inherited-kidney-diseases

For further information of rare renal disorders take a look at the Renal Association RareRenal.org website: http://rarerenal.org/patient-information/

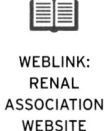

WEBLINK: RENAL ASSOCIATION WEBSITE

HOLISTIC APPROACH TO NURSING CARE

Chronic kidney disease (CKD)

CKD is the irreversible impairment of kidney function measured by a slow decline in glomerular filtration rate. A silent killer and a major public health problem, it currently affects three million people in the UK and there is no cure (Kidney Research UK, 2016). It can occur across all age groups, but becomes more common as age increases. CKD can be caused by a range of disorders and diseases such as diabetes, hypertension, reno-vascular disease, urological problems (including abnormalities of the urinary tract), congenital and childhood kidney diseases, glomerulonephritis and vasculitis. CKD is generally a slow progressive disease with many associated and difficult to treat complications; decline in kidney function is categorised into five stages (Table 28.4). If dialysis or transplantation is not initiated once the patient reaches Stage 5 then death normally occurs.

Table 28.4 CKD stages

Stage	Description	GFR	Treatment
1	Normal kidney function but urine findings, structural abnormalities or genetic trait point to kidney disease	>90	Observation, control of blood pressure
2	Mildly reduced kidney function, and other findings point to kidney disease	60-89	Observation, control of blood pressure and risk factors

(Continued)

Table 28.4 (Continued)

Stage	Description	GFR	Treatment
3	Moderately reduced kidney function	45–59 (3a) 30–44 (3b)	Observation, control of blood pressure and risk factors
4	Severely reduced kidney function	16–29	Planning for established renal failure
5	Very severe, or established kidney failure	<15	Treatment choices and commencement of renal replacement therapy

Source: Kidney Disease Improving Global Outcomes (2013)

Acute kidney injury (AKI)

AKI presents as a decreased urine output, with signs of fluid overload including oedema and shortness of breath, tiredness, nausea and vomiting and potential rashes, oral ulcers and joint swelling. There are three main causes of AKI: pre-renal, intra-renal and post-renal.

GO FURTHER

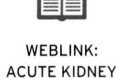

WEBLINK: ACUTE KIDNEY INJURY

Look though the Acute Kidney Injury (AKI) Undergraduate year 3 slide set at www.thinkkidneys.nhs.uk/aki/wp-content/uploads/sites/2/2016/05/UG-nurses-year-three-FINAL.pdf and make notes on:

- pre-renal causes of AKI
- intra-renal causes of AKI
- post-renal causes of AKI.

Stages of AKI

There are three stages of AKI (Table 28.5), where interventions at Stage 1 might include regular monitoring and review, to Stage 3 where immediate interventional treatment is required including intravenous fluid support, medication and possible dialysis treatment.

There are a number of predisposing factors to AKI including: a history of CKD, diabetes, heart failure, sepsis, hypovolaemia, being aged 65 years or over, long-term use of kidney damaging drugs such as non-steroidal anti-inflammatories and some anti-hypertensive medications, use of **iodinated contrast agents** within past week, liver disease, limited access to fluids, e.g. via neurological impairment, deteriorating early warning scores, symptoms or history of urological obstruction and being admitted to hospital for surgery.

Table 28.5 AKI stages

AKI Stage	Serum creatinine criteria	Urine output criteria
1	Increase in serum creatinine of 26 µmol/l or more within 48 hours OR 1.5 to 2-fold increase from baseline	Less than 0.5 ml/kg/hour for more than 6 hours*
2	Increase in serum creatinine to more than 2 to 3 fold from baseline	Less than 0.5 ml/kg/hour for more than 12 hours
3	Increase in serum creatinine to more than 3-fold from baseline OR Serum creatinine more than 354 µmol/l with an acute increase of at least 44 µmol/l	Less than 0.3 ml/kg/hour for 24 hours or anuria for 12 hours

Source: NICE (2014). Reproduced with permission under the NICE UK Open Content Licence.

*This staging was updated by NICE in 2014 to also include an albuminuria category; however, this requires specialist knowledge to interpret, hence the reason for including the more straightforward KDIGO staging.

Prevention

It is an important part of the nursing role to ensure that patients who present with any predisposing factors such as diabetes, hypertension or heart failure, and are at an increased risk of developing CKD or AKI, should receive regular check-ups and monitoring from primary care teams to ensure good management and control. For the rest of the population, reducing the risk can be achieved by living a healthy lifestyle such as: maintaining adequate hydration and drinking approximately 2 to 2.5 litres of non-alcoholic fluid over a 24-hour period; not smoking; maintaining weight within a healthy range; exercising regularly; eating a healthy diet rich in fruit, vegetables and fish; and reduced intake of salt, processed foods and high sugar drinks.

CASE STUDY 28.1: PATIENT JOURNEY (ANONYMISED PATIENT)

KD is a 44-year-old woman. She works full time in the NHS as a carer and is a single parent of a son who is 6 years old and a daughter who is 12 years old. At the age of 42 she began to experience lower back and side pain, blood in her urine and recurrent urinary tract infections. She visited her GP who took blood tests and ordered an ultrasound scan. On asking about her medical history she told the doctor that there was a history of family members having 'bad kidneys'. The ultrasound and blood tests revealed a diagnosis of **autosomal dominant polycystic kidney disease.** Over the last few months she noticed enlargement of her abdomen and increasing pain and episodes of haematuria. Her GP explained that this was caused by cysts bursting and that her latest blood tests had shown a sudden decline in her kidney function with an eGFR of below 15mls/minute. Her GP has also made an urgent referral to a nephrologist at the nearest regional renal unit.

ACTIVITY 28.1: REFLECTION

Using what you have learned from this chapter reflect on the implications of KD's diagnosis for her children and what can be done about this.

After reading about the Multi Professional Team (MPT) (below), reflect on the care and management that will be provided to KD by the nephrologist, pre-dialysis nurse, transplant nurse, dietician, pharmacist, social worker and dialysis nurse (depending on KD's choice of treatment this could be haemodialysis or peritoneal dialysis nurse specialist).

THE MULTI PROFESSIONAL TEAM (MPT)

As the case study demonstrates, living with CKD or established renal failure (ERF) is an arduous and life-changing experience. There are many complexities associated with the pathophysiology of the disease process, the prescribed treatment regimen and the emotional and psychosocial response to this long-term chronic condition. As such, while on placement you will be involved in care and treatment that is assessed and managed by a broad ranging multidisciplinary team who work closely together to ensure the approach is holistic and patient centred. In 2002, the British Renal Society recognised that 'coordinated service delivery requires an integrated multi-professional team with the range of skills, competencies and responsibilities to manage patients throughout their journey of care' (p.6).

While on placement you are likely to work with the following members of the MPT:

- The Nephrologist (renal doctor) – A medical consultant who has specialised in caring for people with kidney disease and kidney failure.
- Nephrology Nurse (renal nurse) – A qualified nurse who has engaged in further study to specialise in renal care. Nephrology or renal nurses can be ward specialists or dialysis specialists or further subspecialise to become renal transplant, anaemia management, pre-dialysis, end of life care, vascular access or renal research nurse specialists.
- Renal Dieticians – These are dieticians who specialise in the nutritional needs of people with CKD or ERF. This is because the diet that must be followed by people with CKD or with ERF is highly specialised and can also require them to drink a limited volume of fluid of between 500 to 750 mls per 24-hour period.
- Renal Pharmacist – Has a high profile within the MPT and helps to manage the complex regime of medications that are often prescribed for renal patients.
- Renal Social Worker – A support person for patients both before and after they start dialysis. Social workers are highly educated and trained to help patients and their families by providing support in all areas of their lives including: emotional, financial, career, lifestyle adjustment and more.
- Renal Psychologist – Psychologists provide assessment and counselling services. They work closely with the healthcare team in the hospital and in the community to contribute to the patients' health and emotional wellbeing.

As a student nurse working as part of the MPT, you may also need to liaise closely with psychiatrists, psychologists or psychotherapists as many patients have mental health issues. Additionally, you may work with physiotherapists as there are many patients with mobility issues, and also with occupational therapists who assist with making reasonable adjustments to people's homes once discharged from hospital.

OPTIONS TO TREAT KIDNEY DISEASE

Depending on the underlying cause, some types of kidney disease can be treated. For example, AKI can be successfully treated by applying a care bundle that includes ABCDE assessment, observation and NEWS score, treatment of underlying causes such as sepsis and the management of fluid status and medications (NHS Think Kidneys, 2015). Often though, CKD has no cure. In general, treatment consists of measures to help control signs and symptoms, reduce complications, and slow progression of the disease. However, if kidneys become severely damaged and CKD Stage 5 is reached then renal replacement therapies are required; these include transplantation, haemodialysis and peritoneal dialysis.

ABCDE assessment of the patient with AKI or CKD

As the kidneys fail and urine production diminishes (the individual becoming **oliguric** or **anuric**), fluid is retained within the body, excessive fluid volume arises and there is also a retention of electrolytes. As a result, excess fluid leaks into the interstitial spaces and forms oedema. At its most severe this can be life threatening leading to pulmonary oedema, respiratory failure and severe hypertension; when it is less severe, this increase in fluid volume can lead to uncomfortable peripheral oedema that inhibits mobility and contributes to hypertension. For the patient maintained on dialysis it is crucial to control the degree of fluid volume disturbance by setting a realistic target weight. Patients diagnosed with AKI or CKD can deteriorate quickly and dramatically, consequently, a systematic approach to assessing and treating them is critical. In 2006, the British Resuscitation Council recommended that clinical staff should follow the airway, breathing, circulation, disability and exposure (ABCDE) approach when assessing and treating critically ill patients to ensure that such critical illness is promptly identified and appropriately managed (Jevon, 2010).

Referring to the principles of the ABCDE approach, assess the following case:

SEE ALSO
CHAPTER 9

CASE STUDY 28.2: MR AKWASI

Mr Akwasi, an 80-year-old gentleman from Ghana, was referred by his GP to A&E. Mr Akwasi is tired but alert and responsive to voice. He has a decreased urinary output and elevation of creatinine from 110 µmol/L to 250 µmol/L. On examination his blood pressure is 170/110, pulse 98 bpm, respirations 20 per minute and weight 70kg. A firm mass was palpable arising above the pubis. He is also diabetic.

Using what you have learned from this chapter so far:

- identify the presenting stage of AKI
- use the ABCDE approach to assess Mr Akwasi's clinical status
- think about the pre-, intra- and post-renal causes of AKI
- identify the most likely predisposing factors for Mr Akwasi's AKI.

Principles of renal replacement therapy

There are three main types of treatment for kidney failure: collectively these are known as renal replacement therapy, but individually these are haemodialysis, peritoneal dialysis and kidney transplantation. Renal replacement therapy is indicated in all of the following:

- fluid overload
- hyperkalaemia
- symptomatic uraemia
- severe acidosis
- removal of toxins.

Haemodialysis (HD)

This form of dialysis removes waste products from the blood by passing it out of the body, through a filtering system (dialyser) often referred to as an 'artificial kidney' and returning it, cleaned, to the body (see Figure 28.5). Blood passes from the body via a specially created vascular access point called an arterio-venous fistula (AVF) to a filtering system. While in the filtering system, the blood flows through tubes made of a membrane that allows the waste products (which are much smaller than blood cells) to pass out through it.

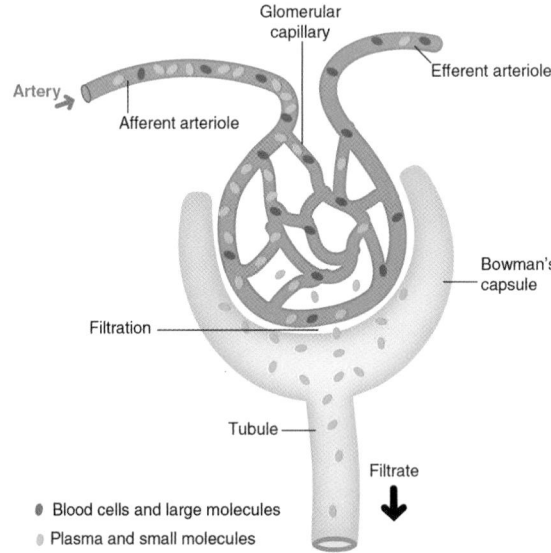

Figure 28.4 Filtration in the glomerulus of the kidney

Source: Boore et al. (2016). Illustrated by Shaun Mercier © SAGE Publications.

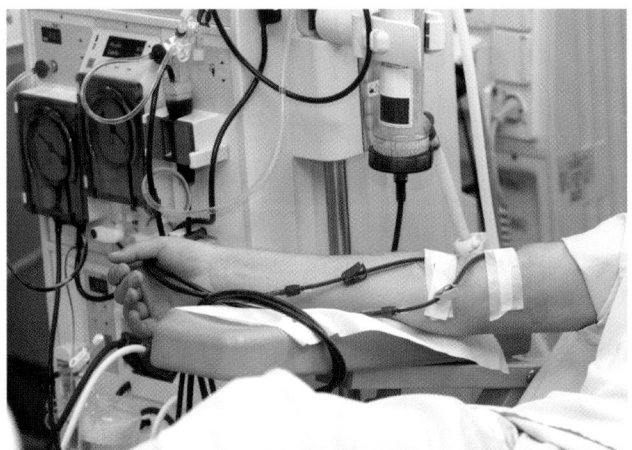

Figure 28.5 Haemodialysis

Source: Shutterstock

Peritoneal dialysis (PD)

With this method, instead of being cleaned by an artificial membrane (dialyser) outside the body, the blood is cleaned inside the body, through the peritoneum. This is the thin membrane that surrounds the outside of the organs in the abdomen. The peritoneum allows waste products to pass through it and is very rich in small blood vessels. By running a dialysis fluid into the peritoneal cavity, through a tube called a PD catheter, and then out again, waste can be filtered from the blood (see Figure 28.6).

For both HD and PD the patient must also learn to adapt to a highly modified diet and a reduced fluid intake in order to help to manage fluid and electrolyte balance.

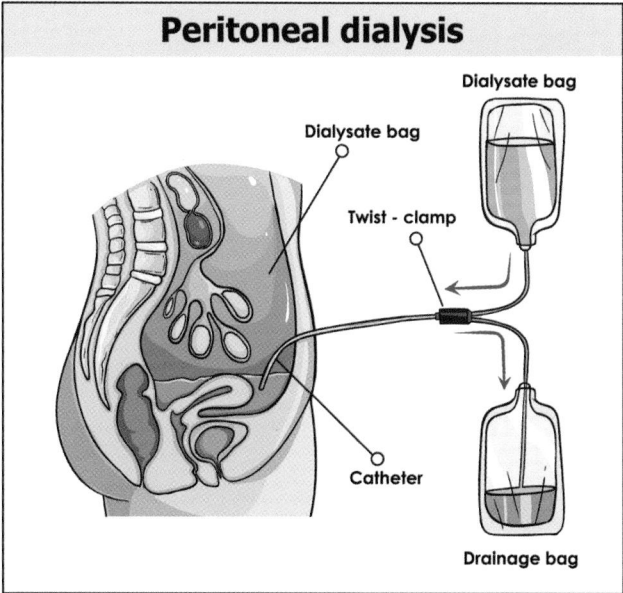

Figure 28.6   Peritoneal dialysis
Source: Science Photo Library

Vascular access

Vascular access is a haemodialysis patient's lifeline and makes life-saving haemodialysis treatments possible. An AV fistula (AVF) is a connection, made by a vascular surgeon, of an artery to a vein (see Figure 28.7). The surgeon usually places an AV fistula in the forearm or upper arm. An AV fistula causes extra pressure and extra blood to flow into the vein, making it grow large and strong. The larger vein provides easy, reliable access to blood vessels. Without this kind of access, regular haemodialysis sessions would not be possible. Untreated veins cannot withstand repeated needle insertions; they would collapse the way a straw collapses under strong suction. However, sometimes the veins are too damaged and an AV fistula cannot be formed, in which case the patient must dialyse via a temporary or permanent catheter that is inserted into the subclavian vein and sits in the right atrium. Infection is a major risk with this type of access, thus the nursing team must take special care when manipulating these during a dialysis session.

An alternative form of vascular access for haemodialysis is the central venous catheter. These can be tunnelled under the skin for more permanent use and with a lower risk of infection, or be non-tunnelled for use in an acute or emergency situation.

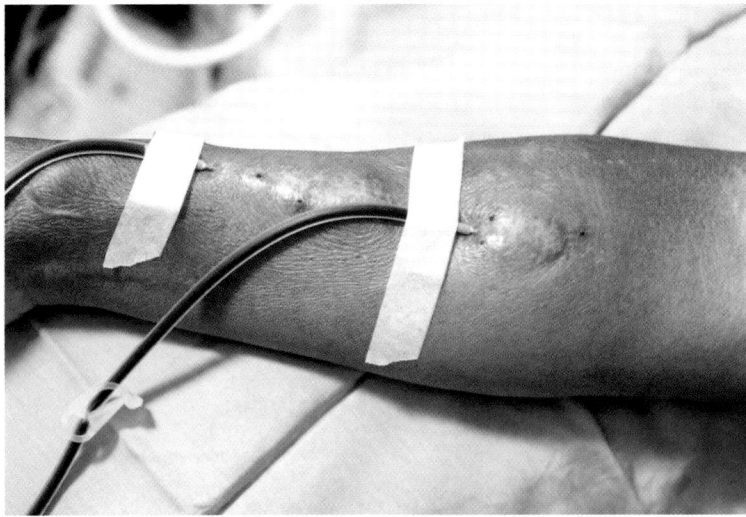

Figure 28.7   Arterio Venous Fistula
Source: Shutterstock

Kidney transplantation

This is a surgical procedure whereby a kidney is removed from a donor patient and transplanted into a recipient patient (see Figure 28.8), who must then take immunosuppressant drugs to prevent the kidney from being rejected. This procedure thus restores kidney function and the patient no longer requires dialysis, and does not have to adhere to a specially modified renal diet or reduced fluid intake. Suitable donor kidneys can be taken from consenting, medically assessed healthy relatives of the recipient (live related donors), consenting medically assessed healthy individuals who are unrelated to the recipient (unrelated live donors) or from individuals who have recently passed away, but who agreed to become a registered organ donor whilst alive (cadaveric donors).

Psychosocial impact of kidney disease

The management of weight, fluid balance, dialysis treatment and a specially modified renal diet for patients with kidney failure have a significant impact on patients' psychological and social wellbeing. This is further complicated by the fact that dialysis is an unrelenting life-long treatment.

Where the patient experiences problems in treatment management there are reports of the patient feeling powerless because treatment is often determined solely by the renal care team instead of involving the patient in a shared decision-making process. But there is evidence to suggest that involving patients in their own care may achieve an improved quality of life and lower mortality rates (Speigel et al., 2007). Self-management courses, often referred to as 'shared-care' programmes, have been developed in parts of the UK. These courses provide renal nurses with the skills to educate and teach patients and their carers to manage aspects of their own care in dialysis units. The programme has enabled patients to gain the confidence and skills to dialyse at home.

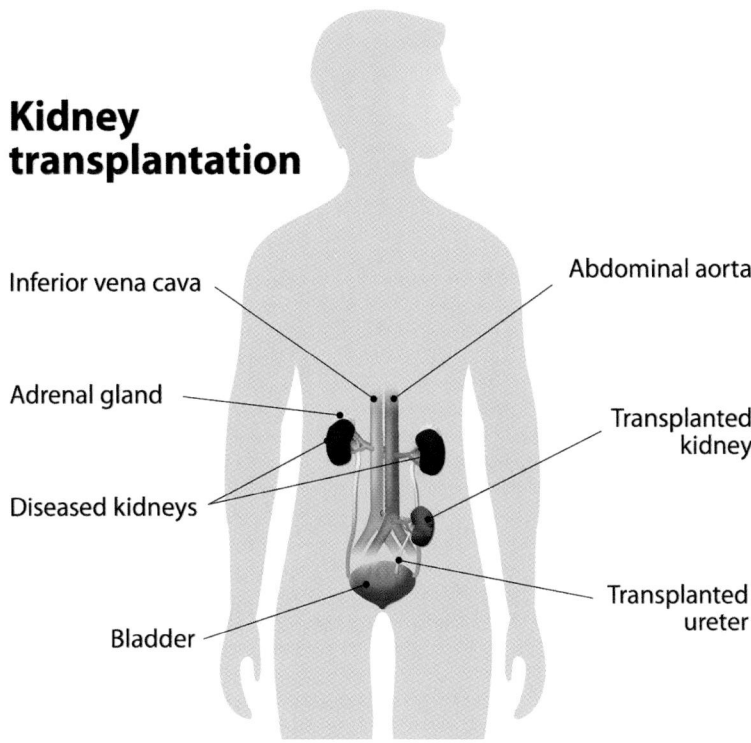

Figure 28.8 Kidney transplantation

Source: Shutterstock

CHAPTER SUMMARY

- Treatment options for renal/urinary system disorders consist of measures to help control signs and symptoms, reduce complications, and slow progression of the disease.
- Management of renal/urinary system disorders can be done medically or surgically and in some instances a combined approach is required.
- Nurses have an important role to play in the prevention, identification and management of renal/urinary system conditions.
- Health promotion has proven benefits for adults living with a renal/urinary condition.

GO FURTHER

Go to https://study.sagepub.com/essentialadultnursing for a further case study related to this chapter. If you are using the interactive ebook, simply click on the book icon in the margin to go straight to the resource.

CASE STUDY: CHRONIC KIDNEY DISEASE

Books

- Daugirdas, J.T. (2014) *Handbook of Dialysis* (5th ed.). Philadelphia: Lippincott Williams and Wilkins. This book provides comprehensive information on both types of dialysis.

- Daugirdas, J.T. (2011) *Handbook of Chronic Kidney Disease Management*. Philadelphia: Lippincott Williams and Wilkins.
  Provides an overview of the complex management of CKD.
- Danovitch, G.M. (2009) *Handbook of Kidney Transplantation* (5th ed.). Philadelphia: Lippincott Williams and Wilkins.
  An excellent book focusing on renal transplantation issues.
- Delves-Yates, C. (2015) *Essentials of Nursing Practice*. London: SAGE
  Page 550 provides a step-by-step guide to performing urinalysis.
- Eaton, C.D. and Pooler, J.P. (2013) *Vander's Renal Physiology* (8th ed.). New York: McGraw Hill.
- Field, M.J., Pollock, C. and Harris, D. (2010) *The Renal System* (2nd ed.). London: Elsevier Health Sciences.
  These books will help you to understand the renal system and gain a fuller appreciation of the consequences of kidney failure.
- Thomas, N. (2014) *Renal Nursing* (4th ed.). New York: Wiley-Blackwell.
  A very good book which focuses on renal nursing.

FURTHER READING: JOURNAL ARTICLES

Journal Articles

Go to https://study.sagepub.com/essentialadultnursing for further free online journal articles related to this chapter. If you are using the interactive ebook, simply click on the book icon in the margin to go straight to the resource.

- El-Sherbini, N. (2016) Nutritional considerations in haemodialysis patients with diabetes. *Journal of Kidney Care*, 1 (4): 178–85.
  This article offers a good insight into the complexity of managing a renal diabetic diet and consolidates the importance of multi-professional support for chronic renal failure patients with diabetes.
- Quallich, S.A., Bumpus, S.M. and Lajiness, S. (2015) Competencies for the nurse practitioner working with adult urology patients. *Urologic Nursing*, September–October 2015, 35 (5): 221–30.
  Although this is an American publication it discusses in detail the urology-specific competencies for urology nurse practitioners that have relevance to the UK.
- Razmaria, A.A. (2016) Chronic Kidney Disease. *JAMA*, 315 (20): 2248. doi:10.1001/jama.2016.1426.
  This article provides a good basic overview of chronic kidney disease. While aimed at patients it offers a good foundation for student nurses new to renal disease.

FURTHER READING: WEBLINKS

Weblinks

Go to https://study.sagepub.com/essentialadultnursing for further weblinks related to this chapter. If you are using the interactive ebook, simply click on the book icon in the margin to go straight to the resource.

- www.britishrenal.org/
  The website of the British Renal Society is a registered charity which aims to coordinate the promotion and delivery of effective, patient-centred care for patients with renal disease.
- www.renal.org
  The website of the Renal Association which is the professional body for United Kingdom nephrologists (renal physicians, or kidney doctors) and renal scientists in the UK.
- www.thinkkidneys.nhs.uk/
  This is a link to the NHS think kidneys campaign to raise awareness of kidney failure.
- www.shareddialysis-care.org.uk/
  This is a link to Yorkshire & the Humber 'Sharing Haemodialysis Care' project.
- www.uhb.nhs.uk/Downloads/pdf/PiKidneyBiopsy.pdf
  This is a sample patient information leaflet on renal biopsies.

- http://library.med.utah.edu/WebPath/TUTORIAL/URINE/URINE.html
  This website provides a clear overview of urinalysis including dip testing and microscopic examination of urine.
- www.renal.org/information-resources/information
  An example of a useful resource for both staff and patients for information about fluid and dietary management on dialysis.
- www.innerbody.com/image/urinov.html
  This is an interactive website which will help you to consolidate your knowledge of normal anatomy and physiology of the renal system.
- www.handwrittentutorials.com/videos.php?id=72
  This is a handwritten tutorial on the gross anatomy of the kidney.

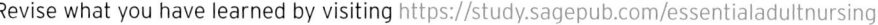

ACE YOUR ASSESSMENT

ONLINE QUIZZES

Revise what you have learned by visiting https://study.sagepub.com/essentialadultnursing

- Test yourself with multiple-choice and short-answer questions
- Do the chapter activities in the book and check your answers online

REFERENCES

British Renal Society (2002) *Recommendations of the National Renal Workforce Planning Group.* Available at: www.britishrenal.org/BritishRenalSociety/files/24/24f2096f-442e-44c3-9ae0-51d9382b5292.pdf. [accessed 9th March 2016)].

Echeverry, G., Hortin, G.L. and Rai, A.J. (2010) Introduction to urinalysis: Historical perspectives and clinical application. *Methods Mol Biol*, 641: 1–12. doi: 10.1007/978-1-60761-711-2_1.

Jevon, P. (2010) Assessment of critically ill patients: The ABCDE approach. *British Journal of Healthcare Assistants*, August 2010, Vol 04, No 08.

Kidney Disease Improving Global Outcomes (KDIGO) (2013) KDIGO 2012 Clinical Practice Guideline for the Evaluation and Management of Chronic Kidney Disease. Volume 3, issue 1, January. Available at: www.kidney-international.org [accessed 26th July 2016].

Kidney Research UK (2016) www.kidneyresearchuk.org/?gclid=CMT6po_ykM4CFRATGwodkbUDEg [accessed 9th March 2018].

Mattson Porth, C. and Matfin, G. (2008) *Pathophysiology. Concepts of altered health states* (8th ed.). Philadelphia: Lippincott Williams and Wilkins.

NHS Choices (2016) *Kidney Cancer.* Available at: www.nhs.uk/conditions/cancer-of-the-kidney/Pages/Introduction.aspx [accessed 9th March 2018].

NHS Think Kidneys (2015) *Recommended Minimum Requirements of a Care Bundle for Patients with AKI in Hospital.* Available at: www.thinkkidneys.nhs.uk/aki/wp-content/uploads/sites/2/2015/12/AKI-care-bundle-requirements-FINAL-12.07.16.pdf_[accessed 9th March 2018].

NICE (2014) *Acute Kidney Injury.* Available at: http://cks.nice.org.uk/acute-kidney-injury [accessed 9th March 2018].

NICE (2015) *Urinary Tract Infections in Adults.* Quality standard [QS90]. Available at: www.nice.org.uk/guidance/qs90 [accessed 9th March 2018].

Preminger, G.M. (2016) *Urinary Tract Obstruction*. Merck and Co., Inc., Manual. Available at: www.msdmanuals.com/en-gb/professional/genitourinary-disorders/obstructive-uropathy/obstructive-uropathy [accessed 9th March 2018].

Renal Association (2009) *UK Renal Registry 12th Annual Report*. Available at: https://www.renalreg.org/reports/2009-the-twelfth-annual-report [accessed 9th March 2018].

Renal Association (2011) *UK Renal Registry 14th Annual Report*. Available at: https://www.renalreg.org/reports/2001-the-fourteenth-annual-report [accessed 9th March 2018].

Renal Association (2013) Available at: www.renal.org/information-resources/the-uk-eckd-guide/ckd-stages#sthash.xEzhI6bU.dpbs [accessed 9th March 2018].

Schmitz, P.G. and Maddukuri, G. (2015) *Kidneys, ureters, and bladder imaging*. Medscape. Available at: http://emedicine.medscape.com/article/2165400-overview [accessed 9thMarch 2018].

Speigel, D.M. et al. (2007) Factors associated with mortality in patients new to haemodialysis. *Nephro Dial Transplant*, 22 (12).

CARE OF THE ADULT WITH AN ENDOCRINE CONDITION

29

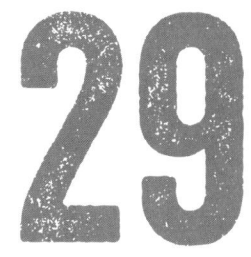

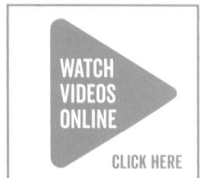

WATCH VIDEOS ONLINE — CLICK HERE

MARK MOLESWORTH AND MOIRA LEWITT

THIS CHAPTER COVERS:

- The regulation of hormone secretion
- Case studies featuring individuals with type 2 diabetes and Graves' disease
- Pathophysiology and clinical characteristics related to diabetes and Graves' disease
- Nursing assessment and clinical investigations
- Nursing care and management.

"

I was first diagnosed with type 1 diabetes mellitus at the age of thirteen. Living with diabetes comes naturally to me, I was able to take the diagnosis in my stride and complete all my ambitions with help and guidance from the diabetes team.

Jemma, aged 25 and has type 1 diabetes

"

"

I hadn't been feeling myself for a few months and knew something was wrong with my body. It was worrying as I didn't know why I felt the way I did. I was eventually told I had Graves' disease.

Pauline, aged 48 and has Graves' disease

"

INTRODUCTION

This chapter focuses on the care of an adult with an endocrine condition. We begin with an overview of hormone regulation, and then move on to focus on two common endocrine conditions: diabetes and hyperthyroidism. Two case studies are presented to support your learning. These go into more detail than the quotes above, but the brief insights shared by Jemma and Pauline are still very useful. In the aftermath of her diagnosis, Jemma learnt to manage her condition in a positive and empowered way with support from the diabetes team. Meanwhile, Pauline highlights the wide-ranging impact that a condition such as Graves' disease can have on a person. The anxiety she felt in relation to inexplicable changes to her body is something that many people will be able to relate to. As a student nurse contributing to the inter-professional team in a range of health and social care settings, it is likely that you will care for people who, like Jemma and Pauline, have been affected by an endocrine condition.

A person with an endocrine condition may come into initial contact with health and social care services in various ways. For example, this might be via an outreach service, a school nurse, while receiving treatment for another condition, or via the emergency department. Often the first point of contact is the person's registered General Practice surgery where a GP or practice nurse will assess and investigate the presenting signs and symptoms. The person may then be treated at the surgery or referred to a wide range of health and social care services depending upon the person's holistic needs. Sometimes, referral to an endocrinologist, a physician specialising in diagnosing and treating patients with an endocrine disorder, is necessary. This chapter will support you to develop your understanding of the nurse's role in assessing and managing common endocrine conditions using patient-centred approaches.

ANATOMY AND PHYSIOLOGY

Endocrine system

The endocrine system consists of a set of glands (see Figure 29.1) and diffuse mechanisms which are responsible for releasing agents that directly or indirectly control many of the processes and responses necessary to ensure life. This gives the endocrine system an undeniable complexity, but it also means it is a feature in many of the health conditions that you will encounter within practice placement settings. The following sections introduce some of the key principles related to the anatomy and physiology of this important system.

Regulation of hormone secretion

The many constituent parts of the endocrine system work alongside those of the nervous system to coordinate the functions of cells, tissues and organs. This is achieved through the release of chemical mediators, called hormones, which have effects on cells throughout the body. The hypothalamus and the pituitary gland are located at the base of the brain and together control many endocrine functions (see Figure 29.2). They are connected via the pituitary stalk and a portal blood system, which enables the hypothalamus to regulate the release of hormones from the pituitary gland. The pituitary gland has two primary sections called the anterior and posterior lobes. The anterior lobe is controlled via stimulating/inhibiting hormones released from the hypothalamus, while the posterior lobe is controlled via nerve impulses, which originate in the hypothalamus.

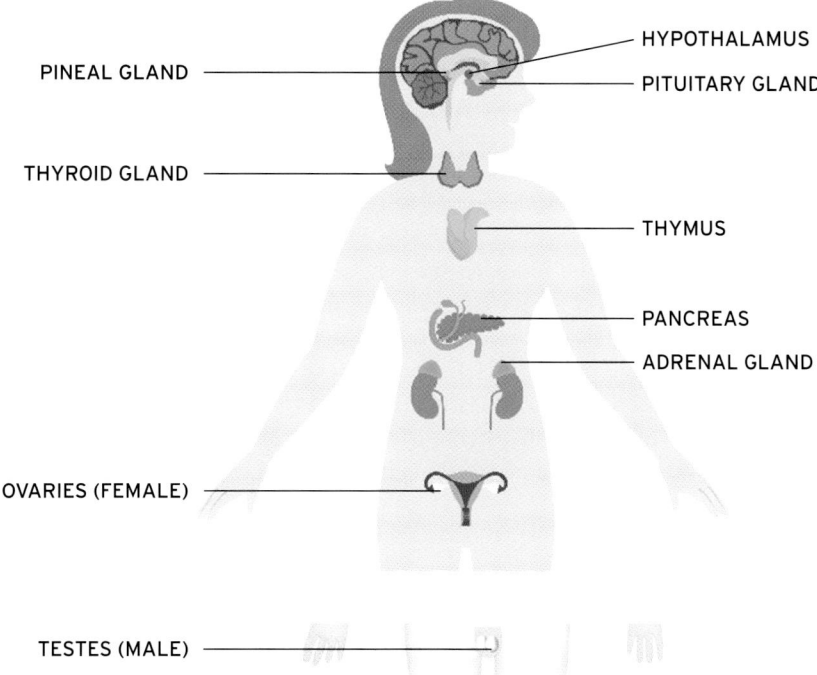

Figure 29.1   The main endocrine glands

Source: Adobe Stock

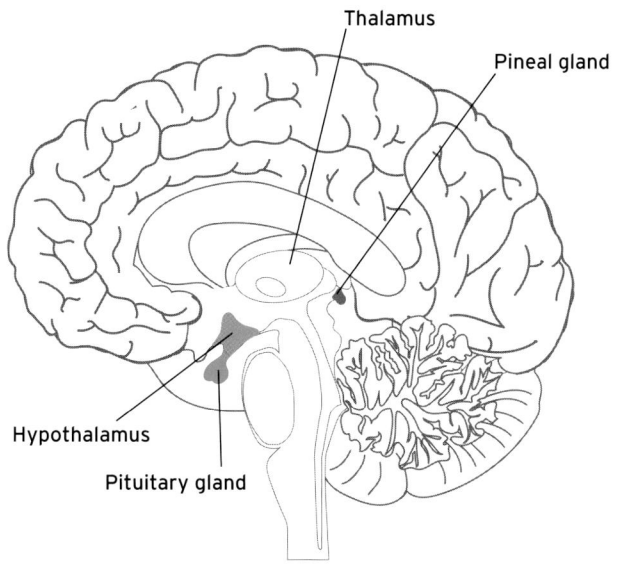

Figure 29.2   Hypothalamus and pituitary gland

Source: Boore et al. (2016). Illustrated by Shaun Mercier, © SAGE Publications.

Hormones are mainly of two types: peptide and protein hormones that are synthesised from amino acids, and steroid hormones that are derived from cholesterol. In general, peptide or protein hormones exert their effects through receptors on the surface of cells, while lipid-soluble steroid hormones act through intracellular receptors. Hormone levels in the bloodstream are tightly regulated at multiple levels, and the pattern of secretion is important for normal physiological activity. Growth hormone, for example, is secreted in pulsatile bursts, and this is important for its proper effect on body growth. Messages from the central and autonomic nervous systems play important roles in regulating hormone secretion. Central effects are important, for example, in determining the secretion of hypothalamic messengers that stimulate or inhibit pituitary hormone secretion. Pituitary hormone secretion is also regulated by feedback of the hormones produced by the target tissues. The pituitary hormones either directly affect the target cells or instruct other parts of the endocrine system to release their hormones. The process is often controlled via a negative feedback system (see Figure 29.3). In this way homeostasis is achieved. If a person develops an endocrine condition then the secretion of specific hormones will be disrupted. This can adversely affect the wellbeing of the individual and may be life threatening in some cases. We will discuss examples later in the chapter.

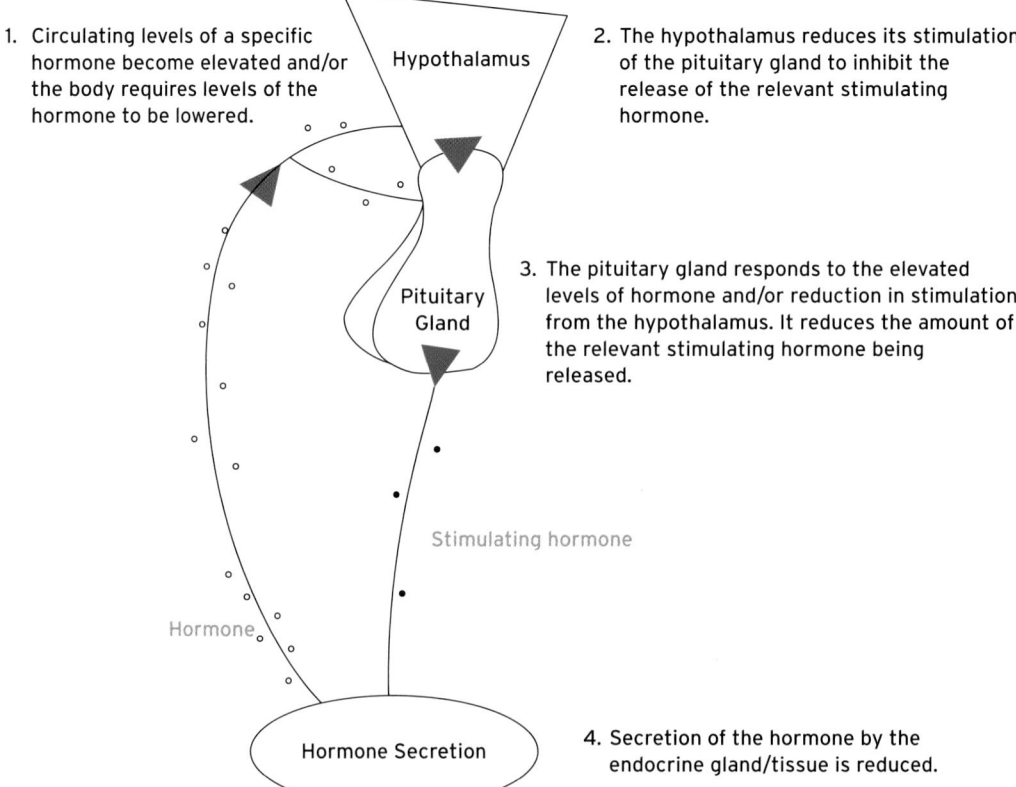

1. Circulating levels of a specific hormone become elevated and/or the body requires levels of the hormone to be lowered.

Hypothalamus

2. The hypothalamus reduces its stimulation of the pituitary gland to inhibit the release of the relevant stimulating hormone.

Pituitary Gland

3. The pituitary gland responds to the elevated levels of hormone and/or reduction in stimulation from the hypothalamus. It reduces the amount of the relevant stimulating hormone being released.

Stimulating hormone

Hormone

Hormone Secretion

4. Secretion of the hormone by the endocrine gland/tissue is reduced.

Figure 29.3   An example of a negative feedback system for control of hormone secretion

© Mark Molesworth

A positive feedback system is used to control the release of some hormones. This is a similar process to the negative feedback system except that, in response to a change in the body, levels of the hormone are increased rather than decreased. A good example takes place during childbirth where the hormone oxytocin is released to stimulate uterine contractions through a positive feedback system.

Care of an adult with an endocrine condition

In the following sections, you will learn about the care of an adult with diabetes mellitus. We begin with a case study then explore the pathophysiology and clinical characteristics of diabetes. This is followed by the nursing assessment, care and management of a person with diabetes. Later in the chapter, a case study featuring Graves' disease is introduced and we discuss the same topics as above in relation to hyperthyroidism.

CASE STUDY 29.1: TYPE 2 DIABETES SCENARIO: RAMESH

Ramesh is a 48-year-old man who lives in a large city with his wife and youngest daughter. He enjoys a gentle walk through the local park at least once a week and is an avid reader. Ramesh knows he needs to lose weight but finds it hard to eat healthy options and get enough exercise. Over the past few months he has been feeling fatigued and his sleep has been poor due to regular visits to the toilet. Recently, his vision has been getting blurry and prescription glasses do not help much. During a routine NHS Health Check his blood sugars were found to be high. After some further tests Ramesh was diagnosed with type 2 diabetes.

- Why did Ramesh need to visit the toilet more frequently?
- What is the most likely cause of the changes to his vision?
- How much exercise should Ramesh aim for each week?

Read through the next few sections to check your answers.

Approximately 4.5 million people living in the UK have diabetes, with 700 new diagnoses each day (Diabetes UK, 2016). Of these cases 10% are type 1 diabetes while the remaining 90% of cases are made up of type 2 diabetes (Diabetes UK, 2016). Type 1 diabetes is usually found in young people, accounting for 90% of diabetes in those aged less than 25 years. Type 2 diabetes is more prevalent among people of African, African-Caribbean and South Asian family origin and can occur in all age groups (National Institute for Health Care and Excellence (NICE), 2015). While not a focus of this chapter, it is worth noting that the incidence of type 2 diabetes among children is increasing.

CRITICAL THINKING STOP POINT 29.1

Did you know that type 2 diabetes was previously referred to as *Non-Insulin-Dependent Diabetes Mellitus* (NIDDM) and type 1 diabetes as *Insulin-Dependent Diabetes Mellitus* (IDDM)? Undertake some research online to try to find out why these names are no longer used.

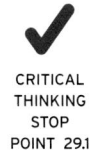

CRITICAL
THINKING
STOP
POINT 29.1

Pathophysiology of diabetes

The pancreas is a large gland that is found behind the stomach. In an exocrine role separate to its endocrine role, the pancreas is responsible for the production and secretion of enzymes which assist with the digestion of food. One of its main endocrine functions is the production and secretion of insulin. This hormone helps to control blood glucose levels by binding to receptors on the surface of cells within the body, enabling a process which allows glucose to move out of the blood and into the cell. Insulin-producing cells are found within small clusters of cells called the islets of Langerhans (see Figure 29.4). The beta cells are responsible for insulin secretion while the alpha cells produce glucagon, which opposes insulin action through increases in glucose production by the liver, and thus blood glucose levels are maintained.

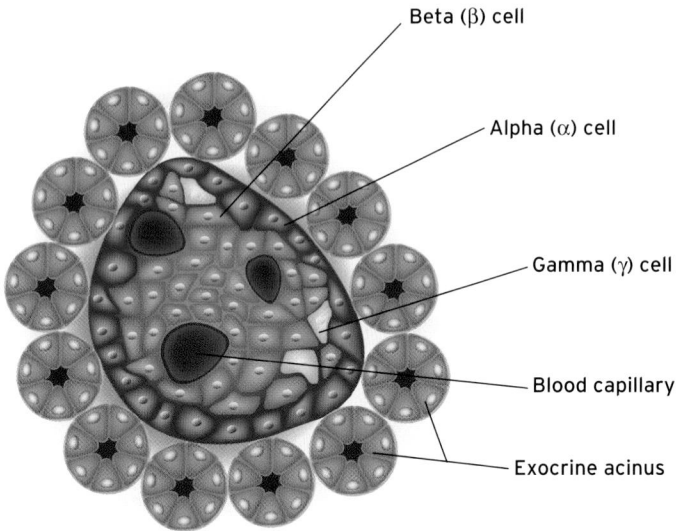

Figure 29.4 Islet of Langerhans

Source: Boore et al. (2016). Illustrated by Shaun Mercier, © SAGE Publications.

In type 1 diabetes the insulin-producing cells in the islets of Langerhans are destroyed through an autoimmune process. This dramatically reduces the body's ability to produce insulin and is life threatening if not treated. Type 2 diabetes results from a more gradual decline in insulin production, along with resistance to the insulin that is produced. You can learn more about the differences between type 1 and type 2 diabetes by completing Activity 29.1. In both type 1 and type 2 diabetes, the cells do not receive the glucose required to function normally and abnormal protein and fat metabolism may occur. Diabetes increases the risk of stroke, heart attack, kidney failure, visual impairment and lower limb amputation. This increased risk can often be mitigated through effective self-management, healthy lifestyle behaviours and access to appropriate support from healthcare professionals.

ACTIVITY 29.1: CRITICAL THINKING

In this activity, you will learn more about the two main types of diabetes. Start by watching this video from Diabetes UK: www.youtube.com/watch?v=X9ivR4yO3DE
Now try to answer the following questions:

1. What role does insulin play in allowing glucose into muscle cells?
2. What causes type 1 diabetes?

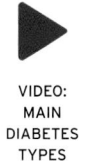

VIDEO:
MAIN
DIABETES
TYPES

3. How does the body remove excess glucose from the blood?
4. What causes type 2 diabetes?
5. What is the main difference in the onset of symptoms between the two main types of diabetes?

Clinical characteristics of diabetes

The clinical characteristics of diabetes usually include the 3Ps: polyuria, polydipsia and polyphagia (see Table 29.1). These symptoms can be severe and develop quickly in type 1 diabetes. A campaign by Diabetes UK (2017) uses the 4Ts to increase awareness among the public about the signs of type 1 diabetes (see Table 29.1). In contrast, a person with type 2 diabetes may remain asymptomatic for many months/years, with symptoms gradually developing if the condition worsens. This is evident in Ramesh's scenario where his condition developed gradually and was only picked up during routine screening. Polyuria results from the body attempting to remove glucose from the blood in urine, raising the osmotic pressure in the filtrate and leading to the production of excess urine. Therefore, patients may need to void urine more frequently. The fluid loss often leads to dehydration, contributing to the excessive thirst (polydipsia) often associated with diabetes. The person's appetite may also increase as a lack of nutrients are able to enter body cells (polyphagia).

Severe insulin deficiency, usually related to type 1 diabetes, can lead to an increase in the amount of fats and proteins being broken down to provide energy. As the body breaks down the fat stored in adipose tissue, there is an increase in fatty acids and their metabolites within the blood. This chain of events can lead to a potentially life-threatening condition called diabetic ketoacidosis (DKA). Patients with type 2 diabetes may develop hyperosmolar hyperglycaemic state (HHS). This is characterised by hyperglycaemia and hyperosmolarity in the absence of significant ketoacidosis, usually occurring when other illnesses and dehydration are present.

Table 29.1 The 3Ps and 4Ts

The classic signs of type 1 diabetes

The 3Ps		The 4Ts
Polyuria	The need to pass urine more frequently.	**T**oilet: going to the toilet a lot.
Polydipsia	Increased feeling of thirst and fluid consumption.	**T**hirst: being thirsty and not able to quench the thirst.
		Tiredness: feeling more tired than usual.
Polyphagia	Increased appetite.	**T**hinner: losing weight or looking thinner than usual.

Source: Diabetes UK (2017)

Diabetes can cause vascular problems with an increased risk that atherosclerosis will develop, causing reduced peripheral circulation and contributing to the higher incidence of heart attacks and strokes. Ramesh may have had high blood glucose levels for many years before diagnosis so will require cardiovascular screening to establish the extent of any damage that is present. Poor circulation increases the risk of ulcers, particularly on the foot or heel, which are difficult to heal. Peripheral neuropathy, which leads to impaired sensation, numbness and weakness, also contributes to the development of ulcers because the person is unaware when prolonged pressure is being exerted on the affected area. Regular foot checks should be completed, normally at annual review as a minimum, and patients should be provided with advice regarding effective foot care. Vascular problems may also affect the blood vessels in the eye, causing diabetic retinopathy. This may explain why Ramesh had been experiencing blurry vision. Diabetic retinopathy may be asymptomatic during the early stages so eye screening at diagnosis, and regularly thereafter, is imperative because visual impairment can often be prevented. It is worth noting that diabetes is just one risk factor for vascular disease, and the management of other risk factors, such as hypertension, abnormal lipid levels and smoking cessation, is necessary.

Nursing assessment of an adult with diabetes

The nursing assessment should go beyond the physical symptoms by using a person-centred approach which aims to understand the individual's experience and needs. It will be important to get as complete a picture as possible as this will assist in supporting the person to manage their condition. In most cases, it will be necessary to assess the person's vital signs, and blood glucose levels should be taken and repeated as appropriate. For a healthy adult, the normal blood glucose levels are 3.9–5.5 mmol/L, except in the period after consumption of food and drink which increase blood sugar levels (Knight et al., 2017). When concentrations of blood glucose exceed normal levels the term hyperglycaemia is used. If this becomes problematic the administration of prescribed insulin may be required, followed by advice on regulating glucose intake as well as support with diabetes medication management if appropriate. When concentrations of blood glucose fall below normal levels the term hypoglycaemia is used. In severe cases, the individual may display behaviours and characteristics which are like that of a person who is intoxicated with alcohol. In this situation, it may be necessary to administer glucose and provide follow-up support and information on managing diabetes effectively.

Clinical investigations for diabetes

Laboratory blood glucose testing is undertaken to establish diagnosis and ongoing screening of diabetes. A glycated haemoglobin (HbA1c) test provides information about a patient's average blood glucose levels over the previous months. The cut off point for diagnosis of diabetes is an HbA1c of 6.5% (48 mmol/mol) (World Health Organization, 2011). Elevated fasted or unfasted blood glucose levels are also indicative of diabetes. Another investigation is the oral glucose tolerance test (OGTT). This involves a person's blood glucose levels being taken before, and after, consuming a drink containing glucose. This indicates how well the body is able to respond to a sharp increase in blood glucose levels and may be used to screen for gestational diabetes, a type of diabetes that develops in the mother during pregnancy and usually resolves following birth. A positive test for glucose in the urine may also indicate diabetes, often requiring further investigation.

A common method of monitoring blood glucose levels is carried out using a glucose meter (see Figure 29.5), a small device that uses a droplet of the person's blood to provide a blood glucose reading. Ensure that you are trained and competent prior to taking a blood glucose reading and always adhere to the manufacturer's guidelines, as well as local policy and procedures.

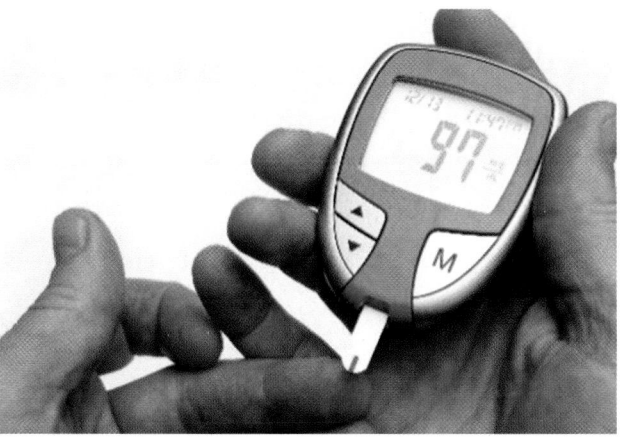

Figure 29.5   A glucose meter

Source: Adobe Stock.

GO FURTHER

If you want to increase your understanding of blood glucose monitoring, consider reading a useful article by Trisha Dunning (2016) called *How to monitor blood glucose*, which is published by the *Nursing Standard* journal. You may be able find this via one of the academic databases provided by your university's library. Alternatively, you can access the relevant information here via the following web address: https://journals.rcni.com/nursing-standard/how-to-monitor-blood-glucose-ns.30.22.36.s45

Ask for assistance from staff at your library if necessary.

WEBLINK: BLOOD GLUCOSE MONITORING

Nursing care and management of a patient with diabetes

A holistic and person-centred approach should be adopted which takes into consideration the physical, psychological, emotional and spiritual needs of the adult with type 2 diabetes. A person who has recently been diagnosed with diabetes may experience a wide range of emotions and is likely to require support during this period. They may also feel overwhelmed by the amount of information they are exposed to following diagnosis. As well as medical and nursing support, they will usually require input from a range of specialists, such as dieticians, ophthalmologists and podiatrists. Remember that patients may experience anxiety, stress and depression requiring specialist psychological support.

It is important to remember that every patient is different in how they understand and deal with diabetes. If the patient needs more support or information then I make them aware that they can book to discuss it with me anytime, thus helping them manage and reduce the potential complications of type 2 diabetes.

Lisa Grant, General Practice Nurse

Nurses are often well placed to support the person's holistic and ongoing care needs within primary care settings. They will often see patients on multiple occasions through routine check-ups (e.g. annual review) and non-routine appointments. A positive and trusting relationship should be developed through effective communication incorporating the use of open questions, listening, observing, summarising and joint goal-setting.

SEE ALSO
CHAPTER 7

HEALTH PROMOTION

Read the information below and then reflect on three ways in which you can ensure your health behaviours are a role model for others to follow.

Nurses have an important role in working with others to promote the health of the individuals within society. Through patient education, providing evidence-based information, raising awareness and helping to deliver national interventions nurses can directly influence the health of individuals and the wider communities within which they work. This may be through traditional methods alongside the increasing area of health promotion via social media and the wider internet (Donnelly, 2017). There is also growing expectation that nurses are role models for healthy behaviours (Kelly et al., 2017). We would argue that nurses also have a role in recognising and reducing the impact of the structural factors that contribute to health inequalities within society.

Health promotion is crucial to reducing the incidence of type 2 diabetes, and ensuring the risk of complications and co-morbidities is minimised. Obesity significantly increases the risk of type 2 diabetes so weight loss is usually desirable. For patients who have been diagnosed with diabetes, weight loss also reduces the likelihood of complications. The weekly physical activity guidelines for adults are a total of 150 minutes of moderate aerobic activity combined with strength exercises on two or more days (NHS Choices, 2015). Ramesh requires support in this area as he finds it hard to get enough exercise. Initially the guidelines may seem like a lot to achieve in one week, so it may be helpful to break the time up into short, regular periods. This might consist of 30 minutes of moderate activity (such as cycling and brisk walking) on five days of the week, for example. Strength exercises incorporating all the muscle groups should also be undertaken on at least two days of the week. The amount of time when a person spends extended periods in sedentary positions (e.g. sitting watching the TV) should be kept to a minimum.

Individuals may benefit from information and support for smoking cessation and safe alcohol consumption. To keep health risks from alcohol to a low level it is safest not to drink more than 14 units a week on a regular basis (Department of Health, 2016). Promoting a healthy balanced diet using resources such as the Eatwell Guide (Public Health England, 2016) can help individuals make better choices about the food and drink they consume. This may be through increasing their intake of fibre (particularly soluble fibre) by eating more whole grain food, for example. Reducing the number of liquid calories consumed is another beneficial change, often achieved by drinking less fizzy drinks and fruit juices, which may contain high levels of sugar.

Self-management is a concept where the person takes ownership of their condition, incorporating a process through which a person becomes empowered to manage their life with diabetes. It is not done by a single action or delivered by one organisation. It is reliant on the person working together with individuals and organisations who offer support, guidance and information. Interventions, such as motivational interviewing, cognitive behaviour therapy and conversation maps, may assist the person to manage their diabetes.

WHAT'S THE EVIDENCE? 29.1

Zhao et al. (2017) carried out a systematic review of randomised controlled trials exploring the efficacy of different theory-based self-management educational interventions for patients with type 2 diabetes. They found that greater patient involvement during the development of self-management educational interventions made them more effective.

All adults with type 2 diabetes should have access to a structured education programme following diagnosis (NICE, 2015; Scottish Intercollegiate Guidelines Network (SIGN), 2010). A popular structured education programme is the 'Diabetes Education and Self-Management for Ongoing and Newly Diagnosed' (DESMOND) which incorporates a suite of different programmes. One of the most popular programmes is the 'newly diagnosed' module, which offers the first steps in self-management education for people with type 2 diabetes. This programme is available UK-wide and typically runs over one to two days. Patients are often referred by their GP or practice nurse following their diagnosis of type 2 diabetes. Patients who undertake the course receive information and support from DESMOND-trained educators, diabetic specialist nurses and dieticians. The curriculum covers areas including understanding what diabetes is, common symptoms, treatment options, blood glucose monitoring (see Figure 29.6), diet, physical activity and long-term complications/screening. A popular alternative to DESMOND is X-PERT Health, which offers a selection of diabetes-related programmes by trained educators. An adult who has been diagnosed with type 1 diabetes may benefit from the 'Dose Adjustment For Normal Eating' (DAFNE) programme, particularly if they are experiencing problems with hypoglycaemia or fail to achieve glycaemic targets (SIGN, 2010). It provides people with skills and knowledge to help them to manage their condition.

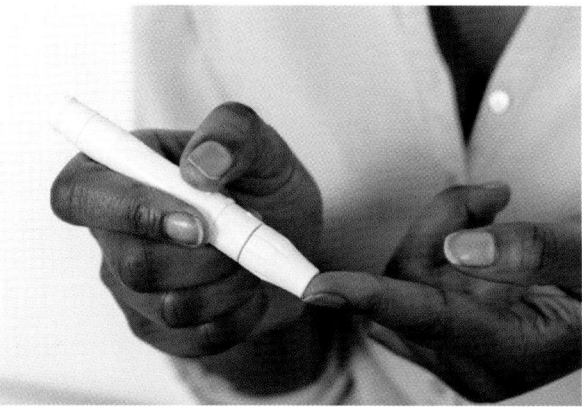

Figure 29.6   A person acquiring a sample of their own blood using a lancing device

Source: Adobe Stock

GO FURTHER

WEBLINK: DESMOND PROJECT

Undertake some further research into the DESMOND project by visiting its website: www.desmond-project.org.uk

Find out more about the programme by clicking on the *About* page. Review the process for becoming a DESMOND educator in the *Professional Development* page. You can also find out which DESMOND Centre/s are closest to your location via the interactive map.

GRAVES' DISEASE

CASE STUDY 29.2: KIM

Kim is 36 years old and lives with her wife in a seaside town. She works as a store manager for a large supermarket. Work is enjoyable, but Kim's real passion is reserved for the pet lizards (a bearded dragon and two geckos) they keep at home. Recently, Kim noticed that she was getting thinner than usual despite eating at least as much as before. She also noticed changes to her mood, becoming noticeably more agitated, restless and anxious. Kim learnt that an autoimmune response called Graves' disease had resulted in her developing hyperthyroidism – an overactive thyroid. Her condition was managed with medications initially but the symptoms persisted. In response, Kim was treated with radioactive iodine and her condition went into remission.

1. Why did Kim lose weight?
2. Why is radioactive iodine sometimes used to treat an overactive thyroid?
3. Name an alternative form of ablative therapy for hyperthyroidism.

Read through the next few sections to check your answers.

In the following sections, we'll focus on hyperthyroidism, another common endocrine disorder. One of the main causes of this condition, Graves' disease, will be introduced. As with type 2 diabetes, hyperthyroidism is another condition where an individual may first present with a range of non-specific signs and symptoms. For this reason, detailed and holistic assessment will assist with the identification of potential problems, which can then be explored through biochemistry and other clinical investigations. While this section focuses on primary thyroid abnormality it is important that you are aware that other disorders (e.g. diseases affecting the pituitary gland) can also influence thyroid function, with or without primary abnormality of the thyroid gland.

Pathophysiology of hyperthyroidism

The thyroid is a butterfly-shaped gland located anterior to the larynx and trachea in the neck (see Figure 29.7). It secretes thyroid hormones, which have wide-ranging effects within the body, including the maintenance of the basal metabolic rate, and regulating growth and development.

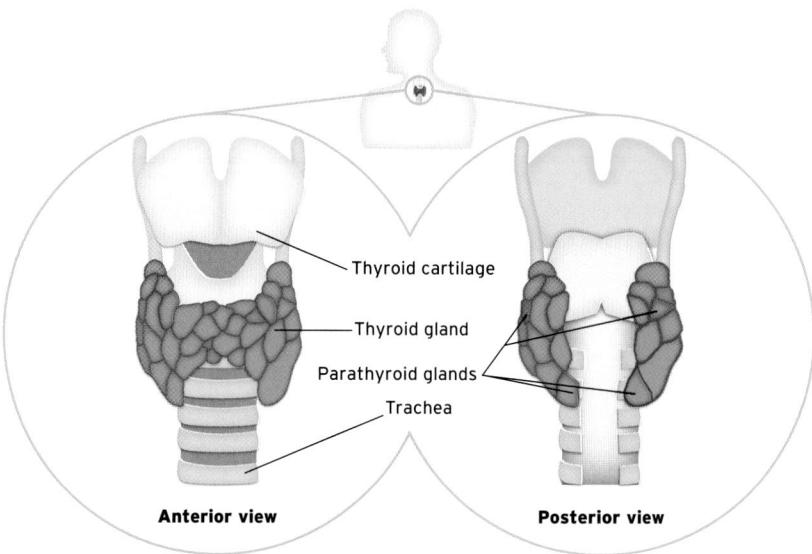

Figure 29.7 Image showing the thyroid gland

Source: Boore et al. (2016). Illustrated by Shaun Mercier, © SAGE Publications

The thyroid produces, stores and secretes two hormones: thyroxine (T4) and triiodothyronine (T3). Iodine is required to produce both hormones and is actively transported into the thyroid follicle, where thyroglobulin plays a key role in thyroid hormone synthesis. T3 is produced by a combination of a tyrosine module that contains iodine at a single site (monoiodotyrosine or T1) with a tyrosine module at two sites (diiodotyrosine or T2), while T4 consists of two T2 molecules. It is this process which explains why the thyroid is dependent upon sufficient levels of iodine.

Production of T3 and T4 is stimulated by the action of thyroid stimulating hormone (TSH), a pituitary hormone that is itself stimulated by thyrotropin releasing hormone (TRH). TRH is secreted from the hypothalamus in response to a negative feedback system (see Figure 29.3) for T3 and T4. TSH stimulates the thyroid to synthesise and release more T4 and, to a lesser extent, T3. Once the thyroid hormones have entered the target cells they stimulate enzymes that are involved in glucose oxidation. Thus, increased secretion of T3 and T4 raises the basal metabolic rate with increased oxygen consumption by target cells and the production of body heat. Thyroid hormones increase the basal metabolic rate, with widespread effects on the cardiovascular system, protein carbohydrate and lipid metabolism of nutrients, the nervous system and other tissues.

Graves' disease is an autoimmune disease that results in hyperthyroidism. It is likely that environmental and genetic factors combine to cause Graves' disease, but the exact mechanism is unknown. It results in an overactive thyroid, which usually becomes enlarged and secretes more T3 and T4 than is required. Cells within the body respond to the increased levels of thyroid hormones accordingly and a broad range of symptoms result.

Clinical characteristics of hyperthyroidism

The main signs and symptoms of hyperthyroidism are shown in Table 29.2. We have contrasted these with hypothyroidism, an underactive thyroid, to demonstrate the different characteristics each bring.

Table 29.2 Signs and symptoms of hyperthyroidism and hypothyroidism

Hyperthyroidism	Hypothyroidism
• Tachycardia	• Bradycardia
• Palpitations	• Fatigue/lack of energy
• Restlessness	• Weight gain
• Moist skin/increased sweating	• Cold/dry skin
• Heat intolerance	• Muscle and joint pain
• Diarrhoea	• Constipation
• Tremors	• Tiredness/sleepiness
• Irritability	• Depression
• Hair loss	• Hair loss

In the case study Kim experienced weight loss, even though she was eating more than normal. This is because her body is using up more energy resulting from the increase in basal metabolic rate caused by hyperthyroidism. Anxiety is a common psychological symptom of hyperthyroidism, particularly where there is a rapid increase in thyroid hormone levels. A related clinical characteristic of hyperthyroidism is an increased heart rate, potentially leading to tachycardia. In many cases the person's skin is excessively warm and they may be more heat intolerant and prone to increased sweating (see Figure 29.8).

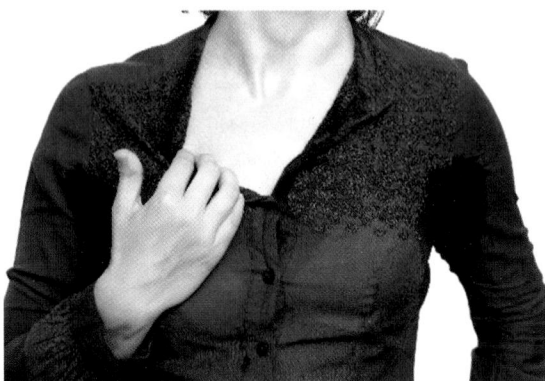

Figure 29.8 Increased sweating and heat intolerance

Source: Adobe Stock.

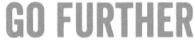

GO FURTHER

WEBLINK: THYROID DISORDER

Visit this website which aims to provide support and information to people with a thyroid disorder: www.btf-thyroid.org

Hair loss is common in hyperthyroidism and eye problems are often present in Graves' disease. Eye problems include the thyroid 'stare' associated with the increased adrenergic tone of hyperthyroidism, and a condition known as exophthalmos which is specific to Graves' disease and is characterised by an abnormal protrusion of the eyeballs (see Figure 29.9). It is caused by an inflammatory process in the tissues behind the eyes. In severe cases, the eyelids may not completely cover the person's eyes when they blink or sleep, potentially drying the conjunctiva and increasing the risk of ulceration and infection.

Goitre is the term used for an enlarged thyroid gland. In Graves' disease, the goitre is diffused in

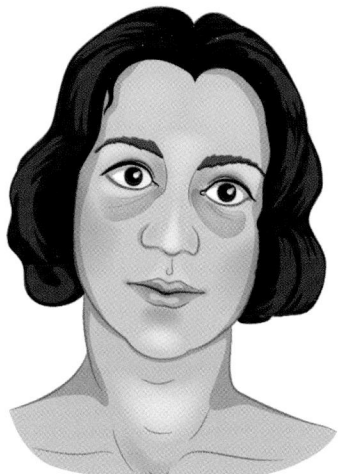

Figure 29.9 A person with exophthalmos

Source: Adobe Stock.

nature – this is the type of goitre likely to be present in Kim's scenario. A multi-nodular goitre (see Figure 29.10) is another common type of goitre which may be associated with hyperthyroidism. In the absence of hyperthyroidism, an enlarged thyroid is called simple goitre. A single thyroid mass or a dominant nodule in a multi-nodular gland may indicate the presence of malignancy.

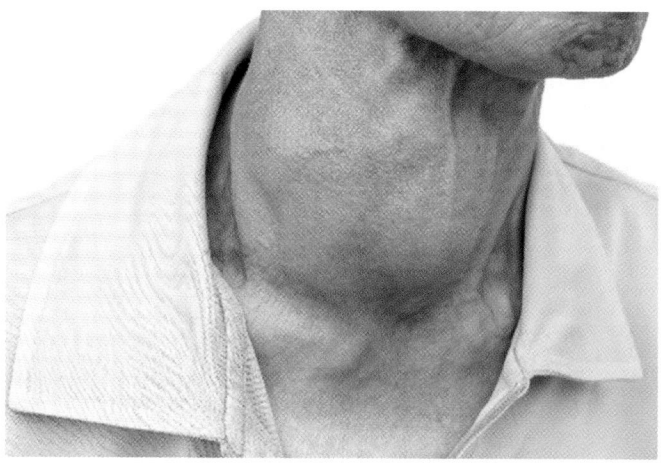

Figure 29.10 Goitre (multi-nodular)

Source: Adobe Stock.

Nursing assessment of an adult with hyperthyroidism

Prior to diagnosis, a person may present with a range of generalised symptoms, which may be attributed to other factors, leading to the underlying hyperthyroidism being missed. A detailed and holistic nursing assessment will assist in identifying potential hyperthyroidism. Endocrine disorders can cluster in individuals and families so a detailed history will often be useful. Baseline clinical measurements should be recorded, remembering that hyperthyroidism can influence a person's vital signs. It is also important to observe for the extent of any tachycardia and to be aware that, in some cases, arrhythmias (e.g. atrial fibrillation) will be present. Body temperature will require to be monitored and you should assess the patient for signs of dehydration and malnourishment. Rarely, there can be an acute onset of severe symptoms, sometimes referred to as a thyroid storm, which is a life-threatening condition requiring urgent treatment.

Clinical investigations for hyperthyroidism

In endocrinology the physical examination, biochemistry and other clinical findings are key to diagnosis. Checking TSH blood concentration level is an important screening process for thyroid problems. Levels are suppressed in hyperthyroidism, and increased in hypothyroidism. Circulating T3 and T4 levels can also be measured. The nature of the goitre or cause of hyperthyroidism may be further explored using ultrasound examination of the thyroid (see Figure 29.11) and scanning techniques.

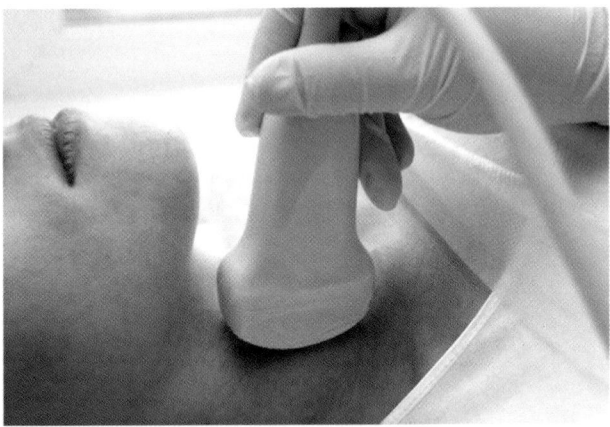

Figure 29.11 Ultrasound of the thyroid examination

Source: Adobe Stock.

Nursing care and management of an adult with hyperthyroidism

A person-centred approach should be taken ensuring that the person can make informed choices about their care and treatment. Sleep can be problematic for a person with hyperthyroidism, so ask them about the type of environment they find most conducive to sleep. Often this will be a quiet and dark room. It is also important to find out if the person is intolerant of heat and whether they require a cool environment (using fans if appropriate), lightweight clothing and bedding. When providing care, it will be necessary to meet the person's dietary needs, remembering that they may require additional calories in the short term. Their fluid intake and output should be monitored, strictly if necessary, and adequate clear fluids provided. Eye care may be necessary to prevent the eyes from drying out and to minimise corneal abrasion.

If the person is anxious or agitated it is important to provide them with reassurance and support. Explain that it is common for a person with hyperthyroidism to experience changes to their mood. Psychological issues may impact on social aspects of the person's life, such as relationships with family and friends and in the workplace. It is often helpful if the person discusses their condition and symptoms with their employer and the people they are close to. Symptoms can be reduced using medications such as beta blockers (e.g. atenolol) and referral to mental health services may be necessary in some cases.

Nurses will provide care to patients undergoing treatment for hyperthyroidism. Where the cause of the hyperthyroidism is likely to remit, medications which aim to lower the production/secretion of T3 and T4 may be used (e.g. carbimazole). In other cases, ablative therapy may be necessary. This may be through the administration of radioactive iodine which is absorbed by the thyroid causing it to shrink, as was the case for Kim. Alternatively, a partial or total thyroidectomy may be carried out. Where the thyroid is removed or no longer produces sufficient hormones the person will require hormone replacement therapy (HRT). Where thyroid function is still present following ablative therapy there is a significant increase in the risk of long-term hypothyroidism in the future.

WHAT'S THE EVIDENCE? 29.2

A Cochrane systematic review undertaken by Liu et al. (2015) found that total thyroidectomy is more effective than subtotal thyroidectomy for the surgical management of Graves' disease. This is because partial removal of the thyroid is associated with a high rate of persistence and recurrence of the disease.

CONCLUSION

We started the chapter by drawing on quotations from two individuals who have personal experience of an endocrine condition. This was followed by a brief introduction to the regulation of hormone secretion, a process which enables our bodies to maintain homeostasis and regulate metabolic rate. We discussed the care of a person with diabetes and the importance of health promotion and self-management before considering the assessment and holistic care of a person with hyperthyroidism. Endocrine conditions are common and we hope the information in this chapter has helped you to develop the skills and knowledge necessary to provide effective evidence-based care to the adult with an endocrine condition.

CHAPTER SUMMARY

- Endocrine conditions are common within the UK population.
- Nurses have an important role to play in the prevention, identification and management of endocrine conditions.
- Health promotion and patient-centred involvement have proven benefits for adults living with endocrine conditions.

GO FURTHER

CASE STUDY: SAFEGUARDING FAMILY CARE

Go to https://study.sagepub.com/essentialadultnursing for a further case study related to this chapter. If you are using the interactive ebook, simply click on the book icon in the margin to go straight to the resource.

Books

- Greenstein, B. and Wood, D. (2011) *The Endocrine System at a Glance* (3rd ed.). Oxford: Wiley-Blackwell. A handy reference for learning more about the endocrine organs and how endocrine conditions are managed within clinical settings.
- Rees, A. and Levy, M. (2017) *Clinical Endocrinology and Diabetes*. Oxford: Wiley-Blackwell. Primarily aimed at undergraduate medical students, this is still an excellent resource for nurses with an interest in expanding their knowledge of clinical endocrinology and diabetes.
- Dunning, T. (2013) *Care of People with Diabetes: A Manual of Nursing Practice*. Oxford: Wiley-Blackwell. A comprehensive guide to diabetes tailored to meet the needs of nurses.

Journal Articles

FURTHER READING: JOURNAL ARTICLES

Go to https://study.sagepub.com/essentialadultnursing for further free online journal articles related to this chapter. If you are using the interactive ebook, simply click on the book icon in the margin to go straight to the resource.

- Nugent, L., Carson, M., Zammitt, N., Smith, G. and Wallston, K. (2015) Health value & perceived control over health: Behavioural constructs to support Type 2 diabetes self-management in clinical practice. *Journal of Clinical Nursing*, 24(15-16): 2201-10. This article undertakes qualitative research with people who have type 2 diabetes. It explores health value and perceived control over health in relation to self-management behaviours.
- Knight, J. and Nigam, Y. (2017) Anatomy and physiology of ageing 7: The endocrine system. *Nursing Times*, 113 (8): 48-51. Use this article to learn more about the effects of aging on the endocrine system.
- Nigam, Y. and Knight, J. (2017) Diabetes management 3: The pathogenesis and management of diabetic foot ulcers. *Nursing Times*, 113(5):.51-4. A useful article discussing the clinical features of diabetic foot along with effective assessment, treatment and patient education.

Weblinks

FURTHER READING: WEBLINKS

Go to https://study.sagepub.com/essentialadultnursing for further weblinks related to this chapter. If you are using the interactive ebook, simply click on the book icon in the margin to go straight to the resource.

- Royal College of Nursing (2018) *Diabetes: Education, prevention and the role of the nursing team*. Available at: www.rcn.org.uk/clinical-topics/diabetes/education-prevention-and-the-role-of-the-nurse. A useful summary of self-management approaches and the prevention of type 2 diabetes with focus on the role nurses play.
- Scottish Intercollegiate Guidelines Network (2010) *Management of Diabetes (SIGN 116)* Available at: www.sign.ac.uk/assets/sign116.pdf This evidence-based publication is a fantastic resource for healthcare practitioners aiming to enhance their practice.
- National Institute for Health and Care Excellence (2018) *Diabetes* Available at: www.nice.org.uk/guidance/conditions-and-diseases/diabetes-and-other-endocrinal--nutritional-and-metabolic-conditions/diabetes. An extensive range of resources and guidelines related to the topic of diabetes.

ACE YOUR ASSESSMENT

Revise what you have learned by visiting https://study.sagepub.com/essentialadultnursing

ONLINE
QUIZZES

- Test yourself with multiple-choice and short-answer questions
- Do the chapter activities in the book and check your answers online

REFERENCES

Department of Health (2016) *How to keep health risks from drinking alcohol to a low level.* Available at: www.gov.uk/government/uploads/system/uploads/attachment_data/file/545911/GovResponse2.pdf

Diabetes UK (2016) *Facts and Stats.* Available at: www.diabetes.org.uk/Professionals/Position-statements-reports/Statistics/).

Diabetes UK (2017) *Do you know the 4 Ts of type 1 diabetes?* Available at: www.diabetes.org.uk/get_involved/campaigning/4-ts-campaign

Donnelly, G. (2017) Promoting health through the internet and social media. *Holistic Nursing Practice,* 31(3): 141–2.

Dunning, T. (2016) How to monitor blood glucose. *Nursing Standard,* 30(22): 36–9.

Kelly, M., Wills, J. and Sykes, S. (2017) Do nurses' personal health behaviours impact on their health promotion practice? A systematic review. *International Journal of Nursing Studies,* 76: 62–77.

Knight, J., Nigam, Y. and Andrade, M. (2017) Diabetes management 1: Disease types, symptoms and diagnosis. *Nursing Times,* 113(4): 40–4.

Liu, Z.W., Masterson, L., Fish, B., Jani, P. and Chatterjee, K. (2015) Thyroid surgery for Graves' disease and Graves' ophthalmopathy. *Cochrane Database of Systematic Reviews,* 25(11).

National Institute for Health and Care Excellence (NICE) (2015) *Type 2 Diabetes in Adults: Management.* Available at: www.nice.org.uk/guidance/ng28

NHS Choices (2015) *Physical activity guidelines for adults.* Available at: www.nhs.uk/Livewell/fitness/Pages/physical-activity-guidelines-for-adults.aspx

Public Health England (2016) *Eatwell Guide.* Available at: www.nhs.uk/Livewell/Goodfood/Documents/The-Eatwell-Guide-2016.pdf

Scottish Intercollegiate Guidelines Network (2010) *Management of Diabetes* (SIGN 116). Available at: www.sign.ac.uk/assets/sign116.pdf

World Health Organization (2011) *Use of Glycated Haemoglobin (HbA1c) in the Diagnosis of Diabetes Mellitus.* Available at: www.who.int/diabetes/publications/report-hba1c_2011.pdf?ua=1

Acknowledgements

Special thanks to Lisa Grant, General Practice Nurse, Dr Cassidy and Partners, Linden Medical Centre, Johnstone, for her assistance with the diabetes information in this chapter.

We gratefully acknowledge the advice and information provided by Laura Smith, Associate Diabetes Specialist Nurse, Managed Clinical Network for Diabetes, NHS Dumfries and Galloway, on the self-management of diabetes and DESMOND programme.

CARE OF THE ADULT WITH AN IMMUNOLOGICAL CONDITION

30

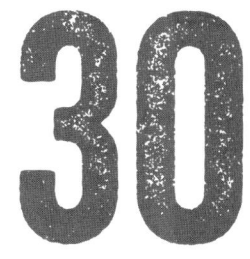

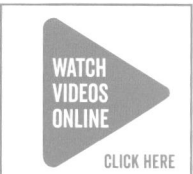

WATCH VIDEOS ONLINE

CLICK HERE

EMILY CARNE AND NICKY OWEN

THIS CHAPTER COVERS:

- The anatomy and physiology of the immune system
- Pathophysiology
- Clinical investigations
- The psychological aspects of immunodeficiency

- Care and management of immunodeficiency
- Monitoring
- Rare disease care provision.

> " Living with a rare disease is tough. Nobody knows what is wrong with you and then when you have a diagnosis, nobody has ever heard of it, let alone knows how to treat it. Nurses and doctors with specialist knowledge feel like a lifeline that connect me to the care and treatment that I need.
>
> **Charlene B-B, patient** "

INTRODUCTION

The immune system is fascinating and incredibly complex in both its structure and function. It has an effect on all the body's other systems and this chapter will provide an overview of how it works and what happens when it doesn't. Due to the highly specialised nature of immunology nursing, it is unlikely that, as a student nurse, you will get an opportunity for placement with a specialist immunology service. This chapter will provide you with a basic understanding of how the immune system works, some of the complications of a defective system and how such complications are managed. The aim is also to provide an awareness of the specialist roles that can await you beyond your initial nurse training and the unique aspects of caring for patients with rare disease.

This chapter will focus on the condition of **immunodeficiency**, which is impairment of the immune response and its symptoms, rather than allergic conditions, which instead, are characterised by an overactive response within the immune system. While primary immunodeficiency remains a relatively rare condition affecting approximately 1:30,000 people, patients with secondary immunodeficiency are increasingly being seen in general healthcare areas. Recent developments in medicines designed to target the immune system to treat diseases such as cancer and autoimmune conditions (widely used in haematology, rheumatology, neurology and gastroenterology) have resulted in an increased rate of diagnosis of secondary immunodeficiency, which can be a side effect of treatment. By considering the management of immunodeficiency you will also learn skills that can be applied in providing care for patients with other rare diseases, such as dealing with the psychological effects of rare disease and also interaction with the 'expert patient'.

As the mechanisms of action within the immune system are varied and highly complicated, it is not possible to cover all of the knowledge needed to provide specialist nursing care within this chapter, but helpful links for further reading have been signposted at the end of the chapter.

ANATOMY AND PHYSIOLOGY OF THE IMMUNE SYSTEM

The following diagram (Figure 30.1) will help you to recognise and revise the key components of the immune system.

The immune system is designed to protect the body from infection and the first defence against such an attack are the mechanical barriers such as cilia, located in the nose, skin, and mucous membranes in the mouth, nose and gastrointestinal tract.

If these external barriers are breached then internal immune defences will be called upon. The internal immune system is divided into two categories: the **innate** and **adaptive** systems; the former being more ancient and undiscerning compared with the more highly evolved adaptive system. A complex relationship exists between the different components of the immune system, which can at first appear daunting. To assist you to learn about this, the following section describes the role and function of the cells and further detailed definition can be seen in Table 30.1. The innate (otherwise known as 'non-specific') system comprises chemicals and immune cells (**leukocytes** or white blood cells) in the blood whose role is to attack any perceived foreign body. These include **neutrophils** and **macrophages** (Table 30.1), which 'engulf' micro-organisms and **eosinophils**, **basophils** and **mast cells** which release toxic agents to attack invaders. Also part of the innate system are **natural killer** (NK) cells which destroy infected cells and have a role in providing knowledge for the adaptive system by posting pieces of the foreign body on their surface

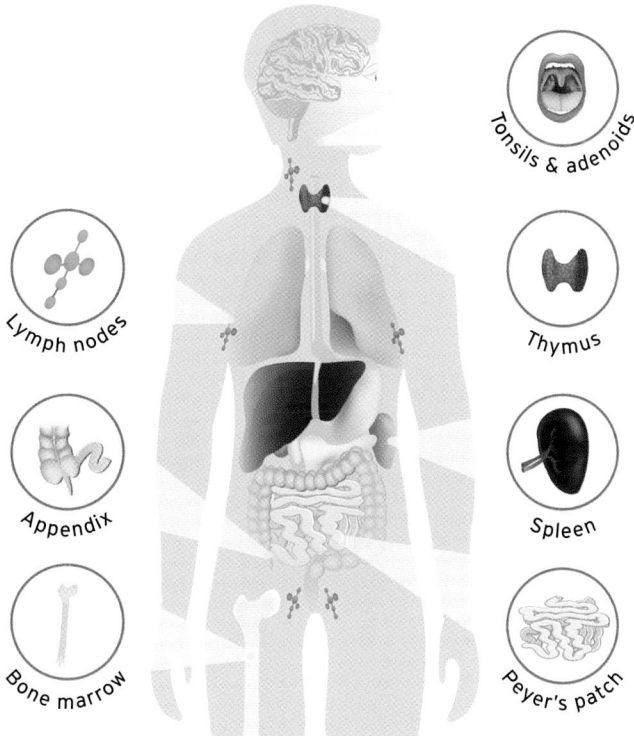

Figure 30.1 The immune system

Source: Shutterstock

and sending chemical messages to the rest of the immune system. Also categorised as innate, is the **complement system** which is a cascade of chemical signals produced to assist the immune system in recognising and destroying pathogens.

The **adaptive (specific) system** utilises a memory system to recognise and target specific foreign bodies, thereby preventing infection. **T helper cells** (see Table 30.1) will attack micro-organisms within the body's cells and signal to the rest of the immune system to mount a response using chemicals called **cytokines**. T cells will also present antigens to **B cells** (Table 30.1) to start the process of future recognition. The first time that a pathogen is encountered by a *naïve* **B cell** (a B cell that has not yet been exposed to an antigen), it will immediately start to change into the type of cell that produces specific antibodies for that pathogen. This will take approximately a week, during which time new *memory* **B cells** (Table 30.1) will also be produced to recognise and take action in subsequent encounters with the same pathogen. Memory B cells are efficient, producing better quality **antibodies** in less time than the original naïve B cells. T cells can also make memory cells which will divide rapidly on encountering an antigen-receptor match, thus communicating (known as 'signalling') to the rest of the immune system that a pathogen has been identified. **Memory cells** remain in our body for a lifetime; this is how we build up a stronger immune system over years of encountering different illnesses and explains why we only get diseases such as chicken pox once. Viruses such as influenza and the common cold are continuously mutating, meaning that on each encounter it is as though the body is dealing with a new illness, with no matching memory cells to tackle the illness early.

ACTIVITY 30.1: CRITICAL THINKING

All immune (white blood) cells are made from haematopoietic (blood stem cells), which originate in the bone marrow, hence the name 'B' cell. The exception to this are the T cells which are made from blood stem cells which have moved to the thymus to mature; hence the name 'T' cell.

The spleen is the largest lymph node in the body and has an important role in storing cells including B cells, producing antibodies and removing antibody-coated bacteria. Consider why a patient who has asplenia (no spleen) may be at greater risk of infection. Why may a patient be vaccinated against common diseases prior to a planned splenectomy? What are the future care implications for a patient who has a splenectomy?

The innate and the adaptive systems are not mutually exclusive; some cells such as the T cell and NK cell have roles in both as shown in Figure 30.2.

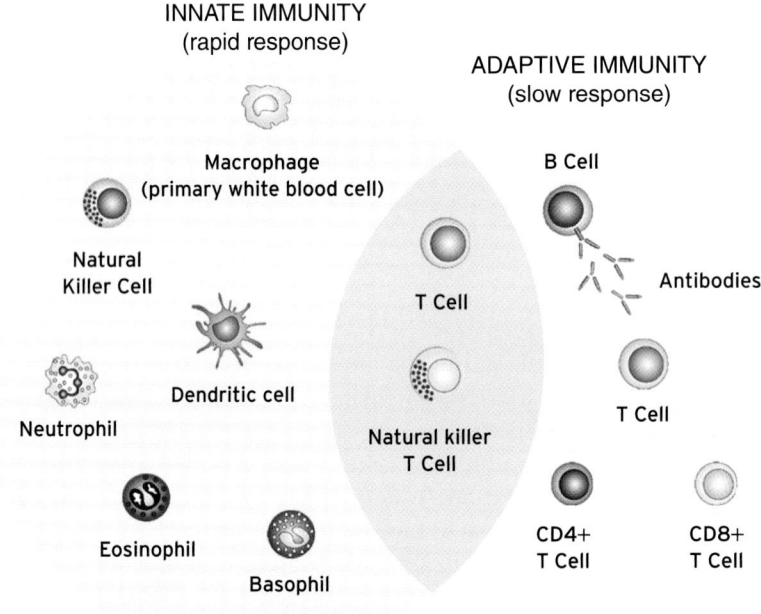

Figure 30.2 Innate and adaptive immunity systems
Reproduced with permission of SpringerNature.

Table 30.1 The role of each white blood cell

Type of cell / component	Category	Description of function	Response speed
Macrophage	Innate	Destroys the foreign body using phagocytosis and signals to rest of the immune system using flags (antigens) on the cell surface	Rapid
Neutrophil	Innate	Destroys the foreign body using phagocytosis	Rapid

Type of cell / component	Category	Description of function	Response speed
Eosinophil	Innate	Destroys the foreign body using phagocytosis - particularly important in parasitic infection	Rapid
Basophil	Innate	Destroys the foreign body using phagocytosis - important in mast cell activation and allergic inflammation	Rapid
Dendritic cell	Innate	Takes up and processes antigen; then present for recognition by T cell	Rapid
Complement system	Innate	A cascade of signals that recruit other immune cells and identify cells for destruction by 'tagging' them	Rapid
Natural killer T Cell	Both	Kills cells that are infected by a virus to stop the virus multiplying. Initially thought of as innate, but now believed to have memory cell characteristics	Rapid
CD4+ T Cell (Helper)	Adaptive	Uses antigen presented by the dendritic cell to signal to the immune system information about the pathogen attack	Slow
CD8+ T Cell (Suppressor)	Adaptive	Kills cancer cells or cells infected with a virus (also signals to the immune system to end the immune response)	Slow
B Cell	Adaptive	Secrete antibodies when activated	Slow
Antibodies	Adaptive	Attach to bacteria and signal to macrophages to phagocytose	Slow

Immune cells travel around the body via blood and lymph vessels. Throughout the **lymphatic system** there are 'meeting areas' where cells gather to activate certain functions, exchange information and make antibodies – the lymph nodes and the spleen. A higher level of activity during an active infection will often cause swelling and pain at adjacent lymph node sites. Following a splenectomy, patients experience an increased risk of serious infection as the immune system is less able to process and get rid of infected cells.

GO FURTHER

For further information about how the immune system works, take a look at the link to the Immune Deficiency Foundation website (a link is provided at the end of the chapter).

ACTIVITY 30.2: CRITICAL THINKING

The innate and adaptive systems are not mutually exclusive and there is communication between all aspects of the immune system to enable the whole cascade to work effectively. This is one of the

ACTIVITY 30.2 ANSWER

(Continued)

(Continued)

reasons that it is particularly difficult to identify the specific area of defect in immune deficiency and can lead to problems in diagnosing and managing these conditions.

- How could collaborative care assist in the diagnosis of a patient with immunodeficiency and which other healthcare professionals will be involved in the process?
- How could you assist the patient with understanding their diagnosis?

PATHOPHYSIOLOGY

There are many reasons why defects in the immune system cause illness, the most common being:

- **Autoimmune disease**: where the body wrongly identifies its own cells as foreign and utilises its own immune response to attack itself.
- **Allergy**: where the body wrongly identifies a benign antigen (such as grass pollen) as harmful and makes an immune response against it (overproduction of antibodies that target the antigen). The symptoms are directly caused by the chemicals released from the mast cells to attack the antigen.
- **Human Immunodeficiency Virus** (HIV) is a virus that infects and destroys helper T cells, preventing the immune system from working properly.
- **Immunodeficiency**: 'a large group of different disorders caused when some components of the immune system (mainly cells and proteins) do not work properly' (IPOPI, 2012).

Immunodeficiency can be further categorised into two groups: Primary and Secondary. Primary immunodeficiencies arise as a result of an intrinsic fault in the immune system and can be inherited or caused by a *de novo* (new) gene mutation. Secondary immunodeficiencies have an external cause such as side effects of medication (e.g. chemotherapy, monoclonal antibodies, immunosuppressive agents or glucocorticoids) or secondary to disease (e.g. leukaemia, lymphoma, myeloma, malnutrition or chronic infection). All immunodeficiency leads to an increased susceptibility to infection and complications due to chronic or recurrent infection.

Primary immunodeficiency (PID) is not one single disease but a group of rare conditions classified by the part of the immune system that is affected. Severe combined immunodeficiency (SCID) affects both T and B cells and is usually diagnosed in childhood due to severity of presenting symptoms. Common variable immunodeficiency (CVID) is an antibody deficiency that mainly affects B cells and is the most common PID, affecting between 1:10,000 and 1:50,000 people (see Table 30.2).

Table 30.2 Primary immunodeficiency classification and features

PID classification	Typical features
Combined T and B cell deficiencies	Increased severity of symptoms due to susceptibility to both viral and bacterial infection.
	Example: Severe combined immunodeficiency (SCID)
Antibody deficiencies	Low numbers of B cells and markedly reduced antibodies
	Example: Common variable immunodeficiency (CVID)
	X-linked agammaglobulinaemia (XLA)
Diseases of immune dysregulation	Altered T cell or NK cell function
	Example: Lymphoproliferative syndrome
	Familial haemophagocytic lymphohistiocytosis

PID classification	Typical features
Congenital defects of phagocyte number or function, or both	Reduced ability of macrophages or neutrophils to clear pathogens due to reduced numbers or function
	Example: X-linked chronic granulomatous disease (CGD)
	Leukocyte adhesion deficiency (LAD)
Defects in innate immunity	Can cause severe defects in lymphocytes (T & B cells) increasing the risk of viral and fungal infections
	Example: Anhidrotic ectodermal dysplasia with immunodeficiency
Auto-inflammatory diseases	Defect of the pathway sensing infection resulting in abnormal inflammation, in the absence of a pathogen
	Example: Familial Mediterranean fever
	TNF receptor-associated period syndrome (TRAPS)
Complement deficiencies	Compromised complement signalling pathway and reduced or delayed immune response
	Example: MBL deficiency
Well-defined syndromes with immunodeficiency	Other illnesses which have a genetic classification and feature immunodeficiency as a symptom
	Example: Wiskott–Aldrich syndrome (WAS)
	Ataxia telangiectasia

Adapted from Al-Herz et al. (2014), reproduced with permission under the Creative Commons Attribution License (CC BY).

Clinical investigations

The defects in the immune system that cause immunodeficiency can be subtle and difficult to identify. Combined with the rarity of the condition, recognition and diagnosis of immunodeficiency remains a significant problem; for example, an average GP is likely to treat only one patient in their whole career. Diagnosis of immunodeficiency is achieved using a combination of medical history, clinical examination and laboratory investigation. The most common clinical feature of immunodeficiency is recurrent, repeated, long lasting or severe infections, usually in the upper and lower respiratory tract, gastrointestinal or urinary tracts.

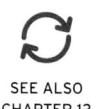

SEE ALSO
CHAPTER 12

WHAT'S THE EVIDENCE 30.1?

Jolles et al. (2014) cite the case of a 19-year-old male who presented to his GP at the age of 4 with a chronic cough, sinusitis and post-nasal drip. He has a tonsillectomy, adenoidectomy, insertion of grommets and a hearing aid. Over the subsequent 15 years he had admissions for pneumonia, suffered 12-15 infections annually, had visited his GP approximately 180 times, and lost 50-60 days of schooling. The average diagnostic delay for Common Variable Immune Deficiency is reported at between 5 and 8 years (Edgar et al., 2014). What strategies could be used to reduce this delay?

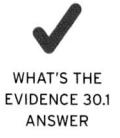

WHAT'S THE
EVIDENCE 30.1
ANSWER

As infections are common without the presence of immunodeficiency, it is important for you to try and differentiate between 'normal' and 'abnormal' infection patterns. Laboratory tests measuring the composition and function of the immune system will indicate immunodeficiency but these are unlikely to be routinely requested by healthcare professionals outside of the specialist team. Diagnosis includes measuring T and B cell numbers and immunoglobulin (antibody) levels. Immunoglobulin level testing will not only indicate the overall number of the main categories of immunoglobulin (IgG, IgA and IgM) but can be used to work out how well the immune system responds to infection using vaccination. For example, you can measure specific antibodies to tetanus in blood serum, then vaccinate the patient against tetanus and re-test 4 weeks later to see if the numbers of antibodies have increased. This indicates how well the immune system is able to recognise the tetanus antigen and mount a response to it.

So what does this mean for patients? Diagnosing immunodeficiency is not difficult; *thinking* of immunodeficiency (and recognising when and how to check the immune system) is. Screening methods such as Guthrie spot analysis for severe immunodeficiency in infants and calculated globulin screening for adults are recommended, as they are useful in identifying immunodeficiency early, but are not currently universally used (Clément et al., 2015; Jolles et al., 2014). Delay in diagnosis can significantly impact ongoing physical health, as early diagnosis can prevent permanent damage caused by recurrent or severe infection and increase success of future treatment (PID UK, 2016). Patients often describe many years of repeated visits to their GP or practice nurse, with unexplained symptoms such as repeated chest infection, colitis symptoms or sinusitis, multiple courses of antibiotics and seemingly 'normal' blood tests. There may be abnormal cell numbers or function, but they are simply not identified by the tests routinely taken by healthcare practitioners. Patients have often been referred to many different specialties, for example haematology, gastroenterology or neurology to try to 'identify the problem'; some even reporting referral for psychological assessment or cognitive behavioural therapy to treat their symptoms (Jolles et al., 2014).

THE PSYCHOLOGICAL ASPECTS OF IMMUNODEFICIENCY

ACTIVITY 30.3
ANSWER

ACTIVITY 30.3: REFLECTIVE PRACTICE

The psychological effect of having a rare disease can go far beyond dealing with everyday symptoms. Consider Charlene's quote at the start of this chapter and take some time to read through some of the patient stories presented on the Primary Immunodeficiency UK website (www.piduk.org/specificpidconditions/primaryantibodydeficiencies/commonvariableimmunedeficiency/cvidpatient stories), taking note of how many times the authors mention not being believed or taken seriously, or report being accused of 'laziness'.

Often, patients with rare disease express relief when given a diagnosis, even if that means having to undertake lifelong, burdensome treatment or deal with deteriorating symptoms or even risk of death.

Consider why this information may be so important to the patient. What different emotions may they feel upon diagnosis and in the subsequent weeks following diagnosis? What could be the reason behind these feelings?

Think about an occasion when you have given or witnessed a diagnosis being given to a patient – did they react as you expected? Compare how you may feel in the same situation and consider why person-centred care is so important.

How may future interactions with healthcare workers be affected by this background of illness or interaction? How could you, as a nurse looking after this patient, help to rebuild trust in healthcare systems?

Inheritance

The causes of primary immunodeficiency (PID) are varied. If you suspect an underlying PID, it is important to ask about family history as there may be clues to an inherited condition; these include a similar history of serious infection, unexplained sudden deaths or diagnosed immunodeficiencies or autoimmune disease.

There are increased risks of genetic defects that cause immunodeficiency in children of closely related parents (known as consanguinity), which can subsequently lead to feelings of guilt or embarrassment within the family. It is important to recognise signs of secrecy within family discussions and help to address these with appropriate referral to genetic counsellors if required. These may include reluctance to disclose information to, or about, family relationships, signs such as moving away from known support networks and living in isolation, or more subtle verbal cues that may be picked up during conversation about inheritance. Disclosure of information may be difficult for the patient and you should address topics with tact and honesty, while allowing the patient time and space to deliberate and reveal information.

With recent rapid growth in whole genome sequencing technology and disease-specific genetic testing, use of such testing in diagnostic practice is now widespread. As nurses, we are expected to understand and use the results of genetic testing in a way that was not possible a decade ago; however, many nurses lack confidence in addressing this with patients. A good understanding of inheritance traits can help you explain many conditions to patients (see Figure 30.3). The genetic causes of primary immunodeficiency can be **autosomal recessive**, **autosomal dominant**, **X-linked** or **spontaneous mutation** of the gene.

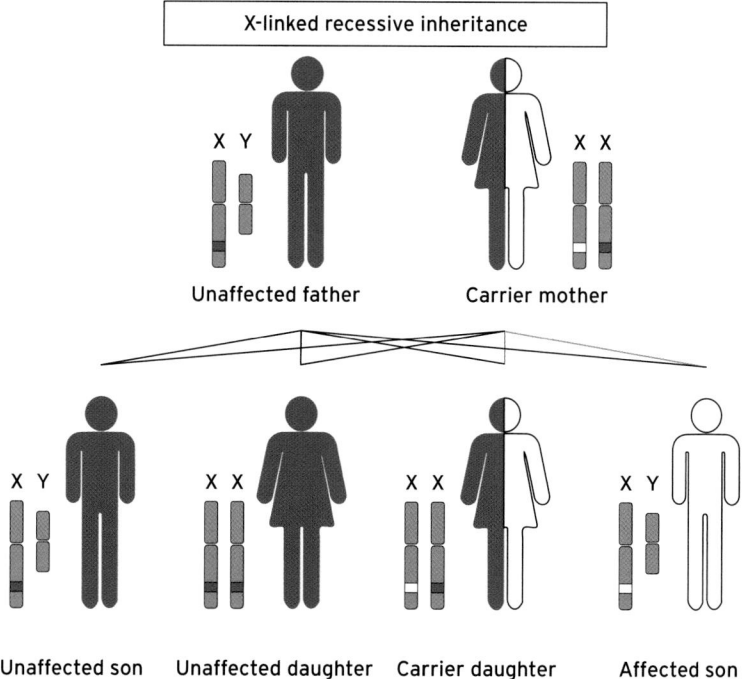

Figure 30.3 Pattern of inheritance

Source: Shutterstock

GO FURTHER

A case study is provided online to help you to better understand the inheritance traits of an X-linked condition and the psychological and social problems that a patient and their family may experience in relation to diagnosis.

Genetic testing for a specific disease can include looking for a particular deletion or rearrangement in a known DNA sequence, which can be relatively easy if there is a suspicion of a named condition for which the pattern of genetic defect is already known. In rare disease with unusual symptoms, the process is more complicated, sometimes requiring the individual's whole genome to be sequenced to look for abnormal patterns. This is not without controversy as other incidental and significant findings about a person's health can be unexpectedly discovered. For example, while looking for an immunodeficiency it is possible that an unrelated finding such as a high-risk genetic pattern for breast cancer could be identified, about which the patient would have been otherwise unaware.

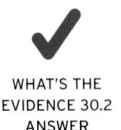

WHAT'S THE
EVIDENCE 30.2
ANSWER

WHAT'S THE EVIDENCE 30.2?

As genetic testing becomes commonplace in nursing care, Seibert (2014: 21) cites the need for nurses to consider the ethical, legal and social implications of such testing:

Beneficence: Generally defined as "doing good to others," beneficence extends to financial and emotional wellbeing, life circumstances, expectations, and personal values.

Non-maleficence: Defined as "doing no harm," non-maleficence includes the risks associated with surveillance and prevention strategies as well as the risks associated with the potential disclosure of personal medical information if other family members are found to be affected.

Autonomy: Respecting individual preference, usually through the informed consent process. Anytime a genetic test is offered, individuals should be fully informed about the risks as well as the benefits of genetic testing and should be able to choose or decline testing. In most cases, patients are asked to make a follow-up appointment to receive their results directly from the nurse practitioner, offering the individual one final opportunity to change their mind by not returning to get their results.

Justice: Equal access to genetic services regardless of ethnicity, financial status, or geographic location.

Privacy: Genetic health information should be protected from inadvertent disclosure to third parties. Genetic privacy can be a challenge because of the hereditary nature of many disorders that often have implications for other family members.

Genetic discrimination: Individuals considering genetic testing are often concerned about employment and/or insurance discrimination.

Think about your own personal feelings: How would you feel about receiving a genetic diagnosis if you were not unwell? Or being informed that you have a statistically higher risk of an illness than the general population? Would you want to know? And would your opinion be different if you could manage that risk, e.g. make a lifestyle change to decrease your chance of developing the disease?

A genetic diagnosis will often have implications for wider family members, whether this is screening for the disease in living relations or considering future family planning. While previously genetic counsellors have been the source of information and explanation, the expansion of gene sequencing as a means to diagnosis now requires non-specialist nurses to also have an understanding of the impact of such testing and potential implications when caring for patients. Feelings of guilt at having passed on a disease and/or fear of future generations inheriting a condition are common and should be acknowledged and discussed (see Case study 30.1).

ACTIVITY 30.4: RESEARCH AND EVIDENCE-BASED PRACTICE

ACTIVITY 30.4
ANSWER

Read: Process and outcome in communication of genetic information within families: A systematic review (Gaff et al., 2007): www.nature.com/ejhg/journal/v15/n10/full/5201883a.html

What are the main themes identified by the systematic review? How could you use these themes to provide person-centred care?

CASE STUDY 30.1: CHRISTOPHER

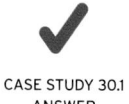

CASE STUDY 30.1
ANSWER

Genetic investigation of undetermined rare disease

Christopher was diagnosed with an unknown immunodeficiency causing low natural killer (NK) cells. A rare malignant growth was identified and treated by an oncologist and he was referred to specialist immunology for further investigation of the cause. The presentation was unusual as he did not present with repeated infection. Christopher comes from a large family with three siblings and during the consultation he disclosed that several of his immediate family have unusual recurrent infections and unexplained malignancies. Christopher has not spoken to two of his sisters for many years following a family argument, but 'hears all of their news' through other family members. In order to try and identify the disease it is necessary for Christopher to have whole genome sequencing, as it is not known in what area the genetic defect may be found. In suspected rare disease it is also helpful to sequence the whole genome of close family members, particularly if symptomatic, as a gene defect pattern is more easily spotted if replicated in other samples. Christopher was referred to genetic counselling for further discussion, prior to making a decision about genetic testing.

- Why may Christopher be reluctant to discuss testing with his family? What could the ethical dilemmas be with regard to contacting the wider family?
- What are the implications for Christopher and his family of possibly finding unrelated risk factors as a consequence of whole genome sequencing?

Consider the importance of communication between healthcare specialties in Christopher's care.

It is not possible to have knowledge about all of the rare diseases that you will encounter throughout your career as a nurse, but it is essential to have an understanding of the psychological impact of inherited conditions. Knowing when and where to refer patients for appropriate support is vital if they are to understand and manage their condition well.

CARE AND MANAGEMENT OF IMMUNODEFICIENCY

The most common classification of PID is antibody disorder (Verma et al., 2013), with the predominant symptom being '**hypogammaglobulinaemia**': *hypo* (low) *gammaglobulin* (immunoglobulins or antibodies) *aemia* (of the blood) – simply put: low antibodies in the blood. The antibodies themselves do not attack pathogens but have the role of alerting the immune system to the presence of invaders. As the previous sections have indicated, there are many different categories of immunodeficiency, but the focus here will be on the management of hypogammaglobulinaemia and your role as a nurse in caring for patients with this condition.

The single most important treatment of hypogammaglobulinaemia is antibody replacement therapy (known as immunoglobulin), the aim of which is to reduce the risk of infection and associated organ damage by artificially 'replacing' the missing antibodies. Immunoglobulin is a fractionated blood product made from pooled plasma obtained from over 5000 carefully screened donors in every batch. There are a number of different manufacturers who each use a slightly different stabilisation and purification technique as well as different donor pools, so care must be taken to minimise risk of reaction by prescribing and administering a single named product and not swapping between immunoglobulin preparations unnecessarily. The treatment is lifelong and is administered either intravenously or subcutaneously; the choice of administration method must be carefully considered, as adherence is key to maintaining health (Ponsford et al., 2015). You should consider each patient as an individual; acceptance of treatment is often determined by the quality of information given and appropriate level of patient-centred care (see Figure 30.4/Table 30.3).

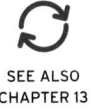

SEE ALSO CHAPTER 13

The replacement dose is initially calculated using weight (0.4g/kg/month) and adjusted based on the clinical response – i.e. the dose can be increased if immunoglobulin levels remain low or if the patient continues to experience high infection levels. Intravenous therapy (IVIg) is administered every 3–4 weeks and subcutaneous therapy (SCIg) is generally given weekly, although regimes can be altered to suit the patient, ranging from daily injection to fortnightly infusion if tolerated (Jolles et al., 2013). The half-life of immunoglobulin in the blood means that the interval between infusions should not be extended to greater than 4 weeks due to the risk of 'wear-off' effect which can leave a patient susceptible to infection. In general, IVIg is given in hospital and SCIg at home. However, it is normal practice for immunology specialist nurses in the UK to train any patient to self-administer treatment at home; even teaching patients to self-cannulate for intravenous therapy if they wish to do so. The choice of treatment option is dependent on many variables (see Figure 30.4) and you should help the patient reach a decision through full and frank discussions. There may be treatment-related reasons for choosing a particular route of administration, but commonly it is lifestyle and social factors that determine treatment choice (see Table 30.3).

While the diagnosis may be made by a doctor, as a nurse it is your role to ensure that treatment choice is correct for each individual. You should pay particular attention to the impact of lifelong treatment from a holistic perspective, including the patient's acceptance of the condition, their relationship with healthcare workers, the impact on their job and family life. This does not mean that the treatment should remain static; once an initial decision is made, life circumstances may change, meaning you should review the treatment options at each clinic appointment. You should use available information, flexibility, compromise and critical thinking to achieve optimum care for individual patients. Have a look at the following table, which lists some of the real-life factors that you should consider when making a choice between IV or SC treatment and hospital or home.

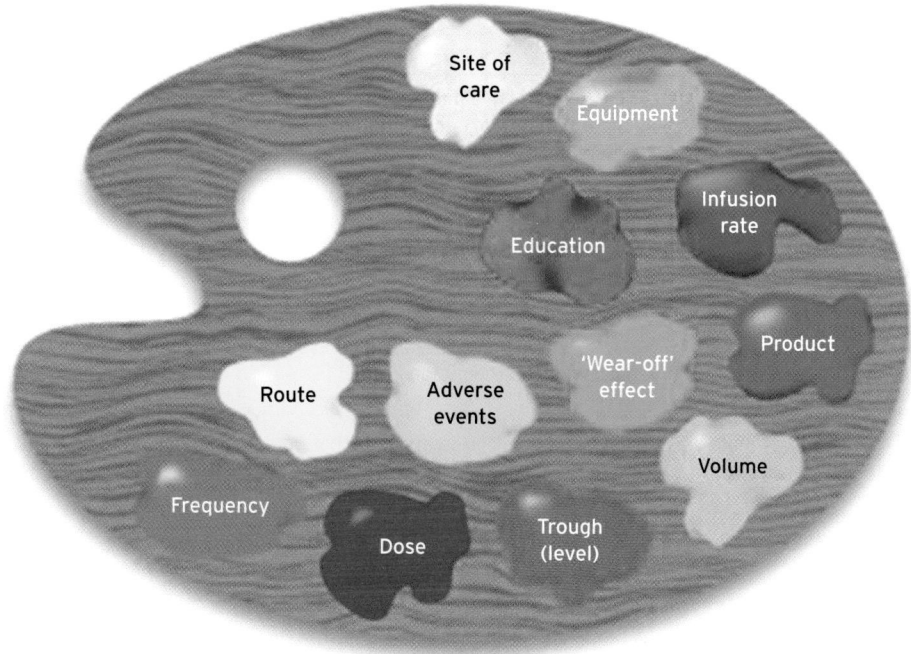

Figure 30.4 Variables in immunoglobulin (IgG) therapy (Jolles et al., 2015)

Reproduced with permission of John Wiley and Sons

Table 30.3 Real-life factors in treatment choice

Practical consideration	Example
Work-life balance	It may be difficult to get time off work to attend regular infusions in hospital, making infusions at home (at a time convenient to the patient) preferable. Other people prefer to make time away from their home life and keep their medical treatment separate
Home environment	The home environment may not be conducive to performing infusions - is the environment clean?
	Are there concerns about the home environment being hectic or unsafe to infuse in? Is there room to store medical supplies? Are there others living with the patient that may pose a risk to safe infusion, e.g. IV drug abusers?
	Are there children at home? Some patients wish to involve their family in treatment by openly infusing to normalise medical treatment, while others prefer to infuse in private
Ability to learn and administer infusions safely	Does the patient have the cognitive ability to understand the risks of self-treatment and to carry out infusions safely? Training programmes are carried out according to strict protocol and formal assessment of technique is undertaken before any home treatment is begun
	Does the patient have the required manual dexterity for drawing up and administering infusions?

(Continued)

Table 30.3   (Continued)

Practical consideration	Example
Venous access	Does the patient have poor venous access? This may prevent home IV administration or make the option of subcutaneous administration more attractive
Adherence	Monitoring of treatment is vital and any patient wishing to administer treatment at home must consent to submitting regular records and blood samples, attending nurse-led clinic appointments and annual home assessment of technique
Flexibility to travel	Does the patient have difficulty travelling to the hospital for 3-weekly infusions? Would home therapy increase quality of life outcomes by reducing the burden of treatment appointments?
Ability of infusion partner to assist	Not all patients are able to administer their own infusions but have a relative or friend who is willing to assist. Is that person in a position to be trained and willing to help? Also see below
Relationship with significant others	Relatives may sometimes wish to help but do not appreciate how assisting with treatment could subtly change the relationship with their loved one. It is important for you to recognise signs indicating that 'carer role' is adversely affecting the relationship and to be prepared to address this
Personal appearance	Subcutaneous treatment can often cause localised lumps under the skin (usually administered to the abdomen or thighs) lasting up to 48 hours. Some patients may prefer to avoid this, choosing IV treatment instead
Fears and phobias	There are all manner of fears and phobias that need to be addressed on an individual basis. A point of note is that needlephobia may differ from patient to patient. One person may be afraid of intravenous needle administration while unconcerned by subcutaneous administration (or vice versa)
Spectrum of responsibility	The way in which patients view treatment and their involvement with administration differs greatly from person to person. Some patients prefer to attend hospital and place the responsibility of treatment on the nurse whereas others prefer to take greater control of their treatment and feel more able to do this at home
Prior experience of healthcare	A broad range of experiences can influence a decision about treatment options. Delays in clinic or mistrust of healthcare professionals could predispose a person to choose home therapy, whereas a positive and supportive hospital environment may have the opposite effect

Once the type and most appropriate location of treatment has been determined, the immunoglobulin treatment should always be initiated in hospital, under the care of specialist immunology nurses. This is due to the risk of reaction, which is greatest in the first few infusions; so you should take care to administer the treatment slowly and with appropriate monitoring. Systemic side effects include headache, nausea, fever, chills, flushing, back ache/myalgia, chest tightness and hypotension, which can be made worse by a too rapid infusion rate. There is a greater incidence of systemic side effects associated with IV administration when compared with SC administration. It is normal to see localised reaction with SC administration such as erythema, itching, blanching and pain, which normally decrease over time. Once stabilised on treatment, infusions will continue in the chosen manner either at home or in hospital with support from you. If treatment is at a local hospital, you may be required to provide training and ongoing support for the local centre. If a patient is at home, support is provided directly to the patient, by regular outpatient clinic reviews, home visits and collection of infusion logs. As a blood product, traceability is a legal requirement, so there must be a robust system of collecting the batch numbers of immunoglobulin that has been administered.

ACTIVITY 30.5: CRITICAL THINKING

From a healthcare provision viewpoint, what are the advantages to offering the option of self-infusions at home?

Monitoring

During regular outpatient appointments, you should provide general health and treatment reviews, including monitoring of blood results such as immunoglobulin levels to guide treatment. Health promotion and monitoring are key elements in this consultation. Avoidance of sources of infection and treatment of infection are the most important aspects in immunodeficiency. You should record the severity and frequency of infections and give treatment as required. Management of immuno-deficiency often includes prophylactic (preventative) broad spectrum antibiotics which are taken continuously, with a supply of 'break through' (different category) antibiotics kept at home and started as soon as the patient has an infection. While it is helpful to obtain a sample for microbiolog-ical testing (e.g. a sputum sample in suspected chest infection) to guide treatment, immune deficient patients need to start treating infection very quickly to prevent prolonged symptoms. Patients are given an individualised pathway to follow on how to manage infection. This is often more aggres-sive treatment (longer, stronger treatment dose) than generally used in patients who do not have immune deficiency; thus patient education and dialogue with the GP or practice nurse looking after the patient is essential.

Nursing a patient with immunodeficiency requires careful cross collaboration of care. As a (special-ist) nurse you would be the main link between primary, secondary and tertiary care and your role would be to liaise with GPs, district nurses, other hospital departments and specialist areas to ensure seamless care. It is not unusual for non-specialist healthcare professionals to lack knowledge about individual rare diseases and require additional information or training to support patients under their care. Some cancers and autoimmune complications are more common in PID and the presentation may differ to the normal presentation; it is imperative that you are able to recognise unusual signs and symptoms and explain to other healthcare professionals regarding the need to investigate seemingly mild or atypical presentation.

Education is crucial in rare disease. People frequently expect nurses and doctors to have knowledge of all diseases, but in reality patients often know more about their rare condition than healthcare professionals working outside of the specialty. Excellent patient information literature is a great place to start learning about rare disease for both patients and healthcare practitioners; it is designed to be easy to understand and presents the most important messages in a simple and candid manner. If more comprehensive or detailed information is required, medical literature is available for further study. Patient forums can also be a helpful learning resource for nurses in order to fully understand the issues that really matter to patients. Anonymous, informal 'chatting' between patients, even in a public arena, may reveal different perceptions or feelings about a disease compared with those revealed in the relatively formal environment of the outpatient clinic. It should be remembered that discussions on forums are not peer reviewed nor evidence based, but a personal expression: a well-informed and knowledgeable site moderator is important. It is crucial that you carefully review any patient information sites before recommendation.

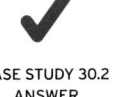

CASE STUDY 30.2
ANSWER

CASE STUDY 30.2: PETE

Immunoglobulin treatment choice

Pete is 36 and has common variable immune deficiency, which was diagnosed four years ago. He lives with his wife and two young children, approximately 50 miles away from his specialist immunology centre. He has been attending the medical day unit at his local hospital for immunoglobulin infusions every 3 weeks. He regularly attends outpatient appointments with the immunology clinical nurse specialist and has recently been reporting more infections, which he feels are due to increased stress levels as he has just started a new job that involves more travel away from home. Following his last appointment it was noted that his immunoglobulin levels have dropped. The immunology nurse contacted the local medical day unit and was told that Pete has been failing to attend some of his infusions and had extended the interval between infusions to 6 weeks on several occasions.

- What could be the cause of Pete's increased frequency of infection?
- How could you support the local day unit in caring for this patient?
- Consider what other treatment options Pete has – what are the pros and cons of each, considering his current lifestyle?
- What role could patient education have in reducing the risk of infection and increasing adherence to treatment?

Rare disease care provision

An interesting aspect of caring for patients with immune deficiency is the problem of raising the profile of rare disease. Your role is not simply the provision of direct care, but to advocate for all patients by ensuring that the problems faced by them are prominent. Greater awareness not only increases the probability of encountering healthcare professionals who have more knowledge of symptoms and treatment but can increase the funding allocated for care. Where resources are limited, it is natural that services which attract media attention have a greater allocation of resources. Smaller groups of patients do not have the political lobbying power of larger groups, so it is important to know how and with whom to engage on their behalf. In 2013, the Department of Health and Rare Disease UK (RDUK) sought to address this by publishing the UK Strategy for Rare Diseases which identified that 3.5 million people in the UK have a rare disease and recognised that collectively, rare diseases are not rare. If you choose specialist nursing as a career, you may be expected to speak to politicians and policy-makers, health managers and commissioners to ensure that patients' care needs are met. This adds another stimulating dimension to your core nursing skills and can lead to a much more comprehensive understanding of healthcare provision and the funding mechanisms of healthcare.

It is important to understand the limitations of knowledge and accept that (in rare disease in particular) you will meet patients who are highly informed – expert patients will often know more about their condition than you do – take time to listen to their stories, they are a great resource to learn from.

During the first year of my nursing degree I was able to do an immunology placement with the specialist nurses. This placement allowed me to learn a lot about Primary Immune Deficiency, that is, the condition, how it affects patients, and the treatment, as well as the communication between healthcare professionals both inside and outside of the locality.

As nursing students, we are reminded throughout our training that the patient is at the core of our nursing practice. This has never been more apparent than throughout my time in immunology. Primary Immune Deficiency patients are patients for life; as a result the relationship between patient and nurse is a close trusting one. This relationship allows the care to be more person-centred and adapted to the changing needs of the patients. From talking to the patients and listening to their stories I developed an understanding of the relief they feel that they are eventually being listened to, after in some cases suffering infection after infection and trying a various array of antibiotics.

It is rewarding as a student nurse, to see the benefits felt by patients when they are given more autonomy regarding their treatment (for example, administration of intravenous and subcutaneous infusions) in diverse locations (primary and secondary care settings). Patients may need to travel for their treatment and it is important therefore that they are given as much independence and support so that they are more able and willing to engage in necessary treatment and management.

Communication through different services such as GPs, consultants and specialist nurses must be effective to ensure the optimal treatment is given to the patient. Immune deficiency patients have a lot of insight into their condition; as a student nurse I am motivated to expand on my knowledge of immunology as a result.

The number of patients suffering secondary immune deficiencies due to receiving chemotherapy is increasing; as students within a constantly evolving profession, we are taught to be aware of altering population demands and related issues within the healthcare system. This placement also alerted me to the impact of relevant recent policy change, such as prescribing of antibiotics for patients, as many immunology patients will often receive them as prophylaxis, or are prescribed them regularly for infections.

By doing an immunology placement I feel I have a better understanding of specific and commonly associated conditions affecting patients. It has also illustrated how person-centred care can be given effectively and demonstrated how effective communication is essential between funding bodies, healthcare professionals, patients and relatives.

Stacey Brinton, student nurse

CHAPTER SUMMARY

- Nurses have an important role to play in the prevention, identification and management of immunological conditions.
- The effective management of rare diseases requires a collaborative and person centred approach.
- A person living with a rare disease is often highly informed about their condition and can provide useful insight to promote effective management of their care.
- Nurses have an important role to play in understanding the psychological impact of inherited conditions and the relevance of appropriate and prompt referral.

GO FURTHER

CASE STUDY: PRIMARY ANTIBODY DEFICIENCY

Go to https://study.sagepub.com/essentialadultnursing for a further case study related to this chapter. If you are using the interactive ebook, simply click on the book icon in the margin to go straight to the resource.

Books

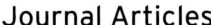

- Ashelford, S., Raynsford, J. and Taylor, V. (2016) *Pathophysiology and Pharmacology for Nursing Students*. (Transforming Nursing Practice Series). London: Learning Matters/SAGE Publications. Designed to provide an integrated introduction to both the biology of the disease and the therapeutic agents that are used to manage them.
- Carver, C. (2017) *Immune: How your body defends and protects you*. London: Bloomsbury Publishing. Although the author is a science writer and researcher this is an informative survey of the immune system.
- Klenerman, P. (2017) *The Immune System: A Very Short Introduction*. Oxford: Oxford University Press. The Very Short Introductions series from Oxford University Press offers this pocket-sized book as the perfect way to get ahead in a new subject quickly.

FURTHER READING: JOURNAL ARTICLES

Journal Articles

Go to https://study.sagepub.com/essentialadultnursing for further free online journal articles related to this chapter. If you are using the interactive ebook, simply click on the book icon in the margin to go straight to the resource.

For an additional learning opportunity about immunoglobulin treatment, please read:

- Jolles, S., Chapel, H. and Litzman, J. (2017) When to initiate immunoglobulin replacement therapy (IGRT) in antibody deficiency: A practical approach. *Clinical and Experimental Immunology*, 188(3): 333–41.
  Then undertake the International Nurse Group for Immune Deficiency (INGID) short online training module entitled *Immunoglobulin Therapy: One size does not fit all*, which teaches you about how to choose the best immunoglobulin therapy for individualised treatment. Available at: https://www.medicaleducation.md/?theme=ingid

FURTHER READING: WEBLINKS

Weblinks

Go to https://study.sagepub.com/essentialadultnursing for further weblinks related to this chapter. If you are using the interactive ebook, simply click on the book icon in the margin to go straight to the resource.

To learn more about the immune system, visit the following webpages:

- Immune Deficiency Foundation (IDF):
  http://primaryimmune.org/about-primary-immunodeficiencies/relevant-info/the-immune-system/
- British Society of Immunology (BSI):
  http://bitesized.immunology.org/

For further information on Immunology Nursing in the UK: The Immunology and Allergy Nurse Group (IANG) www.iang.org.uk

Patient organisations:

- http://piduk.org/
- www.ipopi.org/
- www.geneticalliance.org.uk/
- www.raredisease.org.uk/

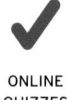

ACE YOUR ASSESSMENT

ONLINE
QUIZZES

Revise what you have learned by visiting https://study.sagepub.com/essentialadultnursing

- Test yourself with multiple-choice and short-answer questions
- Do the chapter activities in the book and check your answers online

REFERENCES

Al-Herz, W., Bousfiha, A., Casanova, J., Chatila, T., Conley, M., Cunningham-Rundles, C., Etzioni, A., Franco, J., Gaspar, B., Holland, S., Klein, C., Nonoyama, S., Ochs, H., Oksenhendler, E., Picard, C., Puck, J., Sullivan, K. and Tang, M. (2014) Primary Immunodeficiency Diseases: An update on the classification from the International Union of Immunological Societies Expert Committee for Primary Immunodeficiency. *Frontiers in Immunology*, 5: 162.

Clément, M.C., Mahlaoui, N., Mignot, C., Le Bihan, C., Rabetrano, H., Hoang, L., Neven, B., Moshous, D., Cavazzana, M., Blanche, S., Fischer, A., Audrain, M. and Durand-Zaleski, I. (2015) Systematic neonatal screening for severe combined immunodeficiency and severe T-cell lymphopenia: Analysis of cost-effectiveness based on French real field data. *Journal of Allergy and Clinical Immunology*, 135(6): 1589–93.

Department of Health (2013) *The UK Strategy for Rare Diseases*. London: Department of Health.

Edgar, J.D., Buckland, M., Guzman, D., Conlon, N.P., Knerr, V., Bangs, C., Reiser, V., Panahloo, Z., Workman, S., Slatter, M., Gennery, A.R., Davies, E.G., Allwood, Z., Arkwright, P.D., Helbert, M., Longhurst, H.J., Grigoriadou, S., Devlin, L.A., Huissoon, A., Krishna, M.T., Hackett, S., Kumararatne, D.S., Condliffe, A.M., Baxendale, H., Henderson, K., Bethune, C., Symons, C., Wood, P., Ford, K., Patel, S., Jain, R., Jolles, S., El-Shanawany, T., Alachkar, H., Herwadkar, A., Sargur, R., Shrimpton, A., Hayman, G., Abuzakouk, M., Spickett, G., Darroch, C.J., Paulus, S., Marshall, S.E., McDermott, E.M., Heath, P.T., Herriot, R., Noorani, S., Turner, M., Khan, S. and Grimbacher, B. (2014) The United Kingdom Primary Immune Deficiency (UKPID) Registry: Report of the first 4 years' activity 2008–2012. *Clinical Experimental Immunology*, 175(1): 68–78.

Gaff, C., Clarke, A., Atkinson, P., Sivell, S., Elwyn, G., Iredale, R., Thornton, H., Dundon, J., Shaw, C. and Edwards, A. (2007) Process and outcome in communication of genetic information within families: A systematic review. *European Journal of Human Genetics*, 15: 999–1011.

IPOPI (2012) *Primary Immunodeficiencies – Diagnosis of Primary Immunodeficiency* (1st edition). December 2012.

Jolles, S., Torgerson, T., Nimmerjahn, F., Schellenberg, R., Helbert, M., Wimperis, J. and Herriot, R. (2013) *Hospital Pharmacy Europe: Immunoglobulin pocket guide*. London: Campden Publishing.

Jolles, S., Borrell, R., Zouwail, S., Heaps, A., Sharp, H., Moody, M., Selwood, C., Williams, P., Phillips, C., Hood, K., Holding, S. and El Shanawany, T. (2014) Calculated globulin (CG) as a screening test for antibody deficiency. *Clinical Experimental Immunology*, 177(3): 671–8.

Jolles, S., Orange, J.S., Gardulf, A., Stein, M.R., Shapiro, R., Borte, M. and Berger, M. (2015) Current treatment options with immunoglobulin G for the individualization of care in patients with primary immunodeficiency disease. *Clinical and Experimental Immunology*, 179(2): 146–60.

PID UK (2016) web page [online]. Available at: www.piduk.org/whatarepids/symptomsanddiagnosis

Ponsford, M., Carne, E., Kingdon, C., Joyce, C., Price, C., Williams, C., El-Shanawany, T., Williams, P. and Jolles, S. (2015) Facilitated subcutaneous immunoglobulin (fSCIg) therapy – practical considerations. *Clinical & Experimental Immunology*, 182(3): 302–13.

Seibert, D.C. (2014) Genomics and nurse practitioner practice. *The Nurse Practitioner,* 39(10): 18–28.

Verma, N., Thaventhiran, A., Gathmann, B. for the ESID Registry Working Party, Thaventhiran, J. and Grimbacher, B. (2013) Therapuetic management of Primary Immunodeficiency in older adults. *Drugs Aging,* 30: 503–12.

CARE OF THE ADULT WITH A MUSCULOSKELETAL CONDITION

31

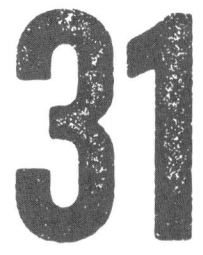

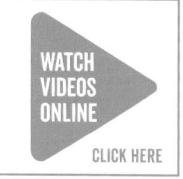
WATCH VIDEOS ONLINE
CLICK HERE

JULIE SANTY-TOMLINSON AND KATHRYN LEWIS

THIS CHAPTER COVERS

- An overview of how a healthy musculo-skeletal system supports and protects the body and facilitates movement
- Effective nursing care to facilitate bone and soft tissue healing and prevent complications

- Assessment and evidence-based care that facilitates patient recovery from orthopaedic conditions, injuries and surgery and prevents associated complications.

I was annoyed with myself for falling and breaking my hip. At first I thought that it would be healed in a few weeks and I'd be able get back to normal life. But getting over the fracture and operation has taken it out of me physically and mentally. I have to take it one step at a time. Immediately after the surgery I had to start mobilising again almost straight away. The nurses and physios helped me to understand how to start to walk again and have been with me every step. Now I'm home I still have to work at slowly walking a bit further and doing things bit by bit. I had a period when I felt quite down.

Mrs Everingham, aged 84

I'd had arthritis for a few years before I had the surgery. The pain was so bad that I didn't really have much choice to have the operation. The pre-assessment staff explained everything that would happen and what it would be like after the operation. That really helped me feel less anxious as I knew what to expect. Although the operation was painful and it was hard to get up and start to walk the first day, the nurses made sure I had the painkillers I needed and they encouraged me by talking me through every stage. I couldn't believe how quickly I was ready for home.

Mr Kalim, aged 77

When I started my orthopaedics placement I was scared of getting it wrong when helping patients to move around. Every movement seemed to be important: from moving around in bed to getting up and walking to the toilet. I saw some orthopaedic surgery in my first week and that helped me understand what patients were going through and why it was important to control their pain so that they can start their rehabilitation. My mentor explained what had happened to each patient and how their healing should progress so that I could understand why we gave the care we did. I loved seeing patients get up and walk after their surgery and then walk out of the hospital when going home.

Andrea, 2nd year student nurse

INTRODUCTION

Nursing adults with musculoskeletal conditions happens in both acute and primary care and involves all age groups. Patients present with both acute and chronic conditions that involve bone, muscle and soft tissues, such as cartilage, tendon and ligaments, either as a result of chronic disease processes or the acute or chronic effects of injury. Many patients require orthopaedic surgery to improve pain and function or stabilise and support healing. Those whose surgery is planned (elective) and those whose surgery follows traumatic injury (urgent/emergency) need different approaches, but the principles are similar. As Andrea's experiences above show, musculoskeletal conditions can have a profound effect on a patient's quality of life, affecting some of the most basic human functions and the nurse has a vital role to play in ensuring that conditions are treated effectively and in a person-centred way. Care of orthopaedic patients is also a multidisciplinary team process that is led by the principles of rehabilitation.

This chapter will focus on the most common musculoskeletal conditions and injuries, considering pre- and post-operative care following surgery and the provision of harm-free care leading to recovery and rehabilitation.

ANATOMY AND PHYSIOLOGY

Overview

The skeleton (see Figure 31.1) provides a framework to support the human body and protects the organs of the pelvis, abdomen, chest and skull. Each bone articulates with at least one other at joints and is attached to muscles and tendons that enable and control movement. Bone also stores and releases minerals and, in the bone marrow, manufactures blood cells (haematopoiesis). Bone is very dynamic tissue with excellent blood supply.

Bone

Bone is specialised tissue made up mainly of a collagen matrix (providing strength) and calcium (providing stiffness). Calcium is absorbed from the diet in the presence of Vitamin D, which is mainly absorbed through exposure to the ultraviolet rays of the sun.

There are three types of cells: osteoblasts (bone builders), osteoclasts (bone eaters) and osteocytes (see Figure 31.2). Bone health and remodelling are facilitated by a continuous interaction between these bone cells and hormones and minerals that is influenced by:

- changes in calcium levels in the blood
- pressure/strain on the bones caused by gravity and the action of muscles and
- hormones (oestrogen, testosterone and growth hormone).

The outer layer of the shafts of long bones (e.g. femur, humerus) provides strength and is formed from cortical (or compact) bone (80%). The ends of long bones and the centre of the vertebrae and ribs are lightweight and are formed from trabecular (or cancellous) bone (20%) (see Figure 31.3). Figure 31.4 demonstrates the microscopic structure of compact bone. Throughout life, bone undergoes a continuous process in which mature bone is replaced with new, to maintain bone structure. This results in replacement of 5–10% of the skeleton each year and the entire skeleton every decade. In youth, bone formation exceeds resorption, so bone mass and strength increase. Peak bone mass is achieved at the age of 20–25 years. At 30–40 years bone mass gradually decreases as bone resorption exceeds bone formation. By the age of 80, total bone mass is around 50% of its peak. When the balance tips towards excessive resorption, bones weaken (osteopenia) and, over time, become brittle and fracture easily (osteoporosis).

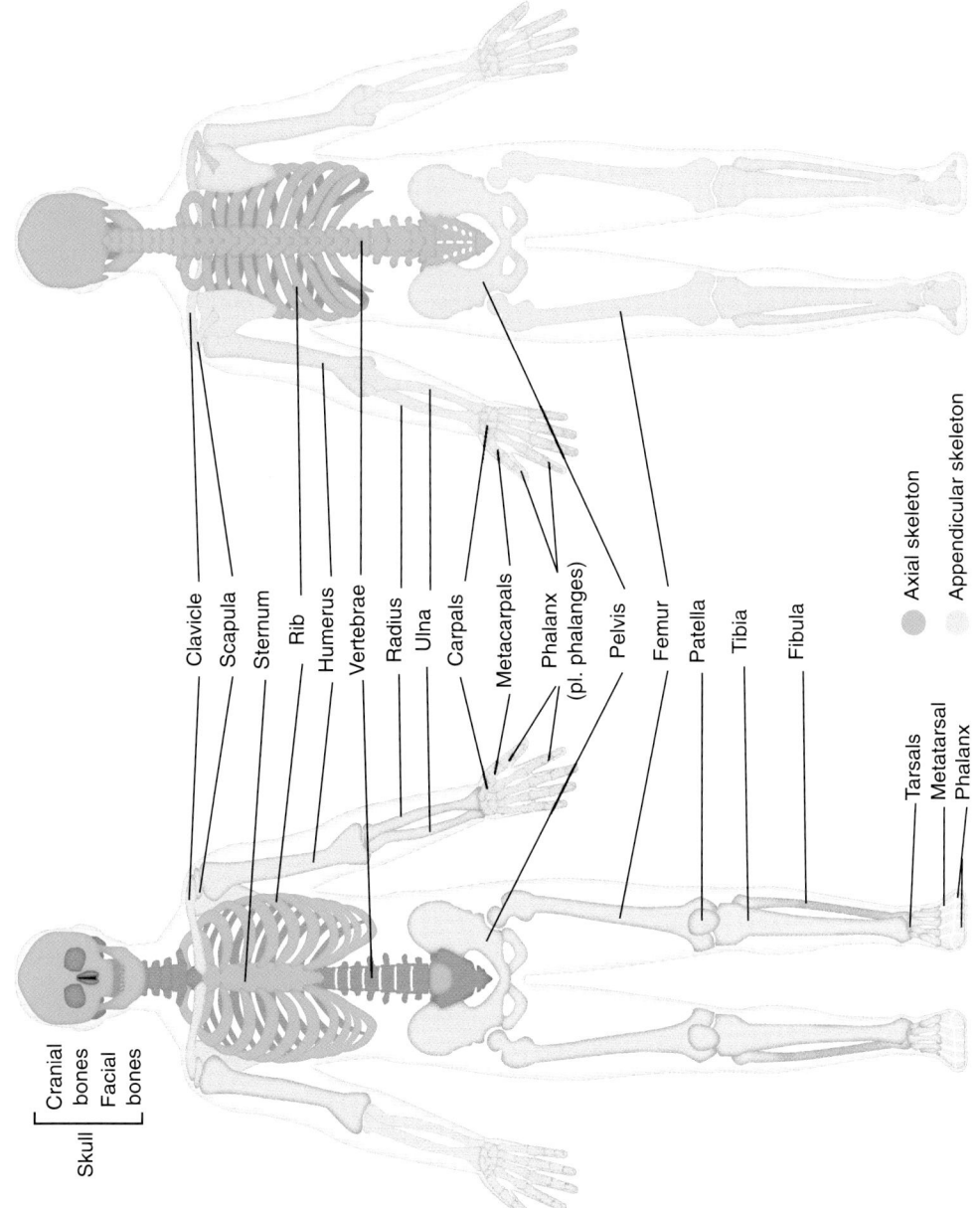

Figure 31.1 The skeleton

Source: Boore et al. (2016). Illustrated by Shaun Mercier © SAGE Publications

BONE CELLS

Osteogenic cells	Osteoblasts
Derived from mesenchymal cells (adult stem cells), they undergo cell division developing into osteoblasts. They are found in the periosteum, endosteum and within the canals that contain the blood vessels.	Bone building cells. They make the bone matrix by synthesising and secreting collagen fibres and other organic components. They also initiate calcification of the matrix.
Osteocytes	**Osteoclasts**
These start as osteoblasts. As they are surrounded by the matrix they are trapped, no longer able to secrete matrix, and become osteocytes. Osteocytes are therefore found in mature bone and are the main cell type in bone. Their function is to maintain the daily metabolic function of bone by ensuring exchange of nutrients and waste products with the blood.	Formed by the fusion of approximately 50 monocytes (type of macrophage, white blood cell) and remove old bone. They are very large, multinucleated and found predominantly in the endosteum. Their plasma membrane is folded into deep ruffles and faces the surface of the bone. It secretes powerful lysosomal enzymes and acids that are responsible for dissolving the protein and mineral matrix. This is known as resorption and is part of normal development, maintenance and repair of bone. Removal of old bone is usually aligned to the production of new bone cells by the osteoblasts.

Figure 31.2 Types of bone cells

Source: Boore et al. (2016). Illustrated by Shaun Mercier, © SAGE Publications

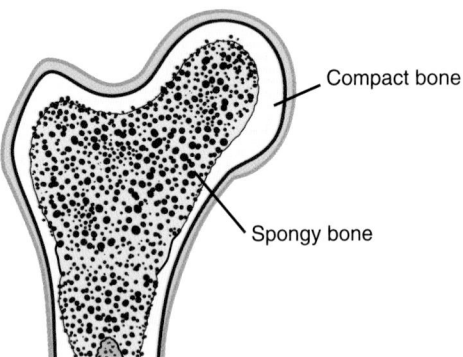

Figure 31.3 Bone tissue

Source: Boore et al. (2016). Illustrated by Shaun Mercier, © SAGE Publications

Joints

There are three types of joints:

- fibrous joints – attaching two bones by fibrous connective tissue, with no joint cavity and little or no movement (e.g. the sutures between the bones of the skull)
- cartilaginous joints – bones are connected by articular (or hyaline) cartilage but have no joint cavity and limited movement (e.g. the symphysis pubis of the pelvis)

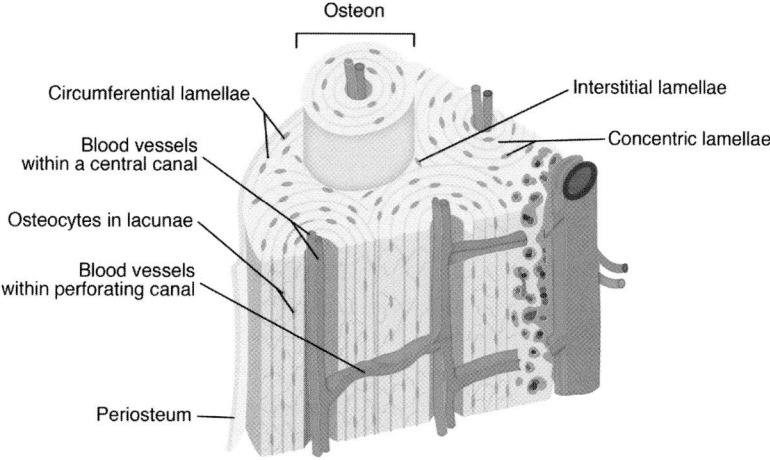

Figure 31.4   Compact bone

Source: Boore et al. (2016). Illustrated by Shaun Mercier, © SAGE Publications

- synovial joints – the most common type of joint; the ends of bones are covered with articular cartilage and the joint cavity is filled with synovial fluid (e.g. hips, knees and joints of hands and feet). (See Figure 31.5.)

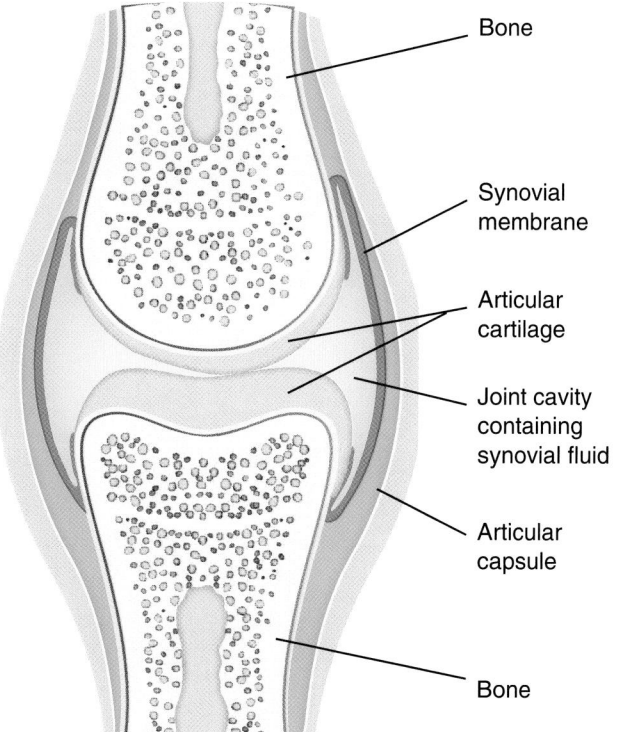

Figure 31.5   Synovial joint

Source: Boore et al. (2016). Illustrated by Shaun Mercier, © SAGE Publications

Articular cartilage is smooth, flexible connective tissue that covers the end of long bones in synovial joints to provide protection, lubrication and shock absorption. It is constantly replaced and remodelled.

Bone healing

When bones are fractured or damaged by disease, the process of healing results in a structure that is as strong as previously (see Figure 31.6). The repair process begins when the bone is damaged; bleeding occurs immediately from the bone ends and the inflammatory process is instigated. In response to inflammatory cytokines, clotting of blood results in a haematoma. Fibroblasts and new capillaries rapidly infiltrate the haematoma, forming a matrix of granulation tissue. Collagen fibres and minerals such as calcium are laid down within the matrix, gradually replacing the clot with fibrovascular tissue known as callus, beginning the stabilisation of the fracture and the formation of new bone. This initial process takes 2 to 3 weeks.

The fibrous tissue is then replaced with new bone that begins to bridge the fracture – a process that takes a further 3 to 10 weeks, depending on the patient's age and general health. The average total healing time for a wrist fracture in a younger, healthy adult patient is around 6 weeks while a fracture of the shaft of the femur or tibia will take around 12 weeks. Bones heal more quickly in youth. Over the following year or two the bone around the fracture site is remodelled by the action of osteoclasts and full strength is regained. Weight bearing on bones as soon as possible is known to facilitate bone repair.

The health care team can support bone repair by ensuring that, initially, movement at the fracture site is minimised, the patient maintains a healthy diet rich in protein, calcium and calories, is well hydrated and mobilises as soon as possible under the guidance of the team.

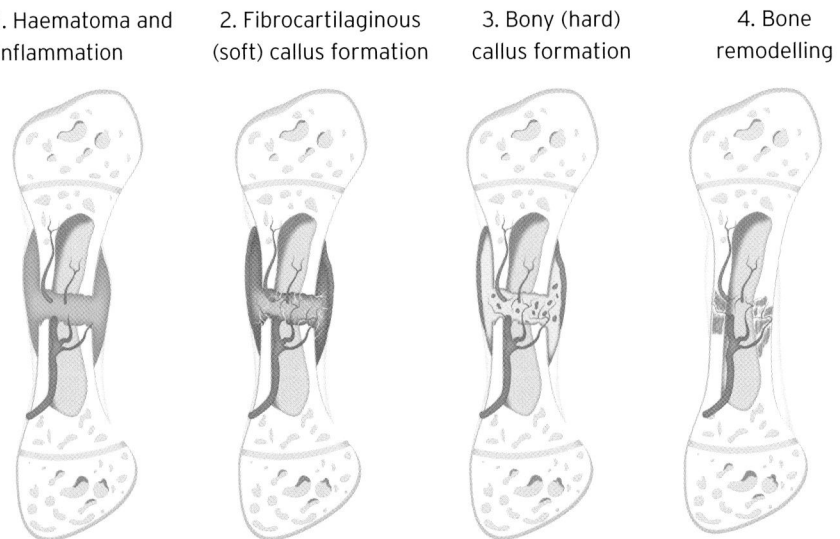

1. Haematoma and inflammation 2. Fibrocartilaginous (soft) callus formation 3. Bony (hard) callus formation 4. Bone remodelling

Figure 31.6   Fracture healing

Source: Illustrated by Shaun Mercier © SAGE Publications

GO FURTHER

This chapter has provided a brief overview of the skeletal system. To develop a more detailed understanding of the entire musculoskeletal system to help direct your learning in practice read Chapter 15, The Musculoskeletal System: Support and Movement in: Boore et al. (2016) *Essentials of Anatomy and Physiology for Nursing Practice*. London: SAGE.

FRACTURES: CLINICAL CHARACTERISTICS AND PATHOPHYSIOLOGY

Fractures occur when there is a break in the continuity of a bone: the term 'break' and 'fracture' are synonymous. Throughout the life span, fractures occur for many reasons, such as an accident/ traumatic event (direct trauma) or from a pathological cause due to weakened bone (indirect). Conditions such as osteoporosis or congenital bone disorders, bone tumours, cysts or infections can result in pathological fractures.

Classifying/describing a fracture helps to plan the most appropriate treatment. Fractures in children are often called 'greenstick' fractures as the bones have not fully developed and are more flexible than adult bones. This can result in an incomplete fracture where the opposite side to the force buckles and is not completely broken. Rapid bone remodelling in children allows for correction of a greater degree of deformity. Other common fracture classifications are listed in Table 31.1.

Table 31.1 Common fracture classifications

Simple	The bone is broken cleanly into two bone fragments In long bones, the fracture may be: • **transverse** – travelling roughly at right angles across the bone • **oblique** – running at an angle across the bone • **spiral** – the fracture spirals around the bone
Multi-fragment (comminuted)	Often resulting from high energy injuries – highly unstable (see Figure 31.7)
Closed or open (compound)	An open fracture; the bone penetrates the skin with high infection risk

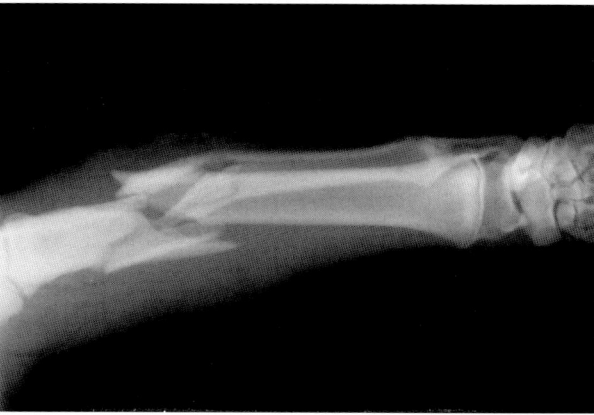

Figure 31.7 Multi-fragment (comminuted) fracture of the radius and ulna

Source: iStock

As the skeletal system ages, different factors contribute to the type of fractures that occur. Young adults sustain most fractures through trauma, in road traffic accidents or sports activities, often due to risk-taking. Older adults are more likely to suffer fractures from falls and may have weaker bones due to osteoporosis (fragility fractures).

The most common signs and symptoms of a fracture are:

- pain
- deformity of the affected area
- swelling
- loss of function.

SEE ALSO
CHAPTER 9

Nursing assessment

No matter what the type of trauma, the immediate care of the injured patient must involve detailed assessment so that appropriate management can be planned. This includes:

- taking a clinical history of the injury (including the mechanism of injury)
- full patient examination
- clinical investigations
- diagnosis and classification of the fracture/s
- planning of fracture management.

A fracture can result in damage to related structures such as arteries and veins, nerves and adjacent soft tissues such as muscles, tendons and ligaments. Undetected, these can lead to permanent functional damage that may be limb threatening. Significant amounts of blood can be lost from bone and surrounding structures. In the early stages of fracture management nursing assessment must, therefore, involve:

- monitoring of wounds and vital signs to detect blood loss/haemorrhage
- monitoring of the neurovascular status of limbs by observing the pain, colour, sensation, warmth and peripheral pulses of the limb distal to the injury.

Clinical investigations

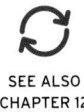

SEE ALSO
CHAPTER 12

X-rays (radiographs) are obligatory in all cases of suspected fracture as images enable the assessment of bone position and are central to planning the correct treatment and care of the fracture. Two or more views are usually required to understand the extent of the injury. Further imaging such as CT (computed tomography), ultrasound and MRI (magnetic resonance imaging) may be required to assess complex/displaced fractures and assist with planning any surgical interventions.

Nursing care implementation and management

Physiological stabilisation of the patient using the ABCDE approach is the initial priority after any injury followed by managing symptoms such as pain and preventing and detecting complications. Once the patient has been assessed and stabilised and the fracture has been diagnosed, fracture management can begin and the patient's individual needs addressed. Fractures can be treated either with or without surgery.

Non-operative methods

Casting and splinting

If surgical intervention is not required, the patient may attend a fracture clinic and be reviewed by a trauma specialist to formulate a treatment plan. The primary objective is to stabilise and support the fracture while healing takes place; this can be done with a sling, splint or cast. Casts are applied by specially trained nurses or technicians. Traditional casts are made from plaster of Paris, but synthetic casts are now freely available and require different application techniques, and they are lighter and more durable than plaster of Paris. The patient will be followed up for the duration of their treatment in the fracture clinic, and the position of the fracture will be x-rayed when required. The patient will be given comprehensive information about caring for their cast, details of who to contact if there is a problem, and advice regarding exercises to avoid joint stiffness and promote circulation. See Table 31.2 for a list of potential complications of casts to consider.

Table 31.2 Potential cast problems

Cracking or breakdown of the cast	Occurs if the patient does not treat the cast as instructed. The patient must allow the cast time to dry and mobilise according to instructions. They should return to the plaster room if problems occur so that the cast can be repaired or reapplied.
Bleeding through the cast	If there is a wound under the cast, this may continue to bleed. Any bleeding through the cast should be carefully observed.
Neurovascular compromise	If the cast is too tight or there is significant swelling, this can impact on the nerve and blood supply to the limb. Colour, movement, sensation, warmth and capillary refill should be observed along with any increase in pain levels - any problems should be treated as an emergency. The limb should be elevated and urgent advice sought from the surgeon.
Pressure injuries (cast sores)	Skin injuries can occur under the cast if there are dents or areas where the cast is too tight. Reports of pain under the cast or any oozing through the cast must be taken very seriously.

Traction

Traction is a pulling force applied using weights and other devices to facilitate healing of fractures by:

- reducing or preventing deformity
- maintaining or gaining correct bony alignment
- securing immobilisation
- relieving pain
- restoring blood flow or nerve supply.

Continued development of surgical techniques has reduced the use of traction systems significantly, but it is still used as a temporary measure to provide pain relief while a treatment plan is formulated or where surgery is not possible.

GO FURTHER

WEBLINK: PATIENTS IN TRACTION

The Royal College of Nursing (2015) provides guidelines for the management of patients in traction. Patients with traction will remain on bed rest so specific attention must be paid to assessing complications of immobility. Take a look at the document to provide you with additional information: www.rcn.org.uk/-/media/royal-college-of-nursing/documents/publications/2015/february/pub-004721.pdf

---

Surgical management

Once a decision is made that surgery is needed, the surgeon will plan the most appropriate method of fixation and the patient will be prepared for the operation, including ensuring they understand what surgery is taking place and what the post-operative plan will be. The care of the patient undergoing orthopaedic surgery is considered below. Table 31.3 lists the different types of fracture fixation surgery.

Table 31.3   Types of fracture fixation surgery

Manipulation under anaesthesia (MUA)	The fracture is realigned under anaesthetic before application of a cast or conducting internal or external fixation.
Internal fixation	There are many methods available to surgically fix a fracture using metal nails, plates or wires. This approach allows early mobilisation and weight bearing, but there is a risk of infection.
External fixation	Pins/wires are inserted through soft tissues into the bone and attached to a bar or ring frame. These techniques are often used for temporary fixation or if the fracture is complex and the soft tissues around the fracture site prevent internal fixation. Particular attention must be paid to the care of the pin/wire sites to prevent infection travelling to the bone.

FRAGILITY FRACTURE: CLINICAL CHARACTERISTICS AND PATHOPHYSIOLOGY

Fragility fractures are the most common reason for admission to an orthopaedic trauma unit and occur following relatively minor trauma to a bone that is weakened by osteoporosis. Osteoporosis is a common disease of later life that leads to weakened bone structure, making fractures more likely. It is an endocrine disease that is three times more common in post-menopausal women than men. People with osteoporosis are often unaware that they have it until they fracture a bone.

The most common fragility fractures are those of the hip (or proximal femur) alongside fractures of the wrist, pelvis, vertebral bodies and humerus. Most patients who sustain fragility fractures are older people who have fallen. They are often frail with a series of other medical conditions (co-morbidities) that make recovery difficult and can lead to loss of independence, complications and, even, premature death. Caring for such patients can be a significant nursing challenge.

Nursing assessment

Older people with fractures require the same initial assessment as any patient who has sustained an injury. However, older people need specific assessment of their general health status (including cardiovascular and pulmonary assessment) and identification of any co-morbid medical conditions.

Assessment of skin integrity, nutrition, hydration and elimination are also particularly important, especially if the patient has had a 'long lie' on the floor following a fall with delayed transfer to hospital. Following admission, patients require detailed nursing assessment as part of a multidisciplinary approach to assessment of the older person.

Clinical investigations

Older patients require the same clinical investigations as other patients with a fracture, but also need a more detailed assessment of physical health status involving additional blood tests, chest x-ray and ECG so that medical problems can be proactively managed. Nurses should work with the medical team, which may include a geriatrician specialised in working with patients with hip fractures or needing surgery, to work towards comprehensive geriatric assessment involving the whole multidisciplinary team.

SEE ALSO
CHAPTER 19

Nursing care and management

Hip fracture is the most common fragility fracture requiring admission to hospital and almost always requires surgery. Older bone heals with difficulty and months of immobility can lead to significant complications and death, so surgical fixation of the fracture is almost always performed so that the patient can remobilise quickly. This type of fracture involves the upper third of the femur and can occur around the femoral neck (see Figure 31.8) or in the trochanteric region (see Figure 31.9). Hip fractures usually require either hemiarthroplasty (replacement of the femoral head with a metal prosthesis) for femoral neck fractures or fixation with a metal screw and plate for proximal femoral/trochanteric fractures. Hip surgery involves a major operation and is a significant physiological challenge for frail older people. This needs skilled nursing care involving surgical, orthopaedic and older people nursing skills.

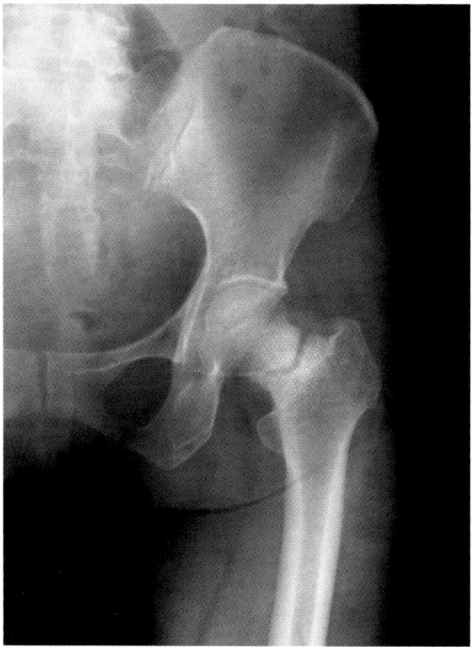

Figure 31.8 Fracture of the neck of the femur

Source: iStock

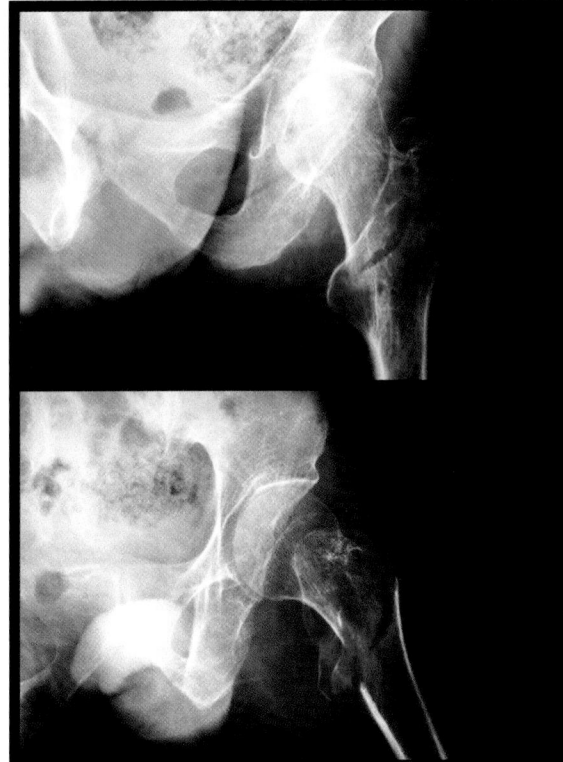

Figure 31.9 Intertrochanteric fracture

Source: iStock

SEE ALSO
CHAPTER 11

A hip fracture is very painful. Effective, regular pain assessment and management are central to both pre- and post-operative care. Poor pain assessment leads to poor pain management and prevents patients from moving, increasing the risk of complications. Sufficient analgesics, paracetamol supplemented with opioids as necessary, should be administered to allow the patient to move around for investigations and nursing care. Femoral nerve blocks are increasingly being used to manage pain following hip fracture. Patients who are cognitively impaired must have a pain assessment conducted that meets their needs.

ACTIVITY 31.1: CRITICAL THINKING

Pain assessment in cognitive impairment

Have you worked with patients with cognitive impairment such as dementia and delirium? Take a few minutes to reflect on what it might feel like to be a patient with cognitive problems who also has a hip fracture and needs surgery. Difficulty retaining information makes it difficult to express pain.

Discuss with your mentor, or local pain team, how you might be able to adapt pain assessment to meet the needs of these patients and involve carers/family.

It is recommended that surgery takes place on the day of or day after admission (NICE, 2011) so that remobilisation can commence as soon as possible. Fasting prior to surgery needs to be minimised and patients should have an intravenous fluid replacement regime in place from admission so that they are well hydrated prior to surgery.

Post-operative care is focused on two main aims:

1.   The prevention and recognition of complications.
2.   Supporting the patient in regaining mobility.

Early remobilisation is essential in preventing complications of immobility and assists in recovery and rehabilitation. Patients usually begin to stand and sit out of bed on the day after the surgery, gradually progressing to taking a few steps and then to walking to the toilet, depending on their capabilities. A remobilisation plan will be recommended by the physiotherapist. Nurses are central in supporting patients both physically and psychologically in their journey towards independence. Pain assessment and management, as well as patient education and support, are central.

Maintaining optimum nutrition and hydration and paying careful attention to elimination, hygiene and comfort along with recognising the specific needs of older people with complex under-lying medical conditions, are fundamental aspects of nursing care that are central to ensuring that patients are supported in their recovery and regaining function. Recognising the risk of pressure injury is essential during this time and, as patients have a large surgical wound, optimal nutrition and hydration are needed. Ensuring good fundamental care is also important in helping to prevent post-operative delirium, which is common in patients following hip fracture surgery.

OSTEOARTHRITIS: CLINICAL CHARACTERISTICS AND PATHOPHYSIOLOGY

There are several types of arthritis – inflammation of joints leading to pain and stiffness ('ARTH' = joint, 'ITIS' = inflammation) – with different causes. The most common is osteoarthritis (OA), the leading cause of chronic pain and disability in the over 70s, affecting around 10% of men and 18% of women over the age of 60 years (Glyn-Jones et al., 2015). The condition affects peripheral synovial joints, most commonly in the hips, knees and hands.

OA can be seen on x-ray as it is characterised by deterioration in and loss of the articular cartilage and changes in the structure and function of the joint that affects the synovium, joint ligaments and the bone near to the joint (subchondral), and can include the growth of bone spurs at the edges of joints. The pathology of OA is not fully understood. It has previously been seen as a 'wear and tear' process in joints that comes with ageing and overuse, but has now been shown to be a complex degenerative disease of synovial joints linked to factors such as inflammatory processes, metabolism and other complex individual factors that appear to prevent the renewal and remodelling of articular cartilage (Mobasheri and Batt, 2016).

OA is more common with ageing, occurs more often in women than men (3:2) and in people who have sustained joint trauma in the past, have been athletes or had an occupation that places stress on joints (e.g. plumber, builder) and those who are overweight or obese. The condition tends to run in families. Although it is thought that OA can, to some degree, be prevented by maintaining a healthy weight and an active lifestyle – in earlier as well as later life – this is not the full picture.

The individual experience varies considerably, but patients with OA usually describe three main features/symptoms:

1. Joint pain – in specific joints, usually starting with one but often progressing to several joints.
2. Joint stiffness – particularly after resting and in the mornings. This can also be associated with grating or grinding when the joint is used (crepitus) and swelling of the joint.
3. Functional impairment – difficulty in carrying out ADLs such as walking, bathing and dressing because of pain and stiffness.

These experiences can lead to several other problems for patients, including sleep difficulties, depression and loss of independence with a significant impact on quality of life.

Nursing assessment

A diagnosis of OA is made if a patient over the age of 45 years presents with joint pain that occurs with activity. Some patients describe morning joint stiffness (NICE, 2014). As part of a generic nursing assessment, a holistic approach to understanding the patient's symptoms and the impact on their ADLs, including employment and leisure, is needed, with a focus on pain and how this impacts on physical and psychosocial functioning.

Clinical investigations

X-ray is useful in understanding the impact of OA on the joint, particularly if referral to a surgeon is likely. However, there is no link between severe joint changes evident on x-ray and the patient's pain and functional levels – appearance of apparently minor changes on the x-ray can have severe consequences for the patient and vice versa.

Nursing care and management

It is important to focus on positive actions the patient can take for themselves that can help to improve pain and function. The main strategies for this as recommended by NICE (2014) are as follows:

- Providing appropriate verbal and written information and discussing this with the patient. Dispelling any misconceptions about progress and treatment and encouraging the patient to take control with regular monitoring, review and support.
- Advising on activity, exercise and positive behaviour change such as engaging in the right kind of exercise including muscle strengthening. This should be in conjunction with appropriate pain management that enables the patient to exercise, and supports them in understanding that the right exercise will not make them worse and that they should pace themselves. Advice about footwear and aids to function such as walking sticks should also be provided.
- Advising about weight-reduction if the patient is overweight or obese, while recognising that both dietary and exercise change are difficult for patients whose mood, motivation and function can be limited by OA.
- Pain management includes offering advice and support about non-pharmacological modes (such as the use of heat and cold) and advice and information about pharmacological options. Patients are usually prescribed oral analgesics such as paracetamol and non-steroidal anti-inflammatory drugs (NSAIDs) or COX-2 inhibitors. Topical preparations and intra-articular injections may also be recommended. Patients need to understand the benefits, limitations and side effects.

In the early stages of OA the focus is self-management. However, before the disease causes significant functional impairment or if non-surgical options prove to be unsuccessful, the GP may refer them to an orthopaedic surgeon for joint replacement surgery (arthroplasty); discussed below. Nurses can help patients to understand what surgery is likely to mean for them.

ACTIVITY 31.2: CRITICAL THINKING

In one of the patient voices at the beginning of this chapter Mr Kalim says: 'The pain was so bad ...". NICE (2014) describes osteoarthritis as a syndrome of 'joint pain accompanied by varying degrees of functional limitation and reduced quality of life'.

Thinking about what you now know about how osteoarthritis affects patients, take some time to reflect on how you imagine this could have impacted on Mr Kalim's daily life prior to his forthcoming surgery. What might the time waiting for his surgery feel like for him?

ORTHOPAEDIC SURGERY

Orthopaedic surgery is required by many patients to stabilise fractures or manage musculoskeletal conditions such as osteoarthritis. Musculoskeletal nursing involves developing surgical nursing skills that are applied specifically to the patient before, during and after orthopaedic surgery. In most cases, surgery involves the insertion of an implant such as a replacement joint (arthroplasty) or a metal fixation device. Specialist operating theatres are used for orthopaedic surgery where airflow and other factors are carefully controlled to minimise the likelihood of infection. Some common orthopaedic procedures include:

Elective/planned procedures

- total joint arthroplasty: joint replacement most commonly of the hip or knee
- ligament repair: e.g. repair of anterior cruciate ligaments of the knee – often done using carbon fibre materials.

Trauma/urgent procedures

- hemiarthroplasty: 'half' a hip replacement performed for some types of hip fracture
- open reduction and internal fixation: fixation of a fracture using metal pins, wires, plates or screws
- manipulation under anaesthetic: to 'reduce' a displaced fracture by placing it in a good position without a surgical incision or insertion of implants, usually followed by application of a cast.

Elective (planned) orthopaedic surgery is arranged in advance and enables the care team and the patient to prepare effectively for the surgery and subsequent discharge; this is less feasible following acute trauma surgery, although some of the same principles can be applied. In many units, patients undergoing elective orthopaedic surgery are managed under the principles of an 'Enhanced Recovery' pathway or programme, particularly for total joint arthroplasty. This evidence-based approach ensures that patients are as healthy as possible prior to surgery and have the best care possible during and after their surgery.

Patient preparation for elective surgery involves attendance for pre-assessment when their general health and fitness for surgery will be assessed by a nurse practitioner and any investigations carried out so that medical problems can be minimised prior to the operation. Patients are also given written and verbal information about the procedure and they are advised how they can prepare for the surgery, what is likely to happen during and after the operation and what needs to be in place for them to be discharged as early as possible. This preparation has been shown to be effective in reducing patient anxiety and improving recovery outcomes.

Post-operative care in the first 24 to 48 hours following all orthopaedic surgery involves the following:

SEE ALSO
CHAPTER 10

- monitoring for the after effects of the anaesthetic
- close monitoring of the wound and vital signs for haemorrhage
- effective post-operative pain assessment management
- monitoring of the peripheral neurovascular supply to operated limbs
- ensuring patients are well hydrated
- supporting optimum nutrition
- prevention and recognition of infection and other complications.

Most patients who have sustained major trauma or undergo orthopaedic surgery report moderate to severe pain post-operatively. Pain management is complex and most units have an acute pain team to support staff and patients in the management of their pain. Regular assessment using an appropriate pain assessment tool is essential. Effective pain assessment and delivery of effective analgesia reduces the physiological and stress response to pain and can reduce complications including cardiac arrhythmias, pulmonary complications, venous thromboembolism and delirium.

As soon as patients are medically stable and their pain is under control they will be supported by the healthcare team in gradually regaining mobility. In most cases, patients need to be able to mobilise to the toilet independently and manage stairs (if needed at home) prior to discharge. Nurses can contribute to achieving this by assisting patients to do as much for themselves as possible within carefully assessed limits.

THE COMPLICATIONS OF MUSCULOSKELETAL CONDITIONS AND ORTHOPAEDIC SURGERY

When caring for a patient with a musculoskeletal injury or condition, the nurse must be aware of potential complications relating to:

- the surgical procedures and fractures
- stasis and immobility.

Surgical complications

A surgical intervention, whether it is to stabilise a fracture or to perform an elective orthopaedic procedure, involves the surgeon outlining to the patient the risks involved. These can include:

- risk of infection (deep infection and surgical site infection)
- damage to adjacent soft tissues (nerve, muscle or tendon)
- complications from the anaesthetic.

The infection risk for elective orthopaedic surgery (e.g. knee and hip hemiarthroplasties) is about 1% (Uckay et al., 2013). This figure can rise for surgery associated with traumatic fractures, especially open injuries, to 5–10%. Preventative measures such as effective hand preparation of the operating surgeon and the use of prophylactic antibiotics have been shown to reduce surgical site infection rates from 4–8% to 1–3%. Other factors that may contribute to a post-operative wound infection can include pre-existing medical conditions such as poorly controlled diabetes, a history of smoking and poor nutrition.

Osteomyelitis, infection of the bone, can occur for many reasons but is a major risk after internal fixation of fractures and other orthopaedic surgery. The main factors that can help prevent infection include standard infection prevention precautions and prophylactic antibiotics. Signs and symptoms of infection include raised temperature, altered blood chemistry and a discharging wound. If an infection is suspected, the patient will return to theatre to have the wound assessed and cleaned. Deep tissue samples may be sent for microbiology and appropriate antibiotics will be commenced. If the infection persists, regular assessment is undertaken by a specialist bone infection unit and treatment may need to continue over two to three years.

Complications of immobility

Patients who are injured or undergo surgery will usually have a period of immobility. There are many complications associated with immobility including the following:

- pressure injuries
- chest infection/pneumonia
- muscle contractures
- venous thromboembolism (VTE), deep venous thrombosis (DVE), pulmonary embolism (PE).

These complications are not unique to the musculoskeletal patient and are an essential part of nursing assessment and care, requiring continuous re-evaluation. Failing to recognise complications can lead to a rapid deterioration of the patient and need for urgent medical attention.

Venous thromboembolism (VTE)

This topic is covered in Chapter 26: Care of the adult with a vascular condition.

SEE ALSO
CHAPTER 26

Compartment syndrome

A serious complication of fractures and limb surgery is compartment syndrome (CS). Bleeding and swelling within a muscle compartment increases the contents of the compartment, resulting in a build-up of pressure. Muscle compartments are encased in dense fascia that cannot expand to allow for swelling. As the pressure within the compartment rises, blood vessels and nerves become compressed, preventing nourishment and oxygen from reaching nerve and muscle cells. This can result in muscle death and nerve damage. If left undiagnosed, the effects of compartment syndrome can have a life-changing impact due to muscle contractures, peripheral numbness and loss of limb function. Early diagnosis is essential to prevent this complication. The main signs and symptoms of CS are listed in Table 31.4.

Table 31.4   Main signs and symptoms of compartment syndrome

Early sign

Pain - the most important early indicator of compartment syndrome; the pain is severe and out of proportion to the injury or surgery and is unresponsive to analgesia. Passive stretching of the affected limb muscles will produce severe pain. Monitoring of the patient for this should be carried out at least hourly for the first 24 h after injury or surgery then reduced to 4 hourly once the patient is stable. Any suspicion of compartment syndrome must be immediately reported to the senior surgeon.

Late signs

Pallor - the skin is white and cool to touch

Paraesthesia - numbness or tingling of the digits

Paralysis - the limb may have little or no active movement

Pulselessness - this is a very late sign. The pulse will decrease as the syndrome persists

If CS is suspected, the patient must undergo a fasciotomy procedure to decompress the compartments. The affected muscle fascia are cut open to release the pressure. Any dead muscle is removed. The wounds are left open and closed surgically at a later date, often using a skin graft to cover the open tissue.

Fat embolism

A serious complication of a long bone fracture is fat embolism syndrome (FES). A fat embolism can occur within 12–72 hours of major trauma including a fracture of a long bone. The exact mechanism is not fully understood. After a fracture, bone marrow fat can escape into the blood stream and fat globules can block a blood vessel in a major organ such as the lungs or brain. The main signs and symptoms include:

- dyspnoea
- petechiae (skin rash)
- hypoxaemia
- cognitive dysfunction.

Prompt treatment is essential to prevent respiratory failure and death. There is no specific therapy for a fat embolism – symptomatic treatment is essential in preventing complications and death. Adequate oxygenation and ventilation can reduce respiratory distress. Early immobilisation of a fracture is the best way to reduce the incidence of fat emboli.

REHABILITATION

Rehabilitation of the patient who is recovering from a musculoskeletal condition, injury or surgery is based on the same principles as for any individual who has experienced a life-changing health crisis. The aim of rehabilitation is to enable people to 'optimize functioning and reduce disability in individuals with health conditions in interaction with their environment' (WHO, 2017). It is 'a process of assessment, treatment and management with ongoing evaluation by which the individual is supported to achieve their maximum potential for physical, cognitive, social and psychological function, participation in society and quality of living' (British Society of Rehabilitation Medicine, 2015: 2).

Recovering from an injury can be complicated, affected by previous experiences, coping mechanisms and life skills and there are many factors that influence recovery. Magee et al. (2009) identified factors such as age, gender and education that influence the outcome of rehabilitation.

Multidisciplinary team (including physiotherapists, occupational therapists and psychologists) input can help the patient to achieve optimal function. Recovery is not always a straightforward journey and various strategies, such as goal setting, can help both the patient and the health professional. Patient motivation is a particularly important aspect of the process and can be affected by the individual's prior experiences of coping with stressful situations. Maslow (1970) suggested that humans are driven to their maximum potential but there will be obstacles that need to be overcome before this can be achieved.

Lack of motivation in the process of rehabilitation can be a barrier to recovery. Tutton et al. (2012) identified that patients living with injury struggled to be hopeful while feeling frustrated with the process of treatment and recovery. Healthcare professionals facilitate the patient's progression, both physically and emotionally, using realistic hopefulness. Recovery from trauma may also require input from psychologists to support the individual through this potentially life-changing event. Patients who have had a traumatic injury resulting in disability experience changes resulting in physiological stress that can impact on their normal coping mechanisms. Emotional reactions following a traumatic incident may affect their ability to assimilate and retain information, so repeating information is important in enabling the patient and family to understand their situation and implications for the future.

Physiotherapists use a range of techniques to maximise the physical function of the patient. These may include:

- muscle-strengthening exercises
- joint mobilisation/continuous passive movement
- assessment for mobility aids
- splinting and casting.

Advice and education are also an important part of the therapist's role to ensure that the patient understands how to continue their rehabilitation. This will include exercises, leaflets and websites of organisations that are available to offer support in the community.

CASE STUDY 31.1: ELLEN

Ellen has sustained a fractured ankle and needs to use crutches while the fracture heals.

- What challenges can you foresee for Ellen? Consider home, work and leisure.
- Which professionals will be required to support her rehabilitation?
- How would this differ if Ellen's age was either 23 years or 72 years?

CHAPTER SUMMARY

- The musculoskeletal system is a complex structure that supports and protects the body and facilitates movement.
- Musculoskeletal conditions can be life changing.
- Nurses have a vital role in providing patient-centred care and preventing complications.
- The multidisciplinary team can deliver a detailed rehabilitation programme to enable the patient to maximise their recovery.

GO FURTHER

CASE STUDY: EVIDENCE-BASED CARE PATHWAY

Go to https://study.sagepub.com/essentialadultnursing for a further case study related to this chapter. If you are using the interactive ebook, simply click on the book icon in the margin to go straight to the resource.

Books

FURTHER READING: JOURNAL ARTICLES

- Clarke, S. and Santy-Tomlinson, J. (2014) *Orthopaedic and Trauma Nursing. An evidence-based approach to musculoskeletal care.* Oxford: Wiley Blackwell.
- Hertz, K. and Santy-Tomlinson, J. (eds) (2018) *Fragility Fracture Nursing.* London: Springer. Available at: https://link.springer.com/book/10.1007%2F978-3-319-76681-2

Journal Articles

Go to https://study.sagepub.com/essentialadultnursing for further free online journal articles related to this chapter. If you are using the interactive ebook, simply click on the book icon in the margin to go straight to the resource.

- Walsh, J.S. (2018) Normal bone physiology, remodelling and its hormonal regulation. *Surgery,* 36 (1): 1-6.

Weblinks

FURTHER READING: WEBLINKS

Go to https://study.sagepub.com/essentialadultnursing for further weblinks related to this chapter. If you are using the interactive ebook, simply click on the book icon in the margin to go straight to the resource.

- RCN (2014) *Peripheral neurovascular observations for acute limb compartment syndrome: RCN consensus guidance.* London: Royal College of Nursing. Available at: www.rcn.org.uk/-/media/royal-college-of-nursing/documents/publications/2014/september/pub-004685.pdf

ACE YOUR ASSESSMENT

ONLINE QUIZZES

Revise what you have learned by visiting https://study.sagepub.com/essentialadultnursing

- Test yourself with multiple-choice and short-answer questions
- Do the chapter activities in the book and check your answers online

REFERENCES

British Society of Rehabilitation Medicine (2015) *Specialist Neuro-rehabilitation Services: Providing for patients with complex rehabilitation needs.* Available at: www.bsrm.org.uk/publications/publications

Glyn-Jones, S., Palmer, A., Agricola, R., Price, A., Vincent, T.L., Weinmans, H. and Carr, A. (2015) Osteoarthritis. *Lancet,* 386: 376–87.

Magee, D,J., Zacharzewski, J.E. and Quillen, W.S. (2009) *Pathology and Intervention in Musculoskeletal Rehabilitation.* St Louis, MO: Saunders Elsevier, p.7.

Maslow, A.H. (1970) *Motivation and Personality* (2nd ed.). New York: HarperCollins.

Mobasheri, A. and Batt, M. (2016) An update on the pathophysiology of osteoarthritis. *Annals of Physical and Rehabilitation Medicine*, 59: 333–339.

NICE (2011) *Hip fracture: management. Clinical guideline [CG124].* Available at: https://www.nice.org. uk/guidance/cg124/chapter/Recommendations#timing-of-surgery

NICE (2014) *Osteoarthritis: Care and management.* Available at: www.nice.org.uk/guidance/cg177/ resources/osteoarthritis-care-and-management-pdf-35109757272517

NICE (2018) *Venous Thromboembolism in over 16s: Reducing the risk of hospital-acquired deep vein thrombosis or pulmonary embolism. NG89.* Available at: www.nice.org.uk/guidance/ng89/resources/ venous-thromboembolism-in-over-16s-reducing-the-risk-of-hospitalacquired-deep-vein- thrombosis-or-pulmonary-embolism-pdf-1837703092165

Royal College of Nursing (RCN) (2015) *Traction: principles and application.* London: Royal College of Nursing. Available at: www.rcn.org.uk/-/media/royal-college-of-nursing/documents/ publications/2015/february/pub-004721.pdf

Tutton, E., Seers, K. and Langstaff, D. (2012) Hope in orthopaedic trauma: A qualitative study. *Journal of International Nursing Studies*, 48 (7): 872–9.

Uckay, I., Hoffmeyer, P., Lew, D. and Pittet, D. (2013) Prevention of surgical site infections in orthopaedic surgery and bone trauma. *Journal of Hospital Infection*, 84 (1): 5–12.

World Health Organization (2017) *Rehabilitation in Health Systems.* Available at: http://apps.who.int/ iris/bitstream/10665/254506/1/9789241549974-eng.pdf?ua=1

CARE OF THE ADULT WITH A HAEMATOLOGICAL CONDITION

32

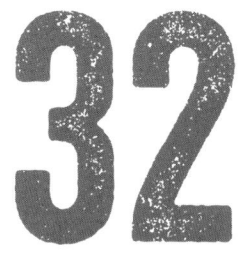

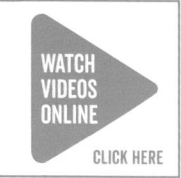

WATCH VIDEOS ONLINE

CLICK HERE

MAURA DOWLING, TERESA MEENAGHAN, AND MARY B KELLY

THIS CHAPTER COVERS

- The role of the blood, bone marrow and lymphatic system in the pathophysiology and diagnosis of haematological conditions
- Common benign haematological conditions of the blood including anaemias, platelet and clotting disorders
- Disorders of the bone marrow including myeloproliferative and myelodysplastic syndrome
- Malignant haematology conditions of the blood, bone marrow and lymphatic system, namely leukaemia, myeloma and lymphomas
- The specific role of nurses as part of the multidisciplinary team in patient assessment, management and evaluation of disease-related and treatment-related side effects
- The nurse's role in empowering patients and their carers through education, health promotion and psychosocial support.

> "Well it did set me back. I couldn't do what I was always doing but you have to face it head on, shake it off and keep living.
>
> **Michael, aged 66 years and has relapsed myeloma**

> "The biggest impact was having to give up work. I loved my work and it was that loss of control/independence I found hard … I had a tough time before I was diagnosed as I lost my daughter in a car accident in Australia so when I survived that I'd survive anything, so I suppose the diagnosis didn't rattle me too much, you just get on with it.
>
> **Patrick, aged 64 years and has chronic myelomonocytic leukaemia (CMML)**

The quotes above from Michael and Patrick illustrate a recurring theme among those diagnosed with a haematology condition and, in particular, a malignant haematological condition; this being a sense of loss associated with their diagnosis and disease management. Although the level and type of loss often varies among individuals, patients often talk about their former self, experiencing loss of identity, loss of value and loss of friendships. Lifestyle changes also occur, accompanied with great sadness and people's ability to participate in life as desired.

Nurses play an important role in recognising the impact of the diagnosis on the patient and their family. Haematology (blood) disorders are often chronic, and many are relapsing and recurring. This means that the patient's needs change over time and they need ongoing support and information.

Blood disorders are complex. In addition to patients coming to terms with their diagnosis, patients may not have even heard of their blood condition and this in itself brings unique challenges. Addressing psychological aspects of fear, anxiety and uncertainty, which accompany a diagnosis of a haematological disorder, is essential. The role of the multidisciplinary team (MDT) is very important in the overall care of patients with a haematology disorder, and nurses are fundamental to the MDT in providing advocacy and support for patients and their carers.

INTRODUCTION

Patients with a suspected blood disorder are usually initially referred to the haematology service, a service that involves many members of the MDT. Most commonly, referrals are from General Practitioners where they find that a simple full blood count has revealed an abnormality in a patient's blood and/or bone marrow; however, referrals also include ENT (ear, nose and throat) where an abnormal lymph gland is detected or from the medical team due to a clotting or bleeding abnormality. As a result, you will often meet haematology patients in a variety of clinical settings and commonly when they are in hospital for another condition or treatment management.

The patient journey begins with an abnormality detected in either the blood, bone marrow or lymphatic system. However, in order to make a confirmed diagnosis, patient 'work up' includes history and physical exam, bloods, bone marrow, lymph node biopsy, x-rays and scans depending on the nature of the abnormality and clinical suspicion. Nurses play a significant role as patient advocate during this stage of investigation. Nurses assist patients by involving them in decision-making and empowering them through education and support. Developing a rapport and providing empathy are key to communicating with patients and ensuring a therapeutic relationship is established and maintained throughout their disease trajectory. As many haematological conditions are chronic in nature and require long-term follow up, the value of the therapeutic relationship cannot be overestimated. In addition, the majority of haematology patients are managed in the outpatient setting, and for those who require admission to hospital their length of stay is minimised. Therefore, close links between the acute and community care teams are essential. Nurses have a significant role in liaising with community colleagues and coordinating discharge planning for patients. All haematology departments will have specialist nursing staff who are further educated in the specialty of haematology. While on placement, you can arrange to meet with these specialists for further knowledge and support.

Disorders of the blood affect many people and can range from simple conditions such as iron deficiency to more complex conditions such as acute leukaemia. It is important that you have an understanding of the range of blood conditions so that you can understand and manage patients' symptoms, treatments and side effects.

Haematology is the study and treatment of blood. It encompasses clinical management of blood disorders, laboratory measurement of cellular components of blood, provision and proper use of transfusion products, and laboratory identification and clinical management of disturbances in haemostasis. Haematology includes the study of the aetiology, diagnosis, treatment, prognosis, and prevention of blood diseases.

Haematology conditions are divided into malignant and non-malignant disorders (see Table 32.1 below). Additionally, they are classified as acute or chronic. Treatment advances for haematological conditions have significantly improved over the past decade. In addition to achieving disease control, symptom management and supportive care measures have resulted in improved quality of life (QoL) for patients and in turn improved patient survival. Observation, clinical monitoring, psychological support and QoL assessment are central to supportive care. Nurses working closely with haematology patients have a unique role in assessing patients' symptoms and providing early intervention.

In this chapter we will explore the common benign and malignant haematology conditions you are likely to encounter in clinical practice (Table 32.1). We will examine these under specific headings such as conditions that occur in the blood, which are non-malignant, and also conditions that are considered malignancies in haematology (Acute leukaemias (Myeloid and Lymphoid)).

Table 32.1 Malignant and non-malignant haematology disorders

Malignant	Non- malignant
Acute leukaemias (myeloid and lymphoid)	Immune thrombocytopenia purpura (ITP)
Chronic leukaemias	Chronic anaemias
Myeloma	Iron deficiency
Lymphoma	Coagulation disorders
Hairy cell leukaemia	Haemochromatosis
Waldenström macroglobulinemia	Haemogloblinopathies
Plasmacytoma	Aplastic anaemia
	Myeloproliferative disorders (MPD) and myelodysplastic syndromes (MDS) (Both conditions can progress to a malignant blood disease)
	Monoclonal gammopathy of undetermined significance (MGUS)

REQUIRED KNOWLEDGE

ACTIVITY 32.1

It would be helpful for you to have a good understanding of the pathophysiology of the blood before you start reading this chapter.

Please look at this YouTube clip, which provides a basic overview of the blood. www.youtube.com/watch?v=_FLjj_Z7SKA

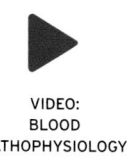

VIDEO: BLOOD PATHOPHYSIOLOGY

SEE ALSO
CHAPTER 12

ANATOMY AND PHYSIOLOGY

Here we will discuss the importance of understanding haemopoiesis. The haemopoietic system is made up of the cells in the peripheral blood, bone marrow, lymph nodes and spleen. You should understand how a defect in these systems results in a haematology disorder, which may be benign or malignant in nature. Here you will also learn the diagnostic tests required to confirm a haematological diagnosis. Nurses are required to understand the rationale for any investigations a patient requires and also how this investigation is completed in order to educate and support patients undergoing such diagnostic tests.

ACTIVITY 32.2
ANSWER

ACTIVITY 32.2: CRITICAL THINKING

List as many investigations as you can think of that would be undertaken to complete a 'work up' on a patient who is suspected of having a haematology condition?

BONE MARROW

All the cells in the peripheral blood originate from stem cells in the bone marrow. These cells maintain active haemopoiesis (the production of blood cells and platelets). The bone marrow is referred to as a factory, which produces all elements of the blood and maintains their numbers within a very strict limit for the life of the individual. In order to maintain haemopoiesis throughout life a pool of resting stem cells is required. These cells, given the appropriate stimulus, can differentiate along specific pathways and so produce the mature cells of the peripheral blood. Each stem cell has the capacity to differentiate into any of the cells in the blood (see Figure 32.2). Abnormalities in a person's full blood count is often the presenting feature in both benign (non-malignant) and malignant blood disorders. A full blood count is a blood biopsy of activity within the bone marrow. However, in order to establish the cause of the abnormality a bone marrow examination is performed.

ACTIVITY 32.3

VIDEO:
BONE MARROW
EXAMINATION

If you get the opportunity on placement, try to accompany a patient who is having a bone marrow (BM) examination.

Look at the video on how a bone marrow examination is undertaken. You can support a patient having a bone marrow examination if you know what the procedure entails. https://www.youtube.com/watch?v=EYd7OnCt7ug

The blood is very complex but if you understand what it is made of and how it works, then you will better appreciate how haematological conditions affect a person and how treatments work.

Blood constantly circulates throughout the body providing the body with nutrients, oxygen and also removing waste. Blood is mostly liquid with numerous cells and proteins suspended in it. The average person has about five litres of blood. A liquid called plasma makes up half the content of blood and contains proteins which help the blood to clot and transport substances through the blood. Blood also contains glucose and other dissolved nutrients. Roughly half the volume of blood is composed of blood cells (red, white and platelets).

- red blood cells: carry oxygen to the tissues
- white blood cells: fight infection
- platelets: help the blood to clot.

First, we need to outline the composition of blood so that conditions discussed in this chapter are more easily understood.

Have a look at the following image illustrating blood composition (Figure 32.1).

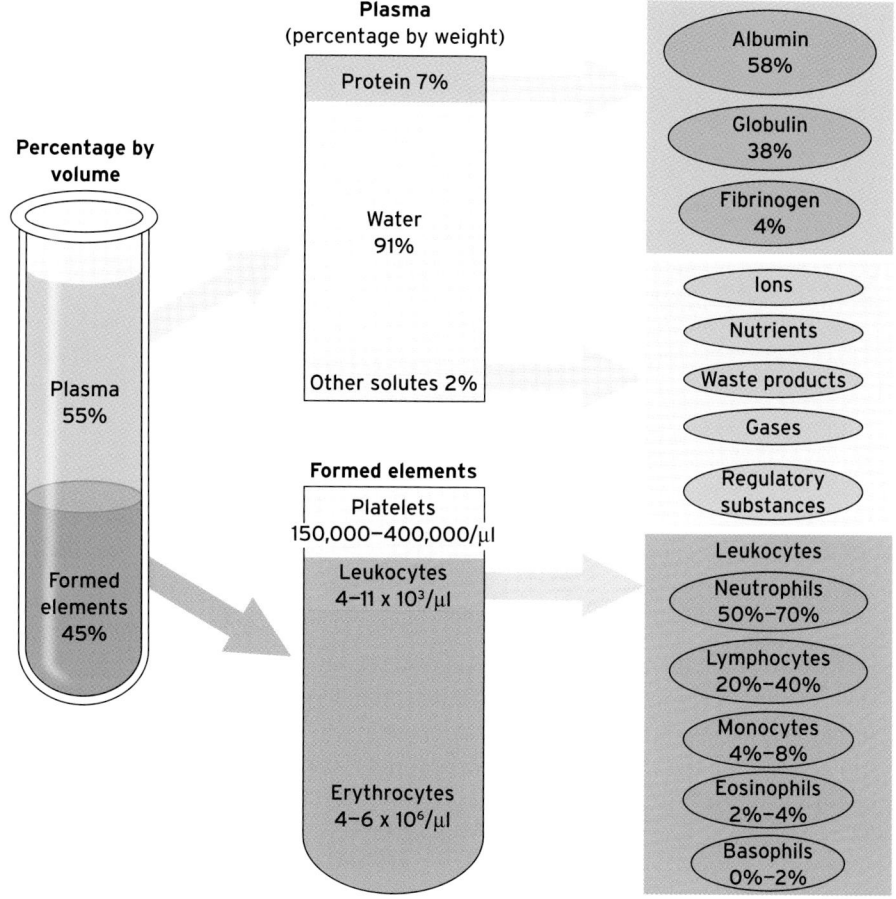

Figure 32.1 Blood composition

(Thibodeau, A., Patton, K. 2004)

Reproduced with permission of Elsevier.

Haematological conditions include a wide range of disorders affecting red blood cells, white blood cells, platelets, blood vessels, bone marrow, lymph nodes, spleen, and the proteins involved in bleeding and clotting. Some blood conditions affect more than one cell type and some do not require treatment (just careful monitoring).

Haematological conditions can be broadly divided into two groups, namely, benign (non-cancerous) blood conditions and blood cancer conditions.

Look carefully at Figure 32.2. You can see that there are two stem cell lines (i.e. myeloid and lymphoid). It is important for you to gain understanding in the broad classifications of leukaemia (myeloid and lymphocytic), which will be addressed later in the chapter.

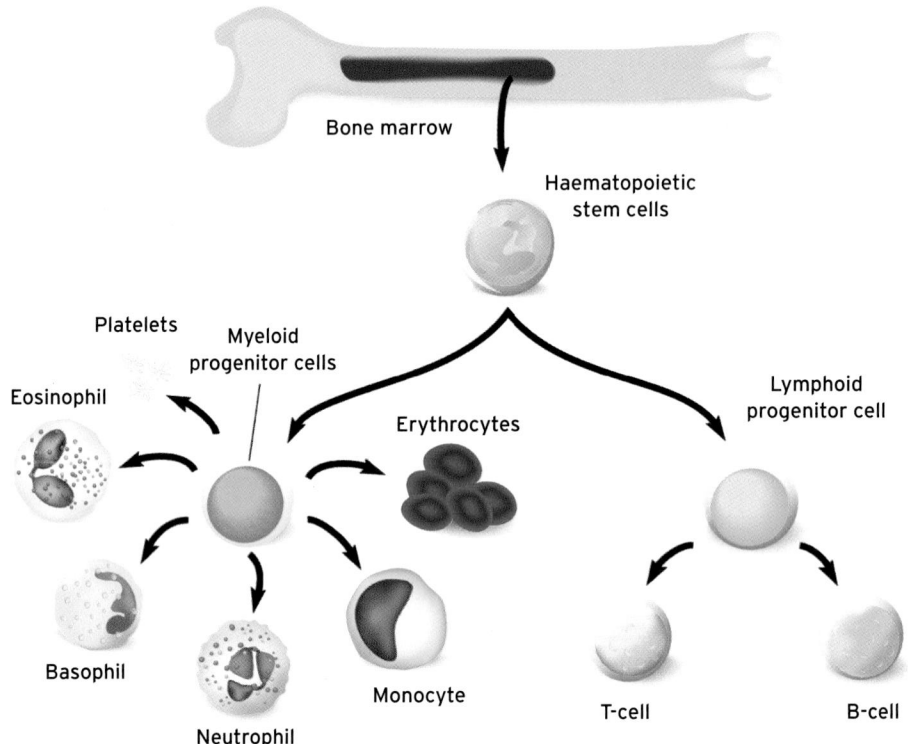

Figure 32.2   Haematopoietic stem cell

Source: iStock

Figure 32.2 does not outline red cell development. The process of red cell production is known as erythropoiesis. This process is stimulated by a reduction in blood oxygen levels. This drop is detected by the kidneys, which release the hormone erythropoietin, which then stimulates red cell production.

You can now see that the blood tells an important 'story' about a person's health and can be the first indication that a disease process is unfolding. This shows how important blood tests are in a patient's diagnostic workup.

LYMPHATIC SYSTEM

The role of the lymphatic system is to protect us from infection and disease. The lymphatic system is made up of groups of lymph nodes throughout the body (see Figure 32.3). They are connected by a network of lymph vessels and are found mainly in the neck, armpit, groin and abdomen. Cancer cells can start in the lymph node or spread via the lymph nodes. If this occurs the lymph node becomes swollen. A lymph node biopsy is required to confirm a diagnosis of cancer in a lymph node/s, e.g. lymphoma. Patients with enlarged lymph nodes will require the expertise of several members of the MDT including nurses, doctors, surgeons and a histopathologist.

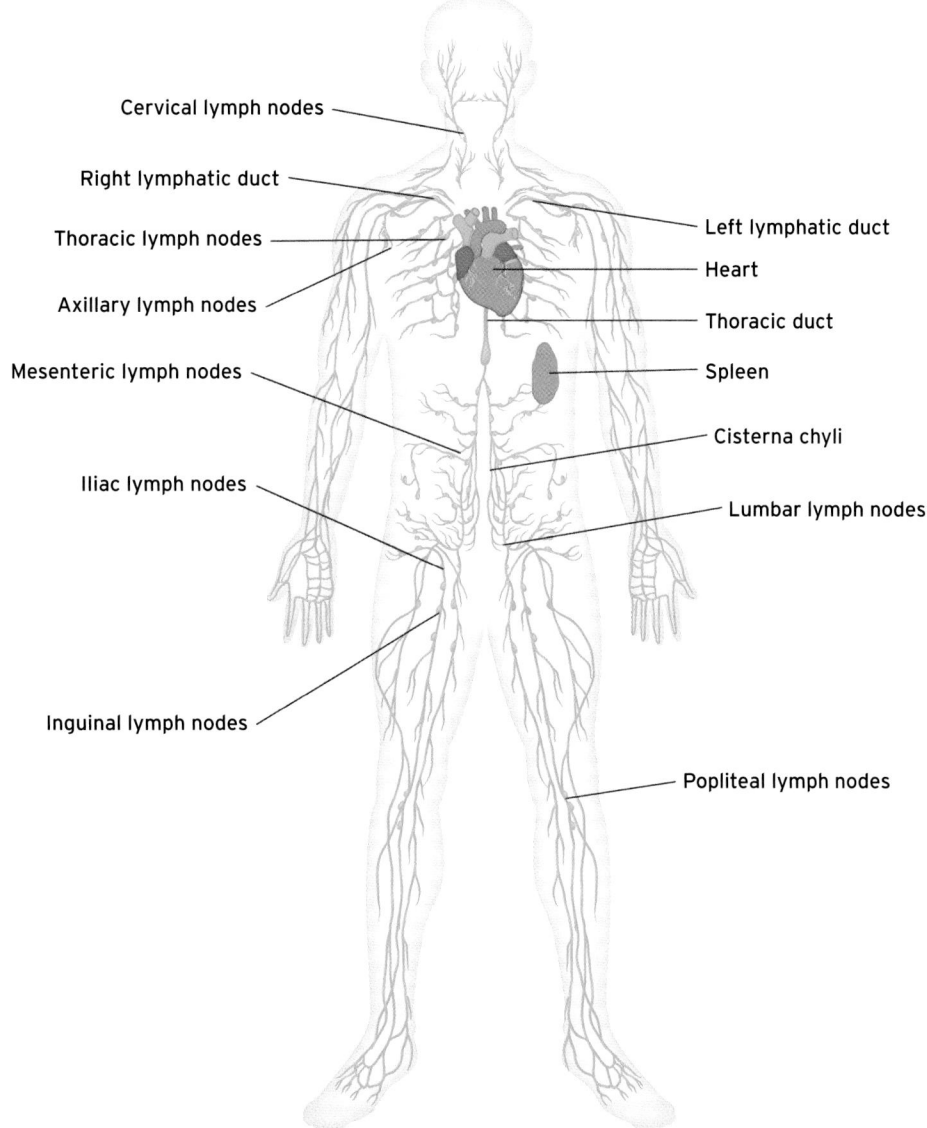

Figure 32.3   The lymphatic system

Source: Boore et al. (2016). Illustrated by Shaun Mercier, © SAGE Publications.

As we mentioned above, a lymph node biopsy is often performed to determine the cause of an enlarged gland. This is undertaken by open incision and patients need to be advised that it takes up to two weeks for the incision to heal and to avoid strenuous activity and exercise until the incision site heals.

Having developed an understanding of the clinical presentation of haematology patients and the diagnostic investigations required for confirmation of a haematology disorder, we will now examine some of the common disorders (both benign and malignant) you are likely to encounter in clinical practice.

RED CELL DISORDERS

There are many red cell disorders and you will most likely care for people with these blood disorders when they are in hospital for another reason (e.g. for elective surgery).

SEE ALSO
CHAPTER 12

Anaemia

Anaemia is diagnosed when a person's haemoglobin (Hb) concentration is below normal. The normal ranges for Hb differ depending on age and sex (11.5–16.0 female; 13.5–17.5 male). Symptoms of anaemia include fatigue, lethargy and shortness of breath.

Anyone diagnosed with anaemia needs further assessment to determine the cause. There are many possible causes of anaemia and these are outlined in Table 32.2. The commonest cause of anaemia is iron deficiency. Iron deficiency anaemia is a condition where lack of iron in the body leads to a reduction in the number of red blood cells. Iron deficiency anaemia like all anaemias warrants further investigation. Clinical investigation includes a patient history, medication history, bleeding history (e.g. heavy menstrual period) and physical examination. Patient assessment will focus on possible causes of malabsorption and blood loss including disease history, diet, medications, bleeding history, weight loss and a change in bowel habit. In addition, the haematology doctor/specialist nurse will perform blood tests and refer the patient to the MDT for special investigations (e.g. endoscopy, bone marrow examination) as appropriate on an individual patient basis. It is important to understand that a male patient does not lose blood 'normally' like a menstruating female, thus women are at higher risk of iron deficiency anaemia. Prompt treatment is important once the cause is established. Treatment is more often with iron replacement, which minimises the patient's symptoms.

It is important for you to be able to recognise symptoms of iron deficiency so that you can assist patients with activities of daily living, give advice regarding a well-balanced diet and encourage patients to have planned resting periods so that patients' symptoms improve.

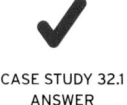

CASE STUDY 32.1
ANSWER

CASE STUDY 32.1: AMY

Amy (pseudonym) is a 19-year-old student who recently attended the university practice nurse with a six-month history of pallor and feeling very tired. She is a vegetarian and is not taking any dietary supplements. Her only history of blood loss is her menstrual periods, which Amy reports as regular but heavy and lasting 5-6 days. Amy had blood tests performed including a full blood count and ferritin. Amy's blood result revealed a low Hb of 9 g/dL. Amy's ferritin level was 2 (the normal range for females is 15-200 ng/mL (=⟷g/L). The ferritin level indicates iron stores in the body and Amy's ferritin store was low. This suggested that Amy has been deficient in iron for some time.

Amy has iron deficiency anaemia and was commenced on ferrous fumarate one daily and advised to return for repeat bloods in 6 weeks.

Critical reflection:

- What are the causes of iron deficiency anaemia?
- What advice do you need to give Amy regarding her iron supplementation and its side effects?
- What dietary advice would you give Amy?
- Does Amy require any further investigations or referrals?

Table 32.2 Anaemias according to cause

Inherited	• Defects of haemoglobin (e.g. sickle cell, thalassaemia) • Defects of red cell metabolism (e.g. glucose 6-phosphate dehydrogenase deficiency) • Defects of red cell membrane (e.g. hereditary spherocytosis)
Acquired	• Reduced red cell production due to nutrient deficiency (iron, vitamin B12, folic acid, vitamin B6) • Bone marrow failure (e.g. associated with acute lymphoblastic leukaemia)
Increased red cell destruction (haemolytic anaemia)	• Immune destruction • Chemical and physical agents • Infections
Systemic illnesses	Anaemia of chronic disease, renal disease, liver disease, cardiac disease

Sickle cell anaemia

Sickle cell anaemia is the most common defect of haemoglobin worldwide, and refers to a group of disorders in which the red blood cell undergoes sickling when deoxygenated. This type of anaemia is most common among those of African descent. The sickle shape makes the red cell both rigid and fragile so it obstructs blood vessels resulting in tissue hypoxia. These misshapen cells also die prematurely resulting in anaemia.

This blood disorder is a major public health concern because it is a chronic disease. Its severity varies across individuals with episodes of wellbeing and symptom free to episodes that require emergency care and intensive specialist medical and nursing management. When a patient experiences an acute episode (e.g. persistent severe pain, severe sepsis), they must seek urgent hospital attention. There are a number of acute episodes that patients can experience; for instance, vaso-occlusive pain (VOC) and **acute chest syndrome (ACS)** (Creary et al., 2015). Other problems that can arise for those with sickle cell anaemia include stroke and leg ulcers.

Supportive therapies include the use of prophylactic penicillin to prevent pneumococcal disease in children, routine immunisations, hydration and narcotics to treat pain from VOC (Quinn et al., 2004). Currently, hydroxycarbamide (referred to in the past as hydroxyurea) is the only disease-modifying therapy recommended for this disease. You need to know about this cytotoxic drug and how it affects patients because it is used for other blood disorders too and you will meet many patients on this medication on placements (see Activity 32.4).

ACTIVITY 32.4
ANSWER

VIDEO:
SICKLE CELL
DISEASE

SEE ALSO
CHAPTER 11

ACTIVITY 32.4

Watch this YouTube video on sickle cell disease. When you get to the end of the chapter, there is a short quiz and some of the questions relate to sickle cell disease. www.youtube.com/watch?v=qe59ar-GZmg

Another condition where the red cell changes shape and is then destroyed prematurely by the spleen is hereditary spherocytosis.

Hereditary spherocytosis

Hereditary spherocytosis is the most common inherited **haemolytic anaemia** among white people. Like sickle cell anaemia, the red cell changes shape (into a spherical shape) and is destroyed prematurely by the spleen resulting in haemolytic anaemia. There is wide variation in disease severity among people. Some people are asymptomatic, and those with mild spherocytosis may show very few signs of the illness. However, those people who experience severe haemolysis of their red cells will be jaundiced, anaemic and have splenomegaly (enlarged spleen), and may develop gallstones (Trompeter and King, 2015). Management of this disease depends on how much haemolysis the person experiences and how the body compensates for the resultant anaemia. Folic acid (needed for red cell production) is given to all patients with mild to moderate disease (Trompeter and King, 2015). The person's ferritin levels (showing iron stores) is normally closely monitored and patients who require regular transfusions are monitored closely for iron levels. Splenomegaly is sometimes present if haemolysis becomes severe. Removal of the spleen increases the red cell life span (to the normal span of 120 days). However, removal of the spleen (or partial removal) is not undertaken until a child reaches at least 6 years of age because of this organ's important role in protecting the body against some organisms.

Now that we have introduced you to anaemia as a result of the red cells changing shape and being destroyed prematurely, we will discuss other causes of anaemia such as B12 and folate deficiency (iron deficiency is also another cause of anaemia and was explored in Amy's case study earlier).

Megaloblastic anaemia

B12 and folate deficiency results in a type of anaemia called megaloblastic anaemia because the red cells are abnormally large and immature, so do not function properly. B12 and folate deficiency can occur for a number of reasons:

1. Pernicious anaemia, an immune disorder where the parietal cells in the stomach are destroyed preventing the body absorbing vitamin B12 in the diet. This is the most common cause of vitamin B12 deficiency in the UK.
2. Although uncommon, a vegan diet or a poor diet over a long time can result in B12 deficiency.
3. Certain medications, such as those used to treat epilepsy can result in less absorption of vitamin B12 in the diet.

The management of most cases of vitamin B12 and folate deficiency is by replacement. In the management of pernicious anaemia, vitamin B12 is given by intramuscular injection for life. To restore folate levels, oral folic acid is prescribed.

Recently, attention is being paid to the finding of a significantly increased risk of gastric cancer among people diagnosed with pernicious anaemia (Vannella et al., 2013). It is now recommended that patients with pernicious anaemia should undergo endoscopy after diagnosis, or if they develop upper gastrointestinal symptoms, to check for any signs of gastric cancer.

Anaemia of chronic disease

You should be aware of anaemia of chronic disease (ACD) (also referred to as anaemia of inflammation because it results from the body's immune system response which affects iron absorption and the production of erythropoietin). You will meet many patients with this type of anaemia on your clinical placements because more and more people are living with chronic disease (Hipkiss et al., 2013). These patients tend to have a systemic illness, haemoglobin level > 9.0 g/dL and usually a raised C-reactive protein (a sign of inflammation). ACD affects nearly all cancer patients at some stage of their disease.

Haemochromatosis

Another condition that you should be aware of is haemochromatosis. Primary haemochromatosis, a genetic condition, results in too much iron in the body. The main treatment for haemochromatosis is venesection (the removal of a unit of blood). Secondary haemochromatosis is caused by too many blood transfusions when treating haemochromatosis. Depending on the level of iron overload, treatment with iron chelation may be required (chelating agents remove iron form the body).

GO FURTHER

See www.youtube.com/watch?v=MxGUAafNSnI
  This link will give you a quick overview of haemochromatosis.

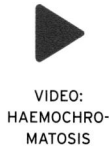

VIDEO:
HAEMOCHRO-
MATOSIS

CLOTTING AND PLATELET DISORDERS

You need to understand normal haemostasis in order to understand clotting and bleeding disorders. (See Go Further Weblink at the end of this chapter.)

Disorders of clotting and platelets can be inherited or acquired (See Table 32.3).

Table 32.3 Clotting and platelet disorders

Inherited	Factor VIII deficiency (Haemophilia A) and Factor IX deficiency (Haemophilia B).
	Haemophilia A is the most common inherited coagulation disorder. This is a sex-linked disease because the factor VIII gene is on the X chromosome. (See Go Further Weblink).
Acquired	Acquired disorders of coagulation can be caused by liver disease, which results in defects of coagulation, platelets and fibrinolysis.
	Another acquired disorder of coagulation is disseminated intravascular coagulation (DIC), where both bleeding and thrombosis may occur. DIC is an emergency and the treatment is aimed at treating the cause (e.g. antibiotics if the cause is sepsis).

> A comprehensive understanding of blood physiology is vital in providing adequate care for those suffering with a bleeding disorder. This became particularly apparent while I was caring for a patient with von Willebrand's disease when on placement in a surgical unit. Von Willebrand's disease is caused by a deficiency in a protein known as 'factor VIII'. This protein is vital for platelet adhesion and its absence impacts negatively on the formation of clots following an injury. A good knowledge of this condition emphasises the need for prophylactic treatment and close monitoring of patients to prevent uncontrolled bleeding after surgical intervention.
>
> **Grace Cosgrove, 3rd year student nurse**

Grace (above) has highlighted the importance of understanding blood physiology when caring for patients with blood disorders. Von Willebrand's disease is due to an inherited platelet function abnormality. Platelet function abnormalities can also be caused by drugs (aspirin and other non-steroidal anti-inflammatory agents). You should also be aware that abnormalities of the vessel wall can be caused by vitamin C deficiency (scurvy) and steroid therapy.

Immune thrombocytopenia purpura (ITP) is another platelet disorder you should know about. This is an autoimmune disorder where the body creates antibodies that attack platelet antigens causing the premature destruction of platelets and persistent thrombocytopenia (low platelets) and this often results in bleeding.

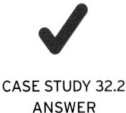

CASE STUDY 32.2
ANSWER

CASE STUDY 32.2: ROBERT

Robert (pseudonym), an 82-year-old man, presented with bilateral intracranial haemorrhages in January 2013. At this time he was taking dual anti-platelet therapy (this is where the person is given aspirin and a second anti-clotting agent at the same time). His platelet count was checked and it was only 1000 (normal platelet count is 150–450,000 per microlitre (mcL)). Robert also had chronic obstructive pulmonary disease (COPD) for the past 15 years. His critically low platelet count indicated that he may have had immune thrombocytopenia purpura but this provisional diagnosis needed to be confirmed and other possible reasons for the low platelet count eliminated.

Robert was treated with two drugs that suppress the immune system. These were high doses of steroid and rituximab (which blocks the activity of that part of the immune system that is causing the attack on Robert's platelets).

Robert also was given an infusion of immunoglobulin (IVIG) and he received platelet transfusions. Platelet transfusion in ITP is not always advised as the autoimmune nature of the disease results in the transfused platelets also being destroyed. However, for patients with severe bleeding transfusion is warranted.

Despite these treatments he only achieved a minimal response. Robert was then treated with TPO (thrombopoietin receptor agonists). This drug therapy increased platelet production by working on the TPO receptors which are found on the megakaryocyte cell surface (the megakaryoctye gives rise to platelets).

Robert continues to receive this treatment each week and his platelet count has returned to normal.

(From UK ITP Association website)

Now that you have an understanding of the causes for anaemia and clotting disorders, we will examine disorders of the bone marrow and lymphatic system.

MYELOPROLIFERATIVE AND LYMPHOPROLIFERATIVE DISORDERS

This group of blood disorders involves all types of malignancies of the blood. Myeloproliferative neoplasms (MPNs) (refer back to Table 32.1) are a group of diseases where there is malignant proliferation of myeloid precursors (precursors are cells that pre-exist before another cell) resulting in too many or too few blood cells being produced. MPNs most commonly seen in practice include the following: essential thrombocythaemia (ET), polycythaemia vera (PV) and primary myelofibrosis (MF) (explained later). There is a strong genetic influence with these conditions; a mutation in the Janus Kinase 2 (JAK) pathway, *JAK2,* is found in the majority of PV patients, and among 50% of both ET patients and MF patients.

A limited number of treatments and interventions are available to treat MPNs. These include venesection (withdrawing blood), hydroxycarbamide (mentioned earlier as used with sickle cell disease), anagrelide (a drug that inhibits the maturation of platelets), interferon (acts on the immune system) and busulfan (an anti-cancer cytotoxic agent) (Tonkin et al., 2012).

Although there are a number of similarities in these blood diseases, each of the MPNs has distinct features. Important diagnostic investigations include specific blood tests including a complete blood film and JAK2 mutation, physical examination and bone marrow examination. It is also important to point out that patients with MPNs are at risk of their blood disorder progressing to become an acute leukaemia (acute myeloid leukaemia (AML)).

In polycythaemia vera, too many red blood cells in the blood cause the blood to thicken and this can lead to clots. This condition is strongly related to a congenital genetic defect (Janiszewska et al., 2016). Most people with this condition are managed by phlebotomy (removing blood) to keep their haematocrit below 45% in males and 42% in females. Haematocrit is the ratio of red blood cells to the total blood cells. These patients are also given low dose aspirin (75 mg daily) unless contraindicated by gastric intolerance or major bleeding. People with a high risk of thrombosis are also given the antineoplastic medicine hydroxycarbamide (also referred to as hydroxyurea, mentioned earlier) to reduce the red cell count, the dose of which is titrated depending on the person's red cell count.

ACTIVITY 32.5

Remember hydroxycarbamide? We mentioned this medicine earlier in the management of sickle cell anaemia. Well, it is also used frequently in myeloproliferative disorders. Look up hydroxycarbamide and make a list of the advice that you would give patients taking this medication.

Essential thrombocythaemia (ET) is a disease where there is an increased cell production of megakaryocytes, which results in frequent thrombotic and bleeding complications. ET is defined as present in a patient with unexplained and sustained very high platelet counts of 450×10^9/L. ET must be distinguished from other causes of raised platelets including haemorrhage, chronic infections, or an iron deficiency. The aim of treatment is to control the platelet count in order to reduce the risk of thrombosis. All patients are educated to reduce cardiovascular risk, by keeping active, well hydrated, stopping cigarette smoking, maintaining a healthy weight, having a good diet and lifestyle and keeping their blood pressure within normal limits. Patients are commenced on aspirin unless contraindicated. In addition, based on established risk factors including age over 60 years, a history of previous thrombosis, or a risk of atherosclerotic disease, cytoreductive therapy (hydroxycarbamide) is considered. Most physicians recommend cytoreductive therapy in cases where the patient's platelet count is over 1500×10^9/L (Beer et al., 2011).

Myelofibrosis (MF) is characterised by bone marrow fibrosis, splenomegaly, anaemia and constitutional symptoms such as fatigue, weight loss, night sweats, pruritus, fever, and bone, muscle or abdominal pain (Mesa, 2009). MF is a debilitating and life-threatening disease with most patients dying as a result of progression to AML or from thrombotic or cardiovascular events (Cervantes et al., 2009). Treatment for MF is aimed at reducing the effects of anaemia and splenomegaly. While transfusion support and folic acid is the mainstay of treatment, hydroxycarbamide can be used for splenomegaly and constitutional symptoms. More recently, drugs which target the molecular JAK2 pathway have been found to have a beneficial effect on splenomegaly and constitutional symptoms; however, there is no clear indication of a disease-modifying effect (Cervantes, 2014). **Allogeneic stem cell transplant** remains the only curative option for MF patients. However, it is associated with high morbidity and mortality, therefore it is usually restricted to eligible patients with higher mortality risks (Cervantes, 2014).

When managing patients with a MPD nurses need to consider individual patient risk factors and tailor patient education to each patient's specific needs. Patients should be advised to ensure they eat a healthy diet and exercise at least 30 minutes every day, five days a week. These lifestyle actions can help in keeping patients strong while coping with a myeloproliferative disorder. Specific dietary advice includes avoiding refined foods, such as white breads, pastas, and especially sugar; eating fewer red meats and more lean meats, cold-water fish, tofu (soya, if no allergy), or beans for protein; avoiding caffeine, alcohol and tobacco and drinking 6 to 8 glasses of filtered water daily.

SEE ALSO
CHAPTER 7

Myelodysplastic syndromes (MDS) are a group of myeloid neoplasms where there are changes in one or more of the blood cells, ineffective blood cell production and a high risk of developing an acute leukaemia, called AML. People with MDS develop the signs of bone marrow failure, which are low white cells (neutropenia), low red cells (anaemia) and low platelets (thrombocytopenia). MDS occurs mostly in older people where the incidence rises rapidly in those over 70 years of age. The management of MDS is to prolong survival and improve patients' quality of life by treating the symptoms of bone marrow failure (Kelly et al., 2015). Treatment includes transfusion support and erythropoietin in selected patients. Erythropoietin helps to raise the Hb level in the blood and therefore reverses the anaemia. Erythropoietin requires close monitoring in the outpatient setting. Those identified to be at high risk of developing AML are treated with immunosuppressive drugs to delay the progress of the disease.

THE LEUKAEMIAS

There are many types of leukaemia and they are generally classified as acute or chronic (see Table 32.4).

Table 32.4 Classification of leukaemia

Lymphoid	*Key points*	Myeloid	*Key points*
Acute lymphoblastic leukaemia (ALL)	– More common in young children. – Survival rates very high for children. – Chromosomal make-up examined to determine prognosis and treatment. Intensive chemotherapy results in pancytopenia (neutropenia, anaemia, thrombocytopenia). – Central nervous system prophylaxis treatment also given (chemotherapy given into the cerebrospinal fluid) to attack any leukaemia cells hiding there.	Acute myeloid leukaemia (AML)	– Vast majority of AML cases are in adults. – Many categories of AML based on the examination of cells. These categories determine prognosis and treatment. Intensive chemotherapy results in pancytopenia (neutropenia, anaemia, thrombocytopenia).
Chronic lymphocytic leukaemia (CLL)	– The most common type of adult leukaemia. – Disease course can be variable with some patients monitored closely and not actively treated and others needing chemotherapy. – People with CLL have a three-fold risk of developing another cancer and an 8-15 fold increased risk of developing a skin cancer. This risk is thought to be because of the way CLL affects the person's lymphocytes and immunity among other factors such as age and chemotherapy treatment.	Chronic myeloid leukaemia (CML)	– Occurs in all age groups but median age is 60 years. – In this leukaemia, a Ph Chromosome (reciprocal translocation between chromosomes 9 and 22) is formed and this results in the unregulated development of tyrosine kinase (BCR-ABL). – Treated by blocking BCR-ABL formation with medicines known as tyrosine kinase inhibitors (TKIs) such as imatinib, nilotinib or dasatinib. – Most patients will experience long survival on a TKI.

ACTIVITY 32.6

Look up tyrosine-kinase inhibitors (TKIs) online at the American Cancer Society site: www.cancer.org/cancer/leukemia-chronicmyeloidcml/detailedguide/leukemia-chronic-myeloid-myelogenous-treating-targeted-therapies

What advice should nurses provide to patients taking this oral treatment for their leukaemia?

ACTIVITY 32.6
ANSWER

VIDEO:
TKIS

Multiple myeloma

Multiple myeloma (MM) is a blood cancer where there is an uncontrolled production of plasma cells (plasma cells arise from B lymphocytes). These plasma cells overproduce immunoglobulins (antibodies) known as a paraprotein which build up in the bone marrow resulting in a variety of effects on the body including anaemia, bone pain as a result of bone lesions, kidney failure, hypercalcaemia, and increased risk of infection. MM is not curable but development in treatments have resulted in control of disease progression and prolonged survivorship. The standard first-line treatment for transplant-eligible patients is high-dose chemotherapy followed by **autologous stem cell transplant (ASCT)** (Atanackovic and Schilling, 2013). MM is a relapsing recurring disorder. A variety of what are known as 'salvage treatments' are used when a patient's disease relapses. One of the challenges for nurses caring for those newly diagnosed with MM is that there is no clear standard of care. It is, therefore, very difficult for patients to make decisions and they often look to nurses for advice.

Tailored exercise is very important for patients with MM because of the damage that the disease can do to bones leading to chronic back pain. Increasing evidence is showing the importance of involving a physiotherapist in designing an individualised exercise plan to strengthen muscles that support the spine.

WHAT'S THE EVIDENCE? 32.1

In a research study (Craike et al., 2013), the benefits of exercise for multiple myeloma patients were reported and these benefits were not just physical.

Reflect on what benefits you think exercise brings to patients with multiple myeloma.

Now read the article and consider if these findings match your own views.

MALIGNANT LYMPHOMAS

Lymphomas are a heterogeneous (diverse types) group of diseases characterised by the presence of malignant lymphocytes which usually accumulate in lymph nodes and cause lymphadenopathy (enlarged lymph nodes). Occasionally, these malignant cells can spill over into blood ('leukaemic phase') or infiltrate organs outside the lymphoid tissue. The key diagnostic test in lymphoma is an adequate lymph node biopsy. The histopathologist examines the lymph node tissue and **immunohistochemistry** and using the WHO classifications for lymphoma makes a diagnosis. Lymphomas are divided into two groups: Hodgkin's lymphoma (HL) where the presence of the Reed-Sternberg cell confirms diagnosis and Non-Hodgkin's lymphoma (NHL) where the Reed-Sternberg cell is absent. Work up for a diagnosis of lymphoma includes blood tests, bone marrow and CT and/or PET scanning. The extent of a patient's lymphoma symptoms can vary widely and a detailed patient history and physical examination is important to determine the effects of the disease and to indicate if treatment is required. Particular attention is given to the presence or absence of B symptoms (this is a term used to describe systemic symptoms of fever, night sweats and weight loss).

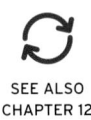

SEE ALSO
CHAPTER 12

Hodgkin's lymphoma (HL)

Hodgkin's lymphoma (HL) is one of the most curable types of blood cancers and accounts for 6% of childhood cancers. It differs from other types of lymphoma by the presence of Reed-Sternberg cells. Approximately 80% of those with HL present with painless supraclavicular or cervical enlarged lymph nodes. In addition, about 35% of children and 75% of adolescents present with symptoms of enlarged nodes in the mediastinum (cough and breathlessness).

Treatment of HL includes radiation or chemotherapy or both. However, long-term consequences of these treatments among survivors are a concern for patients. Current attention is on the late effects on people treated for HL, which include breast cancer and cardiotoxicity (Candela and Thom, 2016). For instance, those treated with radiation for HL before the age of 30 are at a higher risk of secondary breast cancer (Candela and Thom, 2016). Nurses play a significant health promotion role in the care of HL survivors. You should know that these survivors must ensure that they attend for regular mammography and other screening measures.

Non-Hodgkin's lymphoma (NHL)

Non-Hodgkin's lymphoma (NHL) is a group of lymphoproliferative malignancies which behave differently from each other and respond differently to treatment. Because there are so many types of NHL, they are often classified as either aggressive (high grade or faster growing) or indolent (less aggressive). Most NHL affect B lymphocytes. The main treatment options are watch and wait (active surveillance), chemotherapy, radiotherapy and stem cell transplantation.

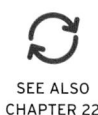

SEE ALSO
CHAPTER 22

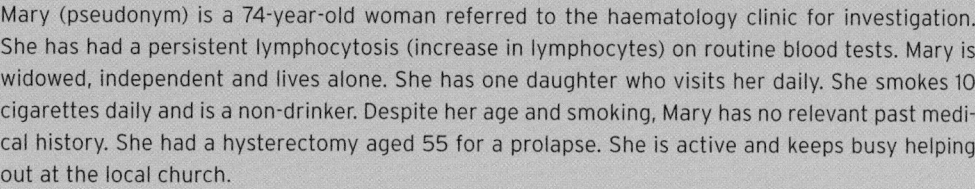

CASE STUDY 32.3: MARY

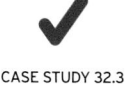

CASE STUDY 32.3
ANSWER

Mary (pseudonym) is a 74-year-old woman referred to the haematology clinic for investigation. She has had a persistent lymphocytosis (increase in lymphocytes) on routine blood tests. Mary is widowed, independent and lives alone. She has one daughter who visits her daily. She smokes 10 cigarettes daily and is a non-drinker. Despite her age and smoking, Mary has no relevant past medical history. She had a hysterectomy aged 55 for a prolapse. She is active and keeps busy helping out at the local church.

She has no allergies. Her only medication is aspirin 75 mg daily. Mary has no B symptoms She had no lymphadenopathy or organomegaly (enlarged organs) on physical examination. Her blood count was Hb 12.7, white cells 22.2, lymphocytes 14.5 and platelets 185. Her blood film revealed a lymphocytosis with smear cells suggestive of chronic lymphocytic leukaemia (CLL). The potential diagnosis of CLL was explained to Mary and the work up investigations required outlined.

She was reviewed in outpatients by her consultant and clinical nurse specialist with her daughter. The diagnosis, prognosis and management of her CLL were explained. Reassurance was provided on the chronic nature of CLL and as she was asymptomatic no treatment was indicated.

- What additional blood investigations would Mary require to confirm her diagnosis?
- What advice should the nurse give Mary regarding her diagnosis following her review at the clinic?
- What health promotion advice does Mary need from the nurse?

ACTIVITY 32.7

Now that you are near the end of the chapter, test yourself with the following questions. The answers can be found on the website.

1. What is a normal platelet count?
2. What cell increases in number following blood loss?
3. Jaundice is a symptom of haemolytic anaemia. True or False?
4. What is the term used to describe a low neutrophil count?
5. Name this type of anaemia where occlusion of blood vessels can occur when the person experiences stress.
6. This surgical procedure is sometimes undertaken in the management of spherocytosis.
7. What is the hallmark sign of a sickle cell crisis?
8. Identify one self-help measure someone with sickle cell can do to keep well.
9. What are B symptoms?
10. A bone marrow is required to diagnose CLL. True or False?
11. Myeloproliferative neoplasms are a myeloid or lymphoid disorder?
12. What is the commonest leukaemia in the western world?
13. What is the characteristic cell found in the diagnosis of Hodgkin's lymphoma?
14. Name a blood condition which immunophenotyping is used to diagnose.

CONCLUSION

Nursing patients with haematological conditions requires an understanding of the blood, bone marrow and lymphatic systems. Many haematological conditions are complex and require prompt intervention. However, the majority are chronic in nature requiring long-term care and follow up.

Greater understanding of the disease processes of haematological conditions has increased the number of treatments available, many of them targeted therapies (drugs that interfere with specific molecules involved in cancer cell growth and survival).

Nurses have a fundamental role in monitoring the symptoms of the patient's disease and controlling side effects to minimise the impact on a patient's daily life. Continuity of care is essential and thus the nurse's role has evolved to include many nurse-led services for this patient group. Understanding patients' lived experience of their blood disease also enhances patient care. If you understand patients' experiences, then you can respond effectively to their needs.

The role of the nurse in the multidisciplinary team management of patients is fundamental. Nurses have a leading role in educating patients about their condition and treatments in order to minimise the impact of their condition on their daily lives. In addition, nurses have a key role in holistically evaluating patient needs and tailoring nursing management to each individual patient. Due to the chronic nature of many haematological conditions, ongoing assessment of patients' changing needs and evaluation of appropriate intervention is required. Nurses must also ensure patients are supported throughout their disease journey. This continuity of care is central to haematology patients' overall positive experience and satisfaction with care.

Support from nurses is especially important when patients need palliative care. Patients with haematological malignancies do know that they will need the help of palliative care services at the final stages of their illness journey. However, for some of these patients, quantity of life is placed ahead of quality of life and they continue to look for treatments right up to the end (McGrath, 2002).

This places significant emphasis on nurses knowing each patient and knowing the 'right' time to introduce a conversation about the role of palliative care in managing their symptoms.

In all areas of clinical practice you will encounter patients with abnormalities in the blood. These abnormalities will range from mild to severe. It is important that you know the normal blood values and always refer to laboratory reports when you are caring for haematology patients on placement. If you have any questions, ask any of the haematology team.

Caring for patients with a haematology condition is one of the most interesting and fulfilling aspects of nursing because it represents the synergy of the art and science of nursing. Because of the chronic nature of haematology conditions, nurses develop unique relationships with patients and their families. Nurses walk alongside patients on their treatment journey and are patients' 'professional friend', and haematology patients value being 'known' by nurses who are knowledgeable and responsive to their ongoing and changing needs.

CHAPTER SUMMARY

- Haematological conditions can be broadly divided into two groups: namely, benign (non-cancerous) blood conditions and blood cancer conditions.
- Haematology disorders are complex and often chronic in nature, and can range from simple conditions such as iron deficiency to more complex conditions such as acute leukaemia.
- Haematological conditions can affect red blood cells, white blood cells, platelets, blood vessels, bone marrow, lymph nodes, spleen, and the proteins involved in bleeding and clotting. Some blood conditions affect more than one cell type and some do not require treatment (just careful monitoring). Nurses therefore require a good understanding of the pathophysiology of the blood in order to effectively care for haematology patients.
- Many blood disorders are relapsing and recurring and nurses support patients on their disease journey. The patient's needs change over time and they need ongoing support and information. Nurses play a key role in monitoring the symptoms of the patient's disease, and controlling side effects of disease and treatment, to minimise the impact on a patient's daily life.

GO FURTHER

Go to https://study.sagepub.com/essentialadultnursing for a further case study related to this chapter. If you are using the interactive ebook, simply click on the book icon in the margin to go straight to the resource.

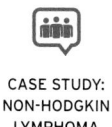

CASE STUDY:
NON-HODGKIN
LYMPHOMA

Books

- Adler, E.M. (2016) *Living with Lymphoma. A Patient's Guide* (2nd ed.). Baltimore, MD: Johns Hopkins University Press.
  This text provides clear and succinct explanations of complex tests (such as serum protein electrophoresis), chemotherapy regimens used across the varieties of lymphoma, monoclonal antibodies and other 'magic bullet' therapies, and stem cell transplant. You will find these aspects of the text particularly helpful in getting to grips with the complexity of diagnosing and managing lymphoma in its various forms.
- Brown, M. and Cutler, T. (2012) *Haematology Nursing*. Oxford: Wiley-Blackwell.
  There are very few specialised haematology texts for nurses so this text is welcome. It is an edited book divided into four sections, which address both non-malignant and malignant blood disorders.

Journal Articles

FURTHER
READING:
JOURNAL
ARTICLES

Go to https://study.sagepub.com/essentialadultnursing for further free online journal articles related to this chapter. If you are using the interactive ebook, simply click on the book icon in the margin to go straight to the resource.

- Dowling, M., Kelly, M. and Meenaghan, T. (2016) Multiple myeloma: Managing a complex blood cancer. *British Journal of Nursing*, 25(16): S18–S28.
  The management of multiple myeloma is constantly evolving. This paper provides the most up-to-date overview.
- King, H. and Myatt, R. (2013) An overview of Non-Hodgkin's Lymphoma. *Cancer Nursing Practice*, 13(1): 31–8. This paper is an excellent overview of lymphoma and clearly explains this complex blood cancer.
- Meenaghan, T., Dowling, M. and Kelly, M. (2012) Acute leukaemia: Making sense of a complex blood cancer. *British Journal of Nursing*, 21(2): 76–83.
  This paper provides a detailed overview of acute leukaemias and the nurse's role in care of these patients.

Weblinks

FURTHER
READING:
WEBLINKS

Go to https://study.sagepub.com/essentialadultnursing for further weblinks related to this chapter. If you are using the interactive ebook, simply click on the book icon in the margin to go straight to the resource.

- www.hematology.org/Patients/Blood-Disorders.aspx
  The American Society of Haematology (ASH) offers a valuable recourse for anyone wanting to know about a blood disorder, with clear information on treatments. The explanations are clear and easy to understand.
- www.youtube.com/watch?v=hb92wr93JrE
  This YouTube computer-generated video presents a very engaging animation of the coagulation process and explains haemophilia. It is only 12 minutes long.
- www.cancerresearchuk.org/about-cancer/type/
  Cancer Research UK site is a great resource which offers simple explanations of the blood cancers. The front page has links to all cancers and it is a very easy site to find information on what you want.
- www.lls.org/lymphoma/hodgkin-lymphoma
  This is the website for the Leukaemia and Lymphoma Society. It offers great detail on these blood cancers.
- www.cancer.org/cancer/leukemia/
  This is an excellent resource from the American Cancer Society for detailed information on all the types of leukaemia, even the very rare ones.
- www.cancer.org/cancer/myelodysplasticsyndrome/index
  The American Cancer Society provides detailed information for multiple myeloma It is also difficult to find information on this blood condition so this website is a great resource.
- www.myeloma.org.uk
  Myeloma UK provides detailed information and support for multiple myeloma patients and is also a great resource for carers and nurses also.

ACE YOUR ASSESSMENT

ONLINE
QUIZZES

Revise what you have learned by visiting https://study.sagepub.com/essentialadultnursing

- Test yourself with multiple-choice and short-answer questions
- Do the chapter activities in the book and check your answers online

REFERENCES

Atanackovic, D. and Schilling, G. (2013) Second autologous transplant as salvage therapy in multiple myeloma. *British Journal of Haematology,* 163(5): 565–2.

Beer, P.A., Erber, W.N., Campbell, P.J. and Green, A.R. (2011) How I treat essential thrombocythemia. *Blood,* 117(5): 1472–82.

Candela, J.L. and Thom, B. (2016) Cardiotoxicity and breast cancer as late effects of pediatric and adolescent Hodgkin lymphoma treatment. *American Journal of Nursing,* 116(4): 32–42.

Cervantes, F. (2014) 'How I treat Myelofibrosis', www.bloodjournal.org. accessed 1/9/2016.

Cervantes, F., Dupriez, B., Pereira, A., Passamonti, F., Reilly, J.T., Morra, E., Vannucchi, A.M., Mesa, R.A., Demory, J.L., Barosi, G., Rumi, R. and Tefferi, A. (2009) Blood Journal. New prognostic scoring system for primary myelofibrosis based on a study of the International Working Group for Myelofibrosis Research and Treatment 113:2895-2901; https://doi.org/10.1182/blood-2008-07-170449

Craike, M.J., Hose, K., Courneya, K.S., Harrison, S.J. and Livingston, P.M. (2013) Perceived benefits and barriers to exercise for recently treated patients with multiple myeloma: A qualitative study. *BMC Cancer,* 13: 319–419.

Creary, S., Zickmund, S., Ross, D., Krishnamurti, L. and Bogen, D.L. (2015) Hydroxyurea therapy for children with sickle cell disease: Describing how caregivers make this decision. *BMC Research Notes,* 8(1).

Hipkiss, V., Benton, S. and Jenkins, K. (2013) Identifying and treating anaemia effectively. *Nursing Times,* 109(38): 20–1.

Janiszewska, H., Bak, A., Hartwig, M., Kuliszkiewicz-Janus, M., Całbecka, M., Jaźwiec, B., Kuliczkowski, K. and Haus, O. (2016) The germline mutations of the CHEK2 gene are associated with an increased risk of polycythaemia vera. *British Journal of Haematology,* 173(1): 150–2.

Kelly, M., Meenaghan, T. and Dowling, M. (2015) Myelodysplastic syndromes: Update and nursing considerations. *Cancer Nursing Practice,* 14(4): 28–37.

McGrath, P. (2002) Qualitative findings on the experience of end-of-life care for hematological malignancies. *The American journal of hospice & palliative care,* 19 (2): 103–11.

Mesa, R.A. (2009) How I treat symptomatic splenomegaly in patients with myelofibrosis. *Blood,* 113(22): 5394–400.

Quinn, C.T., Rogers, Z.R. and Buchanan, G.R. (2004) Survival of children with sickle cell disease. *Blood,* 103(11): 4023–7.

Thibodeau, A., Patton, K. (2004) *Anatomy and Physiology.* (6th ed.). New York: Elsevier.

Tonkin, J., Francis, Y., Pattinson, A., Peters, T., Taylor, M., Thompson, R. and Wallis, L. (2012) Myeloproliferative neoplasms: diagnosis, management and treatment. *Nursing Standard,* 26(51): 44–51.

Trompeter, S. and King, M.J. (2015) Hereditary spherocytosis. *Paediatrics and Child Health (United Kingdom),* 25(8): 381–6.

Vannella, L., Lahner, E., Osborn, J. and Annibale, B. (2013) Systematic review: Gastric cancer incidence in pernicious anaemia. *Alimentary Pharmacology and Therapeutics,* 37(4): 375–82.

CARE OF THE ADULT WITH A DERMATOLOGICAL CONDITION

33

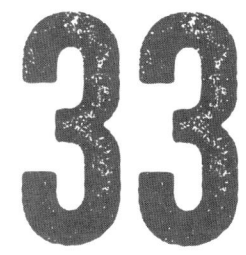

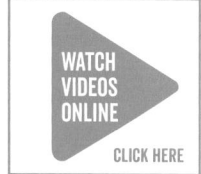

WATCH VIDEOS ONLINE
CLICK HERE

ANDREW EVERED AND LYN BAZLEY

THIS CHAPTER COVERS

- An overview of the anatomy and physiology of the skin
- An explanation of the pathophysiology and clinical characteristics of common skin disorders

- Nursing care of patients with skin conditions
- Discharge planning
- Preparing for your practice.

> "
> My severe acne and scaring on my face has dramatically reduced my confidence and self-esteem. I feel ugly and ashamed, and I don't like people staring at me so I avoid going out of the house as much as I can.
>
> **Patient, All Party Parliamentary Group on Skin (APPGS, 2013)**
> "

> "
> Many known skin conditions can have a significant impact on quality of life for the people who live with them on a daily basis. They can often leave people feeling helpless, anxious, vulnerable and isolated. The greatest achievement as a nurse and patient advocate is being able to provide optimum comfort and support to help alleviate some of the physical and emotional distress caused by their condition and associated symptoms.
>
> **Gill, 3rd year student nurse**
> "

INTRODUCTION

Dermatology is an important but often underemphasised area of nursing practice. It is estimated that in any given year, 54% of the UK population will experience a skin disorder with 14% requiring healthcare intervention (APPGS, 2013). Skin disease can have a profound effect on the physical and psychological wellbeing of the person and, without comprehensive and well-planned care, can affect their quality of life. Understanding the impact skin disease has on the patient can help you deliver holistic care which, as Gill the student nurse stated above, gives you the self-satisfaction that your nursing care is making a positive difference to the patient's life.

This chapter will focus on three common skin conditions: acne, dermatitis and psoriasis; and one less common but serious condition, malignant melanoma. In your practice you will nurse patients with many different physical and mental health conditions and in each experience you will indirectly be caring for their skin. The Nursing Midwifery Council (NMC, 2015) expects all nurses to make safeguarding an everyday aspect of their practice and for dermatology this means not ignoring the medical, emotional and physical care needs of patients and their families. This chapter encourages you to appreciate that in order to deliver good care, you need to consider the holistic implications of the person's skin.

ACTIVITY 33.1
ANSWER

ACTIVITY 33.1: REFLECTION

In your nurse education to date, consider the teaching and practice you have had in relation to the skin. It is likely that you have learnt how to assess your patient's skin to help make a nursing diagnosis, such as checking for cyanosis in the breathless patient or assessing skin integrity for wound care; but not necessarily about diseases of the skin. Take time out to reflect on your understanding of the anatomy of the skin and what it means to your patient when normal skin cell proliferation is disturbed.

ANATOMY AND PHYSIOLOGY OF THE SKIN

The skin is the largest organ of the body covering a surface area of approximately 1.8–2 m² and has several important functions:

- It acts as a protective barrier.
- It supports temperature control.
- It assists in the production of vitamin D.
- It allows for sensation with the external environment through touch, pressure, heat and cold.
- It absorbs and excretes substances.

Dermatology is concerned with the diagnosis and treatment of skin conditions and to fully understand problems of skin disease, it is necessary to appreciate the basic structure and function of the skin. In this explanation the anatomy is described from the innermost layer first, leading through to the outer layer of the skin, following the natural life cycle of a skin cell.

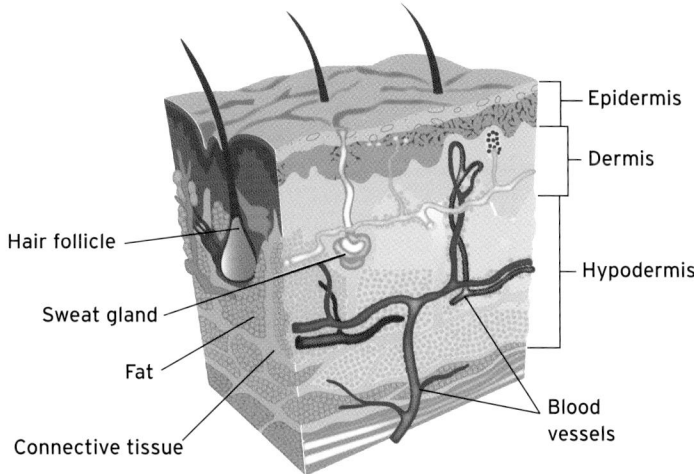

Figure 33.1 Cross section of the skin

Source: Boore et al. (2016). Illustrated by Shaun Mercier, © SAGE Publications.

Subcutaneous tissue

This layer is also known as the subcutis or hypodermis. It contains fat and its thickness will vary between individuals. Connective tissue, nerves and larger blood vessels are also to be found in this layer. Its primary function is regulation of temperature, fat storage and shock absorption.

Dermis

Above the subcutaneous tissue is the dermis. This is the largest layer of the skin making up approximately 90% of the overall skin structure. There is variation in thickness of the dermis depending on body location from the eyelids (0.3 mm) to the back (3 mm). The dermis is the most functional layer of the skin with its papillary layer connecting it to the epidermis and its reticular layer made of collagen and connective tissue giving it strength and elasticity. The dermis contains many specialised structures that assist with maintaining a healthy skin and temperature control. For skin care the most important structures are the sebaceous glands.

Sebaceous glands produce sebum, which is secreted into the hair follicles. Sebum is an oily substance and its function is to keep the surface of the skin supple and hydrated. **Androgenic hormones** control the release of sebum and the amount produced is influenced by hormonal changes. The bacteria *Proprionibacterium acnes* (P. acnes) colonises the sebaceous gland, which is a harmless bacteria under normal circumstances and is thought to have a role in immune regulation.

Epidermis

The outermost layer of the skin is the epidermis, which consists of four layers that represent the different stages of maturation of skin cells.

1.   Stratum basale. This layer is immediately above the dermis and it contains the stem cells from which **keratinocytes** are formed. Melanocytes are present in this layer and it is these cells that produce the pigment that colours the skin and protects it from harmful ultraviolet radiation from the sun. As more keratinocyte cells are produced, the existing cells get pushed into the next layer.

2. Stratum spinosum. The cells in this layer differentiate and flatten. They offer structural support to the skin but also start to produce more keratin that adds strength but also waterproof qualities.
3. Stratum granulosum. Keratinisation of the cells continues in this layer. A superficial layer, the stratum lucidum, is found adjacent with more cells containing melanin. Not all areas of the skin have this layer, for example the eyelids.
4. Stratum corneum. This is the outermost layer and consists of heavily keratinised dead cells. These have a protective function for the lower layers of the skin and also waterproofs the skin. It is this layer where desquamation or shedding of dead skin happens.

The normal life cycle of a skin cell is approximately 28 days in which time it is produced in the stratum basale and is gradually pushed through the layers to the stratum corneum, by which time the cell has flattened and keratinised and is eventually shed from the skin to be replaced by more cells rising to the surface.

GO FURTHER

This brief overview identifies the cell proliferation of the skin and will help you understand dermatological conditions. For a more in-depth understanding of all functions of the skin read: Boore, J., Cook, N. and Shepherd, A. (2016) Skin and temperature regulation. Chapter 14 in *Essentials of Anatomy and Physiology for Nursing Practice*. London: SAGE.

THE PATHOPHYSIOLOGY AND CLINICAL CHARACTERISTICS OF COMMON SKIN DISORDERS

ACNE

Pathophysiology

Acne vulgaris is the most common skin condition worldwide (Williams et al., 2012) and is described as a chronic inflammatory disorder of the pilosebaceous unit. This 'unit' is situated in the epidermis and consists of a hair, hair follicle and sebaceous gland. Sebum is produced in the glands and travels up the hair follicle to the skin; in acne, however, the route to the skin is blocked by keratinocytes, and plugs of **keratin** and sebum become trapped in the skin pores. P. acnes, a harmless bacteria found on the skin, multiplies in the presence of excess sebum causing an inflammatory response which produces pus-filled spots. The factors causing acne are, therefore, excess sebum, abnormal shedding of keratinocytes, proliferation of P. acnes and inflammation.

Acne appears to be influenced by androgenic hormones increasing sebum production and this reflects the prevalence of acne between genders and age. It is most often seen in adolescents and young adults; however, it can persist or even develop in adulthood and older age. Acne appears more prevalent in males than females during adolescence but with changes in the balance of androgens women can predominantly be affected in adulthood (Fisk et al., 2014).

Clinical characteristics

Acne is diagnosed by the presence of comedones and pustules. Comedones are classified as closed (whiteheads) or open (blackheads) and if neither of these is seen then you should consider alternative dermatological conditions. Pustules are often associated with acne and can range from small red spots to yellow pus-filled pimples. Acne appears in areas of the skin where there is an increased production of sebum, most commonly the face, neck, chest and upper back and shoulders.

Nursing assessment

Your assessment of the patient should ensure you have a comprehensive understanding of the patient's symptoms and problems that include both physical and psychological aspects of the condition. This should include family history of acne, medical history including chronic conditions and for women their menstrual cycle and any history of **hirsutism**. Specific questions should be asked regarding their acne such as onset and duration, severity of comedones and presence of pustules as well as distribution on the skin. The patient should be asked to self-assess their acne in relation to previous episodes and they should be allowed to explain how they normally treat their acne, what treatments have worked previously and what exacerbates or irritates their acne. A physical assessment of the patient's skin should be undertaken to assess the current level of distribution and severity.

Clinical investigations

Although diagnosis is made primarily from the physical appearance of the comedones, acne can be categorised by severity of the condition. In mild acne, both open and closed comedones are present but the absence of any further inflammatory response such as pustules or scarring. Moderate acne will have comedones present and will also have the appearance of inflammatory pustules. Severe acne will have an increased presence of comedones and inflamed pustules and may also have evidence of scarring. Your assessment should address the social and personal impact acne has for the patient to determine the psychological impact and possible low self-esteem and social isolation.

Nursing care and management

Most patients can independently care for their acne and the nursing responsibilities are to support any psychological effects of the condition and to promote self-management. Excellent interpersonal skills are needed to ensure that the patient's quality of life and levels of self-esteem are enhanced. Care should include the following:

- An understanding that acne does not indicate poor hygiene. Patients shouldn't be expected to increase their hygiene practices as this can be counterproductive. Skin should be bathed gently as harsh washing will only cause irritation. Cleaning the skin will remove the sebum from the skin surface but does not affect the production of sebum. Hair can be washed more frequently to remove any excess oil.
- Ensure that treatment is started as soon as possible as this will help prevent scarring and improve self-esteem. Assist the patient to apply topical medication if they are unable to reach all the affected areas such as back and shoulders. Encourage the patient to continue the full treatment to ensure medication has time to take effect.
- Advise the patient to use cosmetics and toiletries that are non-comedongenic oil- and alcohol-free as these will reduce clogging of pores or skin irritation.
- Encourage the patient not to pick the spots and pustules as this causes scarring and permanent damage.

ACTIVITY 33.2
ANSWER

ACTIVITY 33.2: CRITICAL THINKING

The sufferer has the unenviable choice of how to manage their acne. To squeeze the spots for immediate improved cosmetic appearance and risk long-term scarring; or leave alone and feel unable to venture out and socialise. Consider how the person must feel having to make this choice and how they may think they appear to others. The Primary Care Dermatology Society has some good illustrations: www.pcds.org.uk/clinical-guidance/acne-vulgaris

DERMATITIS

Pathophysiology

The terms dermatitis and eczema are synonymous and the words are often used interchangeably, although they have a different emphasis as dermatitis implies inflammation and the origins of the word eczema means to boil. It is a skin condition that can be both acute and chronic in nature, and causes inflammation and intense irritation. The aetiology of dermatitis is different in respect of type with the causes being classified in two groups: a) exogenous, those having an external cause; and b) endogenous, those having an internal cause.

With endogenous dermatitis there are genetic factors that contribute to the cause. The Filaggrin gene plays an important role in the protective nature of the epidermis and it is believed that deficiency of this gene has a significant effect on dermatitis (Wedgeworth et al., 2013). **Atopic** dermatitis is a good example of this whereby the immune system is affected elevating immunoglobulin E (IgE) antibody levels, causing patients to often suffer from asthma and allergies such as hay fever and rhinitis.

Exogenous dermatitis is often caused by external irritants to the skin. Contact dermatitis is a common form of this whereby substances that come into contact with the skin cause an inflammatory response. These causes can be through exposure to irritants that are chemical, biological and even mechanical in nature but also through allergic causes whereby the patient is exposed to a substance to which they become sensitised.

It is important to note that the two classifications of dermatitis are not exclusive and a patient may present with a history of both; current research suggests that while there is variation of evidence it is highly probable that the figures are underestimating the true numbers of patients presenting with both types (Aquino and Fonacier, 2014).

Clinical characteristics

Dermatitis affects the protective properties of the skin and ultimately results in damage to the dermis and epidermis. In both classifications the epidermal skin barrier is impaired and, based on the histological changes, the patient presents with several clinical features. Wet dermatitis occurs where there is oedema in the epidermis and vasodilation of the dermis whereas dry dermatitis is caused by dermal extravasation and thickening of the epidermal layer. In both cases the skin is red, inflamed, painful and itchy.

Nursing assessment

Dermatitis can affect all age groups and you are as likely to care for older patients with the condition as you are children and young adults. With older people the dermatitis may be due to physical changes to the body such as venous (gravitational) dermatitis while atopic dermatitis is common in younger people.

Taking a recorded history and completing a body chart to detail the site and distribution of the lesions is important as accurate detail and visual assessment of the condition helps future evaluation of treatment. The patient's age and general health status is needed to ensure important indicators to define type of dermatitis are not missed. These should include any medical illnesses, history of previous skin problems and any family history of skin conditions, allergies or autoimmune diseases. You should also take a social history to indicate any triggers that may exacerbate the condition such as occupation, exposure to chemicals and substances, types of cosmetics and toiletries used, and hobbies that may expose the patient to irritants such as swimming (chlorine) or gardening (sap). Understanding the patient's perception of the problem is also vital as this will enable you to appreciate the impact it has on their activities of daily living, their levels of self-esteem and whether they have access to and comply with treatments.

Clinical investigations

Physical examination of the patient's skin is a defining factor to diagnosis. Dermatitis will manifest visually and the type of inflammation and clinical change to the skin can help classify the type of dermatitis. Wet dermatitis will present with oedema and weeping lesions, and the integrity of the skin is compromised whereas dry dermatitis will have thick scaly skin. Most patients will have inflamed skin, either red or pink in colour and will complain of pain and pruritus. Patients may also describe irritability, loss of sleep and sometimes loss of function in the affected area such as hands and joints.

In atopic dermatitis the patient can undergo allergy patch tests to identify allergens that can trigger the condition. These may also involve skin pricks tests or specific IgE blood tests and are often performed in allergy clinics.

Nursing care and management

The aim of nursing care is not to provide a cure to the patient; where possible the irritating substances or allergens should be identified and removed. However, often these are unknown and so priorities of care are to manage symptoms. Improving the quality of life of the patient and reducing distress will be the focus of the care; this will include managing the itchiness, pain and discomfort that is associated with the condition. The use of emollient therapy and corticosteroids form part of treatment plans and are discussed later in the chapter.

CRITICAL THINKING STOP POINT 33.1

There is a real issue for your nursing practice as the use of soap and gels for handwashing and the use of COSHH substances raise the risk of you suffering from contact dermatitis. The Health and Safety Executive website www.hse.gov.uk/healthservices/dermatitis.htm offers some good advice for protecting your skin.

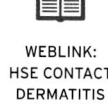

WEBLINK:
HSE CONTACT
DERMATITIS

PSORIASIS

Pathophysiology

Psoriasis is a lifelong chronic condition affecting skin cell production. The normal reproduction and proliferation is accelerated from 28 days to 7 days, which results in the epidermal cells failing to mature properly. The immature cells cause a build-up of keratin in the stratum corneum, which leads to the characteristic silvery scale of psoriasis. In addition to the thickening of the epidermis there is an increased blood flow to the dermis, which encourages inflammatory cells to enter the epidermis giving the red appearance to the psoriatic lesions.

The extent of psoriasis within the worldwide population is not known although self-reporting prevalence ranges from 1.5–8.5% (Danielsen et al., 2013). It is an autoimmune condition and the exact cause is not known but is associated with other autoimmune conditions such as rheumatoid arthritis, Crohn's disease and inflammatory bowel syndrome. There are genetic causative factors with many studies identifying familial tendencies between relatives and especially twins, and also environmental factors which include trauma, infection, sunlight, drugs, alcohol, smoking and stress (Enamandram and Kimball, 2013).

Clinical characteristics

Psoriasis is characterised by red plaques with silvery scales, the extent and thickness of which can be variable. Patients may present with few plaques of several millimetres to coverage on the entire torso or limb. While the lesions can appear anywhere on the body, common sites include elbows, knees and scalp. As scales detach from the skin there can be bleeding.

Nursing assessment

NICE guidelines (2012) recommend that assessment of the patient should be holistic and follow four themes:

- **Disease severity**. The Physician's Global Assessment tool should be used to determine whether the presence of psoriasis is 'clear', 'nearly clear', 'mild', 'moderate', 'severe' or 'very severe'. You should also use a body chart to assess the extent of psoriasis on the body surface especially in difficult to see sites such as soles of feet, scalp, flexures and genitals.
- **Quality of life**. An index or tool is recommended to determine the physical, psychological and social wellbeing of the patient.
- **Whether there is associated psoriatic arthritis**. This condition can appear with only mild skin changes but have severe arthritic symptoms that can have a devastating impact similar to rheumatoid arthritis.
- **The presence of any co-morbidities**. Patients with psoriasis appear to have a higher incidence of health problems and are more likely to suffer from cardiac and digestive disorders, diabetes, obesity and depression compared to the general population.

Clinical investigations

Diagnosis of psoriasis is made by physical examination and history taking. There are, however, several types of psoriasis that can be differentiated by visually examining the skin. Examples include: plaque psoriasis which is the most common form and presents as red patches with silvery flaky scale; guttate psoriasis (sometimes called 'Raindrop' psoriasis) which often occurs 2–3 weeks after a streptococcal throat infection and appears as small red dots on the torso, arms and legs; pustular psoriasis which has blisters that appear on the hands and feet; and a rare and potentially life-threatening form of psoriasis, erythrodermic, which presents over the whole body as very red and burned skin which can peel.

Nursing care and management

Your care needs to be holistic and demonstrate appreciation of the psychosocial implications of the condition. Health promotion in maintaining a healthy skin but also preventing or managing co-morbidities is an important aspect of care. While many patients can self-administer topical treatment, advice on how and when to apply, and education on the different treatments, is part of your role. Some patients will require phototherapy at a dermatology unit where ultraviolet light is administered in a specially designed cabinet. Advice and support is needed for the patients as UV light is generally associated with causing skin cancers; however, carefully measured doses of psoralen and ultraviolet A radiation (PUVA) and ultraviolet B (UVB) are very effective in treating psoriasis. Patients need either skin preparation or oral medication shortly before treatment which may be required three times weekly for several weeks. This can have an impact on their working and family life, which needs to be discussed.

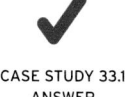

CASE STUDY 33.1 ANSWER

CASE STUDY 33.1: THOMAS

Thomas is 19 years old and lives at home with his parents and his younger sister. His father is a staff sergeant in the army, his mum is a self-employed hairdresser and his sister Claire has just started a health and beauty course at college.

A fit and healthy man, Thomas has plaque psoriasis that is especially evident on his elbows, knees, back and scalp. He uses a range of topical treatments that are normally effective in managing his condition. He does, however, have relapses when stressed. His mother is very supportive and helps apply the lotions but his sister complains of the mess left in the bathroom and on the towels.

Thomas enjoys playing sport and is a member of the local rugby team. He likes to train weekly but does occasionally miss sessions when his psoriasis is too sore and painful.

Thomas works for a well-known supermarket: his role is to accept deliveries and ensure the products are correctly stacked on the shelves. This means occasionally working on the shop floor and giving advice to customers. He prefers to work in the warehouse as he finds that sometime customers react negatively when he is among food products.

Socially, Thomas has a small but supportive group of friends. He doesn't have a girlfriend as he is conscious of how he must appear to others and is anxious about starting an intimate relationship.

1. What are the quality of life issues for Thomas?
2. How could you advise Thomas to help his motivation and self-esteem?

MELANOMA

Pathophysiology

Melanoma is the most lethal form of skin cancer and is often termed 'malignant melanoma'. It occurs when the melanocytes become damaged due to UV radiation. Melanocytes are found between the dermis and the epidermis and their function is to produce the pigmentation that colours the skin, and it is this pigmentation that helps protect the deeper layers of the skin from ultraviolet light by synthesising melanin. When exposed to high levels of UV light either directly from the sun or through the use of sunbeds there is a proliferation of melanocytes, which become malignant. Melanoma often develops at the site of a mole.

Incidence of malignant melanoma is on the increase and now estimated to be the fifth most common cancer in the UK with 14,500 new cases diagnosed each year (Cancer Research, UK, 2015).

GO FURTHER

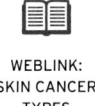

WEBLINK: SKIN CANCER TYPES

In your reading of this condition you will come across basal cell and squamous cell skin cancer. These are common cancers affecting different cells of the skin and termed non-melanoma skin cancer. You can find out more at www.cancerresearchuk.org/about-cancer/type/skin-cancer/about/types-of-skin-cancer

---

Clinical characteristics

Malignant melanoma presents as nodules on the skin surface. These nodules are characteristically irregular and **hyperpigmented**; the cells continue to produce melanin and this gives a variation in colour from light tan to black. There are four types of melanoma that help with diagnosis.

1. Superficial spreading melanoma. The most common form accounting for 75% of cases in patients with white skin. Patients are generally in the 40–50 year group and the lesions appear on sun-exposed areas of the body.
2. Nodular melanoma. Approximately 10–15% of all melanoma cases and affects patients in the 50–60 year group. Lesions are seen on sun-exposed parts of the body and men are twice as likely to be affected as women.
3. Acral lentiginous melanoma. This is the most common form of melanoma in people with dark skin and is more common over the age of 50, affecting men and women equally. Common sites for the lesions are under nails, soles of feet and palms of hands.
4. Lentigo melanoma. This melanoma affects between 4–15% of people in old age and is attributed to long-term sun damage. Due to its slow growth it is often dismissed, maybe as natural aging of the skin, and diagnosis is often delayed until considerable spread has occurred.

Nursing assessment

There will be many situations during your nursing when you will have the opportunity to assess your patients' skin, and not necessarily those with a skin complaint. These opportunities should be used to assess for signs of malignant melanoma and the ABCDE tool is a useful guide (see Table 33.1).

Clinical investigations

To aid diagnosis, treatment and prognosis the affected mole will be reviewed using a dermatoscope, and then if necessary the mole will be excised for a biopsy test. If cancer is present then there are a

Table 33.1 Warning signs of melamona

Asymmetry	Are both sides of the mole similar or is one side more irregular than the other?
Border	Moles should have a smooth border with occasional notches. Are there any jagged or misshapen edges?
Colour	Is there consistency in the colour or does the mole have several colours especially blue, black or red?
Diameter	Moles tend to be small in size, approximately 6 mm. Any unusually large moles are a warning sign.
Evolving	Is the mole changing in size or colour compared to other moles on the skin?

number of tools that can be used to determine the spread of the disease. These tools can be complicated and complex and patients may be given a more simplified version of the spread of the cancer. The TNM tool is a common grading system used in the UK and a simplified version given below (see Table 33.2).

Table 33.2 Grading melanoma

T = Size and extent of primary cancer

N = The number of nearby lymph nodes affected

M = Describes if the cancer has metastasised

The TNM system may then be grouped into 5 stages of malignant melanoma:

Stage 0. The cancer remains in the epidermis and has not spread

Stage 1. The cancer is only 1–2 mm thick, remains in the skin and has not spread

Stage 2. The cancer is growing and may have ulcerated but has not spread

Stage 3. The cancer has spread to nearby nodes

Stage 4. The cancer has spread beyond the primary site and nearby nodes to other organs of the body such as brain, liver or lungs.

Nursing care and management

The priority throughout the care of your patient is the psychological effects of living with cancer. Studies have indicated that female patients with malignant melanoma have similar needs as female patients with other cancers; however, men required more information than those men with other cancers (Passalacqua et al., 2012). The need for a good nurse–patient relationship is evident. Education of the condition and psychological support will underpin all care; however, the nature of discussion will depend on staging and diagnosis. Those patients with stage 4 melanoma will need significantly different and more intense nursing interventions than those with a stage 0 melanoma. Treatments will vary quite considerably from simple education on sun protection advice and self-examination of skin for those with localised melanoma, to advice and support during the uncomfortable period of diagnosis when tests such as biopsies, x-ray, computed tomography (CT) scans and magnetic resonance imaging (MRI) are performed, especially for those with more advanced melanoma. Surgical removal

SEE ALSO
CHAPTER 22

SEE ALSO
CHAPTER 23

SEE ALSO
CHAPTER 10

of the cancerous cells or tumour is a common approach and your nursing care should reflect that of the needs of the surgical patient. In advanced disease you may be involved with care that is managed by the oncology team such as radiotherapy and chemotherapy while in end stage cancer you will be working with the palliative care teams.

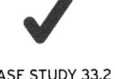

CASE STUDY 33.2
ANSWER

CASE STUDY 33.2: PAULINE

You are on placement with the practice nurse at a busy Health Centre and your current patient is Stephen who is 20 years old and has Down's syndrome. Stephen's main carer is his mum Pauline who had made the appointment as Stephen has been suffering from constipation for the last two weeks.

You have a casual conversation with Pauline while the practice nurse is collecting Stephen's nursing notes and find out that she is 50 years old; a single parent and works part time in a garden centre. She works hard to give her and Stephen a good life and they enjoy outdoor activities and summer holidays abroad that allow Stephen to experience life to the full.

Pauline is wearing a thin white blouse that exposes her shoulders. While she is repositioning Stephen for the physical assessment you notice that on her left shoulder there is a mole about 10 millimetres in diameter. The mole looks irregular around the edges and black in colour.

1. What are your responsibilities in relation to the NMC (2015) expectations of safeguarding?
2. How would you ensure Pauline receives appropriate advice?

NURSING CARE OF PATIENTS WITH SKIN CONDITIONS

Although each skin disease has its own treatments and interventions which require specific nursing care, there are many aspects of care that apply equally to all patients. Having an understanding of these considerations will help you plan holistic patient-centred nursing care.

Topical treatments

For the majority of patients, topical treatment is the main intervention to manage their condition. These treatments are often time consuming, difficult to apply and messy. When discussing topical treatment with your patient consider the following:

- There is a high level of non-compliance with topical treatments as patients are often dissatisfied with the mess involved and time taken to apply the treatments. 'Steroid phobia' about the use of corticosteroids also causes non-compliance and overall young men are more likely than any other group not to comply with therapy instructions (Chella, 2014).
- Treatments are often messy and smelly. Oil- and tar-based treatments can mess and stain baths, towels and clothing. The smell from some of these treatments can also linger on the body and clothing. Many patients need to have a regime for cleaning the bathroom after treatments and having a separate set of clothing for treatment sessions.
- Many treatments need to be applied several times a day and if multiple treatments are being given then time between each to allow for absorption only adds to the length of time needed away from other daily activities.
- Patients may need the support of others to help apply topical treatments. If the skin condition affects hard to reach areas then it is necessary to identify who is available and willing to help.

Emollient therapy

Emollient is a substance that has a softening and soothing effect and it is a staple treatment for all skin conditions. When the epidermis is damaged the skin is more susceptible to water loss and the effects of allergens and irritants. Emollients add a protective layer on the skin that helps minimise dehydration of the skin and irritation. They help make keratinised skin supple, reduce inflammation and can reduce the need for topical corticosteroids; however, they need to be applied in the direction of hair growth to prevent **folliculitis**. The effects of emollients are short lived and need to be applied frequently, liberally and long term and it is not unusual to use up to 500 grams per week. It is important to ensure sufficient amounts are prescribed by the GP so that treatment is not interrupted. You need to ensure the patient has help to apply the lotions to all affected areas and that they understand the need to continue this treatment even when their skin feels healthy.

CRITICAL THINKING STOP POINT 33.2

Emollient therapy is the main physical treatment for skin conditions. It has great impact upon the wellbeing of the patient and their skin. You need to consider how your knowledge and understanding of this therapy can improve the care you give your patient. The British Dermatology Nursing Group (BDNG) has an excellent resource to help you: https://s3-eu-west-2.amazonaws.com/bdngs3/wp-content/uploads/2017/02/EmollientBPG-1.pdf

WEBLINK:
EMOLLIENT
THERAPY

Corticosteroids

Topical corticosteroids are commonly used in skin disease as they have an anti-inflammatory and immunosuppressive effect. They are often used in the exacerbated phases of disease when emollient therapy alone is not sufficient; but they are not a curative measure. Care in applying the solution needs to be taken with some conditions such as psoriasis where inappropriate withdrawal can cause 'rebound' and induce further psoriatic intensity. Instructions on restricting application to a limited number of surfaces such as face, hands and flexures may be necessary. Once the flare-up has subsided corticosteroids should be slowly withdrawn and the patient treated with emollients. Should they need to be used for longer periods of maintenance then there should be rest periods. Corticosteroids are usually applied once or twice daily and commence with the most potent strength that is effective and then reduced as condition improves. Application should be to well-moisturised skin but leave a 30-minute interval after applying emollients to prevent unintentional spread of the corticosteroid. If there are no signs of improvement in 7–10 days then the diagnosis should be reassessed as exacerbation may be due to other causes such as infection.

ACTIVITY 33.3: CRITICAL THINKING

The Finger Tip Unit guide is often used to help patients administer topical steroids. Read what advice the National Institute for Health and Care Excellence (NICE) has to offer you: https://www.evidence.nhs.uk/Search?ps=40&q=fingertip+unit

ACTIVITY 33.3
ANSWER

WEBLINK:
ADMINISTERING
TOPICAL
STEROIDS

QUALITY OF LIFE

> Any activities that need uncovering myself at all, (I live covered from neck to toe, and with makeup on my face) are a no-no as I get stares and people cat calling or moving away from me, thinking I have something catching. This particularly includes swimming, dancing, gym, going to the beach or being out in the sun.
>
> **Patient with acne (APPGS, 2013)**

Healthcare today does not necessarily focus on ensuring absence of illness and disease but acknowledges that the physical, mental and social wellbeing of the population is equally as important. To determine the wellbeing of individuals there is a need to assess their quality of life. While this is a subjective notion, many tools have been developed to score both the negative and positive aspects of a person's health and the impact it has on their life. Within dermatology, tools are available to help assess the impact and severity of specific conditions such as psoriasis upon the patient's life and to determine effectiveness of treatment. These tools ask the patient to score the effect their condition has had on quality of life over a period of time; for example, they may ask the following questions about the impact of their condition over the last week.

- How itchy and sore their skin has been?
- What effect the condition has had on their sleep?
- Whether there have been changes to their social life and leisure activities?
- Whether the condition has caused a change in their dress sense or appearance?
- Whether the patient has suffered any personal relationships and/or sexual difficulties?
- Whether the patient's work or study has been affected?
- Whether the treatments are causing problems with mess or laundering?

WHAT'S THE EVIDENCE? 33.1

WEBLINK: DERMATOLOGY LIFE QUALITY INDEX

What quality of life tools are available for you to use in clinical practice? Have a look at www.cardiff. ac.uk/dermatology/quality-of-life/ and consider how these can enhance your nursing care.

Studies into living with a skin disease have shown that, with all conditions, the person suffers from life issues and that healthcare professionals need to give particular emphasis to the patients' wellbeing when planning care (APPGS, 2013). Self-esteem has a major role to play in the wellbeing of patients and is closely linked to the general health of the individual. People with high levels of self-esteem often have a more positive view on their health and lower levels of anxiety and distress. Low self-esteem is associated with poor health outcomes, emotional distress, and suicidal ideation. The psychological impact is not always related to the severity of the condition and those with relatively minor skin disease can have significantly high levels of emotional dysfunction.

HEALTH PROMOTION

Good practice and sensible skin protection will help promote health and wellbeing for patients with skin conditions. Your role is also to help promote compliance in self-application and it is important that they fully understand how and when to use these treatments.

Some tips on how to advise your patients are set out below.

- Emollient therapy is a continuous treatment, so don't stop applying cream even when your skin appears healthy.
- Avoid trigger factors. Substances such as soaps, detergents and shampoos can cause irritation to the skin.
- Wash wisely. Vigorous scrubbing and abrasive washing only inflames skin conditions. Having a skin disease does not mean dirty skin or poor hygiene. Gentle cleaning of the skin, using emollients rather than soap, is beneficial.
- Be sun safe. Cover up when in the sun with dark-coloured, tight-weaved fabrics. Don't go in the sun at the hottest time of the day and use a high-quality sunscreen.

DISCHARGE PLANNING

For discharge to be effective all aspects of the patient's condition and circumstances must be taken into consideration. Patient education is important to ensure compliance with self-administration of topical treatments and adherence to guidance on oral medication. For many patients their skin condition is a lifelong and chronic condition; this means that while they may well be discharged from a clinical setting, they will probably still be under the care of a dermatologist. To ensure safe continuity of care when being discharged from hospital, consider the following questions:

- Has there been any change to the status of the patient's skin condition during admission?
- How are these changes being communicated to their GP and dermatologist?
- Are there other members of the multidisciplinary team who need to be aware of the patient's hospitalisation and discharge?
- Does the patient have sufficient supplies of emollients to allow good skin care until they can get a repeat prescription?
- Has the patient been educated sufficiently to care for their skin condition?
- Is a district nurse needed in the forthcoming days to help with applying treatments?

PREPARATION FOR PRACTICE
PLACEMENTS 33.1

Many patients will access healthcare services for reasons other than their skin condition and unless you are allocated a placement in a specialist dermatology ward or unit, it is unlikely that their skin will be a priority. In a busy healthcare environment the urgency to treat the current physical illness can lead many healthcare professionals to ignore or place little importance on the long-term skin condition. Some people feel disempowered when in a healthcare setting allowing the healthcare

(Continued)

(Continued)

team to dictate care, which can result in their skin needs being overshadowed or they may feel embarrassed to ask busy nurses to assist in their continuing treatment. The combined stress of their current illness and not being able to follow their skin routine may possibly exacerbate their skin condition and you should consider your role in safeguarding to ensure the emotional and physical wellbeing of your patient.

ACTIVITY 33.4
ANSWER

ACTIVITY 33.4: CRITICAL THINKING

How can you link your knowledge of skin conditions to your practice area and how will you be able to give holistic care? Consider the following:

- Does the nurse assessment allow for skin conditions to be documented?
- How will the institutional regime of the placement area impact on the person's routine of daily skin care?
- Will your patient be exposed to toiletries, chemicals or cleaning products that could cause irritation to their skin?
- Is time management sufficient to allow for assistance applying emollients?
- As a student nurse, to whom can you escalate your concerns if a patient is not receiving best skin care?

WHAT'S THE EVIDENCE? 33.2

The British Association of Dermatologists has a set of quality standards for people with skin conditions.
Quality standards for dermatology: Providing the right care for people with skin conditions. www.bad.org.uk/shared/get-file.ashx?itemtype=document&id=795

Read the principles of care section 1.1.4. What supportive services are available within your local healthcare provider to ensure care is holistic?

Read the patient and public involvement section 2.1.3. Where can you find information about how service users evaluate the care of your local healthcare provider?

WEBLINK:
DERMATOLOGY
QUALITY
STANDARDS

CHAPTER SUMMARY

- Skin disease affects a significant proportion of the UK population.
- Many conditions are long term and require lifestyle changes for effective management.
- The psychological effects of living with a skin disorder can be as devastating as living with other chronic conditions such as diabetes and cardiovascular disease.
- Nurses have an important role in patient education, health promotion and holistic care.

GO FURTHER

Go to https://study.sagepub.com/essentialadultnursing for a further case study related to this chapter. If you are using the interactive ebook, simply click on the book icon in the margin to go straight to the resource.

CASE STUDY: DERMATOLOGICAL ASSESSMENT

Books

- Boore, J., Cook, N. and Shepherd, A. (2016) Skin and temperature regulation. Chapter 14 in *Essentials of Anatomy and Physiology for Nursing Practice*. London: SAGE.
- Delves-Yates, C. (ed.) (2018) *Essentials of Nursing Practice* (2nd edn.). London: SAGE.
- Nicol, J. (2011) *Nursing Adults with Long-Term Conditions*. Exeter: Learning Matters.

Journal Articles

- Howard, S., Hafez, A. and Cream, P. (2012) The lived experience of psoriasis patients: A phenomenological study. *Dermatological Nursing*, 11 (4): 48–55.
- Mooney, T. (2014) Preventing psychological distress in patients with acne. *Nursing Standard*, 28 (22): 42–8.
- Onselen, J.V. (2011) Skin care in the older person: Identifying and managing eczema. *British Journal of Community Nursing*, 16 (12): 577–82.

Weblinks

Go to https://study.sagepub.com/essentialadultnursing for further weblinks related to this chapter. If you are using the interactive ebook, simply click on the book icon in the margin to go straight to the resource.

FURTHER READING: WEBLINKS

- British Association of Dermatologists www.bad.org.uk/
  This is a charity dedicated to promoting good practice in dermatology care.
- National Institute for Health and Care Excellence (NICE) www.nice.org.uk/guidance/conditions-and-diseases/skin-conditions
  This site offers up-to-date evidence-based information regarding guidance and care pathways for best practice.
- Primary Care Dermatology Society www.pcds.org.uk/
  This site has a community-based focus.
- The Psoriasis Association www.psoriasis-association.org.uk/
  This site is a good example of the many patient-focused websites that are condition specific and contains much useful information from people living with the disease.

ACE YOUR ASSESSMENT

Revise what you have learned by visiting https://study.sagepub.com/essentialadultnursing

ONLINE QUIZZES

- Test yourself with multiple-choice and short-answer questions
- Do the chapter activities in the book and check your answers online

REFERENCES

All Party Parliamentary Group on Skin (APPGS) (2013) *The Psychological and Social Impact of Skin Diseases on People's Lives*. Available at: www.appgs.co.uk/publication/the-psychological-and-social-impact-of-skin-diseases-on-peoples-lives-final-report-2013/ (accessed 30th March 2017).

Aquino, M. and Fonacier, L. (2014) The role of contact dermatitis in patients with atopic dermatitis. *The Journal Of Allergy And Clinical Immunology*, 2 (4): 382.

Cancer Research, UK (2015) *About Melanoma*. Available at: www.cancerresearchuk.org/about-cancer/melanoma/about (accessed 30th March 2017).

Chella, C. (2014) Non-compliance in dermatology and its implications. *British Journal of Healthcare Assistants*, 8 (10): 500–5.

Danielsen, K., Olsen, A.O., Wilsgaard, T. and Furberg, A. (2013) Is the prevalence of psoriasis increasing? A 30-year follow-up of a population-based cohort. *British Journal of Dermatology*, 168(6): 1303–10.

Enamandram, M. and Kimball, A. (2013) Psoriasis epidemiology: The interplay of genes and the environment. *Journal of Investigative Dermatology*, 133 (2): 287–9.

Fisk, W., Lev-Tov, H. and Sivamani, R. (2014) Epidemiology and management of acne in adult women. *Current Dermatology Reports*, 3(1): 29–39.

National Institute for Health and Care Excellence (NICE) (2012) *The Assessment and Management of Psoriasis*. NICE CG153. Available at: www.nice.org.uk/guidance/cg153 (accessed 28th July 2016)

Nursing and Midwifery Council (2015) *Introduction to Safeguarding for Adults*. Available at: www.nmc.org.uk/standards/safeguarding/introduction-to-safeguarding-for-adults/ (accessed 30th March 2017).

Passalacqua, S., Di Rocco, Z.C., Di Pietro, C., Mozzetta, A., Tabolli, S., Scoppola, A., Marcgetti, P. and Abeni, D. (2012) Information needs of patients with melanoma: A nursing challenge. *Clinical Journal of Oncology Nursing*, 16 (6): 625–32.

Wedgeworth, E.K., Sharp, H., Powell, A. and Flohe, C. (2013) What's new in eczema? Part 2: Prevention, treatment and management. *Dermatological Nursing*, 12 (1): 10–17.

Williams, H.C., Dellavalle, R.P. and Garner, S. (2012) Acne vulgaris. *Lancet*, 379 (9813): 361–72.

CARE OF THE ADULT WITH A GASTROINTESTINAL CONDITION

34

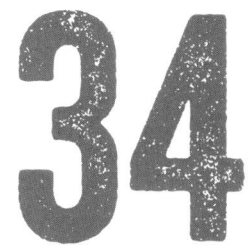

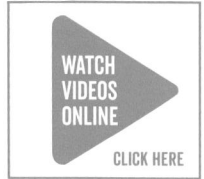

WATCH VIDEOS ONLINE

CLICK HERE

DEBBIE RAINEY AND DEIRDRE MCGRATH

--- **THIS CHAPTER COVERS** ---

- Anatomy and physiology of the gastrointestinal system
- Inflammatory bowel disease

- Patient-centred care
- Care of a patient requiring bowel surgery
- Care of a patient with a stoma.

> "
>
> It was a relief to be diagnosed with Crohn's as I had been so ill with the signs and symptoms for 3 months. But even when I'm in remission I don't feel like I'm in remission. Although there are no signs of active disease I still have pain, fatigue and loose bowel movements. I really thought remission would mean feeling well with no signs and symptoms. The chronic signs are always with me.
>
> **Kelly-Anne, patient**
>
> "

INTRODUCTION

A functioning gastrointestinal system is fundamental to health and wellbeing. Problems with the gastrointestinal system range from mild and self-limiting to severe and life threatening (see Table 34.1). We are all affected at some point during our lives, but as Kelly-Anne suggests, some conditions can be life changing. This chapter focuses on inflammatory bowel disease (IBD), specifically Crohn's disease (CD) and ulcerative colitis (UC). Initially, we will review the anatomy and physiology of the gastrointestinal tract. We will then discuss the pathophysiology and features of IDB. Finally, patient assessment and diagnostic tools will be explored along with the nursing care and treatment.

Table 34.1 GI conditions

Appendicitis

Alcoholic liver disease

Bowel obstruction

Cancer (colorectal, oesophageal, liver, pancreatic, stomach)

Cholecystitis

Coeliac disease

Constipation

Diarrhoea and vomiting

Diverticular disease

Gastrointestinal bleeding

Gastro-oesophageal reflux

Haemorrhoids

Hepatitis

Hernia

Inflammatory bowel disease (IBD)

Irritable bowel syndrome (IBS)

Pancreatitis

Peptic ulcer disease

Peritonitis

ANATOMY AND PHYSIOLOGY OF THE GASTROINTESTINAL SYSTEM

The gastrointestinal (GI) system contains the GI tract (gut) and the accessory digestive organs (see Figure 34.1). It has a number of functions primarily involved with the consumption and processing of food:

- ingestion
- propulsion
- digestion (mechanical and chemical)
- secretion
- absorption
- elimination.

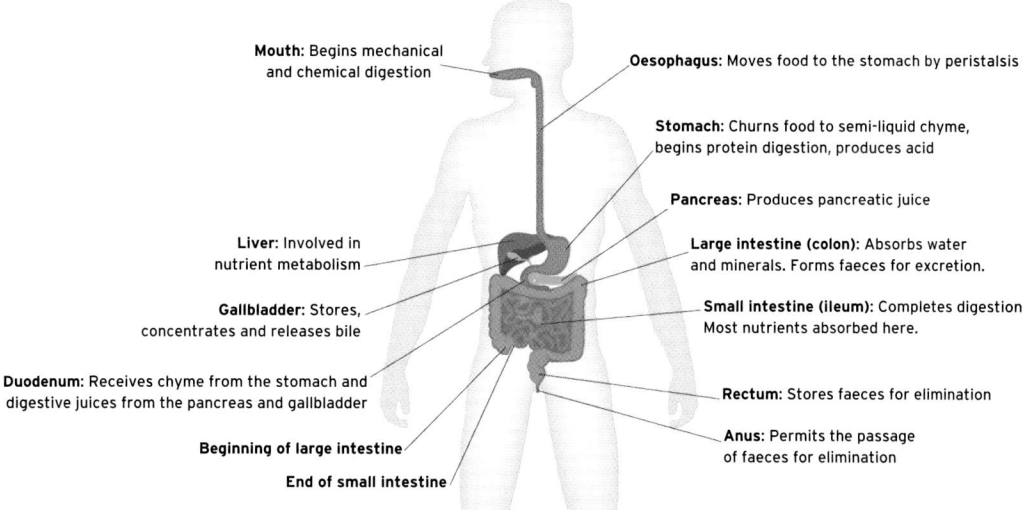

Figure 34.1   The gastrointestinal system

Source: Boore et al. (2016). Illustrated by Shaun Mercier, © SAGE Publications.

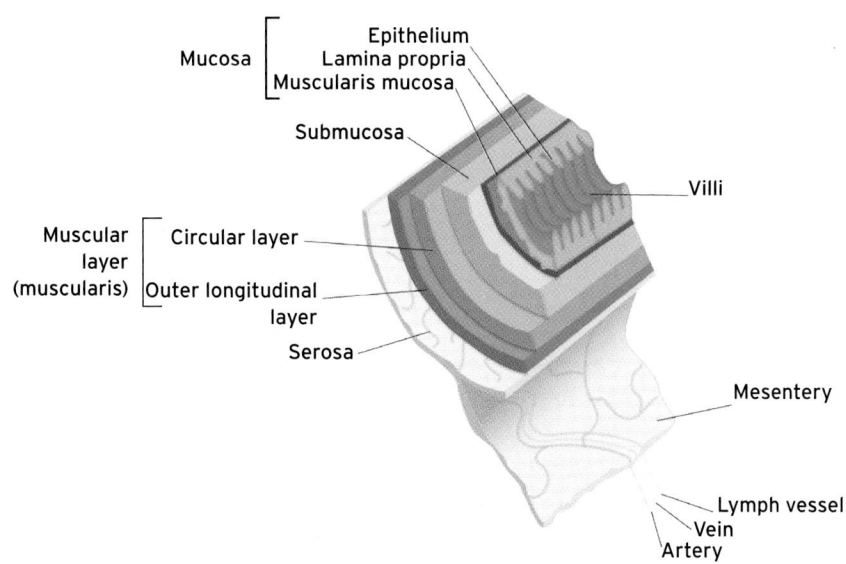

Figure 34.2   A cross-section of the wall of the gastrointestinal tract

Source: Boore et al. (2016). Illustrated by Shaun Mercier, © SAGE Publications.

The GI tract is a 4.5 m continuous tube from the mouth to the anus. It contains the pharynx, oesophagus, stomach, small intestine and large intestine. The wall of the GI tract has four layers: mucosa, submucosa, muscularis externa and serosa (see Figure 34.2). The accessory digestive organs are the salivary glands, liver and pancreas. The majority of the GI system is contained within the abdominal cavity by the peritoneum. This has two layers (visceral and parietal) creating the peritoneal cavity, which contains serous fluid to lubricate the organs. The peritoneum is connected by the mesentery, which secures the abdominal organs in place, provides a route for blood vessels and stores fat. The splanchnic circulation conveys oxygen-rich blood to the organs, but also directs nutrient-rich blood from the gut to the liver for processing.

When food is ingested via the mouth, salivation increases to hydrate and lubricate it with water and mucus. Mechanical digestion is carried out by the teeth, which cut and crush the food. The tongue forces food against the hard palate and mixes it with saliva, softening it and forming a bolus. Chemical digestion begins when salivary amylase breaks down starch (carbohydrates) into smaller glucose molecules. Food is swallowed when the tongue pushes the bolus posteriorly into the muscular pharynx. Peristalsis moves the bolus along the oesophagus, through the cardiac sphincter and into the stomach.

The stomach is an expandable storage sac with three layers of muscle and a mucosal lining folded into rugae. The bolus is subjected to further mechanical digestion by muscular contractions which churn the bolus, breaking it up and mixing it with gastric juices to form a liquid called chyme. Protein digestion is initiated by stomach acid and pepsin. The stomach lining is covered with a protective, tight layer of epithelial cells, which produce mucus and alkaline fluid to prevent damage by stomach acid. Chyme leaves the stomach after 3 or 4 hours via the pyloric sphincter and enters the duodenum.

The liver is the largest gland in the body and has a number of essential functions. Nutrient-rich blood from the gut is processed by hepatocytes (liver cells). 1L of bile, a yellow/green alkaline solution, is produced daily and stored in the gall bladder for secretion into the duodenum. Bile salts emulsify (break up) fats to provide small molecules for enzymatic action, and facilitate absorption. Bile pigments include bilirubin, a waste product of haemoglobin recycling. Other functions of the liver include:

**SEE ALSO
CHAPTER 29**

- carbohydrate metabolism
- fat metabolism
- protein metabolism
- storage, e.g. vitamins, iron, glycogen, protein and fat
- detoxification, e.g. alcohol and drugs
- immunity
- body heat production.

The pancreas has both endocrine and exocrine functions. The endocrine cells, called Islets of Langerhans, secrete insulin and glucagon required for blood sugar control. The exocrine tissue is composed of acinar cells which produce 1.5L of pancreatic juice per day, containing pancreatic digestive enzymes. Like bile, it is an alkaline solution, which helps neutralise acidic chyme entering the duodenum, and provides an optimum pH for enzymatic activity.

The small intestine (small bowel) is the main location for digestion and absorption. It is a 6 m tube, which extends from the pyloric sphincter to the ileocaecal valve and is divided into three sections: duodenum (25 cm), jejunum (2.5 m) and ileum (3.5 m). The small intestine has a huge surface area for absorption due to deep mucosal folds, finger-like villi and microvilli (the brush border). Each villus contains a lacteal (lymph capillary) and a blood capillary bed. 1–2L of intestinal juice is secreted per day from the crypts of Lieberkühn. This is a watery, alkaline solution containing mucus, electrolytes and antibacterial enzymes. The arrival of chyme in the duodenum stimulates the secretion of bile, pancreatic and intestinal juice. Rhythmic peristaltic contractions (segmentation) mix the contents and propel it forward. Chyme takes 3–6 hours to pass through the small intestine. Once each food group has been broken down into small enough molecules, they are absorbed through the small intestine lining into either the blood or lymph capillaries.

**SEE ALSO
CHAPTER 35**

The large intestine (large bowel or colon) stores faeces until it is ready to be eliminated. It is 1.5 m in length and extends from the ileocaecal valve to the anus, but has a larger diameter than the small intestine. It is divided into the caecum, ascending colon, transverse colon, descending colon, sigmoid colon, rectum and anal canal. The appendix is a small finger-like projection attached to the caecum. The mucosa contains mucus-secreting goblet cells and is colonised by bacterial flora. There are no villi, but pocket-like sacs instead, called haustra. Arrival of chyme in the caecum causes the ileocaecal valve to close preventing reflux of bacterial flora into the ileum.

Peristaltic movements are slow and infrequent. Contents take 12–24 hours to pass through the colon. The only digestion occurring is minimal further breakdown by bacterial flora. Remaining water and electrolytes are also absorbed. Arrival of faeces in the rectum initiates the defecation reflex. This causes the sigmoid colon and rectum to contract, and the internal anal sphincter to relax, forcing faeces towards the external anal sphincter. Opening of this is under voluntary control, and defecation is aided by contraction of the abdominal muscles against a closed glottis. Gases occur in the colon from swallowed air and bacterial fermentation. They are released in varying amounts as flatus.

INFLAMMATORY BOWEL DISEASE

Crohn's disease (CD) and ulcerative colitis (UC) are both long-term conditions and the most common forms of inflammatory bowel disease (IBD). It is estimated that IBD affects over 300,000 people in the United Kingdom and the prevalence is increasing. IBD affects people of all ages; however, it is more often diagnosed in the 15–35 age group. The causes of IBD are unclear but probably occur due to the interaction between genetic and environmental factors. There are some similarities between CD and UC, but also some key differences (Table 34.2). Both diseases are associated with abdominal pain, vomiting, diarrhoea, rectal bleeding, anaemia, weight-loss, fever and fatigue. Non-GI symptoms may include joint pain (arthritis), painful red eyes (iritis) and painful red skin nodules (erythema nodosum). The symptoms of IBD characteristically come and go, with periods of severe flare-ups, followed by remission when symptoms improve or disappear. Significant, life-threatening complications include bowel obstruction and/or perforation and an increased risk of developing colorectal cancer. Treatment options include medication, surgery, dietary management and counselling.

Table 34.2 Key differences between CD and UC

	Crohn's Disease	Ulcerative Colitis
Location	Mouth to anus (commonly ileocaecal and terminal ileum region)	Rectum and descending colon
Depth of inflammation	Deep, transmural	Shallow, mucosal
Pattern of inflammation	Patchy or 'skip lesions'	Continuous
Abscesses	Yes	Yes
Stricture (narrowing)	Common	Rarely
Fistula (abnormal connection)	Common	Rarely
Adhesions	Common	Possible following surgery
Stools	Porridge-like, bloody	Blood and mucus
Chance of surgery	70%	20-30%

PATIENT-CENTRED CARE IN IBD

IBD is a chronic disease; therefore, one of the main roles for you as a nurse will be to support the patient and promote health education, ensuring your patient understands the disease, the signs and symptoms and triggers for them, as these can vary from patient to patient. The aim is to enable the patient to live their life with IBD. Matini and Ogden (2015) identified that patients often do not understand the chronicity of the disease. In today's healthcare service there is a strong focus on quality and delivery of care driven by policies and outcome measures. Emphasis is not just on treatment but on improving quality of life. To prevent inequality, IBD standards have been published (NICE, 2015). As a nurse, you need to work as part of the multidisciplinary team (MDT) in assessing and managing care and implementing the standards. A key role for you is to advocate patient-centred care. This entails involving the patient in decision-making and supporting them during this process. One of the IBD standards identified empowering the patient in management of their condition through education and support (Glatter et al., 2014). To assist with implementing the standards of care IBD nurse specialists have been appointed. Their role is multifaceted but they are pivotal in providing ongoing patient-centred care for patients with IBD, ensuring relevant education to patients, families and to other nurses (Hall, 2011). The majority of patients are managed in the community setting and you will likely come into contact with them during clinical placements in GP practices, community nursing, outpatient departments and day procedure units. You will meet patients who are having an exacerbation in A&E or in the acute medical or surgical wards depending on the proposed treatment plan.

WHAT'S THE EVIDENCE? 34.1

WEBLINK:
NICE
GUIDELINES
IBD

Access the NICE guidelines for IBD at www.nice.org.uk/guidance/conditions-and-diseases/digestive-tract-conditions/inflammatory-bowel-disease

Explore the treatment options for CD and UC – what common medications are used?

Look at the sections on patient information and support and consider where you might be involved as a nurse.

PATIENT ASSESSMENT IN IBD

IBD affects many aspects of your patients' lives and each person has different experiences. It is your responsibility as a nurse to ensure that each person receives a holistic individualised assessment. This will enable you to set patient-centred goals and deliver nursing management tailored to meet their specific needs. During assessment it is essential to explore all aspects of the patient's life: biomedically, physically, psychologically and socially. Some parts of the assessment will be undertaken alongside other members of the MDT, particularly diagnostic investigations. Continuous reassessment of their needs is important as these will change depending on the stage of the disease and response to treatment. Key areas of assessment include the following:

- diagnostic investigations
- nutrition and hydration
- bowel function

- pain and discomfort
- knowledge and understanding of IBD
- lifestyle
- psychological impact.

DIAGNOSTIC INVESTIGATIONS

Diagnosis of CD and UC can be difficult. There is no single test and symptoms can be present for some time before presentation. Differential diagnoses such as irritable bowel syndrome (IBS) will be considered. Diagnosis includes history taking (duration, frequency and severity of symptoms), physical examination, blood tests, stool samples and colonoscopy. Blood tests include full blood count (FBC) to check for anaemia, and iron and platelet levels; urea and electrolytes (U&E) and liver function tests (LFT) to assess renal and liver function; and inflammatory markers, such as C-reactive protein (CRP) and erythrocyte sedimentation rate (ESR). Faecal calprotectin is a key stool test, which indicates active inflammation in the intestine. Radiological investigations include x-ray, computed tomography (CT) and magnetised resonance imaging (MRI). A colonoscopy is an examination with a long flexible camera inserted through the anus to inspect the bowel lining, take biopsies (tissue samples), remove polyps (small growths) and dilate strictures. Investigations are also used to assess severity, identify relapse (flare-ups) and response to treatment.

--- **GO FURTHER** ---

Crohn's and Colitis UK (2017) Tests and Investigations for IBD http://s3-eu-west-1.amazonaws.com/files. crohnsandcolitis.org.uk/Publications/tests-and-investigations.pdf

Review this patient information booklet and explore some of the other tests and investigations. How would you support a patient undergoing a colonoscopy?

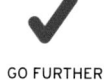

GO FURTHER
ANSWER

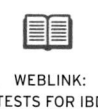

WEBLINK:
TESTS FOR IBD

NUTRITIONAL STATUS

In whatever clinical environment you meet a patient with IBD, they can often be malnourished and dehydrated due to the changes in the digestive tract (see Table 34.3). As part of your patient-centred assessment it is vital that a nutritional assessment, such as MUST (BAPEN, 2003), is completed.

Table 34.3 Causes of malnutrition and dehydration

Malnutrition	
Reason	Cause
Inadequate intake	Patient afraid to eat as may exacerbate condition Nausea
Increased nutritional requirements	Periods of infection or inflammation
Malabsorption	Diseased part of intestine cannot absorb nutrients
Short bowel syndrome	Surgical removal of sections of the small intestine

(Continued)

Table 34.3   (Continued)

Dehydration	
Reason	**Cause**
Inadequate intake	Patient not drinking enough
	Nausea
High elimination	Diarrhoea/vomiting
Ileostomy	Higher water content of stools

DIET

There is no specific recommended diet for patients with IBD. Some patients find certain foods trigger their symptoms such as dairy products, alcohol, spicy food and coffee. However, this varies from person to person and is very individual. To help your patient identify if there are certain foods that exacerbate their condition, you can advise them to complete a food diary. This entails your patient recording their food intake and any symptoms that occur after eating this food. On evaluation of the food diary the two entries can be compared and patterns established. This will enable food triggers to be identified. Patients require a healthy well-balanced diet and a good basis for this is the *Eatwell Guide* (Public Health England, 2016). Your patient may find it easier to have small regular meals rather than three large ones. If your patient is unable to meet their nutritional requirements a referral to the dietician should be made. This will ensure that your patient receives an individualised dietary plan for their own needs.

SEE ALSO
CHAPTER 35

HYDRATION

On assessment, you may identify signs of dehydration (see Table 34.4). During patient education you need to ensure the patient is aware of these, especially during an exacerbation of IBD. To monitor fluid intake, patients should be advised to record the amount and type of fluid they drink in 24 hours. They should be aiming for approximately 2 litres of fluid a day, but should avoid caffeinated drinks, which can contribute to dehydration. During an exacerbation, fluid intake should be further increased to compensate for excess fluid losses.

Table 34.4   Signs of mild dehydration

Dry mouth
Thirst
Headache
Tiredness
Dizzy
Urinating only 2–3 times a day
Dry skin

BOWEL FUNCTION

Bowel-related symptoms are a key feature of IBD. Patients may experience frequent, loose bowel motions containing blood or mucus. Diarrhoea can be explosive and patients may experience incontinence or leakage of faeces. Some patients endure severe abdominal cramps and discomfort associated with the need to pass stools. They may also have tenesmus, the feeling of incomplete defecation. Many have the feeling of urgency, which is commonly associated with UC. This can lead to embarrassment, and some patients may avoid going out due to the fear of not being able to get to the toilet quick enough. To help overcome this, you can advise patients to take spare clothes, cleaning wipes and a plastic bag out with them. They can also be advised to find where the nearest toilets are located prior to going out. Excessive diarrhoea may be caused by a variety of reasons (see Table 34.5) and can lead to excoriation and soreness around the perianal area. You can educate patients to ensure a good level of hygiene, keeping the perianal area dry and clean. They should use a soft disposable wipe and some patients may benefit from applying a barrier cream.

Table 34.5 Causes of diarrhoea in IBD

Side effects of drugs, i.e. antibiotics

Malabsorption of fats

Food sensitivities, i.e. spicy food, too much fibre, caffeine, fructose, artificial sweeteners

Iron supplements

Post small bowel surgery

Post colectomy and ileorectal anastomosis

Bowel function assessment should include a record of stools and bowel habits. A tool such as the Bristol Stool chart (Heaton, 2006) can be used. This assessment can assist in identifying an exacerbation or any potential triggers, especially if other factors have been recorded as well. In conjunction with completing the stool chart the patient can write a diary. In this they should record:

- date
- time
- amount of stool
- type of stool including colour, mucus or blood
- what they have eaten
- other events that have occurred.

When comparing all the entries, patterns can be observed to see if anything particular caused the change in the stool.

PAIN AND DISCOMFORT

The majority of patients with IBD have some type of pain or discomfort. Each patient will experience pain differently. It is essential that an individual pain assessment is undertaken using a validated and appropriate pain assessment tool. Reassessment using the same tool allows comparisons to be made and can identify if analgesics and other interventions are effective. Alternatively, it can assist in determining if the patient's condition is getting worse. A pain assessment tool, such as the one in Table 34.6, can also be used by the patient to keep a diary.

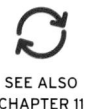

SEE ALSO
CHAPTER 11

Table 34.6 Pain assessment tool

Time of pain - what time did it start, how long it lasted for

Quality - dull, sore, spasmodic, stabbing

Severity - pain level using a score of 1–10

Onset - what was the patient doing before pain came on, i.e. eating

Pattern - is the pain consistent, intermittent

Region of pain - where is the pain, does it radiate anywhere

Relieving factors - what relieved the pain

KNOWLEDGE AND UNDERSTANDING OF IBD

A crucial element during patient assessment is to establish the patient's understanding of their condition. This will enable you to plan and implement patient-centred health education specific for that individual. When you assess their knowledge, it is important to ascertain where they have gained their knowledge from as it may not be a reliable source. Many patients search the internet to gain an understanding of IBD or friends may give advice. As a nurse, you will need to be aware of relevant evidence-based patient-orientated health education websites and leaflets to direct your patient to.

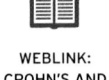

**WEBLINK:
CROHN'S AND
COLITIS UK**

CRITICAL THINKING STOP POINT 34.1

A patient-orientated website that gives a variety of externally validated information on all aspects on IBD is www.crohnsandcolitis.org.uk

Have a look at some of the background information that is available on the website.

How will you, as a nurse, assess the patient's knowledge and understanding of their IBD? What nursing skills will you use to gain the information?

The patient with IBD will need to understand what is occurring pathophysiologically in their body. This will enable them to understand how their body is affected and make them aware of why they have the signs and symptoms of their condition. This will assist them to identify when an exacerbation is occurring. You should educate the patient to contact the IBD nurse specialist or their doctor and seek support if they notice an increase in their signs and symptoms. Before education can begin it is important to assess the patient's health status, ensuring they are well enough to receive information. If they are extremely ill, they may not be receptive. The amount of information given at one time should be limited to ensure that it can be taken in and understood.

LIFESTYLE

It is also important for you, as a nurse, to understand what type of lifestyle your patient leads. In today's society most people have a busy, stressful life. Often people do not recognise their stressors until someone asks them pertinent questions. Stress can cause exacerbations of IBD, so it is important for the patient to identify stressors or lifestyle triggers that cause an increase in signs and symptoms.

Coping strategies to reduce stress need to be incorporated into the patient's lifestyle. These will depend on your patient and are very individualised, but may include interventions such as counselling.

Fatigue is a common symptom that many of your patients with IBD have to contend with and may be related to their lifestyle. During your nursing assessment it is important to identify the causes of fatigue. The patient should be encouraged to keep a dairy of activities and record how they felt afterwards. These can be compared to see if there are triggers that increase their feelings of fatigue. At the same time they can record what they do when they are tired. This information will assist you and the patient to develop a patient-centred plan for how they can reduce fatigue and develop coping strategies. This may include incorporating periods of rest within their day, which can be quite difficult to achieve in everyday life, but is important for wellbeing.

ACTIVITY 34.1: HEALTH PROMOTION ALERT

1. List signs and symptoms that people have when they feel tired and stressed.
2. Think what causes you to feel tired and stressed within your life.
3. Identify how you relieve your feelings of fatigue and stress.
4. How could you apply this information to support your patient or their family?

ACTIVITY 34.1
ANSWER

Another area of your patient's life that can be affected by IBD is their working life. This is due to the disease having cycles of exacerbation and remission. During an exacerbation of the disease, some of your patients will be unable to work. You should encourage patients to discuss their diagnosis with their employers, as this will enable the employer to understand the need to take time off work. It will also allow support and adjustments to be put in place. Some patients may need directing to financial or legal advice.

CASE STUDY 34.1: JULIE

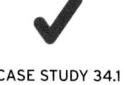

CASE STUDY 34.1
ANSWER

Julie is a 42-year-old married woman. She has four children aged 5, 8, 12 and 14. Her children are very active and enjoy going to many clubs to do various sports. Julie enjoys running and is aiming to complete a marathon at the start of next year. She works four days a week as a personal assistant in a large supplies firm. Often her job is very busy and demanding. Her husband often works away from home for a couple of weeks at a time and she has minimal family support.

For the last six months Julie has felt generally unwell. She has had very bad crampy lower abdominal pain, diarrhoea and has noted fresh blood in her stools. She has lost 6 kg in weight without trying to and her appetite is poor. She feels exhausted after doing very little. After investigations a diagnosis of ulcerative colitis has been made.

- During your assessment of Julie what key information will you want to find out from her?
- Identify what assessment tools can be used to inform your assessment.
- What nursing skills and tools would you use to educate Julie regarding IBD?
- How will you ensure she understands the information you have provided?
- Identify areas in Julie's lifestyle that could potentially cause exacerbation of her IBD.
- Make a list of coping strategies that could be incorporated into her life to help reduce stressors.

PSYCHOLOGICAL

IBD can have a psychological impact on your patient's life as well as the physical symptoms. Some of the key areas discussed previously in the chapter can affect patients psychologically, such as faecal urgency and the risk of incontinence, chronic fatigue or their diet. Linked to these is the effect on your patient's self-esteem and body image. They must cope with changes in physical appearance caused by malnutrition and side effects of drugs, especially steroids. This, in turn, can lead to social isolation due to not wanting to go out or engage in social activities or relationships because of their appearance. This will further impact on how your patient feels psychologically and can subsequently lead to depression. As a nurse it is your responsibility to assess and evaluate how your patient is looking and feeling on each contact to enable the correct support to be provided. You will need to empower the patient to develop self-management skills. Gethins et al. (2011) highlight that patients who have had IBD for a long time can become experts in their own condition.

VIDEO:
SELF-
MANAGEMENT
OF IBD

CRITICAL THINKING STOP POINT 34.2

Watch: https://videos.rsm.ac.uk/video/self-management-of-ibd
   Read: www.rcn.org.uk/clinical-topics/supporting-behaviour-change
   After watching the video and reading the articles, list ways that you could empower your patient
   to self-manage their disease.

WEBLINK:
SUPPORTING
BEHAVIOUR
CHANGE

CASE STUDY 34.2: JULIE

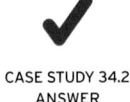

CASE STUDY 34.2
ANSWER

Julie has been seen in the outpatients department by the consultant and the nursing team and the IBD nurse specialist. An assessment has been undertaken and a patient-centred care plan has been commenced.

- Prior to Julie going home, what support and information will you as her nurse ensure she has?

CARE OF A PATIENT REQUIRING BOWEL SURGERY

Some patients with IBD may require a surgical procedure to remove the affected part of the bowel. The reasons for surgery are varied depending on the primary cause of IBD (see Table 34.7). A variety of surgical procedures are used to remove the affected part of the bowel in IBD. Many of the surgical procedures used to treat IBD are also employed with patients who have other bowel conditions.

Table 34.7   Reasons for surgery

Ulcerative Colitis

- Unresponsive to medication
- Perforation of bowel
- Dysplasia (pre-cancerous cells)
- Colorectal cancer
- Chronic continuous severe disease with impaired quality of life

Crohn's Disease

- Unresponsive to medication
- Perianal or intra-abdominal abscesses
- Intestinal stricture and obstruction
- Intestinal perforation
- Fistula

PRE-OPERATIVE MANAGEMENT

Pre-operative care for your patient who requires planned surgery is generally the same care for any patient requiring surgery. However, there are some specific considerations when preparing for bowel surgery.

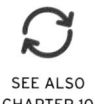

SEE ALSO
CHAPTER 10

Nutrition/hydration

Prior to surgery, many patients will be dehydrated or malnourished due to their IBD and reasons for surgery. Left uncorrected this can cause post-operative complications. During pre-operative assessment, you should assess the patient's nutritional and hydration status using observation skills and assessment tools, i.e. MUST. It is essential to work with the MDT to optimise hydration and nutritional status prior to surgery.

Bowel preparation

Prior to surgery (or colonoscopy) your patient will need to have medication (a powerful laxative and/or enema) to empty their bowel of its contents. This is to prevent bowel contents flowing into the abdominal cavity and causing **peritonitis** during surgery. There are various types of medication that achieve this. Local policy and procedure will direct the MDT in what to prescribe. The medication can be given to your patient at home prior to admission to the hospital. Part of your nursing role is to educate your patient how to take the medication and what is likely to occur. You should advise them to stay near a toilet.

Before I saw my first stoma I didn't know what to expect and felt quite apprehensive. But when I saw one it was OK. I just thought it looked sore because it was so pink looking. But my patient said they didn't feel anything.

Simone, 2nd year student nurse

CARE OF A PATIENT WITH A STOMA

Depending on the procedure, the surgeon may be able to anastomose (join the two ends) of the bowel back together or a stoma may be required (see Figures 34.3 and 34.4). A stoma is formed when the bowel is brought onto the surface of the abdomen to allow stool to be passed. A stoma can be permanent or temporary and the two main types in IBD are an ileostomy or a colostomy (see Table 34.8). If a stoma is required, the patient will need psychological and physical preparation for this. Your patient should be seen pre-operatively by the stoma specialist nurse to enable preparation and education to begin.

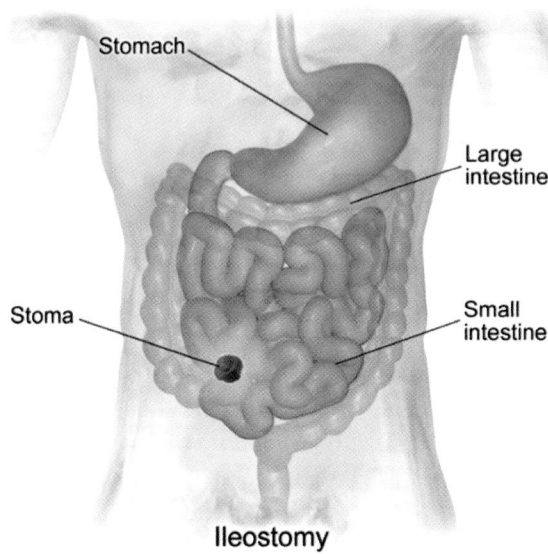

Figure 34.3   Location of a stoma (ileostomy)

© *User:*BruceBlaus, Wikimedia Commons, CC-BY-SA-3.0. Available at: https://commons.wikimedia.org/wiki/Category:Ileostomy#/media/File:Ileostomy.png**.**

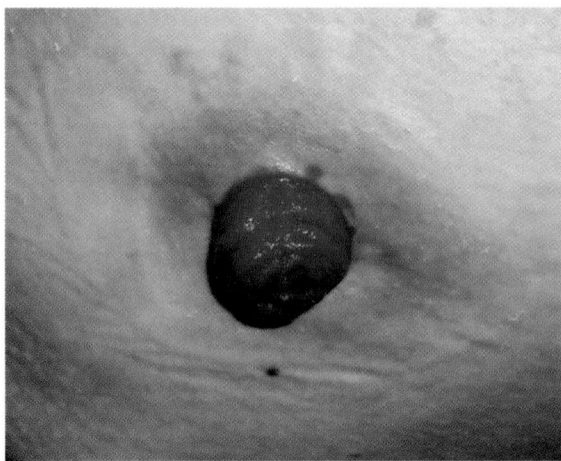

Figure 34.4   Picture of a stoma (ileostomy)

© *User:*Salicyna, Wikimedia Commons, CC-BY-SA-3.0. Available at: https://commons.wikimedia.org/wiki/File:Ileostomy_2017-02-20_5351.jpg

Table 34.8 Differences between a colostomy and an ileostomy

Colostomy
Formed from the colon
Flush to skin
Stool is generally formed

Illeostomy
Formed from the small bowel
Stoma is spout shaped
Stool is of a porridge consistency

CASE STUDY 34.3: JULIE

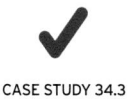

CASE STUDY 34.3
ANSWER

Due to poor response to medication, Julie and the medical team have decided she requires a planned colectomy with ileostomy (subtotal). She has an appointment with the stoma nurse to discuss having a stoma and where to site the stoma.

- What information would you want to know if you were Julie?

Read: Brown, F. (2017) Psychosocial health following stoma formation: a literature review. *Gastrointestinal Nursing*, 15 (3) https://doi.org/10.12968/gasn.2017.15.3.43

- What areas of psychological support and physical care will the stoma nurse provide Julie with?

Read: Cronin, E. (2014) Stoma siting: why and how to mark the abdomen in preparation for surgery. *Gastrointestinal Nursing*, 12 (3) https://doi.org/10.12968/gasn.2014.12.3.12

- What factors will the stoma nurse consider with Julie when siting her stoma?

ACTIVITY 34.2: REFLECTIVE PRACTICE

Read: Wallace, A. (2016) The key factors that affect psychological adaptation to a stoma: a literature review. *Gastrointestinal Nursing*, 14 (6) https://doi.org/10.12968/gasn.2016.14.6.39

Reflect on the differences in nursing care you would need to provide for your patient if they were having planned bowel surgery with formation of a stoma compared to a patient requiring emergency bowel surgery with formation of a stoma.

Think about the pre- and post-operative physical and psychological care.

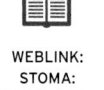

WEBLINK:
STOMA:
PSYCHOLOGICAL
ADAPTATION

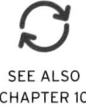

SEE ALSO
CHAPTER 10

POST-OPERATIVE NURSING MANAGEMENT

The nursing care your patient will require post-operatively is overall the same as any patient who is recovering from a surgical procedure. However, there are specific considerations for a patient post bowel surgery.

Fluid balance

An essential nursing skill when caring for a patient post-operatively is ensuring that fluid input and output is measured and recorded accurately. This is especially important if your patient has had an ileostomy. There is an increased risk of dehydration because of the potential for a high fluid output from the watery stool.

Nil by Mouth (NBM)

The majority of patients following bowel surgery will not be allowed to drink or eat until the doctors are satisfied that the peristaltic action of the bowel is occurring. As a nurse, it is important to ensure the patient has mouth care to promote comfort and prevent complications. If the patient is nil by mouth, they will need an intravenous infusion (IVI). While caring for the patient with an IVI, ensure that the cannula is checked for patency observing for redness, swelling and inflammation. Ensure the correct fluid is given as prescribed and that it is running and at the correct rate.

Nasogastric tube

Some patients may return from theatre with a nasogastric (NG) tube in situ. This is to ensure the contents of the stomach are removed. The NG tube can be attached to a drainage bag, which allows the stomach contents to flow out freely. As a nurse, you may need to aspirate the NG tube to ensure that the contents are removed. The surgeon may request this to be undertaken every hour directly following surgery. If your patient is feeling nauseated or is vomiting you can also aspirate the NG tube to alleviate this. It is important for you to record any output from the bag or the aspirate on the fluid balance chart. You will also need to note the colour and type of fluid.

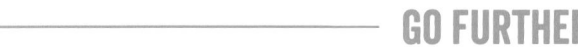

GO FURTHER

For more information on care of an IVI and NG tube, see: Dougherty, L., Lister, S. and West- Oram, A. (2015) *The Royal Marsden Manual of Clinical Nursing Procedures* (9th ed.). Oxford: John Wiley & Sons, Ltd.

COMPLICATION POST BOWEL SURGERY

Your patient is at risk of paralytic ileus. This occurs due to the bowel being handled during the surgical procedure, causing peristalsis to stop. If this occurs, the patient will have nausea and vomiting and their bowel sounds will be absent. Paralytic ileus is treated by resting the bowel. The patient will remain nil by mouth and a NG tube may be inserted if not already in situ.

POST-OPERATIVE STOMA CARE

Post-operatively, it is important to observe the stoma for colour, size and output. All observations should be documented in the nursing notes.

Colour: The stoma should be pink, indicating a good blood supply. The surgeon should be informed if there are any signs of poor blood supply, which is demonstrated by a blueish tinge.

Size: When the stoma is first formed it may be oedematous. Each day post-op the size should reduce. It can take approximately 6–8 weeks for the stoma to get to its final size.

Output: Generally, in the first 24 hours the stoma will not produce faeces. The first output is usually pink/red in colour and liquid. Any output should be recorded on a fluid balance chart.

Skin care: The skin around the stoma needs to be kept dry and clean. Skin is at risk of excoriation due to leakage of faeces on to the skin or reaction to the stoma bags. Skin should be cleaned with water or mild soap and water and dried. There are different products that are specifically designed for use for patients with a stoma if they are prone to, or have, sore skin.

Types of stoma bags: When the patient first returns from theatre the stoma bag will be clear. This is to enable the stoma itself to be observed for colour and size and for the output to be visualised. There are a variety of stoma bags available (see Figure 34.5). Once the stoma has shrunk to its final size, the stoma nurse and the patient can choose the best type of appliance.

Complications: Some patients have complications following stoma formation and will need support from their stoma nurse and the surgeon (see Table 34.9).

Table 34.9   Complications of a stoma

Skin irritation
Ischaemic stoma
Mucocutaneous separation
Stoma retraction
Parastomal hernia
Stoma proplapse

Source: Watson et al. (2013)

GO FURTHER

Read the following article to explore the issues in choosing the correct stoma appliance: Williams, J. (2017) The importance of choosing the correct stoma appliance to meet patient needs. *British Journal of Community Nursing*, 22 (2) https://doi.org/10.12968/bjcn.2017.22.2.58

WEBLINK: CORRECT STOMA APPLIANCE

Applying the stoma bag adhesive

- Ensure the hole in the adhesive is the correct fit around the stoma, to prevent leakage.
- Ensure the skin is clean and completely dry.
- Ensure there is total contact between the adhesive and the skin – light pressure around the adhesive can assist with this.

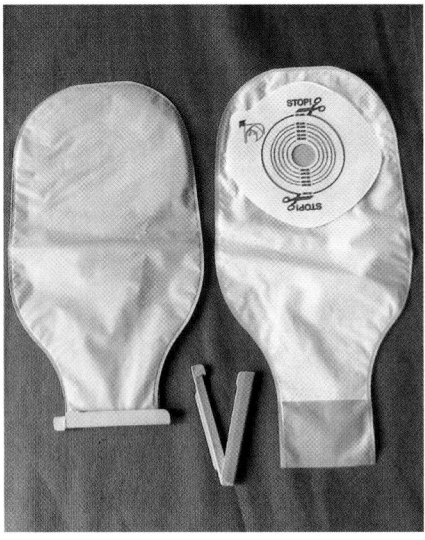

Figure 34.5 Stoma bag

Stoma nurse specialists are really good at helping the patients and teaching us as student nurses. All nurses should spend time with a stoma nurse specialist to learn how to care for stoma.

Ellen, 2nd year student nurse

PREPARATION FOR PRACTICE PLACEMENTS 34.1

During your clinical placement you should endeavour to meet the stoma specialist nurse and discuss their role in caring for patients pre- and post-operatively. If possible, go with them when they meet your patient to observe how they provide education and expert care.

DISCHARGING A PATIENT FOLLOWING BOWEL SURGERY

Discharging a patient home following bowel surgery follows the same principles of safe and effective discharge in general. However, before you can discharge a patient home with a stoma, they will need to be able to care for and change the stoma bag themselves.

ACTIVITY 34.3: REFLECTIVE PRACTICE

Imagine you were being discharged home from hospital post bowel surgery with a stoma.

1. Reflect on what information you would want to know before going home.
2. What concerns do you think you may have?

CASE STUDY 34.4: JULIE

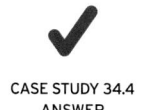

CASE STUDY 34.4
ANSWER

Julie is 5 days post colectomy with ileostomy (subtotal). She has had an uneventful recovery and the consultant would like to discharge Julie home in the next 2 days.

Devise a discharge plan for Julie including:

- a health education plan, to teach Julie about how to change her stoma bag (think about the skills you will use when teaching her)
- follow-up appointments, with whom
- community support
- what products you would need to organise for Julie to take home with her
- information on where to get further ostomy supplies from
- showering or bathing
- skin care
- sexual relations
- wound care and removal of sutures.

CONCLUSION

This chapter has focused on the pathophysiology and management of IBD. Essential anatomy and physiology was reviewed and a range of other GI disorders were identified. Patient assessment and relevant clinical investigations were discussed and many of these are common to other gastrointestinal diseases.

CHAPTER SUMMARY

- GI system disorders are common.
- Health and wellbeing is influenced by a normally functioning GI system.
- IBD are long-term conditions, which can significantly affect physical and psychological health.
- Bowel surgery and the formation of a stoma can be life-changing events.
- Effective patient-centred care and involvement of specialist nurses can empower patients to self-manage their condition.

GO FURTHER

CASE STUDY: CROHN'S DISEASE

Go to https://study.sagepub.com/essentialadultnursing for a further case study related to this chapter. If you are using the interactive ebook, simply click on the book icon in the margin to go straight to the resource.

Books

- Dougherty, L., Lister, S. and West-Oram, A. (2015) *The Royal Marsden Manual of Clinical Nursing Procedures* (9th ed.). Oxford: John Wiley & Sons, Ltd.
  The definitive text on core clinical nursing procedures.
- Pudner, R. (2010) *Nursing the Surgical Patient* (3rd ed.). USA: Elsevier.
  A patient-centred approach to the care of people requiring a variety of surgical procedures.
- Ali, T. and Rubin, D.T. (2013) *Crohn's and Colitis for Dummies. A Wiley Brand.* Oxford: John Wiley & Sons, Ltd.
  An accessible text on IBD.

Journal Articles

FURTHER READING: JOURNAL ARTICLES

Go to https://study.sagepub.com/essentialadultnurding for further free online journal articles related to this chapter. If you are using the interactive ebook, simply click on the book icon in the margin to go straight to the resource.

- Burch, J. (2017) Post-discharge care for patients following stoma formation: What the nurse needs to know. *Nursing Standard*, 31 (51): 41-5.
  This article will help inform your clinical practice about discharging a patient with a stoma.
- Czuber-Dochan, W., Norton, C., Forbes, A., Indira, N., Berliner, S., Darvell, M., Gay, M. and Terry, H. (2014) Assessing fatigue in patients with inflammatory bowel disease. *Gastrointestinal Nursing*, 12 (8): 13-21.
  This article will help you explore the systemic affects of IBD.
- Watson, A.J.M., Nicol, N., Donaldson, S., Fraser, C. and Silversides, A. (2013) Complications of stomas: Their aetiology and management. *British Journal of Community Nursing*, 18 (3): 111-16.
  This article discusses what causes complications with a stoma and how to manage them.

Weblinks

FURTHER READING: WEBLINKS

Go to https://study.sagepub.com/essentialadultnursing for further weblinks related to this chapter. If you are using the interactive ebook, simply click on the book icon in the margin to go straight to the resource.

These are excellent websites with written information and video messages from patients who are living with IBD or a stoma.

- www.crohnsandcolitis.org.uk/news/living-with-ibd-new-videos-launched
- www.colostomyuk.org/
- www.iasupport.org/
- https://s3-eu-west-1.amazonaws.com/files.crohnsandcolitis.org.uk/Publications/ulcerative-colitis.pdf
- http://s3-eu-west-1.amazonaws.com/files.crohnsandcolitis.org.uk/Publications/surgery-for-crohns-disease.pdf

These links will help you to discover more about why your patient may require surgery and the surgical procedures.

- www.dansac.co.uk/~/media/files/dansac/dansac-observation-index.pdf?la=en-gb
- www.dansac.co.uk/~/media/files/dansac/dansac-practical-guide.pdf?la=en-gb
- These websites give more information on the complications of stomas.

ACE YOUR ASSESSMENT

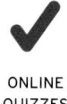

ONLINE
QUIZZES

Revise what you have learned by visiting https://study.sagepub.com/essentialadultnursing

- Test yourself with multiple-choice and short-answer questions
- Do the chapter activities in the book and check your answers online

REFERENCES

British Association for Parenteral and Enteral Nutrition (BAPEN) (2003) *Malnutrition Universal Screening Tool*. Available at: www.bapen.org.uk/pdfs/must/must_full.pdf Accessed 8/3/18.

Gethins, S., Duckett, T., Shatford, C. and Robinson, R. (2011) Self-management programme for patients with long-term inflammatory bowel disease. *Gastrointestinal Nursing*, 9 (3): August.

Glatter, J., Sephton, M. and Garrick, V. (2014) The revised inflammatory bowel disease (IBD) standards and the IBD nurse role. *Gastrointestinal Nursing*, 11 (10): January.

Hall, A. (2011) Recognizing the depth of the IBD nurse specialist role. *Gastrointestinal Nursing*, 9 (8): August.

Heaton, K.W. (2006) *Understanding Your Bowels*. Family Doctor Publications Ltd and the British Medical Association. London: BMA.

Matini, L and Ogden, J. (2015) A qualitative study of patients' experience of living with inflammatory bowel disease: A preliminary focus on the notion of adaptation. *Journal of Health Psychology*, 21(11): 2493–502.

National Institute for Health and Care Excellence (NICE) (2015) *Inflammatory Bowel Disease Quality standard [QS81]*. Available at: www.nice.org.uk/guidance/qs81 Accessed 8/3/18.

Public Health England (PHE) (2016) *Eatwell Guide*. Available at: www.gov.uk/government/uploads/system/uploads/attachment_data/file/528193/Eatwell_guide_colour.pdf Accessed 8/3/18.

Watson, A.J.M., Nicol, N., Donaldson, S., Fraser, C. and Silversides, A. (2013) Complications of stomas: their aetiology and management. *British Journal of Community Nursing*, 18 (3):111–16.

CARE OF THE ADULT WITH A NUTRITIONAL CONDITION

35

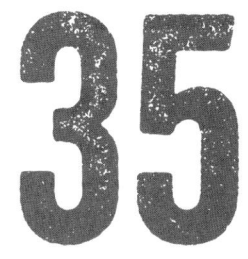

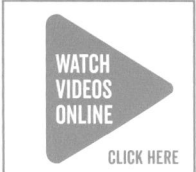

WATCH VIDEOS ONLINE

CLICK HERE

DEBBIE ROWBERRY

THIS CHAPTER COVERS

- Introduction to nutrition
- Macro-nutrients, micro-nutrients and fluids
- An overview of the anatomy and physiology of the GI system
- Fundamentals of nutrition in adults, older adults and impacts on health
- Assessment of nutrition and discussion of malnutrition

- The significance of nutrition with regard to some chronic conditions
- Nutritional interventions.
- Other nutritional considerations – culture, religion and beliefs

> Hello, my name is Charlie, having been a patient in hospital many times over the years I understand how important adequate nutrition is. Being vegan means my choices can be limited making it even more difficult to ensure I eat enough. Offering specific dietary choices would make a huge difference to my stay and I would not feel as much of a nuisance.
>
> **Charlie Edwards (a pseudonym has been used to protect patient confidentiality)**

> Nurses must have 'knowledge of dietary and other factors contributing to ill health, obesity, weight loss, poor fluid intake and poor nutrition to inform practice'
>
> **(NMC, 2015)**

INTRODUCTION

Nutrition is nourishment or energy that is obtained from food consumed or the process of consuming the proper amount of nourishment and energy. It rebuilds and promotes health; therefore, nutrition is vital to patient care. Encouraging healthy eating, a healthy lifestyle and supporting patients to do so is a big part of a nurse's role. All healthcare professionals must be responsible for patients' nutritional needs when ill, for any support to be effective. But the majority of this care does tend to fall to the nursing staff because of the amount of time they spend with their patients and the patient's relatives. This will be a very important part of your role, but bear in mind that these issues can be personal and sensitive at times and you'll need to consider this in order to effectively communicate on this issue. It is, undoubtedly, a difficult role; serving food which all service users like is virtually impossible. However, most hospital kitchens have a variety of menus to cater for all clinical needs as well as personal or cultural preferences; so make it a point to increase your awareness of this when in placement areas.

Nursing students particularly need depth of knowledge regarding nutritional principles and nutritional science in order to understand what patients need, and to provide effective nutritional care as identified by the NMC at the start of this chapter. A 'balanced diet' means different things to different people as will hopefully become clearer throughout this chapter; no one size fits all!

What the plate consists of will vary, but the colours (see Figure 35.3) are a visual reminder that your service users'/clients' plate should be colourful in the food it contains. Values/beliefs and/or cultural/religious aspects can affect the diets people choose, i.e. vegetarian, vegan, kosher, to name but a few.

MACRO-NUTRIENTS, MICRO-NUTRIENTS AND FLUIDS

As mentioned, adequate nutritional intake in the form of a balanced diet is essential in the protection of health and the prevention of ill health. Nutrients are often categorised into two groups: macro-nutrients (see Figure 35.1) (carbohydrates, fats and proteins) and micro-nutrients (see Figure 35.2) (vitamins and minerals) (Kozier et al., 2012).

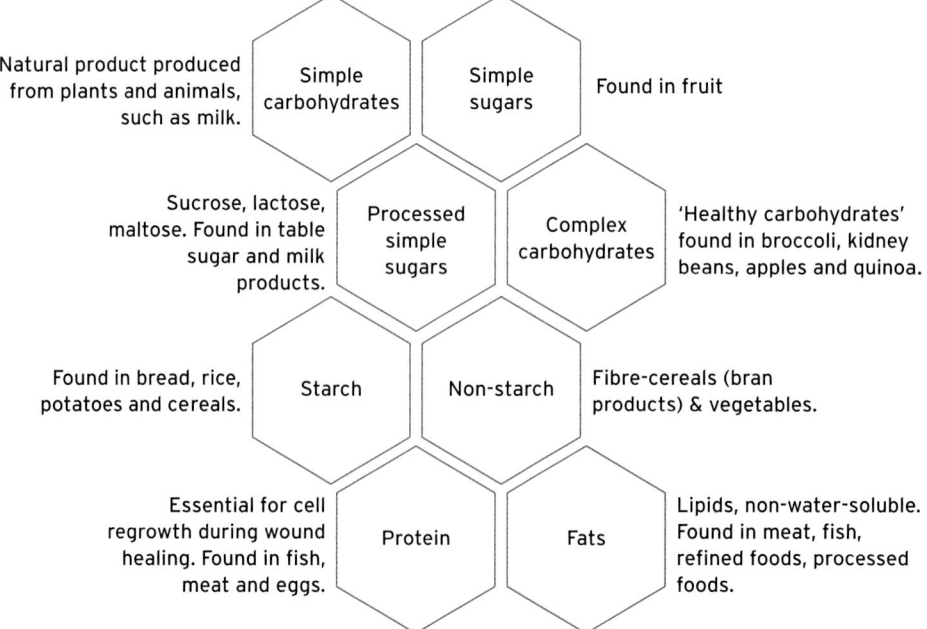

Figure 35.1 Macro-nutrients

GO FURTHER

HIV AND NUTRITION – HIV **(Human Immunodeficiency Virus)** patients often need to increase the protein intake and an understanding of how to do this is very useful. You will find more information surrounding this topic at: www.hiv.gov/hiv-basics/living-healthy-with-hiv/taking-care-of-yourself/food-safety-and-nutrition

WEBLINK:
HIV AND
NUTRITION

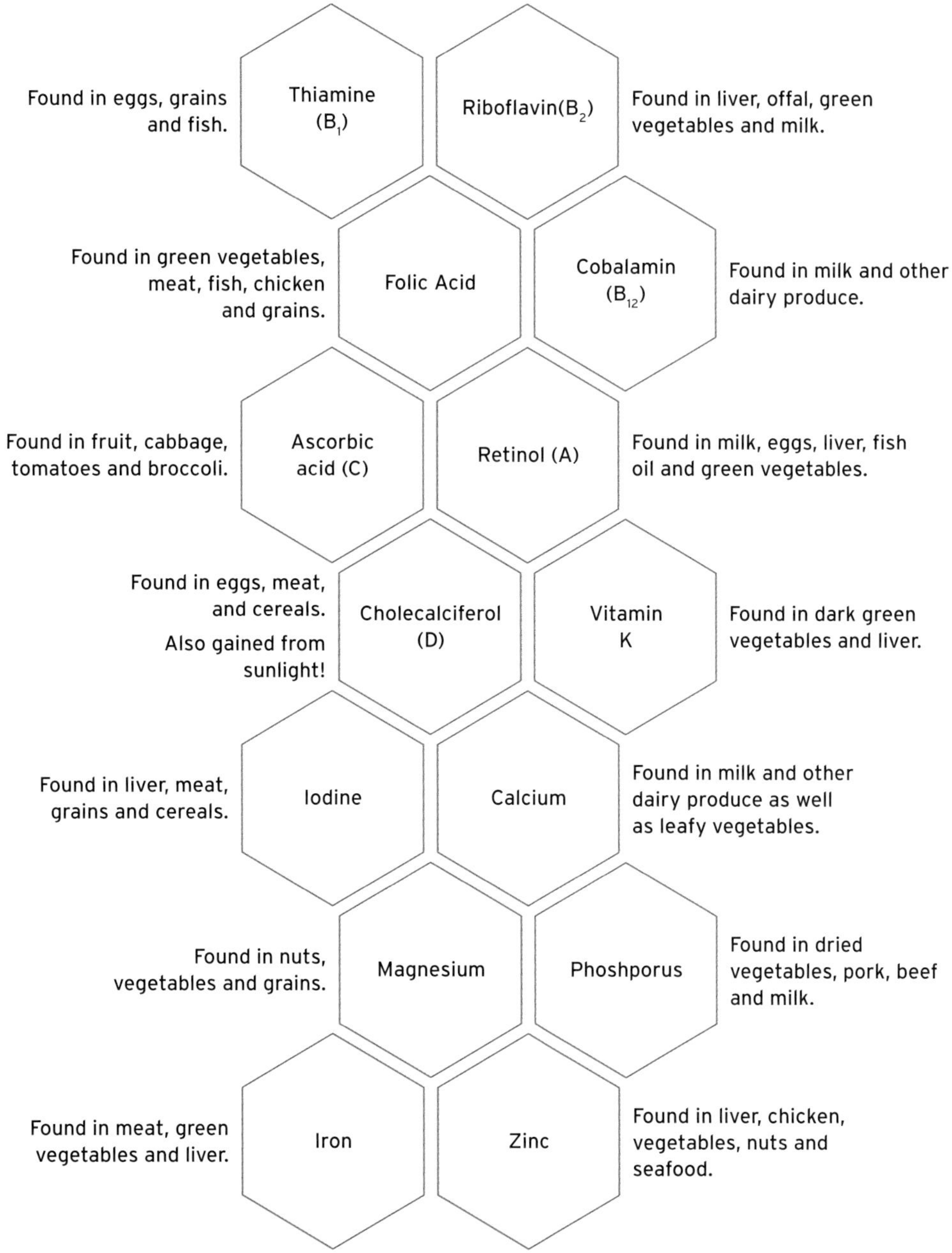

Found in eggs, grains and fish. — **Thiamine (B_1)**

Riboflavin(B_2) — Found in liver, offal, green vegetables and milk.

Found in green vegetables, meat, fish, chicken and grains. — **Folic Acid**

Cobalamin (B_{12}) — Found in milk and other dairy produce.

Found in fruit, cabbage, tomatoes and broccoli. — **Ascorbic acid (C)**

Retinol (A) — Found in milk, eggs, liver, fish oil and green vegetables.

Found in eggs, meat, and cereals. Also gained from sunlight! — **Cholecalciferol (D)**

Vitamin K — Found in dark green vegetables and liver.

Found in liver, meat, grains and cereals. — **Iodine**

Calcium — Found in milk and other dairy produce as well as leafy vegetables.

Found in nuts, vegetables and grains. — **Magnesium**

Phosphorus — Found in dried vegetables, pork, beef and milk.

Found in meat, green vegetables and liver. — **Iron**

Zinc — Found in liver, chicken, vegetables, nuts and seafood.

Figure 35.2 Micro-nutrients

Food preparation must be considered when attempting to preserve the amount of vitamins in foods. The Department of Health releases UK dietary information to help people prepare well-balanced diets.

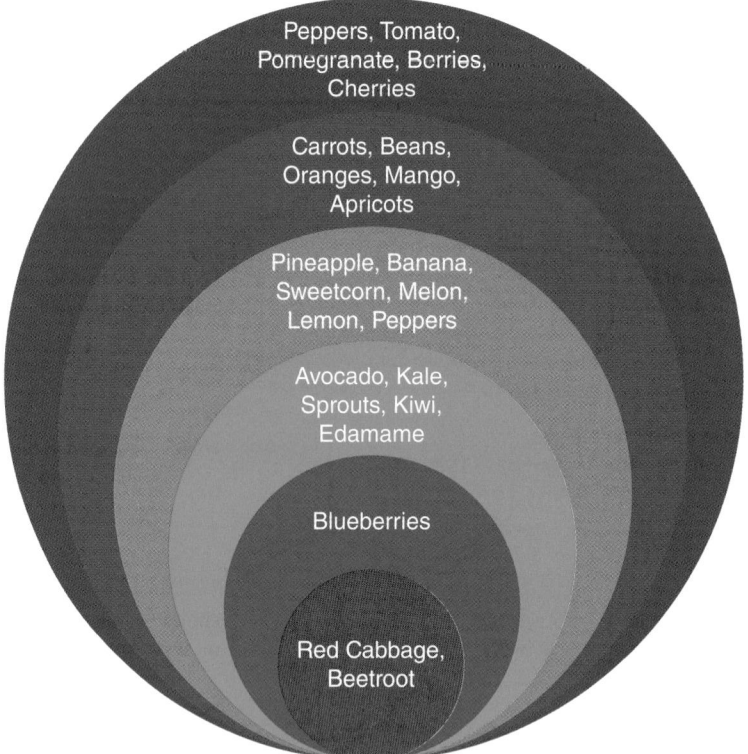

Figure 35.3 A well-balanced diet

Fluids

Water is an essential and, sadly, often forgotten nutrient, making up two-thirds of our body. Maintaining a healthy level of this nutrient is as vital as maintaining a healthy level of all other nutrients. Yet patients still are, or become, dehydrated (Francis, 2013). Without water, survival of life becomes limited and ultimately unsustainable.

Fluid is held in our cells and in the spaces outside the cells: intracellular and extracellular. Water assists us every day as a lubricant for many body parts as well as regulating body temperature: it plays an important role in the transportation of all other nutrients and acts as a solvent for some vitamins (water-soluble vitamins). Helping patients take on board enough fluids is a big part of a nurse's job every day, and accurate documenting of input and output can be difficult to comprehend when first experiencing this in practice. A good understanding of how we lose fluids each day is also useful.

ACTIVITY 35.1: REFLECTIVE PRACTICE

Take a few minutes to list ways in which we lose fluids each day from our bodies.

Fluid loss

We refer to the ways in which we lose fluids as sensible and insensible loss.

| Sensible | loss | →is | Measurable | → Causes: Wounds, urinary output, faeces. |
| Insensible | loss | →is | Unmeasurable | → Causes: Perspiration, respiration. |

You will, over time, learn to recognise thirst in patients. An ideal daily consumption is between 8–12 glasses of water per day (this is an estimate and will alter depending on patients' weight, medical history and time of year). Many hospitalised patients do not drink enough fluids, which drastically increases their risk of dehydration and when we recognise this fully, as staff, we then can begin to understand the importance of the task of offering drinks regularly and often to patients. Water consumption, as mentioned, differs for each person and there will be a variety of factors that need to be considered. Look to deepen your knowledge in practice of maintaining fluid balance and how individualised the process is.

As your journey as a student nurse develops, key signs and symptoms of dehydration that you will learn to recognise will include the following:

- increased to extreme thirst
- raised heart rate
- reduced blood pressure
- a reduction in the frequency of urination
- dry skin with little elasticity
- dry mouth and oral cavity
- dizziness
- confusion in severe cases
- changes in a person's mood
- delirium in some people due to a metabolic imbalance.

GO FURTHER

More details on the importance of macro- and micro-nutrients will require further reading on your part to ascertain a deeper understanding of their effects and significance, and the website *www.nutrition.org.uk* is a good starting place for those wishing to gain an overview.

WEBLINK: BRITISH NUTRITION FOUNDATION

AN OVERVIEW OF THE ANATOMY AND PHYSIOLOGY OF THE GASTROINTESTINAL SYSTEM

Anatomy and physiology of the systems involved in eating and drinking is a good place to start in cementing your understanding of the topic (see Figure 35.4). The digestive system is fundamental to eating and drinking; it is the mechanism of digestion and conversion of all the food and drinks we consume.

Food is first chewed in the oral cavity to start to break it down, in order to increase its surface area so that ultimately oral enzymes can begin to break down the food into an absorbable form. The bolus is then swallowed via the pharynx and oesophagus, and moves along by peristalsis; an action extremely important to the digestive system as it aids movement at different stages and is described as a squeezing action in a rolling wave form. Food is moved into the stomach where digestive acids and muscular contraction of the stomach further break it down. This broken-down food (known as chyme) travels through the duodenum where intestinal fluids help to break it down further. Absorption of essential nutrients occurs when the chyme travels through the small intestine. Nutrients are then transported through the circulatory system via the liver in order that organs receive them in the format required. Peristalsis aids the movement (motility) of the nutrients at each stage and, as mentioned, is extremely important in helping maintain a regular wave-like pattern. Food moving too fast through the system could cause a patient to experience diarrhoea resulting in malabsorption of nutrients or absence of nutrients altogether. The large intestine only absorbs one nutrient – water – making a resulting bulky substance (at this point in the process known as faeces), which travels through the large intestine to the rectum, exiting via the anus for elimination.

While the above system and process can be simplified, many aspects of it rely on other systems to be healthy and working adequately.

If this is not the case, then the mechanism for ingestion and digestion of food and fluids will be affected, therefore ultimately affecting a patient's nutritional status. Some of these will be discussed further in this chapter.

ACTIVITY 35.2

Label the diagram below (Figure 35.4).

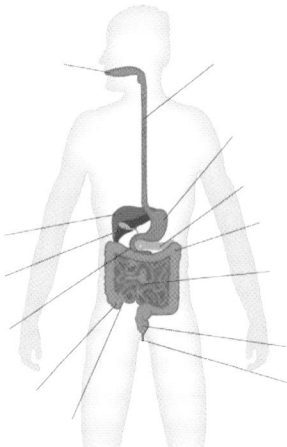

Figure 35.4   The gastrointestinal system

Source: Boore et al. (2016). Illustrated by Shaun Mercier, © SAGE Publications

FUNDAMENTALS OF NUTRITION IN ADULTS, OLDER ADULTS AND IMPACTS ON HEALTH

At approximately 19 years of age, growth and maturation are complete and the focus of most adults is maintenance of a healthy, appropriate weight and of achieving physical fitness. Avoiding excessive weight gain is paramount to health and this is relative to our calorific intake. A guide to daily amounts can be seen in Table 35.1.

Table 35.1   Adult calorie intake

	Daily Calorie Intake – Adults		
	No exercise	Some exercise	Active person
Male	2500 kcal/day	2400-2800 kcal/day	2800-3000 kcal/day
Female	1800 kcal/day	2000-2200 kcal/day	2200-2400 kcal/day

An understanding of healthy foods and exercise habits along with reducing fat intake, eating the recommended amount of fruit and vegetables and staying physically active can help to reduce risk factors for chronic illness later in life. Risks of heart disease, hypertension and diabetes commonly develop between the ages of 40 and 60 years and any attempts at prevention or delay are positive.

Guidelines are often generic and consideration must always be given to those with different needs. For example: lifestyle, excessive physical activity (athletes) or anyone following other dietary choice; vegan, vegetarian, etc., must be considered in order to make the appropriate modifications.

Older adults have specific nutritional needs owing to the physiological changes in organs and tissues as we age (see Table 35.2, after Case Study 35.1). Over the last century, life expectancy has increased dramatically in the main, due to healthier lifestyles, education and significant advances in science and medicine.

Older adults experience a variety of changes that have the potential to affect their nutritional status. Some of these relate to external influences and some more internal, i.e. an increase in the need to take medications as we increase in age, due to chronic illness. Both the sensitivity of the intended effect, and the risk of side effects of medication, increase in the older adult.

Much work has been done on the link between nutrition, age and positive health and an imbalance of nutrition in older adults is a particular problem faced by those caring for this service user group. Attending to positive nutrition, as we know, is vital for health. Certainly, when older adults face hospital admission, nursing and healthcare staff are paramount in providing nutritional information and advice as we are the primary link between the system and the service user, and we must never assume just because someone is older in years, that they have had any interaction with the healthcare system previously. If you remember this, you will help to reduce anxiety in patients and communicate more effectively.

Older adults can experience a range of problems regarding nutritional intake, especially when they are hospitalised. Coping with such stressors in later years can be difficult, anxiety inducing and frightening. Hospitalisation can create such stresses, immediately causing a change in any usual routines they have pertaining to mealtimes and when they usually take fluids. Knowing these routines about your patient as well as **what** they like to eat and drink, **how** they prefer to do it, and any predisposing health issues that may affect nutrition and elimination routines will help you immensely when caring for older adults and maintaining nutrition and hydration (Brown-Wilson, 2013).

CASE STUDY 35.1: NERYS

(A pseudonym has been used to protect the confidentiality of the patient)

When on placement I helped to care for a lady living with dementia. On handover her nutritional status was verbalised as 'feed at risk': this was documented in the notes. I was unsure what this fully meant and spoke with my mentor who explained that for this lady, taking oral nutrition was not always safe and had risks, particularly a risk of aspiration. The advice was

(Continued)

(Continued)

that staff should always feed her to observe and minimise this risk. Assessments deemed that enteral feeding was not in this lady's best interest hence the decision made (with family members) to continue oral feeding even though there was a risk. I had noticed that every mealtime staff did feed the food to her and that she barely ever finished one mouthful, declined most of it and ultimately staff left and took the food away.

I was assigned to feed this lady one mealtime and helped her with yoghurt; I did this as I had observed other staff do by feeding her the food. I noticed that as I did this she constantly reached for the spoon in my hand. I took a chance and handed her the spoon with the yoghurt on instead of doing it for her. She ate it herself and proceeded to do so until the dish was empty.

It was clear to me that this lady wanted to feed herself and not have staff do it for her. I spoke with my mentor and explained this; I asked could she have more variety, could we maybe try finger food? My mentor agreed and reiterated what I should be observing for regards her risk. When hot drinks were offered I also offered some biscuits, dipped them lightly in her cup of tea and handed them to her (three in total), she ate them all. This was the most I had seen this lady take in over a week.

I was confused that 'feed at risk' assumed the patient should be physically fed by staff and that each time refusal to eat is observed it was assumed no more food was wanted by the patient. Ultimately this would mean that nutritional needs of this lady were not met. This lady had no ability to communicate her needs or preferences verbally anymore. However, giving her the choice to take nutrition in her own way, I feel, made all the difference.

Kirsty James, 2nd year student nurse

Table 35.2 Examples of physiological changes

Peristalsis slows down and constipation can be more prevalent.

Reduction in the production of gastric fluids makes it more difficult to digest certain foods and food groups.

Some medications can affect the production of saliva resulting in swallowing difficulties.

Problems chewing can arise from dental issues; loose-fitting dentures or bone deterioration.

Mucosal cells deteriorate; blood supply to the intestine reduces resulting in malabsorption of nutrients.

Ensuring patients take on board a good supply of food and drink is about more than just mealtimes, it should be ongoing and happen when the patient wants it not when we choose to give it to them. Hospital mealtimes can be rigid and induce anxiety in patients living with mental health problems: It is up to us (Nurses) to remove some of the rigidity and barriers and look outside the 'mealtime box'.

Emily Johnson, 2nd year student nurse (Mental Health)

ASSESSMENT OF NUTRITION AND DISCUSSION OF MALNUTRITION

You will need to consult a number of sources when assessing a patient's nutritional status. These will depend upon the setting and environment you are in when conducting your assessment. You will encounter various nutritional assessment tools during your journey as a student nurse and again, these will depend on the placement setting you find yourself in. For example: the MUST screening tool (BAPEN, 2003); Nutritional Risk Assessment of Adult Patients (NRA Welsh Assessment Standards, 2015); Derby assessment tool, (2000), to name a few.

While the variety of tools can be extensive, most work on a similar set of value markers and these may include the following:

- patient's weight and height (BMI)
- any unintentional weight loss
- observations and skin integrity
- appetite/Anorexia/Bulimia
- specific dietary requirements
- lab results (if recently performed)
- medical/Surgical history (particularly if over 80)
- neurological function
- current health state
- psychosocial factors.

Nutritional screening is performed by a qualified healthcare professional, often within the first 24 hours of admission for someone in hospital (always check local policies and guidelines). If a person is then deemed to be at risk, a more comprehensive nutritional assessment may need to be carried out by a registered dietician. Local policy will aid you in any referral needed.

Nutrition for patients is everyone's responsibility. Whether it's a formal assessment or clinical examination; ensuring we document and act upon preferences and choices; making the environment conducive to mealtimes or simply pushing a table or glass closer to a patient so they can reach. All these things make a difference, it also lets the patients know that we take their nutrition seriously. Some placement areas I have visited adopt 'protected mealtimes' and (quite rightly), I have been evicted from the wards/areas during these times to ensure this happens. I can say, I am very careful now to check my watch regularly and exit wards at the right time, I don't want to upset Sister a second time! (lol). I'm proud to work in areas that realise the magnitude and importance nutrition plays to a person and their care.

Thomas Reed, 4th year medical student

CRITICAL THINKING STOP POINT 35.1

Look at some of the value markers (listed above), the importance of them and what they tell us.

Calculating BMI from a patient's weight and height

Using BMI as an indicator requires little training or skill, and for that reason it is valuable, simple and quick to calculate and used by many healthcare professionals (www.nhs.uk/livewell). The problem with relying on BMI is that the weight element assumes excess fat, when in fact other reasons must be taken into account, such as large muscle mass, excess fluid (ascites) or significant limb oedema.

A full top-to-toe, back-to-front examination of your patient's skin is essential when assessing many things, including nutrition. It is vital to gain consent when doing this and essential that you maintain dignity and respect at all times. Nutritional screening and assessment is vital in identifying patients at risk of malnutrition, or who are already malnourished, and consists of a detailed process to identify patient-specific problems and help formulate a plan of care.

On further assessment, Table 35.3 indicates some of the possible problems:

Table 35.3

Imbalance/Deficiency	Signs/Symptoms
Iron	Anaemia: pale, short of breath, reduced immunity, cramps, weakness, weight loss
Vitamin A	Night blindness
Vitamin B	Dry skin, reduced skin turgor
Vitamin C	Bleeding gums, poor wound healing
Vitamin D	Bone pain
Vitamin K	Clotting problems
Protein	Oedema, abdominal ascites, muscle wastage, hair thinning, brittle nails
Riboflavin	Photophobia, grey spots in eyes, red conjunctiva, cracks in mouth
Iodine	Depressed thyroid function: constipation, swollen neck
Fluid deficit	Tachycardia, hypotension, altered consciousness
Calcium/Magnesium	Cardiac problems, peripheral tingling, confusion, hallucinations

> Good nutrition does not only relate to receiving an appropriate calorie intake, but also depends upon a balanced diet. Malnutrition can occur due to inadequate consumption of vital nutrients. It is important, therefore, that regular meals consisting of protein, carbohydrates, good fats, vitamins and minerals are consumed. It is important to ensure that the body receives the essential nutrients it requires.
>
> **Yasmine Alley, 1st year student nurse (Adult)**

OBESITY

Malnutrition refers to undernutrition – not getting enough nutrients – and overnutrition – getting more nutrients than you require. The UK has seen a dramatic increase in an overnourished population (obesity) in recent years and many government and media campaigns have been launched in an attempt to reduce the problem. Excess weight comes with a dangerous increased risk of chronic, long-term health issues. The risk of preventable deaths increases significantly (up to 50%) in obese people compared to a comparable group with a normal weight. The annual financial cost of obesity in the UK is in excess of £7.3 billion (BAPEN, 2016).

The risk of gaining weight can increase with age, but after the age of 60 years, this risk lessens and weight gain is not a natural expectation of ageing; however, genetic influences can play a part as well as other factors (see Table 35.4).

Obesity is an imbalance between energy exerted and calorie intake. If this imbalance continues, the result is weight gain. If the problem were as simple as the explanation, then the solution would be also. Many other factors can influence weight gain; see Table 35.4 for some of these.

Table 35.4   Influencing weight gain factors

Influencing Factor	Result
Chronic illness	Hypothyroidism, depression, Cushing's syndrome are all examples of illness that can heavily influence weight gain.
Medications	Antipsychotics, steroids, antidepressants can cause weight gain. Steroids will increase a patient's appetite.
Family history	Risk can be increased by as much as 33% if there is a family history of obesity, either associated with genetics or lifestyle.
Environment	Poor eating habits, low levels of activity, limited access to transportation.
Psychological	Eating in response to mood and stresses, as well as boredom, sadness and rage.

NURSING INTERVENTIONS

If patients can lose weight, they increase the benefits to themselves and to those around them. Weight loss can, for example:

- lower cholesterol levels
- lower blood glucose
- reduce risk of heart disease and diabetes
- reduce blood pressure.

You should look to work with the patient's own personal motivation to make health changes. Remember to consider food preferences and cultural or religious aspects when addressing nutritional issues. A rise in fad diets and information in the media means many people can be confused when they decide to lose weight. Education and health promotion at this point is vital.

Encourage patients to eat sensible portions but not to avoid food. Dieting doesn't mean no food; reducing calories is proven and safe method of losing weight for most people after relevant assessment. Talk about what to eat – fresh fruit and vegetables where possible, lean meat and high-fibre options and alternatives; and the different ways of cooking food – to steam, grill or bake rather than to fry. Many people need education and guidance on interpreting food labels and information.

Encouraging weight loss must not be prescriptive; the patient needs to be ready and will need guidance and support. Also, look at how they can increase their physical activity. This should be started slowly after consultation with a doctor. It can include simple activities such as increasing household chores or the distance they walk each day.

The waiting list for weight loss surgery is lengthy in most parts of the UK, as the demand is high and the surgery can be costly; £5000 to £15,000. Commitment to the significant lifestyles changes are fundamental to sustaining weight loss. A rigorous nutritional plan will be in place including a carefully controlled, balanced diet and an exercise schedule. While surgery can achieve impressive results, it does not address any mental health problems surrounding the weight gain in the first place.

When caring for dangerously obese patients, always ensure dignity and respect are maintained throughout their care. Community services in many areas can be accessed in order to ensure patients have the correct, safe equipment for their needs and, similarly in hospital, a holistic assessment (not just a BMI calculation) should be conducted in order to access appropriate equipment. Local policy guidelines will give detailed instructions about how to obtain such services and equipment at all hours.

EATING DISORDERS

Undernourished patients also increase their risk of health problems. While most literature looks at how eating disorders affect younger persons, nurses can encounter adults of all ages living with these problems. These nutritional disorders stem from psychological issues rooted in a variety of traumatic events.

Behaviours can include: fasting, obsessive activity regimes and abuse of laxatives and/or diuretics (anorexia nervosa), or eating large portions of food quickly then inducing vomiting and again abuse of laxatives and/or diuretics (bulimia nervosa).

More recently, described behaviours also include: increased eating pace and large quantities of food, sometimes hiding it by eating alone, reaching an out-of-control over-full feeling. This behaviour results in a quiet depression about the episodes, but unlike bulimia nervosa, no induced vomiting occurs (binge eating disorder).

Eating disorders are not gender specific and although often affecting younger females, can occur at any age and need additional specialist nutritional assessment. Long-term effects of eating disorders and under nutrition can lead to chronic ill health including cardiac problems, arrhythmias, and bone problems from long-term calcium deficiency. Electrolyte imbalances increase risks of cardiac problems. Psychological issues underpin some eating disorders and must be taken into account in order to have a positive impact on patients. Treatment given goes beyond restoring nutritional intake and may include behaviour modifications, counselling therapy and psychiatric assessments and interventions.

Malnourished patients and undernourished patients may be at risk of **re-feeding syndrome**. This is a problem that spans many areas of health. This could be when someone purposely does not eat for a length of time. Other examples could be fad diets or eating disorders, unintentional poor nutritional intake or inability to take nutrition. In fact, any episode where little to no nutrition is taken could result in re-feeding syndrome.

Specialised assessment is needed if you feel any patient may be at risk of re-feeding syndrome and strict national and local guidelines must be adhered to (NICE, 2006).

THE SIGNIFICANCE OF NUTRITION WITH REGARD TO SOME CHRONIC CONDITIONS

This section aims to look at the impact of nutrition on some chronic diseases. It will not be possible to cover all of these so further reading will be required in order to have a good understanding of the systems of the body and how each is affected in different ways by nutrition. Some examples are included below.

Table 35.5 Chronic conditions

System	Illness	Symptoms	Dietary Management
Gastrointestinal (GI)	GORD (gastro-oesophageal reflux disease)	Burning pain in the epigastric area. Sour, bitter taste in mouth. Pain radiating to arms and chest. Pain on swallowing, nocturnal salivation causing the patient to cough and choke.	Small, frequent meals. Avoid hearty meals late in the evening/night. Omit known triggers (i.e. pastry, alcohol, caffeine).
	Dumping Syndrome	Occurs post gastric surgery. Abdominal pain, cramping and diarrhoea.	Eat small meals, limit sugar consumption. Lie down for 30-60 mins after eating to delay gastric emptying.
	Coeliac Disease	Abdominal pain. Bloating, weight loss. Pale, loose stools, flatulence. Bone pain, fatigue, dental problems.	Adhere to a gluten-free diet. Research continues into toleration of oats.
	Lactose Intolerance	Bloating, cramps, diarrhoea and nausea.	Avoid lactose in early years. Adults' trial and error of toleration.
	Diverticular Disease	Left-sided, lower abdominal pain, low grade fever, reduced BP, leukocytosis. Haemorrhage if severe.	High fibre diet. Plenty of fluids.
	IBS (Irritable bowel syndrome)	Intermittent cramps, diarrhoea, abdominal pain, constipation, abdominal distension.	Avoid stress; follow a healthy balanced diet, avoid individual triggers, small meals chewed well. Little still known about IBS.
	Crohn's Disease	Tiredness, diarrhoea, left-sided lower abdominal pain, fever, excess fat in faeces, weight loss, nausea, mild bleeding, joints/eye inflammation.	High protein diet, high in calories, small meals frequently, avoid alcohol, caffeine, fizzy drinks, ice, sugars and spicy food.
Cardiac	Coronary Artery Disease	Angina, chest pain, jaw or shoulder pain.	Low cholesterol diet, oily fish, adequate vitamin intake, fat-free options, reduced salt intake.
	Hypertension	'Silent Killer', headache, dizziness, nose bleeds, few symptoms until vascular changes such as clots, CVA and kidney damage occur.	Reduce sodium intake, reduce excess weight, treat underlying cause, reduce alcohol, and increase exercise.
Renal	Renal Calculi	Severe pain in lower back, nausea, vomiting, fever, chills.	Increase fluid intake, restrict oxalate foods such as beetroot, asparagus, chocolate, nuts, soy products and grains.
Endocrine	Type 2 Diabetes	Increased frequency of urination, tiredness, excessive thirst, visual changes, irritability.	Maintain a balanced diet, small meals, avoid processed sugar, increase carbs, and reduce fat and protein. Avoid alcohol.

ACTIVITY 35.3: REFLECTIVE PRACTICE

Think about how culture/religious/belief systems have an effect on nutritional choices.

Nutritional needs in chronic (as well as acute) illness are very important. An understanding and appreciation of the specific changes a condition causes can help significantly in learning the optimal point for nutritional support or nutritional supplementation.

CASE STUDY 35.2: OWEN

(A pseudonym has been used to protect patient confidentiality)

During my time on placement, I helped care for a gentleman with coeliac disease. Many people lean towards gluten-free options in the case of coeliac disease in the hope it helps relieve symptoms.

The gentleman in question suffered significant weight loss since being hospitalised and staff had become very concerned. Hospital food choices can feel limited and he commented that more often than not, he wasn't able to eat the food on offer mainly for fear of becoming unwell. The nurses and healthcare professionals I worked with were extremely supportive of his needs and went to great lengths to resolve the problem.

They liaised directly with kitchen staff and even went in person to the kitchen to come to an arrangement with the staff. This gentleman had recently suffered a myocardial infarction and the nursing staff clearly demonstrated that good nutrition was important in his recovery. Without adequate nutritional intake this gentleman would not have re-gained weight or built up the strength and stamina he needed in order to continue with his treatment and ultimately the cardiac surgery he needed.

Jenna Morgan, 1st year student nurse (Adult)

- How did the team work together to help this gentleman?

NUTRITIONAL INTERVENTIONS

After reviewing the anatomy and physiology drawing of the GI system (see Figure 35.4), you may be able to begin to understand that problems will arise for patients if any section is damaged or altered in any way, and this could cause issues for patients attempting to take in adequate nutrition.

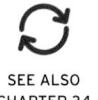

SEE ALSO
CHAPTER 34

CRITICAL THINKING STOP POINT 35.2

Stomas and nutrition

A stoma (i.e. colostomy or ileostomy) is a result of a surgical intervention and has an impact on digestion and absorption. You may care for patients with a 'stoma bag'; a stoma is an opening on the abdominal wall which can divert faeces or urine (depending on the procedure) to the outside of the body. It is worth noting that patients with a stoma have no control over stool or urine elimination. An increased fluid intake is encouraged to compensate for increased fluid loss and patients need education on the altered effects certain foods will have on their body. For example: certain foods will increase odour (garlic, eggs, fish, onions, asparagus); certain foods will block the stoma exit (celery, sweetcorn, mushrooms, peas); certain foods are gas inducing (beans, broccoli, melons, honey, nuts); certain foods will bulk faeces making elimination painful (bread, bananas, cheese, pasta, apples); and certain foods will reduce odour (milk, parsley, yoghurt, herbs, cranberries).

More information can be found here: www.wwl.nhs.uk/Library/All_New_PI_Docs/Audio_Leaflets/Dietetics/Stoma/FT2_healthy_eating_advice_for_people.html

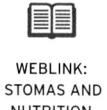

WEBLINK: STOMAS AND NUTRITION

When this is the case, other interventions are needed may often bypass the affected area and access the GI system at a different point to compensate. Some of these interventions will now be looked at and give you some points to consider further in your studies.

Many conditions may affect a patient's ability to chew and swallow (oral cavity and oesophagus) which is crucial for most people when taking in food and drink; neurological deficits will affect this system; acute illnesses, altered conscious levels, physical fatigue and confusion.

When this happens we may look to offer supplementary feeding to patients. Supplementary feeding can be broken down into three categories: - oral supplementary feeding; **enteral feeding** and **parenteral feeding.**

If a patient can take nutrition orally and safely, then they should do so, but if the ability to take in enough nutrients to maintain a balanced diet is impaired, then it may be appropriate to offer supplements.

Oral supplements

The need for oral supplements is likely to be thoroughly evaluated and assessed by either a registered dietician or a clinician or both. These supplements may initially be offered between meals to 'supplement' current nutrition. (Multiple brands are available and it is worth noting that if patients find one brand unpalatable then another can be offered – liaise with the dietician. The products also come in the form of nutrition bars and puddings if the patients do not enjoy the milky or fruit-based drinks.)

Some considerations when caring for patients taking oral supplements:

- Be mindful that some nutritional supplement drinks can cause diarrhoea.
- Supplements should be offered between meals, approximately one hour before the next meal.
- Vary the flavours or brands for patients to avoid boredom. From experience, I have found patients find the drinks particularly more enjoyable when served cold.
- Some patients will need complete nutrition in this way if this is their only intake.
- Patients on a fluid restriction can be offered higher calorific products to reduce volume intake.
- A prescription and guidance from a registered dietician or doctor will be needed; this is usually available after completion of a comprehensive nutritional assessment.

Enteral feeding

Gastric enteral feeding of patients is also referred to as 'tube feeding' and can be via stomach or intestine depending on the location of the problem.

ACTIVITY 35.4: REFLECTIVE PRACTICE

Take five minutes to think of some reasons why patients may need nutritional support.

You may care for patients who have a nastrogastric (NG) tube by way of a feeding method. The choice of enteral feeding tube that the patient has will be dependent on the condition of the GI system, overall physical condition, other medical problems and any risk of aspiration they may have.

NG tubes enter the body via the nose with the tube ending in the stomach, bypassing the oral cavity. Further enteral nutritional intervention can be via a surgical procedure, with a tube surgically inserted into either the stomach (percutaneous endoscopic gastrostomy (PEG) tube) or the intestine (percutaneous endoscopic jejunostomy (PEJ) tube). The choice of tube will depend on multiple factors; for example, is the length of enteral feeding expected to be temporary? NG tubes tend to be used for temporary purposes. Longer than a 4-week period is deemed permanent by clinical staff and an NG tube is less likely to be the option (this is a general rule but exceptions will be made for some cases). Again, as with oral supplements, a registered dietician will be much involved in these patients' care and will carry out a comprehensive assessment and provide a regime that suits the patient and their needs and an appropriate feeding formula liquid.

Options for feeding preparations need to be as varied as an oral balanced diet would be and can include: high protein options, high fibre options, increased calorie options and condition-specific options, i.e. suitable for people with diabetes, renal disorders, or respiratory problems.

The prescribed feeding regime will be available from the dietician; it is also worth being aware, in practice, of local policy as this will give full guidelines and safety considerations for enteral feeding. Regimes are sometimes nocturnal so as to offer minimal interference in the patient's day. There are considerations that must be taken into account when helping patients to take nutrition in this way.

Parenteral feeding

Parenteral feeding refers to the nutritional support we give via intravenous (IV) access for a patient. This option is often for patients whose GI tract is not viable and for whom none of the above options are appropriate. Patients with a normally functioning or part functioning GI tract would be very unlikely to be offered parenteral feeding. Once again, this decision is made with the involvement of the multidisciplinary team and a discussion would take place between dieticians, doctors, nurses, patients (where possible) and family members or significant others before feeding in this way commences.

This type of feeding will be administered via either a peripheral cannula or a central venous catheter. Indications for this type of feeding may include (but are not exlusive to):

- chronic diarrhoea and vomiting
- severe Crohn's disease
- bowel fistulae
- bowel obstructions
- unsuitability to receive long-term enteral feeding.

Parenteral feeding is not only significantly more expensive (up to ten times more expensive than enteral feeding) but also carries more risk; particularly cannula/catheter-related problems such as infection, sepsis, phlebitis, and air embolus.

OTHER NUTRITIONAL CONSIDERATIONS – CULTURE, RELIGION AND BELIEFS

> As a vegan patient, choices offered to me have been limited at times and I regularly decline what's on the menu, meaning I have to rely heavily on family to ensure I have enough to eat and drink. I even have to decline a cup of tea as often there is not a milk alternative available. Consequently I am always eager to be discharged and get home. Having specific vegan choices would make a huge difference to my stay as I would not feel a nuisance to staff and my family but feel also that my choices were valued.
>
> Charlie Edwards, patient

Ensuring patients have an adequate nutritional intake is about more than a healthy balanced diet and sufficient calories. Ensuring they are comfortable, have dignity and are respected when taking diet and fluids are equally important and all are the responsibility of all healthcare professionals who have an involvement in care.

Understanding a patient's cultural, religious and belief choices concerning nutrition not only promotes holistic patient care, but also promotes the possibility that adequate diet and fluids will be taken and nutritional status maintained. Many trusts and health boards will have a helpful local policy that gives advice and guidelines on what foods can and cannot be taken and what must be avoided as well as preparation and significant dates/festivals observed by religious or cultural groups. This information will also give you details on all menus prepared by kitchens and what needs to be done if something different to that is required.

CHAPTER SUMMARY

- Nurses have a very important role in ensuring patients' nutritional needs are met.
- Nutrition is about more than mealtimes, and should be individual and holistic.
- Chronic conditions must be understood in order to ensure nutrition is offered and altered accordingly.
- Education, health promotion, advice and support are ongoing and vital to the role of nursing.

GO FURTHER

Books

- Brotherton, A., Simmonds, N. and Stroud, M. (2010) *Malnutrition Matters: Meeting Quality Standards in Nutrition Care: A Toolkit for Commissioners and Providers in England*. Redditch: BAPEN. Information in Toolkit form of the Standards in Nutrition Care.
- Delves-Yates, C. (ed.) (2018) *Essential Clinical Skills for Nurses* (2nd edn.). London: SAGE. Provides step-by-step procedures.
- Delves-Yates, C. (ed.) (2018) *Essentials of Nursing Practice* (2nd edn.). London: SAGE. Introduces the student nurse to the essentials of nursing practice.

FURTHER READING: JOURNAL ARTICLES

Journal Articles

Go to https://study.sagepub.com/essentialadultnursing for further free online journal articles related to this chapter. If you are using the interactive ebook, simply click on the book icon in the margin to go straight to the resource.

- Chavarro-Carvajal, C. (2015) Nutritional assessment and factors associated to malnutrition in older adults. *Journal of Ageing and Health*. http://journals.sagepub.com/doi/abs/10.1177/0898264314549661
  This article reviews how to determine the nutritional status and factors associated to malnutrition in older adults.
- Mundi, M., Nystrom, E. and Hurley, D. (2016) Management of parenteral nutrition in hospitalized adult patients. *Journal of Parenteral and Enteral Nutrition*. http://journals.sagepub.com/doi/abs/10.1177/0148607116667060
  Despite the high prevalence of malnutrition in adult hospitalised patients, surveys continue to report that many clinicians are undertrained in clinical nutrition, making targeted nutrition education for clinicians essential for best patient care.
- Posthauer, M., Dorner, B. and Friedrich, E. (2014) Enteral nutrition for older adults in health-care communities. *Nutrition in Clinical Practice*. http://journals.sagepub.com/doi/abs/10.1177/0884533614541482
  Review of enteral feeding within a community setting.

FURTHER READING: WEBLINKS

Weblinks

Go to https://study.sagepub.com/essentialadultnursing for further weblinks related to this chapter. If you are using the interactive ebook, simply click on the book icon in the margin to go straight to the resource.

- More information on re-feeding syndrome can be found at the following link: www.youtube.com/watch?v=1572jPnBuZY
- See NICE Guidelines: Obesity: http://guidance.nice.org.uk/cg43
  The prevention, identification, assessment and management of overweight and obesity in adults and children.
- www.NHS.uk/livewell
  NHS choices app to manage your health. Including comparing supermarket ingredients, and audio guides.

ONLINE QUIZZES

ACE YOUR ASSESSMENT

Revise what you have learned by visiting https://study.sagepub.com/essentialadultnursing

- Test yourself with multiple-choice and short-answer questions
- Do the chapter activities in the book and check your answers online

REFERENCES

British Association of Parenteral and Enteral Nutrition (BAPEN) (2016) *Nutritional Care Tool*. Available at: bapen.org.uk

Francis, R. (2013) *Report of the Mid Staffordshire NHS Foundation Trust*. Public HMSO Inquiry Crown copyright.

Kozier, B., Erb, G., Berman, A., Snyder, A., Harvey, S. and Morgan-Samuel, H. (2012) *Fundamentals of Nursing: Concepts, process and practice* (2nd ed.). Harlow: Pearson Education.

National Institute for Health and Care Excellence (NICE) (2006) *Nutrition Support In Adults QS24.* Available at: https://www.nice.org.uk/Guidance/CG32

Nursing and Midwifery Council (NMC) (2015) *The Code: Professional standards of practice and behaviour for nurses and midwives.* London: NMC.

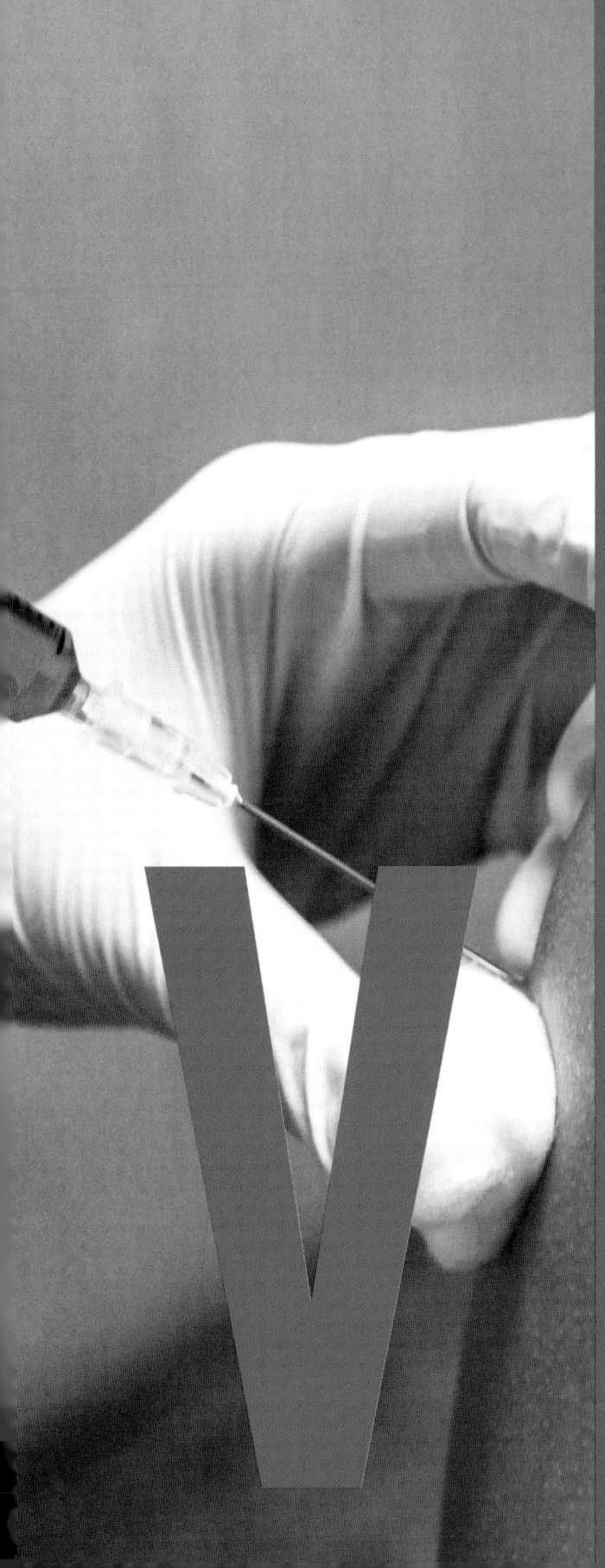

BEING A PROFESSIONAL ADULT NURSE

LEADERSHIP AND MANAGEMENT IN NURSING ADULTS

36

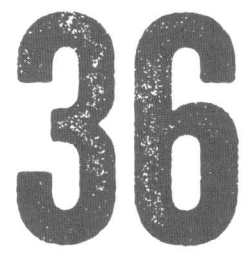

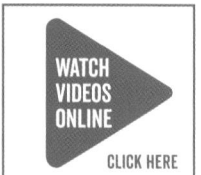
WATCH VIDEOS ONLINE
CLICK HERE

RUTH TAYLOR AND NANCY FONTAINE

THIS CHAPTER COVERS

- The contextual and policy issues affecting nursing leadership
- An overview of leadership theories and management
- Leadership and management in adult nursing practice
- Characteristics, attributes, skills and tools for compassionate leadership.

> "
> A good leader has organisational skills, makes things work well, and keeps everyone happy. Good leadership needs you to have good relationships with staff and for people to feel happy to do what you need them to do. You have to be open to others' views as well. A leader has to be competent and take responsibility and also motivate people. I also think that leadership is about making the standards and values so it goes from the top down – to lead by example is the easy way to say it.
>
> Hannah Leggett, 2nd year student nurse, mental health nursing
> "

INTRODUCTION

The purpose of this chapter is to provide an overview of management and leadership theories in the context of adult nursing. This chapter will give you the opportunity to consider the skills, attributes and characteristics that *you* bring to nursing practice and to consider the areas which you wish to develop. Our starting points are: student nurses are seen as leaders and take on leadership roles as soon as they go into any practice placement; leadership is a vital ingredient to providing the best possible care experience for each and every patient.

Clinical leaders have individual and collective responsibility to create and maintain a positive emotional environment for colleagues and teams so that the working situation is conducive to the delivery of high quality care, optimised safety and enhanced patient experience. It is essential to support a creative environment in which innovation can thrive and improve care. We are going to refer to *you* as the clinical leader as we write: we know that you may well be at the beginning of your nurse education and training, or you may be about to qualify, but it is important that you consider yourself a leader no matter what stage you are at.

Going back to Hannah's quote at the beginning of this chapter, you can see that she has identified some of the key aspects of both leadership and management that are helpful for healthcare practice. She has articulated some of the skills, attributes and characteristics that are important for leadership practice. The chapter will go on to explore these in more depth, and towards the end of the chapter, we will return to some students and 'hear' more about their thoughts on leadership.

CONTEXTUAL AND POLICY ISSUES AFFECTING LEADERSHIP AND MANAGEMENT IN ADULT NURSING PRACTICE

SEE ALSO
CHAPTER 1

There are political drivers and policies that need to be delivered in health. One recent example in England is the NHS *Five Year Forward View* (DoH, 2014). This strategy sets out the focus for change in order to reshape care, make sustainable future improvements in public health and wellbeing, and enable greater engagement with the public. The strategy emphasises enhanced collaborative leadership and ownership of the improvements across all stakeholders, communities, patient groups and frontline staff. The key aim is for services across the different provider organisations to work together to improve pathways for patients. This focus on integrated care has been at the forefront of health policy discussions for some time, but the clear policy direction now appears to be gathering pace. These innovations must be achieved amidst burgeoning financial pressures, fragile social care infrastructure and a reduction in public health spending (Webster, 2015). Analysis predicts that if the health efficiencies and transformation are not implemented then there will be a mismatch of resources and patient need of £30 billion per annum by 2020/21 (DoH, 2014).

A national framework to implement the transformation of health and care was launched by the Chief Nurse for England, Jane Cummings, (*Leading Change, Adding Value*, NHS England, 2016) for nursing, midwifery and care staff and which is aligned to the goals laid out in the *Five Year Forward View* (DoH, 2014). *Leading Change, Adding Value* identifies how you as an individual leader, your team and organisation can deliver the 'triple aim' of:

- better patient outcomes;
- better patient, carer and family experiences; and
- best use of diminishing resources.

The strategy highlights the need for nurses, midwives and care staff to reduce unwarranted variation in health and care outcomes by leading approaches to achieve streamlined consistent care with optimised safety and quality. With creative leadership and focus, the national view is that the three gaps identified in the *Five Year Forward View* (health and wellbeing gap, care and quality gap, funding and efficiency gap) will start to close, in synergy with the delivery of the well-established '6Cs'.

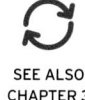

SEE ALSO CHAPTER 3

GO FURTHER

This weblink will take you to the 6Cs so that you can explore the full document: www.england.nhs.uk/wp-content/uploads/2012/12/compassion-in-practice.pdf

WEBLINK: NHS 6CS

Contemporary healthcare is constantly under scrutiny, facing degrees of turmoil and eternally searching for greater productivity and efficiency amidst diminishing resources. However, in times of change, opportunities abound requiring creative, versatile leadership. Clinical leaders need to focus on communicating, motivating, mentoring, investing and innovating staff in order to establish and maintain a climate of transformation and success.

AN OVERVIEW OF LEADERSHIP THEORIES AND MANAGEMENT

This section offers a summary of the key leadership theories and discusses 'management' as part of the role of the nursing leader in adult practice. We take a stance that leadership is the way in which individuals take forward the management requirements of the organisation. So, leadership can be seen as the approach, and management as the tasks and activities. Both are important, and for us it is the development of a leadership approach that is most relevant here so that you are in a position to *manage* the challenges of healthcare practice whatever hierarchical level you are operating in. Consider Activity 36.1.

ACTIVITY 36.1: REFLECTIVE PRACTICE

Reflect on what you know about leadership and management already. Make a list of the characteristics and attributes that you think a 'good' leader needs.

ACTIVITY 36.1 ANSWER

WHAT'S THE EVIDENCE? 36.1

As you were reflecting on your practice in Activity 36.1, you will have identified a number of characteristics and attributes. Heckemann et al. (2015) identified that empathy, empowerment of others (staff and patients), articulation of a vision and direction for an organisation or an area of practice, the ability to motivate and inspire teams, and self-awareness are all considered important attributes for today's leadership context. Heckemann et al. go on to define 'resonant leadership' suggesting that resonant leaders are able to work effectively with teams to enable them to achieve the outcomes that are required for effective practice. Their reading of the existing research in this area seems to demonstrate that resonant leadership leads to improved patient safety and outcomes, as well as enhanced staff wellbeing and satisfaction with the workplace.

Taylor (2009) outlines the theories of leadership as follows:

Great Man theories

You may have heard the expression that 'leaders are born and not made'. Great Man theories arise from a historical perspective where great leaders (usually men) led their (usually) men towards a common purpose. The skills, attributes and characteristics that made up these 'great men' were often defined within the context of social class (often aristocrats), their physical characteristics and personality types, and their age. An example of a leader who helped to define the theoretical stance is Oliver Cromwell.

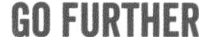 **GO FURTHER**

FURTHER READING: SPECTOR, 2016

Read more on Great Man leadership theories: Spector, B.A. (2016) Carlyle, Freud, and the Great Man Theory more fully considered. *Leadership*, 12(2): 250-60. http://lea.sagepub.com/content/12/2/250.full.pdf+html

Trait theories

Trait theorists assert that leaders have certain inherent traits. According to this theory, it seems that leadership characteristics cannot be learned but are related to particular personalities and behaviours. The problem with trait theories, though, is that just about any characteristic you could think of has been identified as important for good leadership (for example, being assertive, confident and intelligent). Trait theory does not consider the situation in which leadership takes place; nor does it easily enable the actual traits that are required for good leadership to be identified given that so many are cited as important. However, it does give you the chance to think about the multifaceted nature of leadership and to consider which, if any, of the list of traits you possess or would like to develop.

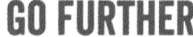 **GO FURTHER**

FURTHER READING: SUDBRACK AND TROMBLEY, 2007

Read more on Trait theories: Sudbrack, B. and Trombley, S. (2007). Lost: A survival guide to leadership theory. *Advances in Developing Human Resources*, 9(2): 251-68. http://adh.sagepub.com/content/9/2/251.full.pdf+html

Situational-contingency theories

As suggested above, the situation in which leadership takes place is important for our understanding of leadership. What these theories suggest is that the situation, the leader, and the follower are all variables that impact on the required approach for leadership. You can probably think of situations where a leader has had to take a strongly directive approach with the followers so as to deal with an emergency situation. In other circumstances you may have seen a leader who has used a more collaborative approach in a situation that demands the 'buy-in' from the followers – for example, in the development of a change in practice such as enhanced visiting hours. Given that different situations require different leadership approaches, could it be said that no one person could encapsulate all the traits (characteristics, skills) to be effective in any circumstances?

GO FURTHER

Read more on Situational-contingency theories in this article that has a military focus but provides analytical commentary which is of interest: Vecchio, R. (2006) The utility of situational leadership theory. A replication in a military setting. *Small Group Research*, 37(5): 407-24. http://sgr.sagepub.com/content/37/5/407.full.pdf+html

FURTHER READING: VECCHIO, 2006

Transactional theories

These theories relate to the way people may be motived by 'reward and punishment'. The basic premise is that the follower does what is asked of them and then is rewarded by pay or in other ways. It is assumed that the follower is responsible for the tasks assigned to them and is, therefore, expected to get on and achieve those tasks. You may be thinking to yourself that there are sometimes things that get in the way of someone's ability to do what is asked of them. For example, in nursing practice it may be that there are staff shortages and it therefore becomes difficult to do what is needed. Transactional theories identify closely with management theories in which delegation and other management skills are important.

GO FURTHER

Read more on Transactional theories: Van Eeden, R., Cilliers, F. and van Deventer, V. (2008) Leadership styles and associated personality traits: Support for the conceptualisation of transactional and transformational leadership. *South African Journal of Psychology*, 38(20): 253-67. http://sap.sagepub.com/content/38/2/253.full.pdf+html

FURTHER READING: VAN EEDEN ET AL., 2008

Transformational theories

Those who aspire to transformational leadership value relationships as a means to the development of practice, in this case nursing. Transformational leadership requires collaboration, participation, sharing, professional development, flexibility (among other attributes). Transformational leaders work to ensure that people are connected and can work together effectively through teams. It could be argued that transformational leadership implies that the leader has particular attributes that make them great (for example, the ability to articulate a vision and bring people with them, possibly through a charismatic approach). However, aspects of transformational leadership seem to address the overarching need to ensure that individuals feel empowered, engaged and connected so as to address the challenges in clinical practice.

FURTHER
READING:
EVERETT AND
SITTERDING,
2011

GO FURTHER

Read more on Transformational theories: Everett, L. and Sitterding, M. (2011) Transformational leadership required to design and sustain evidence-based practice: A system exemplar. *Western Journal of Nursing Research*, 33(3): 398-426. http://wjn.sagepub.com/content/33/3/398.full.pdf+html

Collective leadership theories

The King's Fund is an excellent resource for current debate on leadership in the NHS and health-care sector more widely. West et al. (2014) argue that collective leadership – where everyone in an organisation takes responsibility for its success – facilitates a whole-systems approach to the embedding of good leadership practices within an organisation, rather than an individualised approach. The characteristics of collective leadership include a culture which: values learning, needs lots of challenging dialogue, requires shared understandings of the issues, and enables all who work in that organisation to take individual and collective responsibility (leadership) for safe, effective, high quality and compassionate practice. So, while this is an overarching approach to organisational leadership, you may be able to see that the leadership skills, attributes and characteristics of everyone (including those who are not in defined leadership roles) are crucial to improving practice.

FURTHER
READING:
WEST ET AL.,
2014

GO FURTHER

Read more on Collective leadership: West, M., Eckert, R., Steward, K. and Pasmore, B. (2014) Developing collective leadership for healthcare. King's Fund: London. www.kingsfund.org.uk/sites/files/kf/field/field_publication_file/developing-collective-leadership-kingsfund-may14.pdf

Management

We have identified approaches to leadership and have asserted that these approaches or ways of doing things relate to how healthcare practice is managed. Managers are usually identified through some sort of formal role (for example, ward sister or team leader). Management responsibilities will include but are not limited to:

- budget management
- management of staff, for example rotas
- resource management
- management of the organisation of a shift
- management of staff performance.

In order to undertake these and other management responsibilities, the manager (leader) is more likely to be able to do so effectively when they have certain skills, attributes and characteristics. To go back to resonant leadership: individuals who have the ability to motivate their teams through clearly articulating direction and vision (for example, delivering the best possible care for all patients with compassion), developing individuals and teams, and being a role model, is more likely to be able to manage all aspects of their role effectively. Clearly, the imperative is that care is the best that it can be.

CASE STUDY 36.1

Consider the management of this patient discharge:

You have just taken clinical handover for Mabel, who was admitted following a fall at home. Mabel's family had spoken to the Sister and said that they are concerned about Mabel managing at home.

There is a ward board meeting at 9 a.m. each morning. At the meeting, the patient journey co-ordinator reports that Mabel lives alone in sheltered accommodation. She has a pendant alarm. Previously, Mabel was independent using her Zimmer frame around the flat. Mabel was able to heat up her frozen meals and has a Walsall trolley, which enables her to carry the meal to her chair. Mabel says her daughter is really supportive and makes sure Mabel has bread, milk and snacks which Mabel is able to make for herself. Mabel has a cleaner once a week who also does the washing. The patient journey coordinator reports that she has also discussed this background with Mabel's daughter, Shirley (after gaining consent from Mabel), who reports that her mother 'is amazing and does very well'. Mabel is independent with washing and dressing, although she is starting to struggle with a shower each morning. As a multidisciplinary team, the ward set an expected date of discharge for 3 days' time, and set a plan of investigations, including occupational therapy (OT) and physiotherapy assessments.

Following the board round, during the medical ward round, the consultant tells Mabel that they have planned a number of tests, therapy assessments and are planning for her to be discharged in 3 days. They ensure that Mabel understands this, and is aware that she needs to practise her mobility on the ward to be able to mobilise 20 metres with her Zimmer frame to be fit enough to return home in 3 days' time. Mabel is assessed by the occupational therapist and the physiotherapist. They are concerned that Mabel may need some short-term help at home on discharge as she is not able to walk the full 20 metres, so would be unable to get from her bedroom to her front room chair.

Two days before Mabel's planned discharge date the ward team complete a reablement referral form. This details the activities that Mabel needs help with: mobility practice to be able to mobilise 20 metres with her Zimmer frame. This practice will help Mabel regain confidence in heating, preparing meals and mobilising with these to her dining area. Also the practice will enable Mabel to mobilise independently to the toilet so she does not need to use the commode. Mabel and her daughter both consent to this help and are pleased with the support organised on discharge.

On the day of discharge Mabel is dressed in her own clothes and has her personal care needs met. She has a light breakfast and is transferred to the discharge lounge to wait for her daughter to collect her at 12 p.m. to be home in time for the reablement team to complete their first visit and assessment at 2 p.m.

1. How much of a role has the patient played in helping this to be a well-planned discharge?
2. What is the importance of patients being discharged on the Expected Date of Discharge?
3. What leadership and management skills have been demonstrated in this scenario?

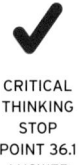

CRITICAL
THINKING
STOP
POINT 36.1
ANSWER

CRITICAL THINKING STOP POINT 36.1

Now that you have read this section on the theory, consider how these theoretical perspectives fit with the current dialogue around nursing leadership for the enhancement of clinical practice. The 'Go further' boxes provide a number of references that you could access to develop your knowledge and understanding about the theory. You could access these as you consider your critical thinking stop point.

LEADERSHIP IN ADULT NURSING PRACTICE

Building on the theoretical perspectives that are described in the previous section, this section begins by summarising the characteristics, attributes and skills for compassionate leadership for adult nursing practice. We acknowledge the challenges associated with the transition from student to qualified nurse, and anticipate that the tools for development that we have identified will, in part, help you to make that transition. We then go on to describe some core aspects of leadership and management that are required for safe, effective, person-centred practice (for example, delegation and people management).

LEARNING TO BE A LEADER

The drivers for improving the quality of care have been described briefly in this chapter, and elsewhere in more detail in the book (Chapter 5, Patient safety). The strong focus on the need to improve the culture and leadership of healthcare practice has been well rehearsed, but in summary, these improvements are needed so that failings as occurred at Mid Staffordshire do not occur again (Francis, 2013). In addition, every nurse on every day that they are in clinical practice has to work to ensure that every interaction with every patient is the best that it can be. We come to this book chapter with the view that this is exactly what people want to do. However, the realities of practice are such that the NHS is under increasing pressure, but it is absolutely essential that all care is of the highest quality and delivered compassionately. The following section offers some views on the characteristics and attributes that could be seen as most important for compassionate leadership. It also identifies some skills and tools that can be used to further develop your leadership. They are not definitive lists but offer you a starting point for your own development.

Characteristics and attributes for compassionate leadership

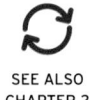

SEE ALSO
CHAPTER 2

- Being person-centred – in relation to patients and those that you work alongside.
- Being visible: 'walking the talk' and being a forward thinker who consistently considers how care and processes for patients and staff could be improved.
- Always leading by example: being a role model who consistently does the right things.
- Being clear about the purpose and direction of the organisation (including at the micro ward level), and feeling involved and 'bought into' that direction.
- Taking personal responsibility: having a proactive approach to problem solving; using errors and omissions as a platform for learning and system improvement.

- Challenging poor standards: escalating issues where appropriate and taking steps to improve standards; adhering to and overtly upholding your Professional Code.
- Having a positive outlook: demonstrating a 'can do' attitude; valuing individuals and teams for their strengths and contributions.
- Good communication at every level: with all patients, carers and families and all members of the health and social care team to get care right first time.
- Empowering others: supporting staff to be creative, taking initiative to be the best you can be and developing future leaders.
- Recognising good practice: always thanking people and taking time to give constructive feedback for specific elements, encouraging deep learning from a positive episode.
- Taking responsibility for your own ongoing learning and personal/professional development.
- Being reflective in a meaningful way (links to resonant leadership).
- Having emotional intelligence which links to the ability to reflect and develop as a person and a practitioner.
- Being able to share your own concerns or challenges in an open and appropriate manner.

SEE ALSO
CHAPTER 3

ACTIVITY 36.2: REFLECTIVE ACTIVITY

Which of the characteristics and attributes do you feel that you need to develop further? What are the challenges that you face in enacting them? What are the benefits (to you, to the patient/carer, to the wider team) of you enacting these characteristics and attributes?

ACTIVITY 36.2
ANSWER

There are many ways in which you can further develop your skills – remember that you will have brought a whole range of skills and attributes into your learning. It is important that you acknowledge them and build on what you do well, while being open-minded enough to acknowledge where you need to improve. Table 36.1 aims to give you some ideas to help you in your personal leadership development.

Table 36.1 Skills and tools for leadership

Skills and tools for leadership

- Sharing best practice with peers and more widely through the evidence-based literature.
- Rewarding others for delivering excellent care: while you may feel that this is out of your hands as a student nurse, telling someone that they have done something well is so important.
- Having coaching as a means for professional development.
- Using action learning sets: an approach where individuals come together in groups to explore work-based issued or concerns, and reflect together on the issues so that the individual can find solutions leading to action.
- Using tools that can facilitate 'knowing self' (for example, the use of tools that indicate your preferences in leadership or team working).
- Taking time and space to do other things that are important to you in your personal life.

TRANSITION

The transition from student to qualified nurse and clinical leader is challenging and a constant source of learning and development. Duchscher (2008) presented the Transition Shock Theory, which described the first four months in professional practice as the most dramatic stage, alongside the three stages of 'doing, knowing and being', during a nurse's first year of practice. Throughout your student experience you rely on mentors to guide and facilitate your learning and this should not change across the span of your career. The first 18 months post registration are vital to your development and extended support is critical for your evolving management and leadership roles (Dyess and Sherman, 2009); you may find that there are differences in what you were learning in the classroom or in textbooks for your leadership role and what it is actually like in practice (Danielson and Berntsson, 2007). To support your clinical leadership development, it is recommended that you explore the NHS 'clinical leadership competency framework' for a range of clinically based examples and scenarios which discuss skill acquisition to meet the leadership challenges, which can be built on throughout your career (see the 'Go further' box at the end of the chapter).

The quote from Emma alludes to the feelings associated with the responsibility that comes with becoming a qualified nurse. You may be thinking about your own transition to being qualified and may have feelings of excitement, but perhaps some anxieties.

Now that I'm qualified I feel a responsibility for the students as I am in charge of how they might practise in the future when I am working with them. I personally found the transition to being a newly qualified nurse quite difficult as my final year placement was in the community and I didn't have the opportunity to delegate for example. I still think it's a jump for everyone because you have all that extra responsibility. You become a leader of that patient's care and there is a lot of responsibility in that. I am enjoying my rotation and am interested to see how I find my next placement which is in elective care and outpatients.

Emma Wolton, a recently qualified children's and young people's nurse

---

ACTIVITY 36.3: REFLECTIVE ACTIVITY

Reflect on Emma's quote in relation to your own thoughts about the process of transition to newly qualified practice. Depending on the stage that you are at on your course, you could use this as an opportunity to set some objectives, which aim to prepare you for that transition. For example, you could discuss delegation with your mentor and find out if there are opportunities for you to practise this skill.

DELEGATION AND PEOPLE MANAGEMENT

Delegation is a leadership/management tool that can be used to develop the skills of less experienced staff as well as demonstrating effective mobilisation of a team. However, ineffective delegation or lack of follow up on the delegated activity can result in errors and omissions. The NMC *Code* (2015) states that nurses are accountable for decisions to delegate tasks. The legal professional responsibility of the nurse undertaking the delegation states:

It is the personal and professional responsibility of each practitioner who delegates activity to ensure that the person to carry out the activity is trained, competent and has the experience to undertake the activity safely (Dimond, 2008: 570).

From a leadership perspective, the key tenets of delegation for you to follow are:

- Delegate the right task under the right circumstances to the right person
- Provide the right direction
- Provide the right supervision
- Assess the effectiveness of the delegation.

GO FURTHER

WEBLINK: RCN: ACCOUNTABILITY AND DELEGATION

The RCN (2015) has a useful guide to accountability and delegation: www.rcn.org.uk/professional-development/accountability-and-delegation

---

CRITICAL THINKING STOP POINT 36.2

It should seem clear that effective delegation is important for good clinical practice. Consider the consequences of ineffective delegation.

CRITICAL THINKING STOP POINT 36.2 ANSWER

PERCEIVED BARRIERS AND CONFLICTS IN CLINICAL LEADERSHIP

One of the most frequently cited barriers to leadership development is a clinical leader's position in the hierarchy, with students and qualified nurses feeling a 'minor player' relative to senior managerial grades, sometimes feeling unable to influence change (Fealy et al., 2011). Further, a common conflict for clinical leaders is learning to balance a managerial function while still needing to remain a visible clinician and demonstrate practice competence to retain credibility (Flood, 2007). You will see this in highly charged areas such as emergency departments or intensive care units, where the management/team leader role may become more dominant, leading to disengagement with staff and creating feelings of isolation from the team, role confusion and a deficiency of credibility in clinical decision-making (O'Shea, 2008). To develop trust and confidence as a clinical leader you must continue to 'walk the talk', reflecting your personal values and behaviours, demonstrating your passion and congruence (Dolan and Holt, 2013).

Managing conflict at work is most likely to occur when staff feel they have been treated unfairly. Leaders and managers must take conflict seriously to ensure there is no disruption in the quality of patient care, poor communication leading to unsafe practice, or an unwarranted negative reputation of the team or service. Some of the common triggers for conflict that you need to watch out for are listed in Table 36.2.

Table 36.2   Most common sources of workplace conflict

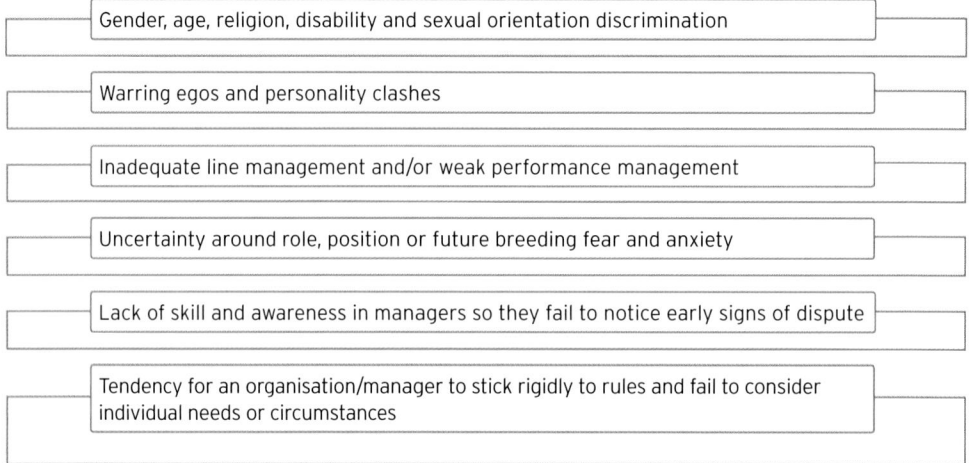

Gender, age, religion, disability and sexual orientation discrimination

Warring egos and personality clashes

Inadequate line management and/or weak performance management

Uncertainty around role, position or future breeding fear and anxiety

Lack of skill and awareness in managers so they fail to notice early signs of dispute

Tendency for an organisation/manager to stick rigidly to rules and fail to consider individual needs or circumstances

Source: Chartered Institute of Personnel and Development, 2008, p.2.

GO FURTHER

WEBLINK:
CONFLICT
MANAGEMENT
AND
RESOLUTION

If you would like to explore conflict management and resolution in nursing in more detail, the America Sentinel University website provides five styles for you to think about: www.americansentinel.edu/blog/2011/07/27/nursing-strategies-common-tactics-for-managing-conflict/

QUALITY IMPROVEMENT AND CHANGE MANAGEMENT

Leadership is at the heart of successful change (Hayes, 2010); however, this does not mean a heroic leadership style dependent on one person, but refers to a 'dispersed' leadership approach (Kings Fund, 2011), in order to cement engagement, ownership and project delivery. Clinical leadership, innovation and quality improvement are inextricably linked and have a core common element, namely bottom-up clinical ownership. Certainly, if you feel included and your ideas listened to and developed, then you are more likely to feel that your role makes a positive difference.

A quality improvement or change management approach that has been found to be useful in developing specific ideas for changes is a process termed Plan-Do-Study-Act (PDSA) cycles (see Figure 36.1). This approach tests a change or group of changes on a small scale to see if they result in improvement. If they do have the desired positive effect, the tests can be expanded, gradually incorporating larger and larger samples until there is confidence that the changes should be adopted more widely (Langley et al., 2009).

The NHS needs people who think of themselves as leaders not because they are exceptionally senior or inspirational to others, but because they can see what needs doing and can work with others to do it (Turnbull-James, 2008). 'Good' leaders display visionary leadership associated with leading change (Daft et al., 2010) through intellectual stimulation, individualised consideration and collaboration. Successful leadership is personified by the success and spirit of innovation evident at organisations such as Apple and Google. For example, Steve Jobs at Apple was described as having 'passion, intensity and extreme emotionalism for achieving perfection' (Isaacson, 2012: 94).

The people who are crazy enough to think they can change the world are the ones who do. (Apple's 'Think Different' commercial, 1997)

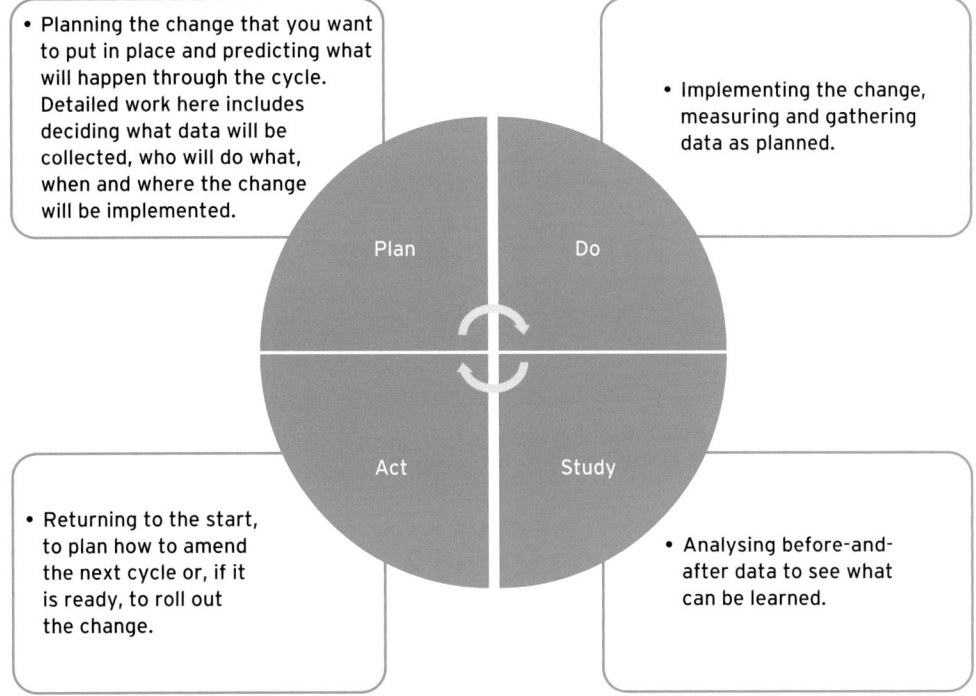

- Planning the change that you want to put in place and predicting what will happen through the cycle. Detailed work here includes deciding what data will be collected, who will do what, when and where the change will be implemented.

- Implementing the change, measuring and gathering data as planned.

Plan   Do

Act   Study

- Returning to the start, to plan how to amend the next cycle or, if it is ready, to roll out the change.

- Analysing before-and-after data to see what can be learned.

Figure 36.1   PDSA process

Finally, in this section, we offer an abridged 'student vignette' which is taken from Taylor and Webster-Henderson's (2016) textbook on leadership for student nurses (where the other student quotes came from also). It offers an insight into what Clare sees as 'good' leadership and illustrates some of the theoretical points we have made in this chapter.

Clare is 27 years old, and in the second year of her adult nursing course:

I think that leadership in nursing practice is probably different to generic nursing leadership and it requires a certain expertise. You need the knowledge-base to lead and an absolute array of communicative and personal skills. You have to be sensitive, compassionate and hard working. I've seen inspirational leadership a multitude of times. One that stands out for me is the second cardiac arrest that I ever saw (my first cardiac arrest was mayhem and it really unnerved me as there was no clear leadership). The deputy sister was so calm and very effective; it was fluid as it should be, and she was the entire reason that it was like that because of how she is. Describing what she did will maybe make what I mean clearer. It was visiting time, the patient was unwell but a cardiac arrest was clearly not expected. The patient was talking to her daughter and went into arrest and the daughter screamed out. I went in with the healthcare assistant and just began to pull the bed out as we've been trained to do. Everyone was there within a few seconds but the moment that the deputy sister was there she just stood at the head end of the bed and just calmly in a normal voice said, "Clare, would you please do this", "staff nurse, would you please do that". So I think it was her calmness, you could see that she was really at ease with the situation.

ACTIVITY 36.4
ANSWER

ACTIVITY 36.4: REFLECTIVE PRACTICE

- Reflect on an example of where you have seen 'good' leadership.
- Make a list of what you consider made the leader 'good'.
- Now reflect on your own leadership skills and think about which of these aspects you can take into your own practice.

CHAPTER SUMMARY

- Leadership skills and attributes can be developed over time and with experience and knowledge gained in different contexts.
- 'Good' and compassionate leadership is needed to address the healthcare challenges in the UK.
- As a nursing student, you can develop your leadership skills from the first day that you are in a clinical placement.

GO FURTHER

Books

- Taylor, R. and Webster-Henderson, B. (2016) *Essentials of Nursing Leadership*. London: SAGE.
  One of the authors of this chapter (Taylor) has edited a textbook on leadership for nursing students (Taylor and Webster-Henderson, 2016). We suggest that you access this book for more detailed information and discussion on the topic area.
- NMC (2015) *The Code: Professional Standards of Practice and Behaviour for Nurses and Midwives*. London: NMC.
  The NMC *Code* is crucial in guiding your leadership practice.

Journal Articles

FURTHER
READING:
JOURNAL
ARTICLES

Go to https://study.sagepub.com/essentialadultnursing for further free online journal articles related to this chapter. If you are using the interactive ebook, simply click on the book icon in the margin to go straight to the resource.

This publication is helpful in enabling exploration of leadership and management in the context of complex healthcare environments.

- King's Fund (2011) *No More Heroes: The Future of Leadership and Management in the NHS*. London: King's Fund.
  This article explores some of the issues that are important for transition to practice.
- Duchscher, J.E.B. (2008) Transition shock: The initial stage of role adaption for newly graduated registered nurses. *Journal of Advanced Nursing*, 65 (5): 1103-13.
  This article focuses on clinical leadership and the things that may act as barriers to development as a clinical leader.
- Fealy, G.M., McNamara, M.S., Casey, M., Geraghty, R., Butler, M., Halligan, P., Treacy, M. and Johnson, M. (2011) Barriers to clinical leadership development: Findings from a national survey. *Journal of Clinical Nursing*, 20 (13-14): 2023-32.

Weblinks

FURTHER
READING:
WEBLINKS

Go to https://study.sagepub.com/essentialadultnursing for further weblinks related to this chapter. If you are using the interactive ebook, simply click on the book icon in the margin to go straight to the resource.

- The NHS Leadership Academy website offers an overview of the programmes that are available for leadership across different levels. www.leadershipacademy.nhs.uk/programmes/

Collective leadership (West et al., 2014):

- This is an excellent resource that looks at the need for organisations to work at developing leadership at all levels.
  https://www.kingsfund.org.uk/publications/developing-collective-leadership-health-care
- The *Five Year Forward View* puts the requirement for leadership into a policy context. If you live elsewhere in the UK or the world, you could look at the relevant policy for health-care.
  Department of Health (2014) *Five Year Forward View*
  www.england.nhs.uk/wp-content/uploads/2014/10/5yfv-web.pdf

ACE YOUR ASSESSMENT

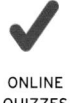

ONLINE
QUIZZES

Revise what you have learned by visiting https://study.sagepub.com/essentialadultnursing

- Test yourself with multiple-choice and short-answer questions
- Do the chapter activities in the book and check your answers online

REFERENCES

Chartered Institute of Personnel and Development (2008) *Leadership and the Management of Conflict at Work*. London: Chartered Institute of Personnel and Development, p.2.

Daft, R.L., Kendrick, M. and Vershinina, N. (2010) *Management*. Andover: Cengage Learning EMEA.

Danielson, E. and Berntsson, L. (2007) Registered nurses' perceptions of educational preparation for professional work and development in their profession. *Nurse Education Today,* 27(8): 900–8.

Department of Health (DoH) (2014) *Five Year Forward View*. Available at: www.england.nhs.uk/wp-content/uploads/2014/10/5yfv-web.pdf

Dimond, B. (2008) *Legal Aspects of Nursing* (5th ed.). Harlow: Pearson Education Ltd, p.570.

Dolan, B. and Holt, L. (eds) (2013) *Accident and Emergency Theory into Practice* (3rd ed.). London: Bailliere Tindall Elsevier.

Duchscher, J.E.B. (2008) Transition shock: The initial stage of role adaption for newly graduated registered nurses. *Journal of Advanced Nursing*, 65 (5): 1103–13.

Dyess, S. and Sherman, R. (2009) The first year of practice: New graduate nurses' transition and earning needs. *Journal of Continuing Education in Nursing*, 40 (9): 403–10.

Fealy, G.M., McNamara, M.S., Casey, M., Geraghty, R., Butler, M., Halligan, P., Treacy, M. and Johnson, M. (2011) Barriers to clinical leadership development: Findings from a national survey. *Journal of Clinical Nursing*, 20: 2023–32.

Flood, A. (2007) *The Clinical Nurse Manager (2): Unlocking the potential of this key role in the transformation of Irish health care*. Unpublished PhD thesis, University of Ulster.

Francis, R. (2013) *The Report of the Mid Staffordshire NHS Foundation Trust Public Inquiry*. Stationery Office, Crown Copyright.

Hayes, J. (2010) *The Theory and Practice of Change Management* (3rd ed.). Basingstoke: Palgrave.

Heckemann, B., Scols, J.M.G.A. and Halfens, R.J.G. (2015) A reflective framework to foster emotionally intelligent leadership in nursing. *Journal of Nursing Management*, 23: 744–753.

Isaacson, W. (2012) The real leadership lessons of Steve Jobs. *Harvard Business Review,* April: 93–102.

King's Fund (2011) *No More Heroes: The Future of Leadership and Management in the NHS*. London: King's Fund.

Langley, G.L., Moen, R., Nolan, K.M., Nolan, T.W., Norman, C.L. and Provost, L.P. (2009) *The Improvement Guide: A Practical Approach to Enhancing Organisational Performance* (2nd ed.). San-Francisco: Jossey-Bass.

NHS England (2016) *Leading Change, Adding Value*. Available at: www.england.nhs.uk/wp-content/uploads/2016/05/nursing-framework.pdf

NMC (2015) *The Code: Professional Standards of Practice and Behaviour for Nurses and Midwives*. London: NMC.

O'Shea, Y. (2008) *Nursing and Midwifery in Ireland: A Strategy for Professional Development in a Changing Health Service*. Dublin: Blackwell Publishing.

Taylor, R. (2009) Leadership theories and the development of nurses in primary health care. *Primary Health Care*, 19(9): 40–5.

Taylor, R. and Webster-Henderson, B. (2016) *Essentials of Nursing Leadership*. London: SAGE.

Turnbull-James, K. (2008) *Leadership in Context: Lessons from the new leadership theory and current leadership practice*. London: The King's Fund.

Webster, R. (2015) What the NHS Improvement Chief Executive must do first. *Health Service Journal*.

West, M., Eckert, R., Steward, K. and Pasmore, B. (2014) *Developing collective leadership for healthcare*. King's Fund: London. Available at: https://www.kingsfund.org.uk/publications/developing-collective-leadership-health-care

DECISION-MAKING

KAREN ELCOCK

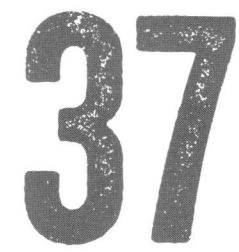

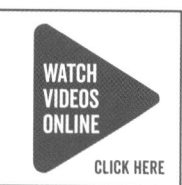

WATCH VIDEOS ONLINE
CLICK HERE

THIS CHAPTER COVERS

- The importance of clinical judgement and decision-making within clinical practice
- Different approaches to problem solving and decision-making
- Sources of information or knowledge that you can use to help you make decisions

- The importance of shared decision-making and the nurse's role in supporting patients through the decision-making process.

> " Making judgements and decision-making in nursing is one of the most difficult tasks to do, but with the right preparation, guidance and training I was able to make the right decision for the patient and their family.
>
> **Louise, 3rd year adult student** "

> " It's all about the patient. Know your limitations and don't be afraid to ask. Always listen to both sides when problem solving, then step back and think about it.
>
> **Kathy Judge, Senior Sister ITU** "

INTRODUCTION

We all make decisions every day; however, as a nurse you will be making decisions that will have implications for patients, yourself and other healthcare professionals and which can be particularly significant if they are the wrong ones. As healthcare becomes more complex nurses are faced with a multitude of decisions every day and often these decisions must be made rapidly. It has been estimated, for example, that acute care nurses can be faced with making a judgement or decision every 10 minutes (Thompson et al., 2013). This is not surprising given the sheer pace of change and the volumes of information with which we are confronted. In order to make the right decision it is essential that you are up to date with best practice and policy to ensure the best outcomes for your patients. This can be challenging. While there will be an expectation that as a registered nurse you are capable of safe and effective care without being supervised, that does not mean that you are expected to know the answer to everything. There will be times when you are unsure what the best course of action is and at these times it is important that you seek advice from other colleagues or access information from appropriate sources. As a registered nurse you will be professionally accountable for your actions, which means that the decisions you make must be based on sound evidence. This chapter will look at some of the theories underpinning decision-making, the resources available to you and the importance of involving patients in the decision-making process.

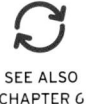

SEE ALSO
CHAPTER 6

THE IMPORTANCE OF CLINICAL JUDGEMENT AND DECISION-MAKING WITHIN CLINICAL PRACTICE

Decision-making and clinical judgement

There is a tendency for problem solving, decision-making and clinical judgement to be used interchangeably; however, they are different (Sullivan and Garland, 2010; Standing, 2017). While the problem-solving process is used to find a solution to a problem, the decision-making process may not always involve a problem but requires choosing from a number of options. Clinical judgement on the other hand is used to guide decision-making through the assessment and evaluation of both objective and subjective data about a patient. For example, making a judgement about whether a patient is at risk of a pressure ulcer will then lead to a decision as to whether any interventions are required to reduce that risk and, if so, which one will be best for your patient. Standing's (2017) most recent definition of clinical decision-making, which she developed from her doctoral research, makes clear your accountability in making these decisions:

> Clinical decision-making applies clinical judgment to select the best possible evidence-based option to control risks and address patients' needs in high quality care for which you are accountable (Standing, 2017: 8).

ACTIVITY 37.1: CRITICAL THINKING

Consider a clinical decision you have made recently. What was the decision about? What judgements led you to that decision?

You may have selected any one of a number of clinical decisions. Thompson and Dowding (2009) identified 11 different types of decisions made by nurses (see Table 37.1) and the range of different decision types demonstrates the range and complexity of decision-making by nurses. Can you see where the decision you described in Activity 37.1 fits?

Table 37.1   Decision types made by nurses

Assessment	Deciding to undertake an assessment or to use a specific assessment tool
Diagnosis	Making a decision based on a collection of signs and symptoms
Intervention/effectiveness	Choosing between two or more potential interventions
Targeting (a subcategory of intervention)	Deciding which patient/client group will benefit best from a specific intervention
Prevention (a subcategory of intervention)	Choosing which intervention may prevent specific health outcomes
Timing (a subcategory of intervention)	Deciding when the best time is to implement an intervention
Referral	Deciding whom to refer a client or patient to for care or management
Communication	Deciding how best to deliver or receive information to or from clients and/or their family
Information seeking	Deciding whether or not to seek further information from another source (e.g. patient/carer/colleague/research)
Service organisation, delivery and management	Deciding which approach to take in organising delivery or managing a service
Experiential, understanding or hermeneutic	Using cues to make a decision as to how another may be experiencing an event

(Adapted from Thompson and Dowding, 2009)

Factors that influence decision-making

There is a range of factors that will influence the decisions you make including the following:

- knowledge
- previous experience
- self-confidence
- ethical codes
- personal values
- patient/client choice
- legislation
- environmental stressors – time, staffing, resources.

Previous experience was identified by Benner (1984) as essential for developing expertise in clinical judgements (see What's the Evidence? 37.1). Lack of self-confidence, which is often seen in the newly registered nurse, can prevent an individual from making decisions in case they may be wrong which is further influenced by concerns regarding their accountability. Ethical codes and personal values will influence where a person's attention is directed to and so influence options chosen. Where the patient has been involved in the decision-making process then their choice will determine the actions to be taken (or not taken if that is their choice). The law may limit the choices open to you or require specific actions to be taken (e.g. health and safety regulations). Environmental stressors can also impact on your decision-making: lack of time, staff or resources may limit the options open to you or can impact on the quality of your decision-making.

ACTIVITY 37.2: CRITICAL THINKING

Consider again the clinical decision you identified in Activity 37.1. What factors influenced your decision?

Whilst Benner's work is over 30 years old, it describes really well how you will be developing the skills and knowledge you need when making clinical decisions and hopefully reassurance that it will become easier as you gain experience.

WHAT'S THE EVIDENCE? 37.1

Benner's (1984) seminal work *From Novice to Expert* was conducted between 1978 and 1981 and looked at the skill acquisition and clinical judgements by senior nursing students, newly graduated nurses and experienced nurses. Healthcare has changed significantly since this research was undertaken with a substantial increase in the amount and calibre of nursing research being published providing a large evidence base which nurses can use to inform their actions; however, Benner's findings still resonate with today's nurses and her model continues to be used by nurse educators and practitioners.

Benner used interviews and participant observation in order to clarify and describe the different characteristics of nurses at different stages of their education and practice and using the Dreyfus model of skill acquisition identified five stages from novice nurse to expert practitioner.

- **The novice stage** – relates to the student nurse who has no experience of an area of practice and, therefore, is taught rules to enable them to perform safely in practice. The rules are general in nature to enable them to be applied to any context; as a consequence, the student nurse's behaviour is limited and inflexible.
- **Advanced beginner (new graduate)** – the nurse is starting to build up experiences that can be used to develop principles to guide actions. The advanced beginner is very aware of their accountability and professional responsibility but still requires some help in identifying priorities and still sees situations in their component parts.
- **Competent stage (1 to 2 years in practice)** – able to set priorities, developing critical thinking skills and is able to predict immediate possible events based on past experience and so better plan for patient needs.
- **Proficiency** – the nurse sees situations as wholes rather than parts and using past experience is able to predict what the expected events will be for the patient, but is able to recognise when the expected doesn't happen. The proficient nurse uses 'maxims' for guidance and is able to adapt to changing situations.
- **Expert** – no longer relies on rules, guidelines or maxims but has an intuitive grasp of the whole, although will fall back on the use of analytical approaches in new situations or where problems occur.

While the model describes a progressive development linked with experience, a nurse who moves from one area of practice to another (e.g. inpatient nursing to community) may move from a higher level to a lower level until experience is gained in that new area of practice.

Looking at the different stages above, think of staff you have worked with. What stage would you put each one at? What are your reasons for making each decision?

CASE STUDY 37.1

The advanced beginner and the expert nurse

John is an 80-year-old patient who was admitted during the night with a chest infection. At handover, the night shift inform the day shift that John has been very restless and keeps getting out of bed and pacing round the ward. He won't keep his oxygen mask on which they feel is contributing to his confusion and restlessness.

Sarah is a recently qualified nurse and John is one of the patients allocated to her for the day. She checks on John and finds him walking round the bay so asks him to return to his seat and places his oxygen mask back on his face. She takes a set of observations, which show his respiratory and pulse rate are slightly raised, his oxygen saturations are at the lower side of normal. During the course of the morning she has to repeatedly return to John to ask him to sit down and replace his oxygen mask and starts to feel quite stressed as he won't comply with her requests to stay by his bed and she is concerned he may fall or come to harm.

Jose, a senior staff nurse, has been working on the ward for five years and sees John walking round the ward. She joins him and guides him back to his bed talking to him as they go. Her immediate impression is that John is well orientated and shows no signs of confusion. She undertakes a set of observations, which are similar to the ones that Sarah took but acceptable given that he has been walking up and down the ward. She also looks at his colour – he is pink and well perfused. She asks him a few more questions to try to determine how orientated he is to time and place and he is able to answer all the questions correctly. At this point Jose intuitively grasps that John's restlessness may be due to other reasons that have not been explored and sits down to talk to him further. Through further questioning she elicits that he had been given sedation during the night but is frightened of falling asleep in case he doesn't wake up so is walking up and down the ward to keep himself awake. Jose explores further his fear of not waking up should he fall asleep, and is able to reassure him that this will not happen and that Sarah will keep a close eye on him while he rests.

In the case study Sarah has followed the directions for John's care regarding observations and oxygen therapy and accepted the night nurse's diagnosis that John is confused, assuming his raised respiratory and pulse rate were due to hypoxia. She has not considered other options for his restlessness. Her main concern has been her accountability should John come to harm. Jose, however, looked at the whole picture and intuitively grasped that neither John's behaviour nor his clinical observations were representative of a confused or hypoxic patient and sought more information to help her make an informed decision. As an expert practitioner Jose was open to other possibilities that Sarah hadn't considered.

DECISION-MAKING MODELS

There are three commonly accepted approaches to decision-making: information processing, intuitive-humanistic approaches and cognitive continuum theory, which combines both the former approaches (Standing, 2017; Thompson and Dowding, 2009).

Information processing

The information-processing model recognises that humans store information in both their short-term and long-term memories. Information stored within the short-term memory is used to trigger retrieval of relevant information from the long-term memory. So, for example, having met a patient and undertaken an initial assessment, the information you have gained from that assessment will reside in your short-term memory. This new information will then trigger retrieval of relevant information from your long-term memory. This information may have been stored there from previous admissions and theoretical learning you have undertaken and will enable you to make judgements about the patient, explanations as to why the patient may be exhibiting certain signs and symptoms or behaving in a certain way. This may result in a number of explanations and preference will be given to the one supported by the greatest evidence. The information-processing approach is one that tends to be more widely used by the less experienced nurse but the ability to generate multiple explanations will depend on the nurse's knowledge base and previous experience. Information processing is an analytical approach to decision-making.

Intuitive

Intuition is described by Benner and Tanner (1987: 23) as *'understanding without a rationale'* and is an approach that is commonly accepted as being used by the expert nurse (Benner, 1984). Intuitive decision-making involves seeing the whole picture rather than breaking a situation down into its component parts (the analytical, information-processing approach) so is a more rapid approach to decision-making and is closely linked to Schon's (1987) reflection in action. The nurse, through their wealth of experience of previous cases, which may be similar, and the knowledge that has been developed over years of practice, is able to see patterns and reject those that don't fit at a subconscious level and come to a decision about the patient's diagnosis or the interventions required.

Cognitive continuum theory

Cognitive continuum theory (Hammond, 1996) recognises that humans use a range of decision-making processes and fits well with the decision-making that takes place in healthcare. Standing (2017) has revised cognitive continuum theory through her research in this area to make it more applicable to nursing (see Figure 37.1). The model shows five modes of clinical judgement from intuitive judgement at one end to the critical review of evidence at the other mapped against the ten perceptions of decision-making by nurses that have been identified by Standing.

The type of judgement that a person will use in a particular situation will depend on a number of factors including the:

- structure of the task in hand – the less structured a task, and more practical and personal it is, the more the judgement used will be towards the intuitive end of the continuum; and
- time available – the more time that is available the more the judgement can be made at the analytical end of the continuum.

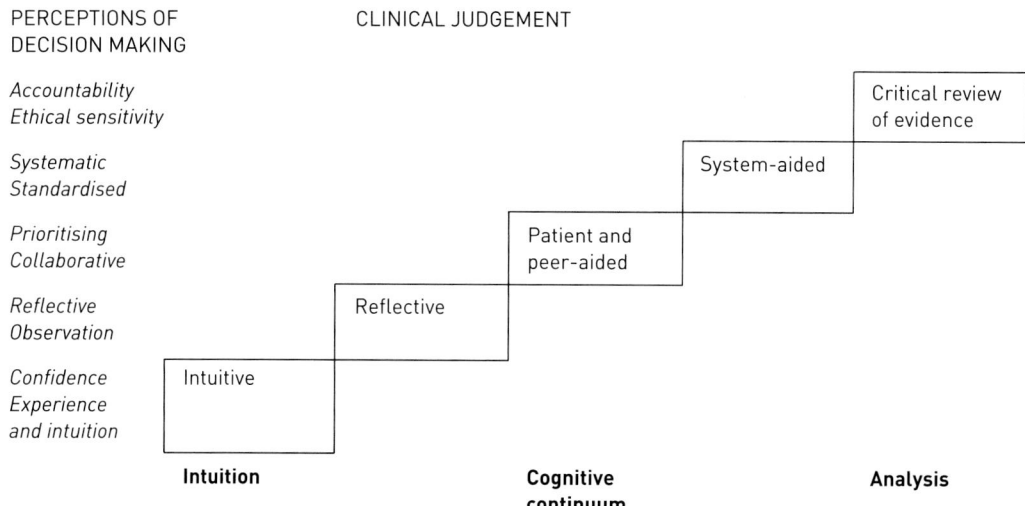

Figure 37.1 A cognitive continuum of five modes of clinical judgement and ten perceptions of decision-making in nursing (Standing, 2017, p.219).

© Mooi Standing. Reproduced with kind permission.

The revised model not only offers nurses an opportunity to consider the different approaches to decision-making that they can use but also recognises the importance of involving the patient in decision-making.

Resources for decision-making

Standing's (2017) model also gives pointers to resources for making decisions:

- Patient and peer judgement – colleagues are probably the first resource that you are likely to use and many patients can equally be a valuable resource, particularly patients with long-term conditions who are usually well informed about their health status and treatments (Corrie and Finch, 2015). In some cases it will be inappropriate for a single person to make a decision and in those situations decision-making will take place through discussion of the relevant members of the multidisciplinary team with (it is hoped) the patient at the centre of the discussion.
- System aided – this includes use of:
  - ○ validated assessment tools
  - ○ clinical guidelines
  - ○ protocols
  - ○ problem-solving frameworks
  - ○ computerised decision analysis systems.
- Critical review of evidence – there is a wealth of research evidence available that can aid the decision-making process and ensure an evidence-based approach to care is taken; however, you need to have effective critical appraisal skills in order to sift out research which is sound from that which is not. This resource will be used where an immediate decision is not required.

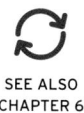

SEE ALSO
CHAPTER 6

SHARED DECISION-MAKING

The principle at the centre of the White Paper *Equity and Excellence: Liberating the NHS* (Department of Health, 2010) is *'no decision about me without me'* (p. 3). The aim of the proposals set out in the paper were to empower patients so that they can share in the decisions about their care. The NMC *Code* (2015) also makes very clear the importance of putting patients at the heart of decision-making. Unfortunately, evidence suggests that shared decision-making is still not widely adopted in practice as discussed in Activity 37.3 which looks at the NHS Inpatient Survey.

ACTIVITY 37.3 ANSWER

ACTIVITY 37.3: RESEARCH AND EVIDENCE-BASED PRACTICE

The 2015 NHS National Inpatient Survey (CQC, 2016) found that 59% of patients felt that they were involved as much as they wanted to be in decisions about their care and treatment, 32% were involved to some extent and only 9% felt they were not involved. However, 17% of patients with a mental health condition and 13% of patients with a learning disability did not feel they were involved in decisions around their care.

- Look this survey up and read through it. Were there any surprises for you?
- Why do you think people with a mental health condition or a learning disability felt less involved in decisions around their care in an inpatient setting?

The sheer volume of information available to patients, particularly via the internet, and the opportunities available for patients to share experiences via discussion forums, social networking sites and mailing lists (O'Grady and Jadad, 2010) means that patients today are far better informed than in the past and are able to take a more active part in the decision-making process. Shared decision-making is at the centre of patient-centred care and so congruent with nursing values and, therefore, should be an aspect of patient care that nurses feel very comfortable with. Makoul and Clayman (2006) identified nine essential elements that should be included during a consultation between a healthcare professional and a patient which Légaré et al. (2014: 7) summarised as:

SEE ALSO CHAPTER 2

- Define/explain the healthcare problem
- Present options
- Discuss pros/cons (benefits/risks/costs)
- Clarify patient values/preferences
- Discuss patient ability/self-efficacy
- Discuss what is known and make recommendations
- Check/clarify the patient's understanding
- Make or explicitly defer a decision
- Arrange follow up.

As a newly registered nurse you may feel that you don't have the experience and/or knowledge to support patients with decision-making. The focus on shared decision-making has generally been on medical treatments and interventions with doctors discussing the different treatment options available to the patient. However, you should be involving patients in decision-making around nursing care interventions, lifestyle choices as well as advocating for the patient where the opportunity for shared decision-making is not being offered by other healthcare professionals. There are a number of resources you can use to help patients you care for become more involved in making decisions about their own care – these can be both web-based and printed materials.

Patient decision aids (PDAs)

While you may not feel confident with being involved in shared decision-making at the moment, there is a range of tools that you can provide for your patients or point them in the direction of, where they are web based. PDAs is a term used to describe a range of tools which prepare patients to make a decision based on evidence, regarding treatments or screening, by providing them with:

- up-to-date information based on best evidence on the different options and the likely outcomes for each (this information can be designed for the healthcare professional to inform the patient and/or be specifically aimed at the patient)
- an exploration of values and what is important to them (e.g. length of life versus quality of life)
- support from a healthcare professional in deciding between the different options (National Steering Group for Decision Support Aids in Urology, 2005).

PDAs usually include one or more of the following:

- information leaflets that include options with benefits/risks/costs for each
- videos
- values clarification exercises to enable patients to identify the desirability of different options
- patient stories of their own experiences with different interventions
- questionnaires to help patients clarify their treatment preference
- guides that the patient can use to help them ask the right questions when meeting with a healthcare professional.

PDAs are not only useful tools for you to use to help a patient with the decision-making process, but also a useful information resource to help you develop your knowledge and understanding of specific health issues. In addition, it has been shown that by involving patients in shared decision-making and using patient decision aids, invasive surgery, high-cost treatments and unnecessary tests can be reduced (Corrie and Finch, 2015).

PREPARATION FOR PRACTICE PLACEMENTS 37.1

Patient Decision Aids

Explore what PDAs may be available that are relevant to your current/next placement and share these with colleagues. There is a range of websites that provide PDAs, such as: https://patient.info/decision-aids or https://decisionaid.ohri.ca/

WEBLINKS

Another resource that you can use and refer patients to is the NHS Choices website which is the largest healthcare online resource with information on over 750 conditions and treatments (Corrie and Finch, 2015).

EVALUATING THE EFFECTIVENESS OF DECISION-MAKING

While it is not appropriate to evaluate every decision you make it is important that you pause at times to review whether the decision you made is the right one where the outcomes are not as expected or you had a degree of uncertainty about the decision. There is a range of methods you can use to do this:

- reflective practice
- peer review and feedback
- clinical supervision.

While on your pre-registration programme you can use both your mentor and your personal tutor at university to discuss and reflect on some of the more challenging decisions you have been confronted with, and how and why you made the final decision you did. This can be valuable in preparing you for your future placements by learning from your decision-making processes and how you can improve these.

It is amazing to make clinical decisions whilst on placement. University prepares you for theory but the best place to practice it is placement. It really builds your confidence to know your mentor trusts you to become involved in decisions and liaise with other professionals to effectively care for the patient's welfare.

Emily Davis, 3rd year adult student nurse

Once qualified, you will have a preceptor who can help you reflect on some of the decisions you make. A reflective diary is a useful tool to record the decisions you make and reflections on the outcomes from them, and you can then use the diary as a prompt when meeting with your mentor, personal tutor or preceptor. It is also good practice for when you have to undertake your **revalidation** with the NMC once qualified. You may also find it helpful to review your entries on a regular basis to identify whether there are any patterns to the decisions you make that have resulted in unexpected outcomes as this may enable you to identify a knowledge deficit or an area for personal development. You may like to identify your decisions by type as set out in Table 37.1.

CHAPTER SUMMARY

- Decision-making is a skill that is developed and refined through experience.
- As you gain more experience you will find that your confidence in your ability to make decisions will increase as will the range of decision-making strategies you use.

- Increased confidence will allow you to involve patients more in the decision-making process, which will enhance their own self-esteem and locus of control.
- Clinical supervision and reflection are important tools to use to learn from the decisions you make in everyday practice.

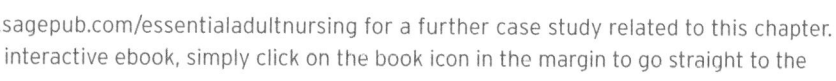

GO FURTHER

Go to https://study.sagepub.com/essentialadultnursing for a further case study related to this chapter. If you are using the interactive ebook, simply click on the book icon in the margin to go straight to the resource.

CASE STUDY: DECISION-MAKING SCENARIO

Books

- Ellis, P. (2016) *Evidence-based Practice in Nursing*. London: Learning Matters/SAGE.
  An excellent book on how to select the best evidence to inform your clinical decision-making.
- Holland, K. and Roberts, D. (2013) *Nursing: Decision-making For Practice*. Oxford: Oxford University Press.
  Aimed at students, this book is useful as it uses common scenarios you will recognise.
- Standing, M. (2017) *Clinical Judgement and Decision-making in Nursing* (3rd ed.). London: Learning Matters/SAGE.
  This is an excellent book on decision-making for nurses with helpful examples applied to practice.

Journal Articles

Go to https://study.sagepub.com/essentialadultnursing for further free online journal articles related to this chapter. If you are using the interactive ebook, simply click on the book icon in the margin to go straight to the resource.

FURTHER READING: JOURNAL ARTICLES

- Légaré, F. and Thompson-Leduc, P. (2014) Twelve myths about shared decision-making. *Patient Education and Counseling*, 96(3): 281-6.
  Explodes many of the myths around shared decision-making.
- Madsen, C. and Fraser, A. (2015) Supporting patients in shared decision-making in clinical practice. *Nursing Standard*, 29(31): 50-7.
  An excellent overview of shared decision-making with the focus on your role as a nurse.
- Stiggelbout, A.M., Pietersea, A.H. and Haes, J.C.J.M. (2015) Shared decision-making: Concepts, evidence, and practice. *Patient Education and Counselling*, 98(10): 1172-9.
  Provides some really helpful communication strategies you can use with patients.

Weblinks

Go to https://study.sagepub.com/essentialadultnursing for further weblinks related to this chapter. If you are using the interactive ebook, simply click on the book icon in the margin to go straight to the resource.

FURTHER READING: WEBLINKS

- Healthtalk.org
  www.healthtalk.org/peoples-experiences/improving-health-care/shared-decision-making/topics
  A wide range of videos of people sharing their own experiences of being involved in the decision-making process covering 50 different health conditions.
- NICE
  www.Nice.org.uk
  See the shared decision-making webpage for excellent guidance and a range of PDAs.
- Shared Decision-making
  www.england.nhs.uk/rightcare/
  An excellent resource for the latest information and resources to imbed shared decision-making and best practice with patients/clients in your care.

ACE YOUR ASSESSMENT

Revise what you have learned by visiting https://study.sagepub.com/essentialadultnursing

- Test yourself with multiple-choice and short-answer questions
- Do the chapter activities in the book and check your answers online

REFERENCES

Benner, P. (1984) *From Novice to Expert: Excellence and power in clinical nursing practice*. Menlo Park CA: Addison Wesley.

Benner, P. and Tanner, C. (1987) Clinical judgment: How expert nurses use intuition. *American Journal of Nursing*, 87: 23–31.

Care Quality Commission (CQC) (2016) *2015 Adult Inpatient Survey Statistical Release*. Available at: www.cqc.org.uk/content/adult-inpatient-survey-2015 (last viewed 4/5/2017).

Corrie, C. and Finch, A. (2015) *Expert Patients*. London: Reform.

Department of Health (2010) *Equity and Excellence: Liberating the NHS*. Norwich: The Stationery Office.

Hammond, K.R. (1996) *Human Judgement and Social Policy: Irreducible uncertainty, inevitable error, unavoidable injustice*. New York: Oxford University Press.

Légaré, F., Stacey, D., Turcotte, S., Cossi, M.J., Kryworuchko, J., Graham, I.D., Lyddiatt, A., Politi, M.C., Thomson, R., Elwyn, G. and Donner-Banzhoff, N. (2014) Interventions for improving the adoption of shared decision-making by healthcare professionals. *Cochrane Database of Systematic Reviews*, 2014, Issue 9. Art. No.: CD006732.

Makoul, G. and Clayman, M.L. (2006) An integrative model of shared decision-making in medical encounters. *Patient Education and Counselling*, 60(3): 301–12.

National Steering Group for Decision Support Aids in Urology (2005) *Implementing Patient Decision Aids in Urology – Final Report*. Oxford: Picker Institute Europe.

Nursing and Midwifery Council (NMC) (2015) *The Code: Professional standards of practice and behaviour for nurses and midwives*. Available at: www.nmc.org.uk/standards/code/ (last viewed 11/5/2017).

O'Grady, L. and Jadad, A. (2010) Shifting from shared to collaborative decision-making: A change in thinking and doing. *Journal of Participatory Medicine*, 2: e13.

Schon, D (1987) *Educating the Reflective Practitioner: Toward a New Design for Teaching and Learning in the Professions*. San Francisco: Jossey-Bass

Standing, M. (2017) *Clinical Judgement and Decision-making in Nursing* (3rd ed.). London: SAGE/ Learning Matters.

Sullivan E. and Garland, G. (2010) *Practical Leadership and Management*. Harlow: Education Ltd.

Thompson, C. and Dowding, D. (eds) (2009) *Essential Decision-making and Clinical Judgement for Nurses*. Edinburgh: Churchill Livingstone.

Thompson, C., Aitken, L., Doran, D. and Dowding, D. (2013) An agenda for clinical decision-making and judgement in nursing research and education. *International Journal of Nursing Studies*, 50 (2012): 1720–6.

LIFELONG LEARNING AND CONTINUING PROFESSIONAL DEVELOPMENT

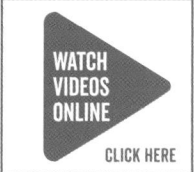

MARIE CERINUS AND CLARE MCGUIRE

THIS CHAPTER COVERS

- Different aspects of lifelong learning and continuing professional development
- Personal, professional and employer perspectives and responsibilities
- Some approaches to your ongoing learning
- Identifying and addressing your learning needs as a qualified nurse
- Your learning and its effect on others.

> " I learned to become a good nurse during my pre-registration programme and I am so looking forward to taking up my first post in the next few weeks. I am a bit nervous too as I know I don't know everything! I'll need to keep learning and meet NMC Revalidation requirements if I want to always be a good nurse – which of course I do! Help, please!
>
> **Amy, UWS student** "

INTRODUCTION

In trying to help Amy and you, this chapter provides some very practical ideas for your **ongoing learning** as an adult nurse. It also addresses clause 22.3 of the NMC *Code* (NMC, 2015):

> … keep your knowledge and skills up to date, taking part in appropriate and regular learning and professional development activities that aim to maintain and develop your competence and improve your performance …

Ongoing learning is an important activity for you as an adult nurse, and this chapter will help you transition from student to qualified nurse by focusing on the ongoing learning required of you as a qualified nurse throughout your career.

The chapter starts by looking at some aspects of **lifelong learning** and **continuing professional development (CPD)** and their similarities and differences to help you better understand these two very commonly used terms. Regulatory body (**NMC**), professional body and employer differences in expectation and responsibilities for your ongoing learning are highlighted. Overall, the emphasis is on helping you to be personally responsible for maintaining and improving your practice through your ongoing learning. Ways to identify and address your learning are suggested, and different learning providers and methods are mentioned. It is shown that cost need not necessarily be a deterrent. The importance of **personal development planning and review**, the key to you identifying and meeting learning needs in the workplace, is emphasised as is the importance of keeping learning records. The chapter concludes with some reflection on how your ongoing learning is and will affect others as your career progresses.

SEE ALSO
CHAPTER 6

DIFFERENT ASPECTS OF LIFELONG LEARNING AND CONTINUING PROFESSIONAL DEVELOPMENT

You will already be aware of many types of learning pertinent to adult nursing. Two of the more common types referred to in the workplace are lifelong learning and continuing professional development (CPD). It is helpful as you embark on your nursing career to look at these terms in a bit more detail.

Lifelong learning, as the phrase implies, is 'the learning we do throughout our life'. The Collins English Dictionary (2012) defines it as 'the provision or use of both formal and informal learning opportunities throughout people's lives in order to foster the continuous development and improvement of the knowledge and skills needed for employment and personal fulfilment'. Lifelong learning is usually, consciously or subconsciously, motivated by the question, 'what do I need?' Some lifelong learning is essential to life (e.g. learning to eat and drink); some can cause life harm (e.g. eating and drinking the wrong things and/or in the wrong amount); and some is for life skills or life fun (e.g. reading a course textbook or reading a magazine article!). So, in lifelong learning:

- some is intentional, some is not
- some is informed (i.e. evidence based), some is not
- some may be good or right, some may not
- some stays current, some does not.

Continuing professional development (CPD), on the other hand, happens throughout your chosen professional life. It should be consciously motivated by the question, 'what does my client group (patients and/or colleagues) need?' In nursing, CPD, although it began in your pre-registration programme, becomes your responsibility once you are qualified. CPD is …

- intentional, a search for maintaining or improving professional competence
- informed, being evidence based wherever possible
- questioning, encouraging pursuit of greater or new evidence, knowledge or wisdom
- good or right if based on the above
- not necessarily current for all our professional life, therefore needs updating.

CRITICAL THINKING STOP POINT 38.1

Can you think of something you have already learned in nursing and which you now need to refresh or update?

CPD, therefore, forms important parts of your lifelong learning journey (see Figure 38.1). It requires you to consciously identify your learning needs, stimulated by caring for and about your patients and colleagues and then take steps to address these. This is quite different from your learning in your pre-registration programme when generic and specific skills and knowledge were set before you, based on the requirements for registration as a nurse within the United Kingdom as determined by the regulator (NMC).

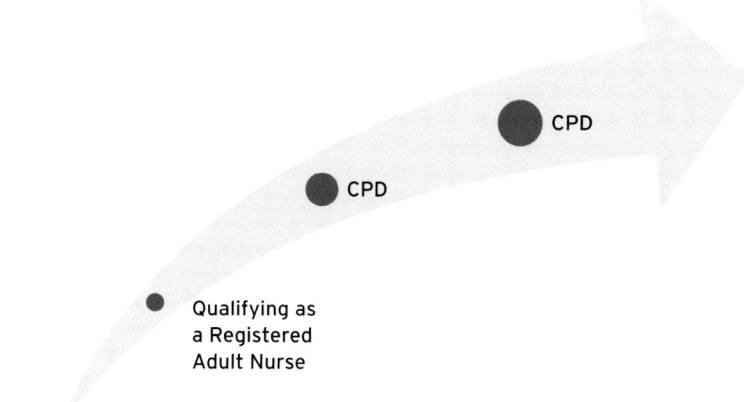

CPD

CPD

Qualifying as
a Registered
Adult Nurse

Figure 38.1 Lifelong learning with CPD

Now, as a qualified nurse, you need to maintain the core professional knowledge and skills required of an adult nurse as set by the NMC by keeping them up to date. You also need to grow new knowledge and skills if the evidence base or your work context of practice changes, or if you aspire to a new post or to promotion. It's also worth noting that in some areas the NMC specifies further standards for some post-registration programmes (see Go Further section).

Associated with your ongoing learning there are a couple of other terms that would be useful to know. For example, if the need to learn is enshrined in law it is deemed 'statutory' and must be undertaken. Fire safety training is a good example of statutory learning. However, if learning is a requirement of your employer it is usually deemed 'mandatory', 'compulsory' or 'essential' and this too will have to be undertaken. An example of mandatory training is safeguarding.

While participation in statutory or mandatory training may be obligatory for you in your work place, and it is part of your lifelong learning, not all of it may form part of your CPD as set out by the NMC in its **Revalidation** guidance (NMC, 2016). The NMC clearly describes which mandatory learning can be included as CPD. In brief, any mandatory training not directly related to your practice, such as health and safety training, should not be included. Any mandatory training necessary to your scope of practice can be included.

WEBLINK:
NMC
REVALIDATION
GUIDANCE

GO FURTHER

NMC Revalidation Guidance http://revalidation.nmc.org.uk/

Fundamentally, to value a learning opportunity as CPD, you need to consider the learning content and its evidence base, its utility, its implementation, its sustainability and overall its relevance, borne out by **critical reflection**, to your practice as an adult nurse. And so, you have to do more than participate in learning opportunities – you have to learn and apply, reflect and review from a professional perspective. Remember, CPD learning is never coincidental, it is purposeful in respect of your professional practice and it takes your energy, engagement and effort!

Overall, therefore, while lifelong learning is useful to the professional nurse and it may be a requirement of your employment, it is CPD that is essential, a point reinforced by the NMC. Fortunately, there is a range of people and organisations with differing perspectives and responsibilities, including your employer, to help you with your lifelong learning and CPD and these will be highlighted in the next section. First though, we start with you!

ACTIVITY 38.2

CRITICAL THINKING STOP POINT 38.2

Think of any training undertaken by nurses with whom you have worked. Would you view this as lifelong learning or CPD and why.

PERSONAL, PROFESSIONAL AND EMPLOYER PERSPECTIVES AND RESPONSIBILITIES

The most important person in any learning situation is you as the learner! This personal importance and associated responsibility builds on themes and concepts introduced in Delves-Yates (2018), in Chapters 7 and 8. Now, as an adult nurse rather than a student, you need to continue to work at: understanding yourself; being kind to yourself; and developing yourself into an independent and professional learner. As true as that was when a student nurse, it is also true once qualified and throughout your whole career.

As highlighted above, once qualified, you must work within NMC requirements and, within the United Kingdom, the policies of your respective **devolved health administrations**. In employment you must also work within the demands and expectations of your employer, whether that is the

NHS, independent or voluntary agencies or further and higher education, for example. With such a range of expectations and demands, it is important that you continue to address your **resilience** so that you are ready to respond in a positive and meaningful way.

Personal resilience was required of you as a student nurse and more resilience will be required as you pursue your career, especially when you consider some of the potential demands: reconciling patients', colleagues' and managers' needs; balancing work and home commitments; and improving your practice and keeping yourself updated. The following activity will help you with this.

ACTIVITY 38.1: REFLECTIVE PRACTICE

Review Chapter 8 in Delves-Yates (2018) and using Table 8.1, consider which activities you, as an adult nurse, could undertake to increase your resilience.

ACTIVITY 38.1
ANSWER

The regulator (NMC)

As has been mentioned, your professional regulator, the NMC, makes clear the requirements for continuing registration as an adult nurse through its Revalidation process. This professional process, for which each nurse has personal responsibility, was introduced on 1 April 2016 and help is easily to hand on the NMC Revalidation Microsite. Although revalidation with the NMC is only required every three years, it covers the preceding three-year period. Over and within each three-year period you must gather the required evidence and make appropriate arrangements to complete the process and so remain on the professional register.

While the NMC, as regulator, is pivotal in informing your CPD requirements as part of the Revalidation process, it does not detail the CPD you need to do nor how to access it – that is for you to determine based on your area of practice. CPD must be informed by your registration as an adult nurse, your current employment (the patients you work with and the context in which you work) and your personal career aspirations. Your employer may help.

SEE ALSO
CHAPTER 3

Employers

Employers of nurses, such as the NHS, are required to ensure their staff are properly prepared for their role. While you have professional responsibilities for maintaining your underpinning registration with the NMC, employers may help with this as they normally exercise their responsibilities in relation to staff learning very seriously. The extent to which they do depends on their policies and procedures around staff learning.

Main examples of employer responsibilities for learning provision emanate from legislation including the Health and Safety at Work Act (1974) and subsequent regulations. It generally covers areas such as: induction, fire safety; prevention and management of violence and aggression; and manual handling. It may also include legislative or policy requirements such as: adult and/or child protection (safeguarding); data handling and confidentiality in keeping with the Data Protection Act 1998, and any subsequent information governance requirements. Other areas may reflect national healthcare policies or programmes of the home nation of your place of work as they apply to your role, such as the Patient Safety or Health Improvement programmes, or your employer's adoption of other UK standards such as those issued by the UK Resuscitation Council in respect of adult and child resuscitation and anaphylaxis for example (www.resus.org.uk). As highlighted above and in the NMC published guidance, not all of this learning can be included as CPD for Revalidation purposes. While all such lifelong learning is important, you need to discern what, if any, constitutes CPD for you.

Employers also need to make sure there is access to learning opportunities in tasks and techniques related to being an employee within their organisation. These may include using clinical or other electronic systems; clinical and critical incident reporting systems; human resource (HR) processes; or concern and complaint management. Also, as part of succession planning for promoted posts, access to leadership and management learning, higher academic study or advanced practice programmes may be supported. Your employer, therefore, is an important source of learning opportunity. Another source could be your chosen professional body or trade union.

Professional body or trade union

As well as advocating for learning opportunities and access to them for their members from employers and others, all the different professional bodies or trade unions provide a range of learning advice and resources to their members. It would be a worthwhile activity if you are a member of a professional body (e.g. the Royal College of Nursing) or a trade union (e.g. UNISON) to find out what learning opportunities or support are currently available, how to access them and how you could best utilise these for your lifelong learning or as part of your CPD.

National organisations

National NHS-funded organisations exist to support learning and development in each of the four devolved health administrations of the UK. The four organisations are: Health Education England; NHS Education for Scotland; Learning@Wales; and Northern Ireland Practice and Education Council for Nursing and Midwifery, and their respective websites are worth exploring for free and easily accessible resources.

In addition, there is a range of national charities with very extensive learning resources. Examples pertinent to adult nurses include Asthma UK (www.asthma.org.uk/), Dementia UK (www.dementiauk.org/) or Diabetes UK (www.diabetes.org.uk/).

Again, explore what is available to you, usually free of charge.

WHAT'S THE EVIDENCE? 38.1

Explore the website of your home nation learning organisation for further learning resources:

1. England: Health Education England (http://hee.nhs.uk/)
2. Scotland: NHS Education for Scotland (www.nes.scot.nhs.uk/)
3. Wales: Learning@Wales (http://learning.wales.nhs.uk/)
4. Northern Ireland: Northern Ireland Practice and Education Council for Nursing and Midwifery (www.nipec.hscni.net/)

WEBLINKS

Higher education institutions

Universities across the UK offer a range of programmes at various academic levels but they all cost money. Often employers have arrangements in place so that some of these may be accessible free of charge to you or partially supported in some way. Financial and/or protected learning time support is usually focused on programmes considered by employers to be essential for people in their workforce (e.g. mentorship, non-medical prescribing, child protection). Remember, universities, colleges, charitable and other organisations may also offer some funding support.

CRITICAL THINKING STOP POINT 38.3

- Find out if your potential or actual employer has a partnership arrangement in place with any educational institutions and for what. Are any of these relevant to you?
- Find out what programmes are provided by your local higher educational institutions and which, if any, may be relevant to you now or in the future. What are the access and funding arrangements?

SOME APPROACHES TO ONGOING LEARNING

As can be seen from the above, learning opportunities may be presented or made available in a variety of ways, some at a cost but many are free. As an adult nurse, for your lifelong learning and CPD, you need to be alert to these learning opportunities, actively seeking participation in those appropriate to you professionally, occupationally or personally. You also need to appreciate your individual **preferred learning style** and consider the various ways of learning that arise so that, where possible, you can best match the two.

As an individual and shaped by your personality, early exposure and ongoing experience of learning, you will have a preferred learning style. This does not mean you only learn in that one way but, in knowing your own preferences, you can be more aware of how you need to engage with a learning opportunity regardless of it being presented in your preferred style or not. It would be worthwhile for you to review Delves-Yates (2018) Chapter 2 and then complete Activity 2.1. A further activity on preferred learning styles is included in the accompanying web resource to this chapter.

Reflecting the diversity of preferred learning styles, opportunities to learn are presented in a variety of different ways. Classroom based; e-learning and e-resources; reading; on-the-job; peer and team activities; undertaking research; using social media; and receiving and providing support and supervision are some of the more common approaches (see Figure 38.2).

In whatever form the learning opportunity is presented it should comprise the presentation of information, some interactive element and some personal reflection. This so-called blended approach results in more effective learning for more people. What you need to find is the approach that best suits you as an individual. If what best suits doesn't exist or if it is something new (e.g. a webinar or using **social media** for learning), you need to exercise your own responsibility in making that approach work for you.

Advancement in technology in recent years provides further varied opportunities for learning. Social media is one example that could enhance your learning, allowing, for instance, the exploration of research evidence to support your professional practice. You must engage responsibly with social

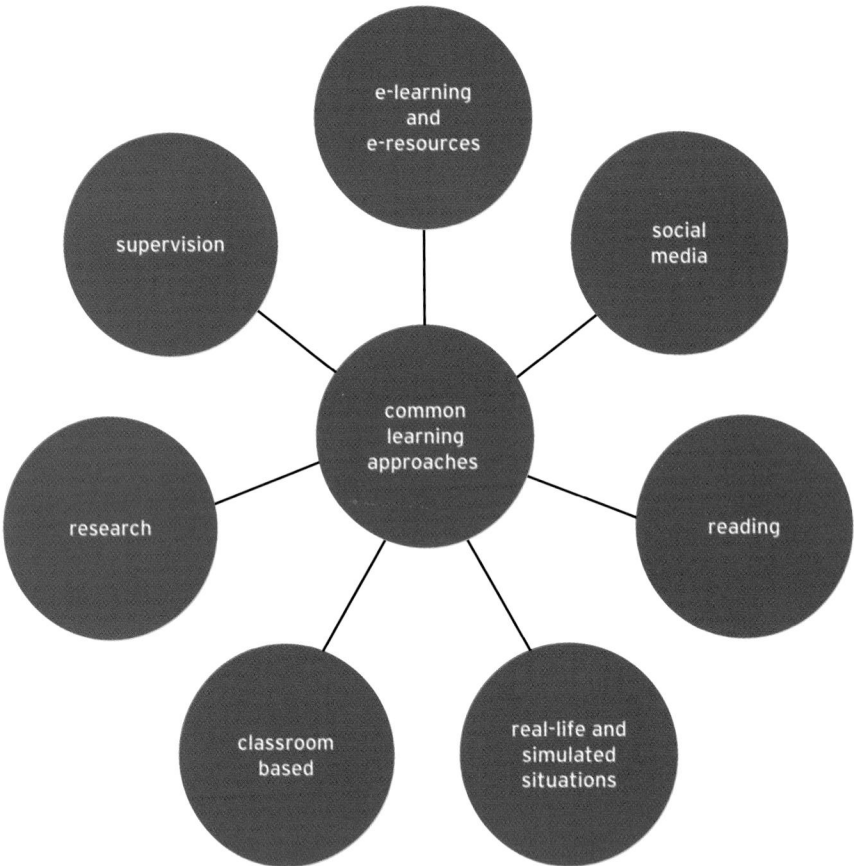

Figure 38.2 Common learning approaches

media, always being mindful to maintain professional standards as indicated in the NMC guidance on the use of social media – a useful resource for all registrants (www.nmc.org.uk/globalassets/site documents/nmc-publications/social-media-guidance.pdf).

CRITICAL THINKING STOP POINT 38.4

- Review the NMC guidance on using social media responsibly. Consider your current social media activity in relation to the guidelines. Are you using social media responsibly?
- Identify at least one opportunity to utilise social media in supporting your lifelong learning or CPD.

And so you can see a range of learning opportunities can and are provided and, while learning as an outcome of that provision requires your active engagement, it starts with you identifying your learning need and making appropriate plans to have that need addressed.

IDENTIFYING AND ADDRESSING YOUR LEARNING NEEDS

Addressing your ongoing learning as an adult nurse requires taking some concrete action. When you are in employment your employer, as previously mentioned, may have policies and processes to support this. You must find out about these and fully participate. This will contribute to the NMC requirements for Revalidation. If you are not in employment you must continue to address your learning as part of the ongoing Revalidation process required by the NMC as your professional regulator.

The most common approach taken is that of personal development planning and review. In whatever way this is approached, you must maintain continuous records as evidence of learning identified and undertaken. For **CPD** purposes, you will also need to demonstrate the outcome or impact of this learning on yourself, your patients or your colleagues.

While different employers may have slightly different titles, details and documentation, personal development planning and review is a simple process of reviewing your learning needs, based on the work you are currently doing or aspire to do, and then taking planned steps to address them. While employment can give a direct focus for identifying your learning needs, being out of employment can also focus your mind on what you need to get into or return to employment.

An underpinning framework can be of use to help identify learning need. The current NMC pre- and/or post-registration education standards can be used or indeed most employers will use a generic framework such as the *NHS Knowledge and Skills Framework* (Department of Health, 2004) or a national framework such as *Leading Change, Adding Value* (NHS England, 2016). Other areas may focus on specific job requirements, or competency or capability frameworks pertinent to your job role. Such frameworks specify the knowledge, skills and attributes needed to work in certain areas. You can use these to consider if you have any deficits in your competencies or capabilities or if you have areas in which you would be keen to improve. From this identification of learning need, plans using some of the learning approaches previously mentioned can then be made to address the need.

ACTIVITY 38.2
ANSWER

ACTIVITY 38.2: CRITICAL THINKING

Find out what framework, if any, is used locally for personal development planning and review?

In addition to identifying and addressing your learning needs as an adult nurse, it is important that you keep appropriate and relevant records. As can be seen from the NMC Revalidation Microsite, maintaining records has been made easy through the provision of recording documents. In addition, your employers may have documentation (electronic or hard copy) that you must use to comply with local policy and process. As an individual, you may also use a personal professional portfolio.

The advantage of maintaining your own personal professional portfolio is that you can retain all your own records of learning across your career, wherever that career takes you. It is as comprehensive as you need it and want it to be and it can be used to draw down evidence required by your employer (current and potential) or the NMC at any given point in time as long as your portfolio contains the information required by the NMC.

What you record must be within legal and professional parameters. It follows that if you are required to share any of your records at any point (e.g. to comply with NMC Revalidation or to complete records required by your employer) such sharing must also be within these parameters.

ACTIVITY 38.3: CRITICAL THINKING

- Access the NMC Revalidation Microsite and download the documents required for revalidation. Make sure you are clear about the kinds of records you will need to keep for professional purposes.
- Find out if your employer or future employer has any documentation you could use. Will this fulfil NMC requirements or do you need to keep additional records for that purpose?
- Is there an electronic portfolio you could start to use that would help you maintain your own and any required records?

Remember, in addition, for CPD purposes, you are required to provide evidence of outcome or impact of your learning. Fundamentally, the question to be answered is 'what difference, if any, has this learning had on you, your practice, your patients'? In some situations, this evidence may be quite concrete – for example, *'I can now administer medicines intravenously which I couldn't do before. I know what's involved, all the safety features and so on, and I feel confident in the actual task having undertaken a period of theoretical learning followed by supervised practice and assessment through which an experienced colleague has deemed me competent. The outcomes for my patients will be better as there will be no delay in getting the right medicine to them at the right time in the most effective way'.*

Other learning, however, may not have such concrete outcomes or impact. This is particularly so when learning has been about our behaviours – for example, *'How will I, my patients or my colleagues know if I am benefitting from supervision or that my communication or leadership skills have been developed or improved?'* Just because such learning may appear less tangible does not mean there are no outcomes or impact. One excellent way of demonstrating learning outcomes or impact is to share your learning with others and/or seek their feedback and then complete a reflective account. Considering the impact of your learning on others, directly or indirectly, is also important to your ongoing learning as an adult nurse.

Your Learning and Others

CASE STUDY 38.1

John, qualified for 8 years, has recently been appointed to a Senior Charge Nurse post in emergency medicine. Since qualifying John focused his CPD on the clinical skills and knowledge required of an adult nurse working in this sphere of practice. More recently, in preparation for his promotion, John has undertaken various forms of management and leadership development as he is acutely aware that, while he needs to maintain his clinical skills, he also needs to be able to manage and lead his nursing team. John said, 'I am confident about my own learning and practice and I have been a mentor to many students. I am aware now though that I have further formal responsibilities with regard to my team and their learning, including being our professional lead for revalidation and using local learning policies and processes for staff learning while delivering care and managing finite resources. While not taking my eye off my own clinical learning and practice, I have shifted my ongoing learning focus in recent times to better reflect my scope of practice.'

From your own learning experience, can you identify at least three ways your CPD might benefit others?

As can be seen from John's experience, your ongoing learning as an adult nurse, while personally driven (derived from your practice), may benefit others too.

Chapter 39 addresses the nurse as educator and it can be seen that through your own personal learning, you can also help others to learn. While your professional priority is for your patients to benefit from your learning, there are a variety of ways in which you can help your colleagues to benefit too. A key area is in the practice of **supervision**.

SEE ALSO
CHAPTER 39

Supervision in adult nursing takes many forms, e.g. mentorship, preceptorship, clinical, educational and/or management supervision. Regardless of form, basic principles apply in supervision: through providing supervision to others you are aiming to share your learning in ways that result in them learning from you; in receiving supervision from others you are aiming to share in their learning.

Supervision may be very practical – learning a new or changed clinical skill, using new or changed equipment, administering or applying new or changed medications or dressings. It may be more cognitive – understanding the evidence base behind these changes or searching for answers to your questions through research, for example. It may also be pastoral – for instance, supporting a colleague who is going through difficult times, helping your team to address workload challenges and demands, or dealing with very worried or concerned patients and their families.

In all forms of supervision there are at least three dimensions (derived from the seminal model espoused by Proctor in 1986): ensuring quality in your day-to-day practice; identifying and undertaking the underpinning learning required for your practice and its improvement; and addressing personal support needs recognising the emotional demands of caring. A supervisory role in adult nursing may be a formal role (for example, as a senior charge nurse or team leader) or more informal within your employment role (mentor, preceptor, link nurse or nurse in charge). In any such situation, you need to consider all three of these dimensions of supervision to maximise effectiveness and so learn or share your learning.

While the majority of adult nurses will have a lifelong career as an adult nurse (registered nurse or staff nurse, for example) some careers may progress into more senior positions. Every employer will have their own job roles and titles and structural hierarchies to reflect career progression; however, what is common is that the more one progresses into senior roles, the greater the demand on one's supervisory skills. Career progression comes with enhanced responsibilities for much wider or more advanced areas of practice and, therefore, you will need to take steps to address your learning to reflect the knowledge and skills required. Fundamentally, these may include advancing your clinical practice into areas beyond that of your initial registration; or advancing your management or leadership into promoted posts; or advancing your practice into teaching roles in clinical practice or education; or developing your role as a nurse researcher, for example. In each and all of these situations or comparable others, your learning needs will grow in range, in level and in depth to support your developing professionalism and the expected supervisory practices and underpinning competencies and capabilities of that role. The following activity will help you consider the extent to which an established career framework can be useful in helping you identify learning that will benefit you and others as your career progresses.

GO FURTHER

Explore a relevant career framework and consider what it indicates regarding your future learning as an adult nurse: NHS employers: https://www.healthcareers.nhs.uk/career-planning/resources/careers-nursing or The NHS Scotland Post Registration Career Development Framework for Nurses, Midwives and Allied Health Professionals: www.careerframework.nes.scot.nhs.uk/

WEBLINKS

CHAPTER SUMMARY

- Learning in your pre-registration programme is the beginning – ongoing learning will continue to be very important throughout your nursing career.
- Ongoing learning will be stimulated by yourself, your patients, your colleagues and your work situation.
- There is a range of learning opportunities and resources for you to seek out.
- Your ongoing learning will benefit yourself, your patients and colleagues including future nurses.

GO FURTHER

CASE STUDY: EMPLOYER LEARNING RESOURCES

Go to https://study.sagepub.com/essentialadultnursing for a further case study related to this chapter. If you are using the interactive ebook, simply click on the book icon in the margin to go straight to the resource.

Journal Articles

FURTHER READING: JOURNAL ARTICLES

Go to https://study.sagepub.com/essentialadultnursing for further free online journal articles related to this chapter. If you are using the interactive ebook, simply click on the book icon in the margin to go straight to the resource.

Read any/all of the following for further deliberation on ongoing learning in nursing:

- Clark, E., Draper, J. and Rogers, J. (2015) Illuminating the process: Enhancing the impact of continuing professional education on practice. *Nurse Education Today*, 35(2): 388–94.
- Draper, J. and Clark, L. (2016) Managers' role in maximising investment in continuing professional education. *Nursing Management*, 22(9): 30–6.
- Kemp, S.J. and Baker, M. (2013) Continuing Professional Development – Reflections from nursing and education. *Nurse Education in Practice*, 3(6): 541–5.

Weblinks

FURTHER READING: WEBLINKS

Go to https://study.sagepub.com/essentialadultnursing for further weblinks related to this chapter. If you are using the interactive ebook, simply click on the book icon in the margin to go straight to the resource.

The NMC and RCN websites have helpful information and resources including:

- Safeguardging: https://www.rcn.org.uk/clinical-topics/safeguarding
- Revalidation and CPD: http://revalidation.nmc.org.uk/welcome-to-revalidation
- Additional post-registration standards: https://www.nmc.org.uk/standards/standards-for-post-registration/

ACE YOUR ASSESSMENT

ONLINE QUIZZES

Revise what you have learned by visiting https://study.sagepub.com/essentialadultnursing

- Test yourself with multiple-choice and short-answer questions
- Do the chapter activities in the book and check your answers online

REFERENCES

Collins English Dictionary – Complete & Unabridged (2012). Digital Edition accessed online on 11/07/2016 at: www.dictionary.com/browse/lifelong-learning

Delves-Yates, C. (ed.) (2018) *Essentials of Nursing Practice* (2nd ed.). London: SAGE.

Department of Health (2004) *The NHS Knowledge and Skills Framework (NHS KSF) and the Development Review Process*. London: Department of Health.

NHS England (2016) *Leading Change, Adding Value. A Framework for Nursing, Midwifery and Care Staff*. NHS England.

NMC (2015) *The Code: Professional standards of practice and behaviour for nurses and midwives*. London: NMC.

NMC (2016) *Revalidation*. Available at: http://revalidation.nmc.org.uk/welcome-to-revalidation.

Proctor, B. (1986) A cooperative exercise in accountability. In Marken, M. and Payne, M. (eds) *Enabling And Ensuring*. London: Council for Education and Training in Youth and Community Work.

THE ROLE OF THE NURSE AS TEACHER AND EDUCATOR

39

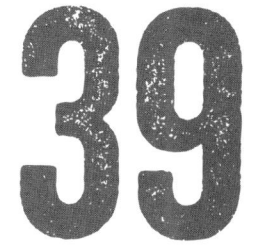

HELEN WALKER

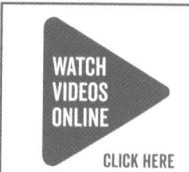

WATCH VIDEOS ONLINE
CLICK HERE

THIS CHAPTER COVERS

- The wider professional nursing role as a nurse educator
- Preparation for practice
- Potential challenges to teaching
- How we educate others effectively
- Interaction with others
- Importance of using an evidence-based approach
- Teaching technology and using technology to teach.

> " I just wish someone had been there to tell me how to deal with the situation properly, I might not have had to come back into hospital if I'd known what to do ... but they never said anything.
>
> **Marion, patient** "

> " I can't understand why they don't listen to me ... I know what he likes better than they do.
>
> **Janice, carer** "

INTRODUCTION

This chapter offers guidance on nurses as teachers and educators. It is important as a student that you are aware of the principles of teaching and the different methods we can use to communicate information to people. You may think this is a somewhat peripheral part of your overall role, but you might be surprised how often you will find yourself as a staff nurse in an educational role, teaching patients, fellow colleagues of all disciplines, care assistants, students or carers. What we are saying is that you are often expected to be more than 'just a nurse'. There is also an expectation that you will adopt an educational role at an early stage in your career – as a student – because you are equipped with the knowledge to guide care assistants and sometimes even liaise with patients or carers, gathering or passing on information when more senior staff are busy. Patients and carers are keen to be informed but they also want to be listened to: you are perfectly positioned to undertake this liaison role as part of your job. This will become an integral component of your working week and be extended once you are qualified. You may also want to take your career in an educational direction.

The **NMC** *Standards of Proficiency for Registered Nurses* (2018) clearly articulate the role of the nurse as a supervisor/teacher. It is stated that the student must be able to:

- support and supervise students in the delivery of nursing care, promoting reflection and providing constructive feedback, and evaluating and documenting their performance;
- demonstrate the ability to challenge and provide constructive feedback about care delivered by others in the team, and support them to identify and agree individual learning need
- contribute to supervision and team reflection activities to promote improvements in practice and services.

THE WIDER PROFESSIONAL NURSING ROLE AS A NURSE EDUCATOR

Given the expectation that you will be required to impart knowledge, the importance of offering accurate and factual knowledge cannot be underestimated. Within the role of a nurse educator you will be expected to have a sound knowledge base, in order that you can effectively teach others. We can consider nurse educators in different contexts, for example, in educational settings or in clinical practice. Good teaching is not confined to university; it is equally evident in clinical practice. It is worth noting that nurse educators in higher education settings need to maintain strong clinical skills (Beck and Ruth-Sahd, 2013) in order to keep in touch with current practice. The same rule applies to nurses in clinical settings; they need to continue to check emerging theories associated with their area of practice.

More recently, there has been a spotlight on graduate nurses having to learn to care, in response to media coverage highlighting poor practice. Caring is often referred to in the nursing literature and is regarded as a complex concept, yet caring transcends every aspect of nursing, including nursing education (Brown, 2011). It is suggested that a fundamental question arising from the evidence base relating to teaching and learning about care is not whether students are able to learn how to care, but how educators design teaching and learning situations that facilitate students to learn more effectively (Costello and Haggart, 2008).

A teacher has a particular set of skills, perhaps similar to mentorship; for example, good interpersonal communication, ability to be supportive and good attention to detail. Mentorship also offers you an opportunity to teach new staff. There is a considerable body of literature on mentorship, yet little is written about mentorship models (Jacobson and Sherrod, 2012). The ability to motivate others as well as being able to convey concepts to others working at different levels and of differing capabilities is equally important, as is helping colleagues, fellow students and carers to overcome difficulties. You may find that you have particular strengths and personal qualities in this area, if so teaching may be something you might consider in the future.

PREPARATION FOR PRACTICE

In preparation for clinical practice you and your fellow students will learn how to teach one another, commonly during clinical skills sessions. Commonly during clinical skills sessions. You will, for example, learn how to give an injection – this kind of information can be passed on to a person with diabetes. You will also be asked at some point to present information to small groups as part of a peer assessment; this skill can also be used when passing on information to families or carers. You may be expected to provide health education material and general advice, perhaps for over or underweight patients or people with cardiac problems. The giving of information related to diet, exercise, smoking, drinking and general wellbeing are well within your capabilities as a student.

ACTIVITY 39.1: CRITICAL THINKING

ACTIVITY 39.1 ANSWER

- What experience do you have of teaching others? What other skills do you possess that would enable you to teach others? Do you feel equipped to do so?
- Take some time to devise a short teaching activity on health promotion advice for someone who is overweight and recovering from a cardiac arrest.

POTENTIAL CHALLENGES TO TEACHING

We must acknowledge that there may be barriers or challenges to teaching effectively, such as: language differences; attitudes towards authority figures; ability to accept diagnosis; and working with people who have learning difficulties or hearing/sight impairment. Language difficulties can sometimes be overcome through the use of interpreters (if available) or specialist technology that can be used to translate information into another language. The reluctance to listen and accept information from professional staff is something we must accept, but it is important not to let this deter us from continuing to try and offer assistance to aid comprehension. Often people are unable or perhaps not ready to accept a diagnosis, or they are simply in a state of shock, and thus, not ready to learn. We need to be patient and hope they will perhaps engage with others at a different point in time. As a student, it is often advisable to seek out some written information – with the permission of a trained member of staff – that offers a brief explanation relating to the condition, e.g. diabetes, then make plans to come back and discuss or explain the situation in full at a later time point, with someone who is knowledgeable about the condition. It is important not to be offended if the patient is quite dismissive at the early stage of diagnosis: this is quite a common reaction. Observe and note the non-verbal reaction of the patient as well as what is actually said.

ACTIVITY 39.2: CRITICAL THINKING

ACTIVITY 39.2 ANSWER

How do you think fellow professionals will view student intervention, i.e. in an educational role? If the attitudes were less positive how would you manage your way around a situation such as this?

As an adult nurse you will see many people with a learning disability in acute hospital and community settings. Working with people who have a learning disability means that information must be presented very clearly and communicated at a slower pace in order that they can understand fully. It is usually better if people with a learning disability are accompanied by someone who can also hear any instructions and repeat them later if necessary. People with a hearing impairment often use British Sign Language (BSL) as their first language; therefore, English is their second language and they may not always understand over-complicated terminology. NHS hospitals are often criticised for the poor service provision and inability to meet the needs of this population.

Since we aim to meet the needs of the entire population to the best of our ability, we should perhaps make the extra effort to learn the basics in BSL.

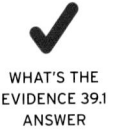

WHAT'S THE
EVIDENCE 39.1
ANSWER

WHAT'S THE EVIDENCE 39.1?

If we look at the number of people who have a hearing impairment, we can accept our ability to communicate using BSL will become more important for practitioners in the health service. In the United Kingdom, there are 50,000 children with hearing loss, 11 million people will experience some form of hearing loss with almost a million experiencing profound hearing loss, and it is estimated that this figure will rise to 15.6 million by 2035 (Action on Hearing Loss, 2015). It has been estimated that between 15,000 and 24,000 people use sign language as their main language (Emond et al., 2015). Two million people in the UK are living with sight loss with 360,000 registered as blind, and there are 25,000 children who are blind or partially sighted. The number of people with sight loss could rise to four million by 2050 (Access Economics, 2009; Royal National Institute of Blind People, 2014). The group of people who will contribute to the rise in sensory impairment are the elderly population, which is due to expand significantly in the next 15 to 20 years. This requires a whole range of issues to be addressed by health and social care as a consequence of sensory impairment.

- Do you have a basic working knowledge of BSL?
- If not, how do you think you would manage a situation that required someone to use BSL?

We all learn differently, but I'm not sure people realise that, I sometimes don't 'get it' when people explain something to me at first, I need to think about it for ages and practise it, then it makes sense.

James, student

HOW WE EDUCATE OTHERS EFFECTIVELY

There are many different methods through which you can pass on information and teach others, yet the most commonly used strategy continues to be the lecture in the formal academic setting. This more traditional teaching style is known as a didactic method and can be applied just as readily in any clinical setting to teach fellow students, care assistants, patients and carers. There are distinct advantages of using this method, namely: information can be passed on to large numbers of people at any one time in a cost-effective manner; a considerable amount of information can be covered quickly; new material and complex issues can be presented, explained and discussed quite readily. The disadvantages are that people do not always engage during these sessions, because they process information at different levels; also participants are also less likely to learn problem-solving skills using this approach. Current thinking tends to focus on active and collaborative learning. Active learning is thought to help educators shift from a teacher-centred to a person-centred approach, which in turn tends to encourage independence in learning, creative problem-solving skills, and critical thinking (Schaefer and Zygmont, 2003).

Educators can use questioning strategies to develop critical thinking. Lower level questioning does not promote critical thinking because people rely mainly on their memory to recall information. A simple recall of information does not enhance your understanding of the information in a meaningful way. It takes higher level questioning to facilitate the development of critical thinking because it is aimed at higher cognitive levels, which involves application, analysis, synthesis and evaluation. Educators should, therefore, pose stimulating questions in order to help create meaningful active learning instead of just prompting the simple recall of knowledge from their audience. Positive role modelling can be a very effective strategy when you want others to learn with you.

ACTIVITY 39.3: CRITICAL THINKING

- If you were to educate a family or group of carers, which approach (in theory) could you use?
- What things do you need to consider in order to get your message across effectively?

ACTIVITY 39.3
ANSWER

In addition to the range of teaching styles, you also need to be aware that learning styles differ. Be cognisant of this. There are many different theories that relate to the way we learn – Experiential Learning (Kolb and Kolb, 2005), Conceptual Learning and Problem-based Learning to name but a few.

GO FURTHER

Businessballs is a useful website providing overviews on teaching and learning for managers. See: www. businessballs.com/kolblearningstyles.htm for an overview on Kolb's learning styles.

WEBLINK:
KOLB'S
LEARNING
STYLES

When we look at the supporting evidence, learning styles that balance experiencing and conceptualising are more adaptable and flexible in learning contexts. Adaptive flexibility in learning style is predictive of highly integrated and complex levels of adult development. The learning style specialising in experiencing showed higher levels of skill development in interpersonal skills and lower levels of skill development in analytic skills; while the reverse is true for the learning style specialising in conceptualising (Mainemelis et al., 2002). In problem based learning (PBL), problems encountered in clinical settings are presented first before students learn clinical concepts (Hsu, 2004). Problem-based learning promotes active learning through self-directed learning, self-appraisal, development of clinical problem-solving skills and teamwork: it also requires the student to have discipline. PBL also improves clinical reasoning skills, increases the retention of learned material and enhances self-directed study (Whitfield et al., 2002).

Often, we learn by simply listening. A short article by a student nurse (Byrne, 2013) relates to how he sat by a patient's bedside and listened to her story, learning much more than he could have through running through his admissions checklist.

ACTIVITY 39.4 ANSWER

ACTIVITY 39:4: REFLECTIVE PRACTICE

When was the last time you stopped and listened to a patient and took their advice?

INTERACTION WITH OTHERS

Interaction with the wider multidisciplinary team, junior staff or students and families and carers is something nurses across all fields will need to consider. The responsibility for teaching others often falls on nurses, but we need to be careful because there are rules that guide the amount of information we share. We need to be mindful of patient confidentiality and only share information when we have consent to do so.

——————————————— GO FURTHER ———————————————

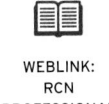

WEBLINK: RCN PROFESSIONAL DEVELOPMENT

The rules and regulations surrounding consent are designed to protect the patient and must be adhered to. Guidance on consent can be found on the Royal College of Nursing Website. See: https://www.rcn.org.uk/professional-development/publications/pub-006047

Members of the wider multidisciplinary team often approach nurses for information. Junior medical staff, for example, are on a six-month rotational programme and at the beginning of their placements you may witness them approaching experienced registered nursing staff for advice on prescribing patterns. It may seem unusual for nurses to be offering advice to medical staff regarding their core role, but nurses can and do provide sound advice if drawn from a solid evidence base, presented carefully with professional judgement. As a student, it is important you watch and learn how to pass on important information such as this, while also considering how you would respond if asked the same questions one day.

More so now than ever, a significant proportion of nurses are completing a postgraduate nurse prescribing course that enables them to fulfil a more specialist role. This equips them with a greater depth and breadth of knowledge that they can utilise to enhance their clinical practice. This is perhaps something you might want to consider for the future, after you have completed your undergraduate training.

Many nurses engage in what they would consider fairly routine activities throughout their working week, but what is routine for you is not necessarily routine for a carer or a student. We need to be mindful of this when delivering information and not skimming over critical details because they seem obvious and trivial to anybody – they often are not.

CASE STUDY 39.1: LUCAS

CASE STUDY 39.1
ANSWER

Lucas is normally an energetic 3 year old who 'has the energy of a million and the appetite of a horse' according to his mother, Karen. He is always running about inside and out 'helping' his mum and dad with whatever tasks they opt to do. Following on from the long summer holiday he returned to his local nursery in Glasgow. When the weather turned colder he seemed to pick up 'a touch of the cold' and was coughing and sneezing. Unusually for him he was off his food and was distinctly less boisterous and energetic, sitting on a chair rather than running around. One night his mother was reading him a bedtime story and could hear a cracking in his chest when he was breathing, but not wanting to be alarmist did not contact the GP. Over the period of the next week he gradually became more tired and lethargic, he was coughing constantly through the night, to the point he was almost making himself sick. Karen went to wake him up one morning because he had not yet surfaced and it was 8 o'clock ... most unusual. His breathing was really laboured when she did wake him and he could hardly gasp a breath. His face was flushed. Karen called the GP immediately but was advised to go to Accident and Emergency (A&E) in Glasgow since it was the weekend. As it transpired he was not given a diagnosis, because he was under the age of 5 and the tests for asthma cannot be confirmed.

Describe what you would do when a child is brought to A&E in a breathless state such as this.

- How much information do you offer at this early stage?
- Thinking ahead, how do you teach the parents to deal with this situation effectively?

After having taught something we need to stop and take stock of how well it went. The ability to self-monitor and self-evaluate is crucial, as is an ability to reflect on your own skills as a teacher, these are seen as key ingredients in achieving teaching excellence (Kreber, 2002). Self-reflection generally enables you to assess your performance, consider what you need to do to progress or develop and enhance your own skills that can in turn be passed on to others. It allows time to consider what went well and what could have been done differently to maximise impact.

THE IMPORTANCE OF USING AN EVIDENCE-BASED APPROACH

SEE ALSO
CHAPTER 6

Due to advances and increased complexity of healthcare practice and a limited lifespan of useful information, the healthcare system has had to change rapidly (Russell et al., 2007). Nursing has changed dramatically over the years, especially in the Adult field; technological advances have led to radical changes in practice. It is no longer the case that nurses simply accept what has always been done in the past, we have a responsibility to improve our practice and are now more motivated to do so. Nurses are more able to engage in research themselves and grow the evidence to support their practice. This, in turn, creates a more confident workforce.

The use of evidence-based practice has enabled nurses to stand alongside other professions within the multidisciplinary team on an even footing, and encouraged the emergence of Clinical Nurse Specialists, Advanced Practitioners and Consultant Nurses, so there are many routes for personal progression. One of the greatest advantages of using evidence-based practice is that it allows you to vigorously defend your actions if the occasion arises. One of the contributory factors that has led to this surge in the use of evidence-based practice is the necessity for nurses to engage in baccalaureate level education.

Recent research evidence supports the improvement in practice as a consequence of lower patient–to–nurse ratios, a higher proportion of nurses with baccalaureate level education and better nurse working environments being associated with lower mortality rates (Aiken et al., 2011). The changing culture moving towards lifelong learning has further promoted attendance in postgraduate courses. Often, these educational programmes need to be quite generic to meet the needs of healthcare agencies. This presents challenges to universities because of the demand for flexible programmes to be offered in a variety of models (Fitzgerald et al., 2013).

There is considerable evidence to support early intervention in clinical practice. Being alert to early warning signs is something we learn more effectively while out in the field. More experienced practitioners are quicker to pick up on early signs and symptoms and, therefore, well placed to pass on this valuable information to junior staff. As a student, it is important that you are aware of this and stress to junior staff the importance of early detection, thus preventing major trauma. Advantages of a preventative rather than reactive approach are well documented and fairly self-explanatory, yet despite the strong rationale people often delay assessment or treatment until a critical point is reached. An example of how a major situation can be averted is highlighted in the Case study below. Although this situation relates more to someone with a mental disorder, that you will find as a student that you may well come across situations such as this, and you will need to know how to deal with them.

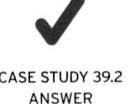

CASE STUDY 39.2
ANSWER

CASE STUDY 39.2: AVRIL

It was last year, the week before my thirtieth birthday. I was alone when I went to A&E; it was a cold dark miserable winter night. I was hungry because I hadn't eaten for two days and I had just split up with my boyfriend. I knew I couldn't face my life without him. I was near hysterical by the time I saw the nurse in triage and couldn't stop crying. I had been here many times before, but this time I needed her ... I needed someone to believe me ... my family had all given up. I couldn't stop shaking. She noticed the burn marks on my arms as soon as I took off my jacket and the lacerations on my wrists were quite deep this time ... I had opened old wounds ... I just hoped and prayed she wouldn't give me one of her looks ... you know ... when people are disgusted with you. Instead she was kind and gentle and tended to my wounds with care and attention. She gave me her time and although we sat in silence I felt that she understood, she didn't make me explain myself.

What do you think you could say to support someone in a situation like this?

Although most things can be taught within the graduate programme at University, dealing with a situation when someone presents with challenging behaviour, such as that displayed by Avril, is probably something you only really learn in a live situation. As a student, it is important that you learn not to judge others and effectively pass this on to those around you. The difficulty may be dealing with existing prejudices of others, for example, care assistants, who are less well informed about the impact something they say they can have on vulnerable people.

WHAT'S THE EVIDENCE? 39.2

People with a diagnosis of borderline personality disorder regularly appear at Accident and Emergency units as their first point of contact with NHS services, commonly in a distressed and highly emotional state. This heightened state of emotion, sometimes bordering on hysteria, is characteristic of someone with this diagnosis, as is poor self-esteem and low self-worth. Personality disorders are best understood as unusual or extreme personality types, which cause suffering to the person or others and hinder interpersonal functioning (Department of Health, 2011). Various strategies need to be explored in order to manage people with this diagnosis in order to try and prevent regular repeat visits. It is also useful to engage with carers as a means of offering support to both parties. A simple alternative strategy to self-harm by burning can be taught very quickly, in that, if you hold an ice cube against the skin instead of a cigarette or hot knife/spoon, it has a similar impact but is less damaging to the skin.

TEACHING TECHNOLOGY AND USING TECHNOLOGY TO TEACH

SEE ALSO
CHAPTER 1

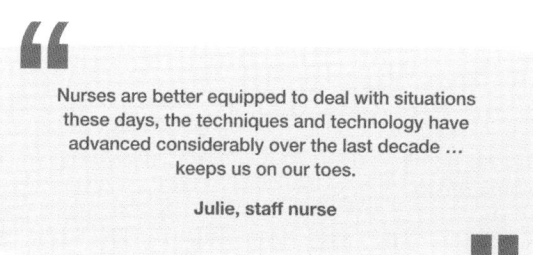

> Nurses are better equipped to deal with situations these days, the techniques and technology have advanced considerably over the last decade ... keeps us on our toes.
>
> **Julie, staff nurse**

Technology moves at a pace and practitioners often struggle to 'keep up' with the radical changes, yet it is thought that technological advancements involving mobile technologies can transform how people interact and communicate with each other (Scottish Government, 2013). 'Telehealth', 'Telemedicine', 'e-health' and 'mHealth' are used interchangeably in clinical practice to describe the exchange of health information at a distance using technology between or relating to a patient and their healthcare provider (Wootton, 2012). The use of technology can be a real advantage if introduced carefully and taught properly, enabling others to achieve their specified goals. Many studies have examined the issue of acceptance and technology adoption in health services around the world. Nurses have been slow to accept, adopt and lead on the use of telehealth in their job roles, however the advantages to patients can be quite remarkable, if they can find a strategy that suits them. An example is using educational apps with prompts to assist with compliance with prescribed medication. This is useful for people who are prone to forgetting to attend to their health. For people with borderline personality disorder this can be a really useful strategy that can be taught quickly. Another example of ways telemedicine can be helpful is in a situation where people require their condition to be monitored, such as someone with chronic obstructive pulmonary disease. The condition can be managed at home and taught via telemedicine.

CHAPTER SUMMARY

- Educational and teaching strategies have changed over the years: some traditional methods are still practised in formal settings, but new and more student-focused approaches tend to be adopted now. A few different approaches have been highlighted throughout the chapter and examples of what to do and how to use your teaching skills have been included as a guide.
- Some hurdles and potential barriers to teaching and learning have been presented in order to make you think creatively and problem solve, ensuring your message is relayed appropriately.
- There is an emphasis on your role as a professional person and a reminder that you have a responsibility to seek out the best available evidence to support your clinical practice in order that you can justify your chosen course of action with sound judgement. Ignorance is not a defence. You can teach this good practice through role modelling.
- Technological advancement means that everyone continues to learn. You need to keep yourself up to date with current information and new technology, and consider what circumstances will enhance learning.
- Finally, some basic principles should be adhered to, such as: afford time to the patient when he/she asks for information/support; involve the carer where appropriate – advise and support them too; be respectful; demonstrate a compassionate caring attitude; consider the wider context and prepare the patient for future eventualities; incorporate education within the plan of care for the patient and ensure it is implemented and evaluated.

GO FURTHER

CASE STUDY:
ELDERLY CARE

Go to https://study.sagepub.com/essentialadultnursing for a further case study related to this chapter. If you are using the interactive ebook, simply click on the book icon in the margin to go straight to the resource.

Books

These books all offer a useful insight to students for teaching, supervising and mentoring in practice, with some valuable examples to draw upon.

- Dolan, B. and Hinchliff, S. (2017) *The Practitioner as Teacher* (4th ed.). London: Churchill Livingstone.
- Gopee, N. (2015) *Mentoring and Supervision in Healthcare* (3rd ed.). London: SAGE Publications Ltd.
- Stuart, C.C. (2013) *Mentoring, Learning and Assessment in Clinical Practice: A Guide for Nurses, Midwives & Other Health Professionals*. London: Churchill Livingstone.

Journal Articles

FURTHER
READING:
JOURNAL
ARTICLES

Go to https://study.sagepub.com/essentialadultnursing for further free online journal articles related to this chapter. If you are using the interactive ebook, simply click on the book icon in the margin to go straight to the resource.

- Oelofsen, N. (2012) Using reflective practice in frontline nursing. *Nursing Times*, 108 (24): 22-4.
- Singh, M.D., Pilkington, F.B. and Patrick, L. (2014) Empowerment and mentoring in nurse academia. *International Journal of Nursing Education Scholarship*, 11 (1): 1-11.
- Taylor, J., Coates, E., Brewster, L., Mountain G., Wessels, B. and Hawley, MS. (2015) Examining the use of Telehealth in community nursing: Identifying the factors affecting frontline staff acceptance and Telehealth adoption. *Journal of Advanced Nursing*, 71 (2): 326-37.

Weblinks

FURTHER
READING:
WEBLINKS

Go to https://study.sagepub.com/essentialadultnursing for further weblinks related to this chapter. If you are using the interactive ebook, simply click on the book icon in the margin to go straight to the resource.

- Audit Scotland (2011) A review of Telehealth in Scotland, prepared for the auditor General for Scotland. www.audit-scotland.gov.uk/docs/health/2011/nr_111013_telehealth.pdf
- Scottish Government (2013) See Hear: a Strategic Framework for Meeting the Needs of People with a Sensory Impairment in Scotland. *www.scotland.gov.uk/Publications/2013/04/2067*

Bazian report: RCN Mentorship Project 2015:

- www.rcn.org.uk/professional-development/publications/pub-005472
- A RCN publication on mentorship models outside the UK

The Collaborative Learning in Practice (CLIP) Project:

- https://healthacademy.lancsteachinghospitals.nhs.uk/collaborative-learning-in-practice-toolkit
- A project in the East of England on an alternative approach to supporting students in practice, which has attracted a lot of attention.

ACE YOUR ASSESSMENT

Revise what you have learned by visiting https://study.sagepub.com/essentialadultnursing

ONLINE QUIZZES

- Test yourself with multiple-choice and short-answer questions
- Do the chapter activities in the book and check your answers online

REFERENCES

Access Economics (2009) *Future sight loss (UK): The economic impact of partial sight and blindness in the UK adult population.* Available at: www.rnib.org.uk/sites/default/files/FSUK_Report.pdf [accessed 02 03 2018].

Action on Hearing Loss (2015) *Facts and figures on hearing loss, deafness and tinnitus.* www.actiononhearingloss.org.uk/how-we-help/information-and-resources/publications/research-reports/hearing-matters-report/ [accessed 02 03 2018].

Aiken, L.H. (2011) Nurses for the future. *New England Journal of Medicine,* 364 (3): 196–8.

Beck, J. and Ruth-Sahd, L. (2013) The lived experience of seeking tenure while practicing clinically: Finding balance in academia. *Dimensions of Critical Care Nursing,* 32 (10): 37–45.

Brown, L.P. (2011) Revising our roots: Caring in nursing curriculum design. *Nursing Education in Practice,* 11: 360–4.

Byrne, G. (2013) Listening is a vital part of care, but how many of us have time? *Nursing Standard,* 27: 28.

Costello, J. and Haggart, M. (2008) The nature of nursing: Can we teach students how to care? *CARE,* 2: 41–55.

Department of Health (2011) *Working with Personality Disordered Offenders: A practitioner's guide.* London: Ministry of Justice National Offender Management Service.

Emond, A., Ridd, M., Sutherland, H., Allsop, L., Alexander, A. and Kyle, J. (2015) The current health status of the signing deaf community in the UK compared with the general population: A cross-sectional study. *BMJ Open.* Available at: http://dx.doi.org/10.1136/bmjopen-2014-006668. [accessed 02 03 2018].

Fitzgerald, L., Wong, P., Hannon, J., Solberg Tokerud, M. and Lyons, J. (2013) Curriculum learning designs: Teaching health assessment skills for advanced nursing practitioners through sustainable flexible learning. *Nurse Education Today*, 33: 1230–6.

Hsu, LL. (2004) Developing concept maps from problem-based learning scenario discussions. *Journal of Advanced Nursing*, 48(5): 510–18.

Jacobson, S.L. and Sherrod, D.R. (2012) Transformational mentorship models for nurse educators. *Nursing Science Quarterly*, 25 (3): 279–84.

Kolb, A.Y. and Kolb, D.A. (2005) Learning styles and learning spaces: Enhancing experiential learning in higher education. *Academy of Management Learning and Education,* 4 (2): 193–212 doi: 10.5465/AMLE.2005.17268566

Kreber, C. (2002) The scholarship of teaching: A comparison of conceptions held by experts and regular academic staff. *Higher Education*, 46: 93–121.

Mainemelis, C., Boyatzis, R.E. and Kolb, D.A. (2002) Learning styles and adaptive flexibility. *Management Learning*, 33 (1) : 5–33 doi: 10.1177/1350507602331001

Nursing and Midwifery Council (2018) *Standards of Proficiency for Registered Nurses.* Available at: www.nmc-uk.org

Royal National Institute for the Blind (2014) *Sight loss statistics postcard.* Available at: www.rnib.org.uk/sites/default/files/Sight%20loss%20stats%20postcard.pdf [accessed 02.03 2018].

Russell, A.T., Comello, R.J. and Wright, D.L. (2007) Teaching strategies promoting active learning in healthcare education. *Journal of Education and Human Development,* 1 (1): 386–92.

Schaefer, K. and Zygmont, D. (2003) Analyzing the teaching style of nursing faculty. *Nurse Education Perspective*, 24 (5): 238–45.

Scottish Government (2013) *Digital Scotland 2020.* Available at: www.scotland.gov.uk/Publications/2013/02/9054/0 [accessed on 02 03 2018]

Whitfield, C., Mauger, E., Zwicker, J. and Lehman, E. (2002) Differences between students in problem-based and lecture-based curricula measured by clerkship performance ratings at the beginning of the third year. *Teaching and Learning Medicine*, 14 (4): 211–17.

Wootton, R. (2012) Twenty years of telemedicine in chronic disease management - an evidence synthesis. *Journal of Telemedicine and Telecare,*18: 211.

GLOSSARY

Absorption In pharmacology (and more precisely pharmacokinetics), absorption refers to the movement of a drug from the site of administration to bloodstream. Absorption comprises of numerous stages. Initially, the drug is introduced via a particular route of administration (orally, subcutaneously, intramuscularly, etc.) and in a specific dosage form such as a tablet, capsule, solution and so on.

Acidosis is an excessively acid condition of body fluids or tissues.

Acute chest syndrome (ACS) is defined as an acute illness characterised by fever and/or respiratory symptoms, accompanied by a new pulmonary infiltrate on chest x-ray

Adaptive immune system The secondary response of the immune system, characterised by the generation of antibodies and T cells that specifically target antigens.

Adjuvant analgesics Drugs that have weak or non-existent analgesic action when administered alone but can enhance analgesic actions when co-administered with known analgesic agents.

Adjuvant chemotherapy Adjuvant chemotherapy is treatment given after primary treatment, such as surgery.

Albumin A protein made by the liver that keeps fluid from leaking out of blood vessels, nourishes tissues, and transports hormones, vitamins, drugs, and substances such as calcium throughout the body.

Allergy A condition caused by hypersensitivity of the immune system to something in the environment that is usually harmless.

Allogeneic stem cell transplant A transplant using stem cells (early blood cells) from another person (a donor) is called a donor stem cell transplant.

Analgesia The inability to feel pain, the effect of analgesics.

Analgesic A drug that is used to achieve pain relief or analgesia.

Androgenic hormones These are responsible for the male features in humans. More prevalent in men, they do occur in smaller amounts in women. There are several different groups of androgens with dihydrotestosterone causing the increased sebum levels in acne.

Antibodies (also known as an immunoglobulin). Large, Y-shaped proteins that are used by the immune system to neutralise pathogens such as bacteria and viruses.

Anticholinergics An anticholinergic agent is a substance that blocks the neurotransmitter acetylcholine in the central and the peripheral nervous system.

Antihistamines A type of pharmaceutical drug that opposes the activity of histamine receptors in the body. Usually used to treat allergies.

Atopic Means there is a genetic predisposition towards an allergic disease that is usually harmless in the rest of the population.

Autoimmune disease A condition characterised by an abnormal immune system response, which attacks the body's own cells and tissues.

Autologous stem cell transplant (ASCT) Stem cells are removed from your body before chemotherapy treatment, and then returned afterwards.

Autosomal dominant A condition caused by inheriting one mutated gene from one (usually affected) parent.

Autosomal recessive A condition caused by inheriting two mutated genes, one from each carrier parent.

Basophil A type of granulocyte found in the blood.

B cells (also known as B lymphocytes). A type of white blood cell of the lymphocyte subtype.

Brachytherapy This is a form of radiotherapy where radioactive seeds or sources are placed in or near the tumour, giving a high radiation dose to the tumour while reducing the radiation exposure in the surrounding healthy tissues. The term 'brachy' is Greek for short distance.

Bradypnoeic Hypoventilating, low respiratory rate.

BRCA 1 and BRCA2 These are known as tumour suppressor genes, genes that protect the cell from one step on the journey to developing cancer. Harmful mutations in the BRCA 1 and BRCA 2 genes may produce a hereditary breast-ovarian cancer syndrome in affected persons.

Bronchodilator reversibility test is used to distinguish asthma from other causes of obstructive lung disease.

Bronchospasm is constriction of the air passages of the lung caused by spasmodic contraction of the bronchial muscles.

Case-based reasoning uses past experiences (cases) to understand and solve new problems.

Cheyne–Stoking An abnormal pattern of breathing often seen in people who are at the end of a protracted period of dying. It is characterised by several deep breaths followed by some very shallow breaths or no inspiration at all for several seconds.

Clonorchis sinenis This is known as the Chinese liver fluke. It is a human liver fluke (a parasite) that lives in the liver of humans, and is found mainly in the common bile duct and gall bladder, feeding on bile.

Clubbing is a deformity of the finger or toe nails associated with a number of diseases, mostly of the heart and lungs.

Complement system A cascade of response of the immune system, which enhances the ability of antibodies and phagocytes to attack pathogens.

Contextual Cognitive Behaviour Therapy (CCBT) A form of behavioural and cognitive behavioural therapies based on acceptance and commitment therapy and mindfulness-based approaches. Its aim is to develop the patient to a better understanding of their pain and to minimise pain-related distress, physical and psychosocial disability, depression, anxiety, mobility, effect of rest and acceptance of pain. It appears most effective for patients suffering with longstanding and complex chronic pain conditions, and may be particularly suited to multi-problem cases characterised by change-resistant behaviour patterns.

Continuing Professional Development (CPD) The learning through which professionals evidence their maintenance and enhancement of their knowledge and skills.

Continuous Positive Airway Pressure (CPAP) A method of applying mild air pressure continuously via a machine, used for patients who are able to breathe spontaneously but whose airways require support to remain open.

C-reative protein A plasma protein which increases in level in response to inflammation.

Critical reflection Questioning of beliefs, values, knowledge and behaviours to continually improve as a nurse.

CT (Computed tomography) A CT scan takes many x-ray images from different angles to produce cross-sectional (tomographic) images (virtual 'slices') of specific areas of a scanned object, allowing the user to see inside the object without cutting. Other terms include computed axial tomography (CAT scan) and computer aided tomography.

Cytokines Proteins that stimulate or inhibit the differentiation, proliferation or function of immune cells. These substances are secreted by certain cells of the immune system and have an effect on other cells (for instance, interferon, interleukin and growth factors).

Devolved health administrations The name given to the responsibility for all health matters in each of the four countries of the UK (England, Northern Ireland, Scotland and Wales).

Differential diagnosis Determining between two different diagnosis which have similar signs or symptoms

Diffusion is the movement of molecules or atoms from a region of high concentration to a region of low concentration.

Diplopia Double vision (medically known as diplopia) is seeing two images of a single object. The two images may be one on top of the other, side by side, or a mix of both.

DNA DNA stands for 'deoxyribonucleic acid'. This is a self-replicating material which is present in nearly all living organisms as the main constituent of chromosomes. It is the carrier of genetic information.

DNACPR Do Not Attempt Cardio-Pulmonary Resuscitation.

Down's Syndrome Also known as trisomy 21. A genetic condition that typically causes some level of learning disability and certain physical characteristics.

Dysarthria Dysarthria is a condition in which the muscles you use for speech are weak or you have difficulty controlling them. Dysarthria often is characterised by slurred or slow speech that can be difficult to understand.

Dysphagia Difficulty swallowing (dysphagia) means it takes more time and effort to move food or liquid from your mouth to your stomach.

Elimination In pharmacology the elimination of a drug relates to any one of a number of processes by which a drug is eliminated from the human body either in an unchanged form (unbound molecules) or modified as a metabolite.

Emotional intelligence The ability to recognise and manage your own emotions and the emotions of others.

Enteral In nursing, enteral administration is food or drug administration via the gastrointestinal tract.

Enterotoxigenic bacteroides fragilis (ETBF) ETBF is a toxin that causes diarrheal disease.

Entonox The brand name for nitrous oxide, which is an inhaled gas, used as pain medication (can be used with other medications for anaesthesia). Commonly used in childbirth and in the emergency setting to manage pain from fractures and dislocations

Eosinophils A type of white blood cell with a role in fighting parasites, inflammation and allergic reaction.

Epidemiology A branch of medicine which studies the incidence, distribution, and possible control of diseases and other factors relating to health.

Epidermal growth factor receptor (EGFR) EGFR is a cell surface protein that binds to epidermal growth factor. About 15% of patients with non-small cell lung cancer have mutations to the EGFR. Some research studies have shown that mutations to the EGFR may predict whether certain types of drugs can help treat lung cancer.

Ethnography A qualitative research methodology concerned with how people interact in groups

External beam radiation (EBRT) This is the delivery of tightly targeted radiation beams from outside the body. A course of EBRT involves several daily treatments (fractions) over a few days to a few weeks.

Folliculitis Infection of the hair follicles.

G-CSF (Granulocyte-colony stimulating factor) Granulocyte-colony stimulating factor is a glycoprotein that stimulates the bone marrow to produce granulocytes and stem cells and release them into the bloodstream. This strengthens the patient's immune system while they are having chemotherapy and reduces their risk of infection. G-CSF is given as an injection under the skin. It can have some side effects, such as bone pain, itchy skin, or a fever. These are not usually severe, and lessen after G-CSF treatment stops.

Genomics A study of the complete genetic material of an organism which can help doctors choose the treatments which are most likely to be effective for each individual.

Grounded theory A qualitative, inductive research approach used to generate theories in the area of human interaction

Haemolytic anaemia is a condition in which red blood cells are destroyed and removed from the bloodstream before their normal lifespan is over

Haemoptysis is the coughing up of blood or blood-stained mucus from the bronchi, larynx, trachea or lungs.

Helicobacter pylori This is a gram-negative bacterium found usually in the stomach.

Helminths are also commonly known as parasitic worms, which live on or in a human or another animal and derive nourishment from the host.

Hemiparesis Hemiparesis is weakness of one entire side of the body. Hemiplegia is, in its most severe form, complete paralysis of half of the body. Hemiparesis and hemiplegia can be caused by different medical conditions, including congenital causes, trauma, tumours, or stroke.

Hepatic portal vein A blood vessel that carries blood (including drugs) from the gastrointestinal tract, gallbladder, pancreas and spleen to the liver.

Her2/neu HER2 is an oncogene, so named because it has a similar structure to human epidermal growth factor receptor. Amplification or over-expression of this oncogene has been shown to play an important role in the development and progression of certain aggressive types of breast cancer. (Neu is so named because it was derived from a type of neural tumour.)

Hirsutism Excessive growth of hair on the body in areas not expected. The term is often associated with abnormal hair growth in women.

Histological The study of organic tissues.

Hospital Passport Assists people with learning disabilities to provide hospital staff with important information about them and their health when they are admitted to hospital.

Human Immunodeficiency Virus (HIV) A chronic, potentially life-threatening virus that affects the immune system.

Hypercapnia Abnormally elevated levels of carbon dioxide in the blood.

Hyperpigmentation Increased colouration of the skin often due to increased pigment melanin.

Hypogammaglobulinaemia An immune disorder characterised by reduced gammaglobulins (immunoglobulin), including antibodies that help fight infection.

Hypoxia Low oxygen in the tissues.

ICE The application of communication skills to StAR values by asking patients about their **I**deas, **C**oncerns and **E**xpectations.

ICE-StAR ICE stands for ideas, concerns and expectations so enquiring about these when looking at a person's strengths, aspirations and resources (StAR).

ICP Integrated Care Pathway (which became Individual Care Priorities after 2011).

Immunodeficiency Conditions in which the immune system's ability to fight infectious disease is compromised or absent.

Immunohistochemistry (IHC) A powerful microscopy-based technique for visualising cellular components in tissue samples

Immunotherapy Immunotherapy is treatment that uses certain parts of a person's immune system to fight their cancer. This can be done by: 1. Stimulating the person's own immune system to work harder or smarter to attack cancer cells; 2. Giving the person immune system components, such as man-made proteins.

Innate immune system The first response of the immune system, mediated by cells able to destroy and engulf a large range of foreign organisms.

Inotropic drugs Medicines that alter the force of the heart's contractions. Either positive – to strengthen – or negative – to weaken the force.

Intestate Dying before the writing of a will.

Intrathoracic pressure refers to pressure within the pleural cavity

Intraventricular or intraparenchymal Surgically catheters placed within the brain's ventricular or parenchymal system to monitor intracranial pressure.

Keratin A protein that provides strength to skin, hair and nails.

Keratinocytes The most common form of skin cells , they produce keratin.

KRAS A mutation of a KRAS gene is an essential step in the development of a number of cancers. One in four people with cancer has inherited the KRAS variant. KRAS variant carriers face an increased risk of developing pre-menopausal triple-negative breast cancer, ovarian cancer, non small cell lung cancer (NSCLC), and colorectal cancer. Approximately 30–50% of colorectal tumors are known to have a mutated (abnormal) KRAS gene, indicating that up to 50% of patients with colorectal cancer (CRC) might respond to anti-epidermal growth factor receptor (EGFR) antibody therapy. However, 40–60% of patients with wild-type KRAS tumours do not respond to such therapy.

LCP Liverpool Care Pathway.

Leukocytes White blood cells, which include neutrophils, basophils, eosinophils, lymphocytes, NK cells and monocytes.

Lifelong learning The learning we do throughout life.

LPA Lasting Power of Attorney.

Lymphatic system A network of tissues and organs throughout the body that help rid the body of toxins, waste and other unwanted materials and transport the fluid containing white blood cells.

Macrophage A large phagocytic cell, which also functions as an antigen-presenting cell.

Malignant Hyperthermia A rare inherited disorder of the skeletal muscle characterised by increased metabolism and core body temperature. A fatal medical emergency (Gwinnutt and Gwinnutt, 2012).

Mast cell An 'allergy' cell with receptors for IgE, which when activated by an antigen will degranulate and release a number of mediators including histamine and leukotriene.

Medicines optimisation Engaging with individual patients to get their medicines right for them, making sure they are happy with that and checking that others involved in their care know.

Memory cell T- and B-cells produced during a primary immune response and that are 'primed' to mediate a secondary immune response to the original antigen.

Metabolism Drug metabolism is the metabolic breakdown of drugs by living organisms, usually through specialised enzymatic systems.

Meticillin-resistant Staphylococcus aureus (MRSA) is a Staphylococcus aureus which is resistant to the antibiotic meticillin

Motion artefact is movement which causes disruption to the collection of patient data.

Myocardial ischaemia or infarction Occurs when blood flow to the heart is reduced, preventing it from receiving enough oxygen usually as a result of a partial or complete blockage of the coronary arteries. Symptoms usually include a feeling of pressure/tightness on the chest, chest pain, pain in the left arm, jaw and/or neck.

Naïve cell A mature T- or B-cell that has not yet been activated by initial encounter with antigen.

Natural killer cell A lymphocyte that can recognise and destroy virally infected cells and control some forms of cancer.

NCPC National Council of Palliative Care.

Nephropathy Kidney disease

Neuromuscular junction A chemical synapse formed by the contact between a motor neuron and a muscle fibre.

Neutrophil A circulating phagocyte that enters tissue early in an inflammatory response.

NMC The Nursing and Midwifery Council, the professional regulator for Nursing and Midwifery in the UK that sets the standards that nurses and midwives must meet in their working lives, ensures that nursing students and student midwives have the right education at the start and throughout their career and keeps a register of all nurses and midwives in the UK.

Nociceptive pain A chronic pain which is caused by damage to body tissue and usually described as a sharp, aching, or throbbing pain. Can be due to benign pathology; or by tumours or cancer cells that are growing larger and crowding other body parts near the cancer site. Nociceptive pain may also be caused by cancer spreading to the bones, muscles, or joints, or that causes the blockage of an organ or blood vessels.

Non-Invasive Positive Pressure Venitilation (NIPPV) This is positive pressure ventilation delivered through a tight-fitting mask used as an approach instead of invasive ventilation.

NRAS The NRAS gene is an oncogene.

Nystagmus A condition of involuntary eye movement, acquired in infancy or later in life that may result in reduced or limited vision.

Oncogenes Proto-oncogenes are normal genes that, when mutated in certain ways, become oncogenes: genes that cause a cell to become cancerous.

Ongoing learning The process through which nurses plan their ongoing learning based on a review of learning need.

OPG Office of the Public Guardian.

Opioid A Class A drug that acts on the nervous system to relieve pain, i.e. morphine, fentanyl.

Opisthorchis viverrini A food-borne parasite that attacks the bile duct.

Parenteral A method of getting nutrition through your veins, total parenteral nutrition or peripheral parenteral nutrition. The parenteral route is any route that is not enteral.

Percussion Use of tapping on a patient's chest wall. It can identify fluid, or excessive air in the lungs.

Peritonitis Inflammation of the thin layer of tissue that lines the inside of the abdomen called the peritoneum.

Personal development planning and review The process through which nurses plan their ongoing learning based on a review of learning need.

Personal protective equipment Equipment that will protect the wearer from health or safety risks e.g., masks, helmets and gloves.

Pharmaco-therapeutics The study of the therapeutic uses and effects of drugs.

Pharmacodynamics The branch of pharmacology concerned with the effects of drugs and the mechanism of their action.

Pharmacokinetics The branch of pharmacology concerned with the movement of drugs within the body.

Pharmacovigilance The practice of monitoring the effects of medical drugs after they have been licensed for use, especially in order to identify and evaluate previously unreported adverse reactions.

Phenomenology A qualitative research methodology used to identify and describe phenomena as perceived by the participants

Phenothiazines One of a group of tranquillising drugs with antipsychotic actions thought to act by blocking dopaminergic transmission (messages sent using the substance dopamine) within the brain.

Polypharmacy The concurrent use of multiple medications by a patient. Polypharmacy is most common in the elderly, affecting about 40% of older adults living in their own homes.

Population health management Improving health outcomes across whole populations using multiple interventions.

Positron Emission Tomography (PET) An imaging test that helps reveal how a person's tissues and organs are functioning. A PET scan uses a radioactive drug (tracer) to show this activity. The tracer may be injected, swallowed or inhaled, depending on which organ or tissue is being studied by the PET scan.

Post intensive care syndrome A collection of health problems that remain following survival of critical illness.

Prader Willi Syndrome A genetic disorder due to loss of function of specific genes. In newborns symptoms include weak muscles, poor feeding and slow development. There is also typically mild to moderate intellectual impairment and behavioural problems.

Preferred learning style Accounting for differences in ways of learning and which ways appeal to us most.

Principles reasoning combined with case-based reasoning principles reasoning provides a values base to the reasoning process e.g. considering concepts such as autonomy, beneficence etc.

PRN *Pro re nata*   (Latin meaning 'when necessary').

Rapid sequence induction   Used when a patient is at risk of aspiration and involves use of cricoid pressure.

Reasonable adjustments Reasonable adjustments include removing physical barriers to accessing health services, but importantly also include making whatever alterations are necessary to policies, procedures, staff training and service delivery to ensure that they work equally well for people with learning disabilities.

Red flags   signs or symptoms that may occur that indicate something more serious may be occurring.

Resilience The ability to adapt or recover and become stronger.

Revalidation The process which the NMC requires every nurse to follow to maintain their professional registration.

Root cause analysis (RCA) A systematic approach that investigates a problem or incident to discover the true cause of the problem and identify the actions to ensure it does not happen again.

Safety netting   Information given to patients about what to do if their condition does not improve or deteriorates.

Safety Thermometer   A local improvement tool that can measure, monitor and analyse patient harms and 'harm-free' care.

Screening   Cancer screening is a way to find cancer before any symptoms appear in the body. Finding cancer this early saves lives. Breast, cervical and bowel cancer screening programmes are common worldwide.

Silent myocardial infarction   A myocardial infarction with few or no symptoms.

Social media   Computer-based technologies that allow for creation and sharing of information.

Spontaneous mutation   A condition caused by a mutation that occurs spontaneously during DNA replication.

StAR values   The strengths a patient may have (rather than just focusing on their problems), their aspirations (expectations of treatment and outcomes) and the resources available to them including their own internal resilience.

Sterile field   An area around the site of surgical incision. It includes all the furniture covered with sterile drapes and all the personnel who are gowned and gloved.

Supervision   Overseeing a person or activity to ensure relevant standards are met.

Surgical emphysema   is when gas or air is present in the tissues, most commonly in the neck as a result of leakage from the lung.

Syncope   A temporary loss of consciousness; fainting.

Systemic isotope therapy A form of radiation therapy where the patient swallows or receives an injection of a radioactive substance, such as radioactive iodine or a radioactive substance bound to a monoclonal antibody.

Systemic lupus erythematosus (SLE) An autoimmune disease with inflammation of the joint, skin and other organs.

T helper cell A type of T cell that helps other cells in the immune response by recognising foreign antigens and secreting cytokines that activate T and B cells.

Tacit or craft knowledge is knowledge from personal experience, often linked with intuition

Tactile fremitus Vibration felt through the chest wall when a patient is asked to vocalise.

Targeted agents Cancer therapies that block the growth and spread of cancer by interfering with specific molecules that are involved in the growth and spread of cancer. These type of agents are sometimes referred to as 'precision medicines'; precision medicine uses information about a person's genes and proteins to prevent, diagnose and treat cancer.

Titrated Where the dose of a drug is calculated against individual aspects, i.e. weight, to produce the most effective outcome. At times the administration of an analgesic may be administered in small amounts until the desired outcome is achieved using the least amount of drug.

Trisomy The presence of one chromosome additional to the normal homologous pair.

Tumour markers These are substances that are produced by cancer or by other cells in the body in response to cancer or certain non-cancerous conditions. Most tumour markers are made by normal cells as well as by cancer cells; however, they are produced at much higher levels in cancers. Tumour markers can be found in the blood, urine, stool, tumour tissue or other tissues or bodily fluids of some patients with cancer. Most tumour markers are proteins.

Type A adverse drug reaction Reactions which result from an exaggeration of a drug's normal pharmacological action, e.g., bleeding when given warfarin.

Utilitarianism an ethical view that an action is right if it does the most good for the greater majority.

Ventilation is the exchange of air between the lungs and the atmosphere so that oxygen can be exchanged for carbon dioxide in the alveoli.

Volition the power to make your own decisions

X-linked A condition caused by the mutation in a gene on the x chromosome.

INDEX

Note: page numbers in **bold** indicate Glossary entries